CURRENT GERIATRIC THERAPY

Timothy R. Covington, Pharm. D.
Associate Professor and Chairman,
Clinical Programs and Services
West Virginia University Medical Center
Morgantown, West Virginia

J. Ingram Walker, M.D.
Assistant Professor of Psychiatry
  and Senior Fellow,
Center for the Study of Aging
  and Human Development
Duke University Medical Center
Durham, North Carolina

1984
W. B. SAUNDERS COMPANY
Philadelphia / London / Toronto / Mexico City / Rio de Janeiro / Sydney / Tokyo

W.B. Saunders Company: West Washington Square
Philadelphia, PA 19105

1 St. Anne's Road
Eastbourne, East Sussex BN21 3UN, England

1 Goldthorne Avenue
Toronto, Ontario M8Z 5T9, Canada

Apartado 26370—Cedro 512
Mexico 4, D.F., Mexico

Rua Coronel Cabrita, 8
Sao Cristovao Caixa Postal 21176
Rio de Janeiro, Brazil

9 Waltham Street
Artarmon, N.S.W. 2064, Australia

Ichibancho, Central Bldg., 22-1 Ichibancho
Chiyoda-Ku, Tokyo 102, Japan

Library of Congress Cataloging in Publication Data

Main entry under title:
Current geriatric therapy.

1. Geriatric pharmacology. I. Covington, Timothy R.
II. Walker, J. Ingram (John Ingram), 1944–
[DNLM: 1. Drug therapy—In old age. 2. Geriatrics.
3. Therapeutics—In old age. WT 100 C9755]
RC953.7.C87   1984   615.5'8'0880565   83-20040
ISBN 0-7216-2743-9

Current Geriatric Therapy   ISBN 0-7216-2743-9

© 1984 by W.B. Saunders Company. Copyright under the Uniform Copyright Convention. Simultaneously published in Canada. All rights reserved. This book is protected by copyright. No part of it may be reproduced, stored in a retrieval system, or transmitted in any form or by any means, electronic, mechanical, photocopying, recording, or otherwise, without written permission from the publisher. Made in the United States of America. Press of W.B. Saunders Company. Library of Congress catalog card number 83-20040.

Last digit is the print number: 9   8   7   6   5   4   3   2   1

CONTRIBUTORS

JAMES R. BOYD, M.S. PHARM.
Assistant Clinical Professor, St. Louis College of Pharmacy, St. Louis, Missouri. Editor-in-Chief, Facts and Comparisons Division, J.B. Lippincott Company, Philadelphia, Pennsylvania.

THOMAS J. CALI, PHARM. D.
School of Pharmacy, University of Maryland, Baltimore, Maryland.

TIMOTHY R. COVINGTON, PHARM. D.
Associate Professor of Clinical Pharmacy and Chairman, Clinical Programs and Services, West Virginia University Medical Center, Morgantown, West Virginia.

CHARLES C. DEPEW, PHARM. D.
Pharmacist, Medical-Surgical Intensive Care Unit Pharmacy, Stanford University Hospital, Stanford, California.

RONALD P. EVENS, PHARM. D.
Associate Professor, Department of Clinical Pharmacy, and Vice-Chairman for Academic Affairs, College of Pharmacy, University of Tennessee Center for the Health Sciences. Consultant in Drug Information, W.F. Bowld Hospital (University of Tennessee) and Le Bonheur Children's Medical Center, Memphis, Tennessee.

HARRY A. GALLIS, M.D.
Associate Professor of Medicine and Assistant Professor of Microbiology and Immunology, Duke University School of Medicine. Attending in Infectious Diseases, Duke University Hospital, Durham, North Carolina.

DAVID W. HAWKINS, PHARM. D.
Associate Professor of Family Practice and Pharmacology, University of Texas Health Science Center at San Antonio, San Antonio. Associate Professor of Pharmacy, University of Texas at Austin College of Pharmacy, Austin, Texas.

ROBERT H. HOY, PHARM. D.
Associate Professor of Clinical Pharmacy and Vice-Chairman of Clinical Programs and Services, School of Pharmacy, Charleston Division, West Virginia University Medical Center, Charleston, West Virginia.

ARTHUR I. JACKNOWITZ, PHARM. D.
Professor of Clinical Pharmacy and Director, Drug Information Center, School of Pharmacy, West Virginia University Medical Center, Morgantown, West Virginia.

PETER P. LAMY, PH.D., F.A.G.S.
Professor and Director, Center for the Study of Pharmacy and Therapeutics for the Elderly. Chairman, Department of Pharmacy Practice and Administrative Science, School of Pharmacy, University of Maryland at Baltimore. Consultant, Veterans Administration Medical Center, Baltimore, Ft. Howard, and Perry Point, Maryland. Consultant, Veterans Administration Medical Center, Washington, D.C.

JAMES W. LINMAN, M.D.
Professor of Medicine, John A. Burns School of Medicine, University of Hawaii, Honolulu, Hawaii.

ALLAN A. MALTBIE, M.D.
Associate Professor, Department of Psychiatry, and Chief, Psychiatric Consultation Liaison Program, Duke University Medical Center, Durham, North Carolina.

ELLIOTT L. MANCALL, M.D.
Professor and Chairman, Department of Neurology, Hahnemann University, Philadelphia, Pennsylvania.

RICHARD A. MATTHAY, M.D.
Associate Professor of Medicine and Associate Director, Pulmonary Section, Department of Internal Medicine, Yale University School of Medicine, New Haven, Connecticut.

MORRIS NOTELOVITZ, M.D., PH.D.
Professor of Obstetrics and Gynecology and Director, Center for Climacteric Studies, University of Florida College of Medicine, Gainesville, Florida.

CHARLES D. PONTE, PHARM. D.
Assistant Professor of Clinical Pharmacy and Family Practice, Schools of Pharmacy and Medicine, West Virginia University Medical Center, Morgantown, West Virginia.

CARL B. SHERTER, M.D.
Associate Clinical Professor of Medicine, Yale University School of Medicine, New Haven. Director, Pulmonary Disease Service, Waterbury Hospital Health Center, Waterbury, Connecticut.

IRMA H. ULLRICH, M.D.
Professor of Internal Medicine, West Virginia University School of Medicine. Attending Physician, West Virginia University Medical Center, Morgantown, West Virginia.

J. INGRAM WALKER, M.D.
Assistant Professor of Psychiatry and Senior Fellow, Center for the Study of Aging and Human Development, Duke University Medical Center, Durham, North Carolina.

MARSHA WARE, B.S.
Research Associate, Center for Climacteric Studies, and Medical Student, University of Florida College of Medicine, Gainesville, Florida.

FRANK J. WEINSTOCK, M.D., F.A.C.S.
Clinical Assistant Professor of Ophthalmology, Ohio State University College of Medicine, Columbus. Senior Attending Staff, Aultman Hospital, and Active Staff, Timken Mercy Medical Center, Canton, Ohio.

FOREWORD

People 65 years of age or older compose 11 per cent of the United States population. These citizens receive more than $45 billion yearly in health care benefits. Costs of nursing home care have risen to $21.6 billion annually, and if the trend continues, this expense will approach $76 billion by the end of this decade. A recent study under the auspices of the Institute of Medicine of the National Academy of Science estimates that from 7,000 to 10,300 primary care geriatricians will be needed by 1990 to provide care for the elderly.

The elderly take 25 per cent of the prescription drugs sold in this country, yet they experience 50 per cent of all adverse drug reactions. Medication errors have been detected in two-fifths to three-fifths of elderly people receiving drugs. In two separate studies, almost 20 per cent of the admissions to the geriatric service of a general hospital were directly attributable to drug complications.

Several factors contribute to drug therapy dilemmas in older people. With advancing age the proportion of body fat increases, serum albumin levels diminish, creatinine clearance rates decline significantly, body water content decreases, drugs are metabolized in the older population at rates different from the younger population, recommended dosages are often prescribed on the basis of the needs of younger adults, and older people take more drugs simultaneously, often mixing over-the-counter drugs with prescription drugs. In addition, drug misuse has been attributed to an unclear explanation of how the medicine is to be taken.

Covington and Walker emphasize the need to be more familiar with drug therapy in the elderly. As medical priorities shift with changes in the age structure of the population, knowledge of geriatric drug therapy becomes more critical. Covington and Walker's book is a clear, concise, and comprehensive volume which represents an excellent contribution to the expansion of the pharmacotherapy knowledge base of health practitioners serving geriatric patients.

EWALD W. BUSSE, M.D.
J.P. Gibbons Professor of Psychiatry
Associate Provost and Dean Emeritus
Medical and Allied Health Education
Duke University Medical Center

CONTENTS

Part One
THERAPEUTIC DILEMMAS

Chapter 1
THERAPEUTIC DILEMMAS IN THE ELDERLY 3
James R. Boyd

Chapter 2
MODIFYING DRUG DOSAGE IN ELDERLY PATIENTS 35
Peter P. Lamy

Part Two
PHARMACOLOGICAL MANAGEMENT OF COMMON DISORDERS IN THE ELDERLY

Chapter 3
PSYCHIATRIC DISORDERS 75
J. Ingram Walker and Timothy R. Covington

Chapter 4
PULMONARY DISEASES AND DISORDERS OF RESPIRATION .. 104
Carl B. Sherter, Charles C. Depew, and Richard A. Matthay

Chapter 5
CARDIOVASCULAR DISORDERS 140
Robert H. Hoy and Charles D. Ponte

Chapter 6
GASTROINTESTINAL DISORDERS 178
Arthur J. Jacknowitz

Chapter 7
INFECTIOUS DISEASES IN THE ELDERLY 239
Harry A. Gallis

Chapter 8
BONE AND JOINT DISORDERS 277
Ronald P. Evens and David W. Hawkins

Chapter 9
ANEMIAS 307
James W. Linman

Chapter 10
ENDOCRINE DISORDERS 328
Irma H. Ullrich

Chapter 11
RENAL DISEASE 366
Thomas J. Cali

Chapter 12
NEUROLOGIC DISORDERS 385
Elliott L. Mancall and Timothy R. Covington

Chapter 13
MANAGEMENT OF POSTMENOPAUSAL WOMEN 405
Morris Notelovitz and Marsha Ware

Chapter 14
PAIN MANAGEMENT 422
Allan A. Maltbie

Chapter 15
OPHTHALMIC DISORDERS 435
Frank J. Weinstock

Index 451

PART ONE

THERAPEUTIC DILEMMAS

CHAPTER 1

THERAPEUTIC DILEMMAS IN THE ELDERLY

James R. Boyd

The goal of achieving rational drug therapy has been aggressively pursued by health professionals over the past decade. In spite of the many advances in pharmacotherapy, the geriatric patient remains a "therapeutic orphan," owing to a general lack of basic knowledge concerning the unique drug therapy requirements of this age group and inadequate communication and application of existing knowledge. Rational drug therapy should attempt to achieve the maximal therapeutic benefit while minimizing undesirable consequences of medication. This is significantly more difficult in the geriatric patient because of multiple factors that obscure accurate diagnosis, limit the therapeutic options available, and increase the number of potential therapeutic hazards.

Diagnostic problems include the atypical presentation of many diseases, the difficulty in differentiating signs of disease from changes associated with the aging process, and the differentiation of symptoms of multiple chronic diseases that coexist in the typical patient. Once an accurate diagnosis is achieved, selection of the drug or drugs of choice is frequently difficult because of potential drug-disease interactions, which may severely limit the therapeutic options in patients with multiple chronic conditions. Furthermore, altered responses to drug therapy in the aged may result from both physiological and pathological changes.

Polypharmacotherapy increases the possibility of a number of therapeutic hazards, which may be particularly problematic in the elderly. There is an increased frequency of adverse drug reactions in this age group due to increased sensitivity to drugs and greater exposure to drugs over longer periods of time. Polypharmacotherapy also increases the risk of adverse consequences from drug-drug, drug-food, and drug-laboratory test interactions. Additional therapeutic hazards include noncompliance, self-medication, and misuse or abuse of medications.

Inaccurate diagnosis, improper drug selection, and untoward effects of drug use present significant therapeutic dilemmas in the care of the geriatric patient. Unless the physician can appreciate and properly interpret the interrelationships among this complex of variables, therapeutic misadventures may lead to additional problems, which further obscure an accurate diagnosis and detract from rational therapy.

DILEMMAS IN DRUG THERAPY: WHO IS RESPONSIBLE?

The literature is abundant—physicians, pharmacists, nurses, and other disciplines have clearly identified various dilemmas in drug therapy. Each group has developed convincing arguments (by virtue of education, experience, proximity to the patient, or legal restrictions) that their profession should assume the responsibility for solving any number of patient related problems (e.g., monitoring response to drug therapy or providing instruction on the use of medications). Proof of Newton's third law of motion* can be found easily in the responses to these arguments: Physicians may resist pharmacists' meddling in the "doctor-patient relationship," pharmacists may not believe that nurses know about the drugs a patient may be taking, and nurses may feel that they are the only ones who can communicate with a patient.

In spite of editorial cajoling, it appears that little has been done to apply collectively the knowledge we have gained in solving various therapeutic dilemmas. What is clearly needed is less rhetoric and more action at the level of primary patient care. Furthermore, it would seem that an interdisciplinary approach, coordinating the efforts of all professionals involved in health care, would benefit the patient. It is unfortunate that the "health care team" remains largely an elusive academic concept rather than a reality of health care delivery.

THE PARADOX OF DRUG THERAPY

Drug therapy represents an interesting yet perplexing paradox, which is perhaps more significant in the elderly than in any other patient population. Advances made in pharmacotherapy over the past 50 years have virtually eliminated acute infectious disease as the primary cause of mortality. Pain and discomfort can be alleviated. Many chronic diseases can be treated in a manner that permits full functional participation in society. Both longevity and the quality of life can be significantly improved. At the same time, unbridled enthusiasm for "a pill for every ill" fails to recognize that even under ideal circumstances, adverse drug reactions, toxic reactions, and therapeutic failures occur. Used improperly, via irrational prescribing or intentional or unintentional misuse or abuse, drugs contribute to both morbidity and mortality.

This chapter attempts to identify some of the therapeutic dilemmas unique to the elderly that place them at increased risk to the hazards of inappropriate or suboptimal pharmacotherapy. An awareness of these potential problems is essential for the rational application of specific therapeutic principles.

---

*For every action or force there is an equal reaction in the opposite direction.

MEDICATION CONSUMPTION PATTERNS

An understanding of medication consumption patterns in the elderly patient is essential to the design of an optimal therapeutic regimen, one that will minimize the risk of untoward responses. Polypharmacotherapy, noncompliance with prescribed regimens, self-medication with "home remedies," and drug misuse and abuse, individually or collectively, may lead to undesirable or even life threatening consequences. The physician and the pharmacist must avoid contributing to these problems and maintain a high index of suspicion to prevent, detect, and remedy these potential problems.

Polypharmacotherapy

The disproportionately high consumption of drugs by the elderly is well documented. It is estimated that the over-65 population, which represents 11 per cent of the United States population, consumes in excess of 25 per cent of all drugs prescribed.[1] Data from the 1977 National Health Care Expenditure Study reveal that persons 65 years of age and over average 10.8 prescriptions annually. In the 77.4 per cent of this group who received at least one prescription, the average number of prescriptions is 14.0 annually.[2] Institutionalized patients may be taking eight to 12 different medications concurrently; examples of individuals taking 20 to 30 drugs at the same time have been cited.

The most obvious reason for multiple drug therapy in the elderly is the prevalence of multiple chronic diseases amenable to drug therapy. Over the past 50 years medical, economic, and social factors have contributed to a significant increase in longevity. As a consequence, there has been an increase in the incidence and prevalence of chronic diseases associated with aging. Multiple diseases in the elderly are the rule rather than the exception. It is not surprising that the elderly take more drugs and take them for longer periods of time than their younger counterparts.

It is important for health care professionals to appreciate both the extent and the potential consequences of polypharmacotherapy. Unfortunately many physicians fail to recognize the extent of drug use by their patients. This is particularly true when a patient receives prescriptions from several physicians. In one study, in-depth medication histories of 58 hospitalized patients identified 193 prescription drugs (3.3 per patient), compared to 38 prescriptions (0.66 per patient) documented by the physician in the patient's chart.[3] A carefully structured and well executed interview is essential to accurately document a complete medication history. Inquiry should be made concerning nonprescription as well as prescription drug use.

Multiple drug therapy cannot be avoided. However, it must be recognized that each drug added to a therapeutic regimen increases the potential for adverse effects, multiplies the potential for drug interactions, increases the probability of noncompliance or abuse, complicates further diagnosis and therapy, and adds to the cost of health care. Therefore, it is essential to recognize factors contributing to unnecessary drug use.

Prescriber Impact

Improper and irrational prescribing may occur for a number of reasons. Diagnostic problems, particularly the atypical presentation of some disease states in the elderly, may lead to improper diagnosis and therapy. Therapeutic failure should suggest a re-evaluation of the diagnosis prior to institution of alternative therapeutic modalities.

The pressures of a busy practice may tempt the physician to omit critical steps in the diagnostic workup. There are, no doubt, instances in which no legitimate attempt is made to establish a diagnosis, particularly for complaints that might be regarded as "trivial" in comparison with patients who seem to be "really sick." Diagnosis by prescription contributes to unnecessary drug exposure and can lead to unwarranted assumptions regarding drug efficacy.

Provided an accurate diagnosis has been established, drug-disease interactions (contraindications), drug-drug interactions, and adverse reaction potential must be considered in selecting the proper drug(s). Concurrent conditions and drug therapy may severely limit the therapeutic options available; failure to recognize potential therapeutic hazards may lead to more problems than are solved, however. Selection of the "drug of choice" at any given time requires constant effort to maintain an awareness of recent developments in pharmacotherapy. The practicing physician cannot be expected to keep up with all advances in experimental therapeutics; however, one should be aware of therapeutic approaches that become standards of practice. Sources of objective therapeutic information should extend beyond the advice offered by pharmaceutical manufacturers' detailmen and drug advertisements in the periodical literature. Several reference books and periodicals focusing on current topics in pharmacotherapy are listed in Table 1–1.

Deliberate overprescribing, especially the use of psychotropic drugs in institutionalized patients, has been a frequent point of criticism. In a study of the use of tranquilizers in a long term care facility, there was no statistically significant correlation between level of anxiety and the use of tranquilizers. Factors found to have a significant relationship to the use of tranquilizers included being female, having a "low mental status," and being judged unfriendly to the staff.[4] Although psychotropic drugs may be of significant clinical benefit, they should not be viewed as substitutes for consultation, caring, and companionship.

The placebo is perhaps one of the most powerful and most frequently used therapeutic options available to the physician. A review of published placebo controlled studies demonstrates a significant number of therapeutic successes as well as adverse effects. There are perhaps situations in which placebos are appropriate. However, rarely are true placebos prescribed; more commonly drugs of dubious therapeutic merit (and, it is hoped, minimal

TABLE 1–1. Current Drug Information Resources

Periodicals
Clinical Pharmacology and Therapeutics
    St. Louis, The C.V. Mosby Company
Drug Therapy: The Journal of Clinical Therapeutics
    New York, Biomedical Information Corporation
Drugs
    New York, ADIS Press
The Medical Letter on Drugs and Therapeutics
    New Rochelle, The Medical Letter Inc.
Rational Drug Therapy (Pharmacology for Physicians)
    Philadelphia, W.B. Saunders Company

References
AMA Drug Evaluations. Ed. 5
    Chicago, American Medical Association, 1983
Current Therapy (Annual)
    Conn, H.F. (Editor)
    Philadelphia, W.B. Saunders Company
Facts and Comparisons
    Kastrup, E.D., and Boyd, J.R. (Editors)
    St. Louis, Facts and Comparisons, Inc., 1984
Handbook of Drug Therapy
    Greenblatt, D.J., and Miller, R.R.
    New York, Elsevier North Holland, 1979

toxicity) are used to avoid detection of the placebo intent of the prescription. The use of pharmacologic agents for the sole purpose of producing a placebo effect presents potential therapeutic hazards that should be avoided. It is not difficult to appreciate the physician's desire to spend 30 seconds writing a prescription rather than the 15 minutes that might be required to arrive at a definitive diagnosis and provide consultation and patient education. Unfortunately prescription writing, to signal the termination of the physician-patient encounter, has become a ritual in the minds of many patients and physicians.

Patient Expectations

Patients themselves contribute to the writing of unnecessary prescriptions. This attraction to the use of nostrums is not a recent phenomenon:

The desire to take medicines is perhaps the greatest feature that distinguishes man from animals (Sir William Osler, 1891).

The patient's expectation of a solution to all problems via a prescription may represent a more formidable obstacle than treating a physical illness. To many, the receipt of a prescription serves as a necessary process to acknowledge and legitimatize the illness. Patients appear to derive great satisfaction from comparing pills (or incisions); however, little pride is derived from quitting smoking, an exercise program, or a diet.

Previous experience, or the experience of a friend or relative, may lead the patient to make his own diagnosis and devise therapeutic recommendations. It is not uncommon for an assertive patient to request a specific prescription medication by name. Improper presentation or interpretation of information disseminated in the news media may also result in exaggerated expectations and a demand for a specific drug. A press release for a new but not unique nonsteroidal anti-inflammatory drug sent thousands of patients to their physicians to obtain prescriptions for the new "cure for arthritis." The physician must exercise care to avoid succumbing to such demands.

The use of multiple drugs by the elderly patient is an unavoidable reality. Care must be taken to avoid drugs or drug combinations that may interact adversely in a given patient. The primary care practitioner must view the whole patient rather than react to or attempt to treat isolated complaints. The avoidance of any nonessential medication is a contribution to improved patient care.

Summary

Polypharmacotherapy is frequently a necessity in the elderly patient because of the prevalence of multiple chronic disease states. When essential and properly monitored, such therapy can be safe and effective. However, because of the increased hazards of untoward responses due to drug interaction, adverse effects, noncompliance, and the potential for misuse and abuse, attempts should be made to eliminate unnecessary drug exposure. The prescriber must be vigilant to avoid undue temptation to utilize the prescription as a substitute for a proper diagnosis, consultation, and education.

Self-medication

The use of nonprescription drugs in self-medication has come a long way from the days of such nostrums as snake oil, swamp root, and wahoo bitters. The availability of safe and effective products, such as acetaminophen, tolnaftate, chlorpheniramine, and more recently topically applied hydrocortisone products, insures the consumer a convenient and economical means of dealing with many minor problems. Beyond legitimate nonprescription drugs of proven value, self-medication may include the use of a variety of substances ranging from innocuous "home remedies" to potentially dangerous compounds, such as Laetrile and dimethylsulfoxide (DMSO).

It is doubtful that the typical physician appreciates the full extent of self-medication use by his patients. In one study of nonprescription drug use in the elderly, use of 74 per cent of the products was unknown to the patient's physician.[5] The elderly patient appears to be less likely to seek professional help and is more likely to self-medicate for a number of seemingly minor ailments.

As with prescription drugs, nonprescription products are capable of causing adverse effects, including drug reactions, drug interactions, and the masking of symptoms of disease. One study of hospital admissions secondary to adverse drug reactions indicated that 18 per cent of such reactions were caused by nonprescription drugs.[6] Careful inquiry into self-medication habits is an essential element of a patient's medication history.

Mass Media Impact

Consumer advertising in many forms has been successful in making the proprietary drug industry a multibillion dollar industry. Although few would question the necessity for nonprescription medications, the manner in which such products are marketed can lead to their excessive and inappropriate use. Objective assessment of commercial claims will identify few inaccuracies; however, implied benefits frequently extend beyond rational uses. Furthermore, the lack of information concerning limitations and potential adverse effects of products insures that there will be insufficient balanced information for the patient to make an intelligent risk-benefit analysis.

Over the last two decades television has exerted a tremendous influence on society. In spite of the occasional noncommercial health related public service message, the preponderance of information broadcast appears to be "pro drug use." One analysis of commercial television found 10 times as many messages urging the use of pills or other remedies than there were against drug use and abuse.[7] It is not surprising that the consumer feels compelled to maintain a completely stocked medicine chest to combat "tired blood," the drip-drip-drip of stomach acid, irregularity, diarrhea, hacking cough, and tension headache, to mention only a few. The impact of Madison Avenue on consumer attitudes toward health and expectations from nonprescription medication cannot be underestimated. Withdrawal of patients from physical dependency on laxatives, nasal decongestants, and nonprescription sedatives can present a significant medical problem.

Although certain activities of the FDA and FTC have led to limited restrictions in the claims made in advertising, we cannot expect marketing efforts to become totally objective and educational in nature. Therefore, physicians and pharmacists must assume a major responsibility for providing accurate and helpful information to assist the patient in the rational use of nonprescription drugs. Of particular importance in the pharmacy are the proximity and accessibility of the pharmacist to the patient seeking an over the counter product. The community pharmacist has a great professional opportunity and obligation to provide guidance to patients in the use of these products.

Over the Counter Drug Use by the Elderly

As with prescription medications, the elderly tend to consume a disproportionately large percentage of nonprescription medications. In one study of ambulatory elderly patients, 80 per cent had used nonprescription medication during the previous year and 44 per cent had used a nonprescription medication during the previous week.[5] Women are generally found to consume a greater number of both prescription and nonprescription drugs than men.[8] It is rather consistently observed that advertising is the greatest influence on nonprescription drug selection. The elderly may be particularly susceptible to the influence of modern advertising techniques.

The most frequently used types of nonprescription medications include laxatives, antacids, analgesics, vitamins, and cold preparations. Although the use of these categories of medications may be easily understood and appropriate, the potential for laxative dependence, drug-drug interactions, and untoward cardiovascular effects from sympathomimetics and anticholinergics in cold preparations graphically illustrates the need for professional concern about the use of these products.

Myths and Fallacies

Beyond the use of legitimate nonprescription drugs, the elderly are also prone to the use of "quack remedies." Lack of knowledge and understanding is one of the principal reasons a patient is susceptible to quackery. Disenchantment with the impersonal attitudes of the medical care establishment may also lead the patient to seek unorthodox methods of dealing with health problems. In either event, compassion and consultation are required if the patient is to be expected to derive benefit from the best of therapeutic recommendations.[9]

The patient who fails to obtain significant relief or promise of hope for debilitating or fatal conditions may be driven to rely on quackery by fear and desperation. It is understandable that any alternative offering a glimmer of hope will be attractive to such patients. Furthermore, patients are unlikely to consult with health professionals who react to unorthodox methods with casual disregard, or who fail to demonstrate a genuine interest or neglect to provide a satisfactory response to the patient's concerns.

A comprehensive enumeration of unorthodox alternatives to traditional health care methods could consume an entire book. The following examples include a number of the more common unproven remedies currently in vogue.[10-12]

Cancer Quackery. Approximately 50 per cent of all cancer patients use or at least contemplate the use of quack cures.[10] Beyond monetary waste, the time lost in making an accurate diagnosis and providing responsible care may be critical to the success of therapy. Laetrile is by far the most notable and controversial cancer "remedy." In spite of the deluge of testimonials and case reports attesting to its curative powers, not one scientifically controlled and documented study has been published to suggest any value of this agent. The social and political pressure to make Laetrile available has been so strong that legislation has been introduced in many states to circumvent the Federal Food Drug and Cosmetics Act in an attempt to make the agent legal for use within the state.

Various vitamins are also advocated as cancer cures when given in megadoses. Vitamin A has been used in doses of up to 3,000,000 I.U. daily. Such doses far exceed recognized toxic doses and no beneficial effects have been established. Vitamin E, another potentially toxic oil soluble vitamin, has also been advocated for use as a cancer cure, to prevent aging, to improve virility, and undoubtedly for other wondrous effects. In addition to its reputed effects in aborting or attenuating the common cold, Pauling has suggested that vitamin C is beneficial in palliating cancer related symptoms and in prolonging survival. Neither claim has been substantiated in placebo controlled studies.

Pangamic acid, which has been referred to as vitamin B_{15}, is not a recognized vitamin and has no established use. Although it is generally available via "health food" outlets, little is known concerning this substance, and its safety has not been established.[13]

Proteolytic enzymes, another panacea from the health food industry, has likewise been advocated in cancer therapy. Most commonly administered by enema, the enzymes are claimed to lyse cancer cells and prevent metastases. Some other bizarre "remedies" include a diet consisting solely of grapes or grape juice and the use of coffee enemas.

A number of diets have been promoted for cancer victims. Such diets usually require extremes in intake of certain components and avoidance of other foodstuffs. No dietary adjustments have been proven to be of any benefit in cancer therapy. Adequate nutrition is important to all patients; any fad diet that neglects balanced intake of essential nutrients, vitamins, and minerals may be hazardous.

Arthritis "Cures." It has been estimated that for every dollar spent for legitimate research on arthritis, $25 is wasted on quack remedies. Annual expenditures for such useless and potentially harmful remedies approach one billion dollars. For those not afflicted, it is difficult to fully appreciate the pain and suffering that arthritic conditions inflict on over 30 million Americans. The chronicity of the disease and the lack of an acceptable level of relief from conventional medical therapy drive thousands of arthritis sufferers to seek some form of "miracle cure."

The voice of quackery holds great appeal with guarantees of "amazing instant relief" via a "secret natural formula," which promises a "doctor tested scientific breakthrough." It is easy to understand how the uninformed patient can be enticed into a trial of a remedy that offers hope.

Products with exaggerated or unproven claims usually do not last long when sold in interstate commerce or via the mail. Yet in spite of federal efforts, many products exist long enough to fleece a large number of patients. Furthermore, persistent and desperate patients knowingly participate in black market activities to obtain their favorite cure from Mexico, Canada, or other foreign sources.

Electronic and electromagnetic devices have been particularly prevalent among arthritis remedies. Such devices include the Palorator, the Gonsertron, the Magnetron, the Diapulse Electro Magnetic Energy Generator, and Solarama Microthermal Panels. None of these devices has any proven value. Arthritic dietary recommendations have included therapeutic fasting and diets rich in fresh fruits, raw vegetables, herb teas, and of course several "natural" grain foods.

A hormonal arthritis remedy, usually including prednisone, estrogen, and testosterone, has been sold under the names of Leifcort, Hormone Balance Treatment, Balanced Hormone Treatment, Holistic Balance

Treatment, and Rheumatril. These products are most frequently promoted via transient clinics, frequently set up in hotel rooms. Patient acceptance of this remedy is understandably quite high because of the dramatic effect of the steroid, in spite of the obvious risks.

"PROven" is a combination of cobra and krait snake venoms popularized in recent years in Florida for the treatment of rheumatoid arthritis and multiple sclerosis. As with other nonconventional remedies, no evidence is available to substantiate the safety or efficacy of this product.

Dimethylsulfoxide (DMSO), a highly publicized "miracle drug," continues to be the source of both scientific and political controversy. Considerable evidence exists to suggest that DMSO is an effective analgesic; however, the drug does not appear to have any significant anti-inflammatory effect. Because of the lack of commercial interest, few well controlled studies have been performed to serve as the basis for sound scientific evaluation of either the safety or efficacy of this drug. Unfortunately media exploitation and the sensationalism of the DMSO story have led to widespread human use of the commercial solvent, chemical grade, and veterinary sources of DMSO. Because of DMSO's capacity to serve as a carrier, thus enhancing transcutaneous absorption of other substances, the use of nonpharmaceutical grades of this agent exposes the patient to unwarranted risks.

Coffee Enemas. Although the use of "therapeutic enemas" appears to have been common for decades, the coffee enema is a rather recent development. No rationale for the use of coffee enemas can be identified; however, their use appears to be advocated for cancer, arthritis, the common cold, and undoubtedly other maladies. It is difficult to understand the persistence of this type of therapy, since no significant commercial interest would appear to be involved. At least two deaths have been reported that were attributed to fluid and electrolyte imbalance related to the use of coffee enemas.[15]

Gerovital H3. Developed and promoted by the Aslan Clinic in Rumania, Gerovital offers the promise of the "fountain of youth." The product, which is a 2 per cent procaine hydrochloride injection, has been promoted to retard the aging process and alleviate many of the chronic diseases common to the elderly. In the United States a similar product is available in Nevada. There are no scientific data supporting the efficacy or safety of this product.[16]

Chinese Herbal Remedies. A variety of Chinese herbal remedies, most commonly with the name "chuifong toukuwan," have been promoted in the United States as cures for arthritis, rheumatism, and other painful conditions. Although the product labeling lists only herbal ingredients, FDA studies have identified indomethacin, hydrochlorothiazide, and chlordiazepoxide in these products. At least one death has been attributed to their use.[17]

Summary

Self-medication, with legitimate nonprescription drug products or quack remedies, must be the concern of all health care professionals. Patients require objective guidance and assistance in deciphering the claims made for proprietary products to insure proper product selection. Pharmacists who advise patients about the selection of nonprescription products must consider the patient's medical history and concurrent prescription drug therapy. Physicians must not neglect inquiry into the patient's use of nonprescription remedies as a part of a complete medication history. Patterns of nonprescription drug use may provide clues to subacute medical problems, which the patient fails to mention because of the apparent triviality of the condition.

The use of unconventional or quack remedies may be more difficult to elicit from the patient. Preventive therapy for patients resorting to such means would seem to include the establishment of an open and trusting dialogue. The professional who offers information, understanding, and hope is least likely to lose a patient to charlatans.

Compliance with Prescribed Regimens

Over the past decade it has become increasingly evident that noncompliance is a significant impediment to optimal health care delivery. Depending upon the definition used to distinguish compliant from noncompliant behavior, studies have documented noncompliance rates ranging from 25 to 90 per cent in various patient populations. The magnitude and significance of this problem demand that all health care professionals make concerted efforts toward understanding and improving compliance. Although it is unrealistic to expect all patients to follow all advice precisely, an appreciation of the incidence and clinical consequences of noncompliance and an understanding of the factors that may contribute to noncompliance can lead to the design of therapeutic regimens and patient education efforts that can significantly improve compliance with prescribed regimens.

Compliance in health care delivery can simply be defined as the extent to which the patient's behavior conforms with medical advice. Although drug therapy has been the most extensively studied aspect of compliance, noncompliance with dietary regimens, exercise plans, the use of tobacco, and alcohol consumption have been the subjects of considerable concern and study. It is important to avoid the assumption that noncompliance is solely the fault of the patient. Both the therapist and circumstances beyond the control of the patient can significantly contribute to noncompliance.

Literally hundreds of studies have been published in recent years on the subject of noncompliance with drug therapy. A comprehensive review, compilation, and analysis of the literature on the subject of compliance can be found in *Compliance in Health Care* by Haynes, Taylor, and Sackett.[18] The following discussion will review the key factors necessary to understand the compliance problem and suggest mechanisms that can improve compliance.

Types of Medication Errors

Noncompliance with prescribed drug therapy includes four general types of problems (Table 1–2). The first opportunity for noncompliance after the physician issues a prescription order is for the patient to fail to have the prescription filled. Since most studies of compliance have been designed to follow up on patients after a prescription has been dispensed, there is little data available to estimate the incidence of unfilled prescriptions. In one study of 134 patients who received 380 prescriptions, 24 prescriptions (7 per cent) were never filled.[19] There appear to be two major factors that contribute to the problem of unfilled prescriptions—the cost of the prescription and failure to appreciate the necessity or benefit of the medication. Although Medicaid programs provide coverage for prescription drugs for the indigent, the Medicare program for the elderly does not provide prescription drug coverage. Fixed incomes during times of rampant inflation may well place the elderly in the position of being "medically indigent" inasmuch as they may not be able to meet the costs of health care services beyond basic insurance benefits. Lack of understanding or appreciation of the necessity and benefits of therapy may also contribute to not having a prescription filled. Considerable education and persuasion may be required to convince the patient of the value of a prescription.

TABLE 1–2. Types of Medication Errors

1. Failure to obtain prescription
2. Improper administration of medication
3. Premature discontinuation of medication
4. Taking inappropriate medication

Improper administration or errors of self-medication have been well documented (Table 1–3). Errors of dosage include both over- and underdosing. An increase in the dose is often related to the belief that if one tablet is good, two will be better. Decreasing the dose may be used in an attempt to conserve an expensive prescription. Errors in frequency of administration include the omission of a dose or the taking of extra doses. Such errors commonly arise from a lack of understanding of ambiguous directions. Directions to take a drug "with meals" fails to recognize that not everyone eats the usual three meals per day. The elderly patient may also be at greater risk of omitting or repeating a dose because of a failing memory.

Errors in the timing or sequencing of medication administration are also common. The direction to take a medication "four times daily" fails to communicate the need to spread out the doses of certain medications over a 24 hour period. For drugs for which proper administration intervals are important (e.g., theophylline), time intervals (every six hours around the clock) or specific times (6 A.M., 12 noon, 6 P.M., and 12 midnight) should be specified. The designations "before meals" or "after meals" also fail to clearly specify appropriate consumption. When food may significantly affect the action of the drug, directions should specify "with food" or "on an empty

TABLE 1–3. Errors in Medication Administration

1. Incorrect dosage
2. Improper frequency of administration
3. Improper timing or sequence of administration
4. Wrong route or technique of administration
5. Taking medication for wrong purpose

stomach—one hour before or two hours following meals." Although specific dosing times are desirable, a schedule that fails to coincide with the patient's daily routine may lead to noncompliance.

Administration of a drug by the wrong route or by an improper technique may not be common but does occur. A patient with an earache may not easily comprehend the rationale for a decongestant nose drop prescription, and therefore he may instill the drug into the ear. Any prescription that requires any technique beyond the simplest swallowing of a tablet deserves a full explanation and demonstration to insure the patient's comprehension.

Knowledge of the purpose of the medication is of particular importance when patients are taking multiple prescriptions. Specific notations on the prescription label as to the name and purpose of the medication will eliminate confusion when a patient is instructed to "increase the sugar pill to three a day, decrease the blood pressure medication to once a day, stop taking the antibiotic, and take the arthritis pills only when needed."

Premature discontinuation of a medication is a common problem. Apparent resolution of an infection when the patient begins to feel better or becomes afebrile commonly leads to premature discontinuation of antibiotic therapy. Exacerbation, reinfection, and the emergence of bacterial resistance may result. Drug therapy of the asymptomatic hypertensive patient exemplifies a situation in which the patient may actually feel worse as a result of the medication, thus leading to poor compliance. Abrupt discontinuation of some medications (propranolol and corticosteroids, for example) can lead to serious consequences beyond the lack of therapeutic response. Clearly, education is essential to impress upon the patient the importance of continued therapy, the expected therapeutic response, anticipated untoward reactions, and the consequences of premature discontinuation of therapy.

The use of an inappropriate medication may occur for many reasons. Failure of the physician or pharmacist to limit refills of prescriptions may result in continuation of a drug that is intended to be discontinued. When a patient is switched from one drug to another, he should be clearly instructed to discard any unused drug remaining from the discontinued prescription. Hoarding of unused medication and reuse of old prescriptions are particularly common in the elderly. Similarly, the sharing of medication with relatives and friends who appear to develop similar illnesses is not uncommon.

Clinical Consequences of Noncompliance

With noncompliance rates estimated to be in the range of 25 to 50 per cent, the clinical consequences of this problem should not be underestimated. The possibility of noncompliance should be a major consideration in every case of therapeutic failure. Undetected noncompliance may lead to unnecessary therapy with more potent agents, which have a greater potential for adverse effects. A sudden improvement in compliance following unnecessary dosage increases may result in toxicity or other untoward effects. Beyond the obvious results of a poor therapeutic response, noncompliance may have significant long term economic implications as a result of increases in both morbidity and mortality. A poor therapeutic response secondary to poor compliance may also lead the practitioner to erroneous conclusions concerning the efficacy of the prescribed regimen.

Correlates of Noncompliance

Our present level of understanding of the problem of compliance does not provide clear or easy solutions. Several studies have demonstrated that physician estimates of compliance are poor.[20,21] A number of factors have been found to be associated with noncompliance in various studies (Table 1–4). An appreciation of these factors may help one to

TABLE 1–4. Factors Associated with Noncompliance

A. Disease factors
  1. Diagnosis
  2. Severity
  3. Symptomatology
  4. Degree of disability
  5. Duration of illness
  6. Clinical response
B. Characteristics of therapy
  1. Duration of treatment
  2. Number of prescriptions
  3. Frequency of dosing
  4. Side effects
  5. Cost
C. Patient factors
  1. Age
  2. Satisfaction with provider
  3. Education
  4. Income
  5. Socioeconomic status

identify those patients most likely not to comply.[18]

Several disease related factors appear to be associated with compliance behavior. Patients with mental or emotional problems tend to be less compliant than other patients. The severity of the disease, as perceived by the patient, may influence compliance; patients are more likely to comply when the disease represents a significant threat to their wellbeing. Similarly, the severity of symptoms and the degree of disability have a positive correlation with compliance. The duration of the illness is negatively associated with compliance, as is the degree of clinical improvement.

Several characteristics of the therapeutic regimen generally appear to correlate with compliance. The duration of treatment, the number of drugs, and the frequency of dosing are all directly associated with poor compliance. The occurrence of side effects will also lead to a decrease in compliance. As mentioned previously, cost may represent an obstacle to compliance; several studies have documented that the greater the cost, the lower the level of compliance with drug therapy.

Patient related factors have also been studied. Although there is some controversy, there is evidence to suggest that the elderly may be poorer compliers than other age groups. If not directly related to age, this generalization would appear to be true from the standpoint that the elderly have an increased incidence of multiple chronic diseases and therefore consume a greater number of medications for longer periods of time. Socioeconomic status (income and education) also appears to correlate with compliance in some studies, low socioeconomic status correlating with poorest compliance rates.

Studies of provider-patient interaction show that "satisfaction with the provider" is associated with better compliance. Such factors as waiting time, time spent with the provider, and the attitude of the provider may all contribute to the patient's satisfaction and, consequently, compliance.

Treating Noncompliance

Although there are no easy or guaranteed solutions for noncompliance, a number of steps can be taken to improve compliance. It is useful to regard compliance as a logical progression of the patient having the *ability,* the *knowledge,* and the *desire* to comply. The design of therapeutic regimens and patient education efforts should address each of these factors.

As has been discussed previously, complicated regimens that include multiple drugs, multiple dosing times, and inconvenient administration intervals detract from compliance. In order to design a therapeutic regimen within the limitations of the patient's ability to comply, regimens should be as simple as possible. Consideration should be given to the patient's life style and patterns of living (e.g., meals, rest). Dosage schedule simplification by the use of fixed drug combinations or sustained release dosage forms may offer a therapeutic compromise pharmacologically or pharmacokinetically; however, improvements in compliance may far outweigh any disadvantages. Coordinating medication administration with meals as an aid in remembering may be of greater advantage than taking the medication under ideal fasting conditions.

Lack of clear understandable directions will preclude compliance with the therapist's intentions by even the most capable and most willing patient. Adequate directions for a prescription should specify the dose, frequency, and timing of administration (preferably including specific times), the route of administration, and the name and purpose of the medication. This information should be given to the patient in writing via the prescription label. Patients do not retain such information when given only verbal instructions. If both the prescriber and dispensing pharmacist provide verbal reinforcement of clearly written directions, a significant contribution to improved compliance will have been made.

Influencing the patient's desire to comply with the prescribed medication regimen may represent a more formidable task. Although data are limited, there is reasonable evidence that the more the patient knows and understands about his disease and therapy, the higher the level of compliance. It is important to stress the benefits of therapy, especially when no significant symptomatic effects are obvious. In addition, the patient should be apprised of the potential consequences of noncompliance. Establishing an open dialogue with the patient and encouraging questions to avoid misinterpretation and uncertainty are essential in establishing trust in the therapist. The patient should be made to view his role as assuming an active part in effecting a positive therapeutic outcome.

Patient Education Materials

In recent years a number of patient education publications have been developed. These publications are useful as guides to key elements of information that should be covered in counseling the patient. Such information usually includes proper administration, timing with respect to meals, foods and other medications to avoid, and common precautions such as "may cause drowsiness." A more detailed approach to education about drugs is provided by printed pamphlets or sheets written in common terminology designed for the patient. Although quantities of pamphlets on numerous drugs can be obtained from several sources, the most practical method of distributing such materials is by photocopying from a single compilation. When using preprinted materials, space should be reserved to write in patient-specific information as the need arises. Information provided by these sources usually provides information about the action of the drug, expected therapeutic benefits, precautions to observe during therapy, and warnings concerning the more adverse reactions. Table 1–5 lists a number of patient education resources that are commercially available.

Patient package inserts, which are required by the United States Food and Drug Administration for selected prescription drugs, represent a regulatory response to the patient's desire and need for drug information. Proponents of mandatory patient package inserts argue that patients have a need and a right to drug information and that such information is not generally provided by physicians and pharmacists. Opponents of mandatory patient package inserts argue that to be effective, drug information must be personalized to meet the needs of the individual patient and that the provision of appropriate information is a clinical judgment best left to the practitioner. Specific fears have been voiced that the emphasis on adverse reactions in patient package inserts may contribute to noncompliance.

In 1980 the FDA initiated a program that would have ultimately led to mandatory patient package inserts for all prescription medications. However, this rule was later withdrawn in response to strong political opposition, because of uncertainty over the cost versus the benefits of the program, and in recognition of increased voluntary efforts. Should pharmacists and physicians fail to seize this opportunity to voluntarily meet this recognized consumer demand, the threat of FDA intervention will undoubtedly return.

Compliance Aids

A number of medication calendars, personal patient profiles, and unique packaging devices have been developed to aid in compliance. Simply asking the patient to record each dose taken on a calendar will serve as a reminder and encouragement to take the medication regularly. Medication calendars can easily be made to include the name(s) and time(s) for taking each drug daily.

Special packaging has proven helpful for oral contraceptives, corticosteroids, and several antibiotics. Although such packaging may increase the cost of the medication, the benefits of improved compliance may be well justified. Similarly, fixed dosage combination drug products and sustained release dosage forms may simplify administration schedules and therefore enhance compliance.

Intelligent Noncompliance

Weintraub[23] has presented an interesting discussion of intelligent noncompliance. Examples include patients who discontinue digoxin therapy without negative consequences or patients who reduce their dosage because of adverse effects of therapy. In such instances intelligent noncompliance is appropriate because the drug therapy regimen is inappropri-

TABLE 1–5. Patient Drug Education Materials

Drug Consultation Guide
    Maudlin, R.K., and Young, L.Y.
    Hamilton, Illinois, Drug Intelligence Publications, Inc.
Consumer's Guide to Prescription Product Information
    Smith, D.L.
    Willimantic, Connecticut, Pharmex
Medication Teaching Manual. A Guide for Patient Counseling
    Washington, D.C., American Society of Hospital Pharmacists, 1983
Medication Guide for Patient Counseling
    Smith, D.L.
    Philadelphia, Lea & Febiger, 1981
United States Pharmacopeia—Dispensing Information
    Rockville, Maryland, United States Pharmacopeial Convention, Inc., 1983
Instructions for Patients
    Griffith, H.W.
    Philadelphia, W.B. Saunders Company, 1982
Advice for the Patient
    Rockville, Maryland, United States Pharmacopeial Convention, Inc., 1983

ate. From this perspective it is essential to recognize that considerations of compliance should be subordinate to appropriate prescribing practices. Compliance-ensuring strategies should not be devised to insure that patients follow an inappropriate drug therapy regimen.

Summary

In spite of sophisticated advances in health care delivery, noncompliance with prescribed therapy remains a significant impediment to successful outcomes. The elderly patient is at high risk of noncompliance for a number of reasons. Health professionals must make concerted efforts to prescribe a simple and easy-to-follow medication plan, provide clear directions for the proper method of administration, and reinforce the benefits of following the prescribed regimen. Patient monitoring must include an assessment of compliance to determine accurately the value of therapy. Perhaps more than in any other aspect of health care delivery, the problem of noncompliance offers an opportunity for an interdisciplinary effort. Professionals in pharmacy, medicine, and nursing can coordinate and reinforce efforts to improve the quality of patient care.

Drug Dependence in the Elderly

Medication consumption patterns span the spectrum from proper drug use to misuse, abuse, and dependence. The previous discussions have covered the topics of basic patterns of the use and misuse of both prescription and nonprescription drugs. The topic of drug and substance abuse and dependence in the elderly represents a relative void in our understanding of medication consumption patterns.

In spite of massive efforts focused on the problems of drug abuse over the last two decades, little attention has been given to these problems in the elderly. Because of the emphasis placed on drug abuse in the teenage and college age populations, one might be led to the conclusion that such problems are limited to these age groups. The limited data available relating to the prevalence of drug abuse tend to indicate that abuse is less common in the over-65 population. However, it is clear that abuse does occur in the elderly, that abuse is probably less likely to be detected in these patients, and that the geriatric patient is at a great risk of harm from abuse.

Use of Illicit Drugs

Illicit or illegal substances include cocaine, the opiates, principally heroin, and the psychedelic drugs, which include marijuana, mescaline, peyote, and LSD. Virtually no data are available relating to the use of psychedelic drugs in the elderly. Since these substances represent a relatively recent phenomenon in drug abuse, it is reasonable to assume that their use in the elderly is rare.

A limited amount of data is available concerning opiate abuse in the elderly. Capel and Stewart[24] estimate that 5 per cent of the patients in methadone maintenance programs are 45 years of age or older, and Pascarelli and Fischer[25] estimate that 1 per cent are over 60 years of age. These estimates seem to confirm that the incidence of opiate abuse is lower in the older age groups. Several suggestions have been offered to account for these findings. Winick[26] suggests a "maturing out process" that occurs with age and with increased length of addiction. It is also probable that a significant proportion of addicts do not survive to continue their addiction into the geriatric years.

As with all statistics dealing with drug abuse, known cases represent only the "tip of the iceberg." It is suggested that the streetwise older addict may escape identification by maintaining a lower profile than the younger addict. In contrast to the use of heroin by the younger addict, the older addict is more prone to the use of pharmaceutical opiates such as hydromorphone (Dilaudid), morphine, oxycodone (Percodan), and codeine.[24] Although the prevalence of opiate abuse in the elderly appears to be lower than in other age groups, most investigators anticipate that the number of older addicts will increase in the coming decade.

Abuse of Prescription Drugs

Abuse of prescription medications may range from inadvertent misuse to intentional abuse and occasionally leads to psychological or physical dependence. As previously discussed, the elderly consume a disproportionately large percentage of all prescriptions. Medications with a potential for abuse, including sedative-hypnotics, antipsychotic drugs, antianxiety drugs, and strong analgesics, are among those most commonly prescribed for the elderly.

Since the source of these medications is

through prescription, it is impossible to ascertain the extent of abuse as compared to legitimate use. As with younger patients, physicians should maintain a high index of suspicion to detect the patient who may fake symptoms in order to obtain a prescription for a drug subject to abuse. Furthermore, the prescriber should avoid contributing to drug dependence by avoiding unnecessary prescriptions, and pharmacists should monitor drug utilization via patient drug profiles for abuse patterns in drug consumption.

Alcohol Abuse

In general, alcohol abuse appears to occur most commonly in the 35 to 50 year age group.[27] Alcohol consumption tends to decrease in the elderly.[28] As with opiate abuse, this may represent a "maturing out" process as well as increased mortality in chronic alcoholics. Although the prevalence of alcohol abuse may be lower in the elderly, it is estimated that 2 to 10 per cent of the general population 55 years of age and over suffer from alcoholism.[29] In one study 44 per cent of the patients over age 60 admitted to a psychiatric institution had an alcohol abuse problem.[30]

The elderly alcoholic patient represents a significant challenge owing to difficulties in the diagnosis of alcohol abuse, difficulties in treatment and rehabilitation, and medical problems secondary to or exacerbated by alcohol abuse. Wood,[29] in reviewing problems in the diagnosis of alcoholism in the elderly, points out that many of the clinical, behavioral, and psychological symptoms of alcoholism occur frequently in elderly individuals who do not have a drinking problem (gastritis, anemia, insomnia, depression). Therefore, alcohol abuse may be overlooked in evaluating the geriatric patient. Failure to recognize and treat the alcoholic patient may lead to a variety of secondary medical problems. The effect of alcohol on drug therapy must also be considered because of the potential for interaction with a number of drugs.

Summary

Drug abuse among the elderly can be a significant medical problem, which is likely to go unrecognized. Research is needed to gain an understanding of the drug abuse patterns in the elderly and to identify related problems that may be unique to this segment of society.

Physicians must be alert to identify and deal with drug abuse problems in the elderly patient.

ADVERSE DRUG REACTIONS

In the broadest sense, any unintended effect as a result of drug administration can be considered an adverse drug reaction. Such a definition would include effects resulting from noncompliance, medication administration errors, toxic effects from intentional or accidental overdosage, toxicity or therapeutic failure due to drug-drug interaction, and therapeutic failures as the result of inappropriate prescribing. Although such events are undesirable occurrences, they result from improper application of the drug and therefore should be distinguished from untoward effects that are directly attributable to the drug. The World Health Organization defines an adverse drug reaction as "any response to a drug that is noxious and unintended and that occurs at doses used in man for prophylaxis, diagnosis or therapy." Untoward effects excluded from this definition include toxic effects resulting from accidental or intentional overdosage or drug abuse. Also therapeutic failure, which may result from medication errors, noncompliance, inadequate dosage, bioavailability problems, or improper drug selection, is not generally considered to be an adverse drug reaction.

Documentation of Adverse Drug Reactions

The topic of adverse drug reactions consumes an increasing proportion of the medical literature each year. However, the data on adverse drug reactions are incomplete, unrepresentative, uncontrolled, and lacking in operational criteria for identifying adverse drug reactions. No quantitative conclusions can be drawn from the reported data in regard to morbidity, mortality, or the underlying causes of such reactions, and attempts to extrapolate the available data to the general population would be invalid and perhaps misleading.[31] In spite of the emphasis on defining and documenting the incidence of adverse drug reactions, the data available remain inadequate.

Sources of drug information often provide extensive lists of adverse reactions reported to have been attributed to an individual drug. However, it is likely that few of the reported reactions have been adequately documented as drug related events. There are numerous problems encountered in confirming a causal relationship between a drug and an adverse reaction. Multiple drug exposure, effects of concomitant disease, and "placebo reactions" all serve to cloud the issue of documentation. The following criteria are helpful in classifying adverse drug reactions:[31,32]

Definite: A reaction that follows a reasonable temporal sequence from administration of the drug or in which the drug level has been established in body fluids or tissues, that follows a known response pattern to the suspected drug, and that is confirmed by improvement on stopping or reducing the dosage of the drug (dechallenge) and reappearance of the reaction on repeated exposure (rechallenge).

Probable: A reaction that follows a reasonable temporal sequence from administration of the drug, that follows a known response pattern to the suspected drug, that is confirmed by dechallenge, and that could not be reasonably explained by the known characteristics of the patient's clinical state.

Possible: A reaction that follows a reasonable temporal sequence from administration of the drug and that follows a known response pattern to the suspected drug but that could have been produced by the patient's clinical state or other modes of therapy administered to the patient.

Doubtful: Any reaction that does not meet the foregoing criteria.

Unfortunately, most reports of adverse drug reactions fail to include enough information for proper classification.

FDA Adverse Drug Reaction Program

The FDA Division of Drug Experience maintains a voluntary reporting program that gathers data relating to adverse drug reactions. In order to aid in the dissemination of information about such reactions, physicians, pharmacists, and other health professionals are urged to report all instances of significant reactions. The types of reactions of greatest interest include new and unexpected reactions not mentioned in the labeling; serious, life threatening, or fatal reactions; unusual increases in the number and severity of reactions; and potential associations with congenital anomalies. Information that is particularly helpful in evaluating reports includes the temporal relationship of the drug to the reaction, whether the reaction decreased when the suspected drug was removed (dechallenge), whether the reaction recurred when the drug was reintroduced (rechallenge), and information relating to concomitant diseases that may have caused the effect and other drugs used concomitantly. Reports should be sent to the Division of Epidemiology and Drug Experience (HFD-210), Food and Drug Administration, 5600 Fishers Lane, Rockville, Maryland 20857.

Incidence of Adverse Drug Reactions

Accurate data relating to the incidence of adverse reactions would be extremely valuable in making risk-benefit assessments. Although the benefits of therapy usually can be estimated, the probability of the occurrence of an adverse effect is difficult to estimate. Most estimates of the incidence of specific adverse reactions are based on small samples of patients in controlled studies. Extrapolation of such data beyond the conditions of the study cannot be justified. Over-reporting may result from inadequate documentation of a causal relationship to drug administration. Under-reporting undoubtedly occurs, since few primary care physicians are likely to publish instances of adverse reactions; furthermore, it is likely that many minor (and some major) adverse reactions are unrecognized.

Published estimates of the incidence rates of adverse reactions in hospitalized patients range from 1.5 to 35 per cent.[33,34] Karch and Lasagna[31] estimate that the incidence is between 6 and 15 per cent in hospitalized medical patients, with a much lower incidence on other services; they further estimate the incidence of fatal adverse drug reactions to be in the range of 0 to 0.31 per cent in medical patients. Another study of hospitalized patients suggests that women are more apt to suffer adverse reactions (38 per cent) than men (30 per cent). In this study 4.3 per cent of the reactions in women and 5.8 per cent of those in men were reported as being "severe." Two deaths (0.1 per cent) were reported to result from adverse drug reactions.[35]

Limited data suggest that adverse drug reactions occur more frequently in the elderly. In one study of hospitalized patients the incidence of adverse drug reactions was 15.4 per cent in patients over 65 years of age compared to 6.3 per cent in those under 60 years of age.[36] A higher incidence of adverse reactions in the elderly may be attributed to the greater use of drugs, increased sensitivity to drug effects, impaired homeostatic mechanisms, and decreases in renal and hepatic function.

Mechanisms of Adverse Effects

Adverse reactions may be classified by mechanisms as pharmacologic, allergic, or idiosyncratic. Adverse pharmacologic reactions are predictable dose related effects that can be expected to occur in all patients if the drug is given in high enough doses. These reactions may be further characterized as either "toxic effects" or "side effects." Toxic effects are the result of extensions or exaggerations of the primary (desired) action of the drug. Orthostatic hypotension from guanethidine and hypoglycemia associated with sulfonylureas are examples of toxic pharmacological reactions that commonly occur. Although the term toxicity is usually associated with overdosage, such reactions can occur at usual therapeutic dosages in a small percentage of patients. The elderly patient is especially likely to experience toxicity at usual dosages because of an increased sensitivity to drugs as well as decreased renal and hepatic elimination.

Side effects are differentiated from toxic effects as being undesired secondary pharmacologic actions that are inseparable from the desired action of the drug. Antihistamine induced sedation and the anticholinergic effects from tricyclic antidepressants are typical examples of side effects. Both side effects and toxic effects can be minimized by dosage reduction.

Allergic or hypersensitivity reactions are the result of antigen-antibody interaction. Such immunologically mediated reactions may range in severity from a minor rash to anaphylaxis and death. Prior exposure to the antigenic agent (drug) is required, and time must elapse for the production of antibodies. Hypersensitivity reactions include immediate (anaphylaxis) and delayed (serum sickness) reactions. Although the initial reaction may be unexpected, careful documentation of previous drug experience should prevent the recurrence of such reactions. Atopic individuals should be considered at high risk for the development of drug allergy. Precautionary measures, including patient observation and the availability of resuscitation equipment, epinephrine, corticosteroids, and antihistamines, are essential and can be life saving in the event of an acute hypersensitivity reaction.

Idiosyncratic reactions are rare, unpredictable, and often severe and are not dose related. Such reactions are frequently difficult to diagnose. A number of genetically determined reactions are generally classified as idiosyncratic reactions. These include such anomalies as glucose-6-phosphate dehydrogenase deficiency, which may lead to hemolytic anemia in patients exposed to oxidant drugs (e.g., primaquine) and the precipitation of acute intermittent porphyria by a number of drugs (e.g., barbiturates). Tables 1-6 and 1-7 list drugs known to precipitate these conditions in susceptible patients.[37–42]

TABLE 1-6. Drugs That May Precipitate Hemolysis in Glucose-6-Phosphate Dehydrogenase Deficiency

Analgesics
   Aspirin
   Phenacetin

Anti-infectives
   Chloramphenicol
   Nalidixic acid
   Nitrofurantoin
   PAS
   Sulfonamides

Antimalarials
   Chloroquine
   Dapsone
   Primaquine
   Quinacrine

Diphenhydramine
Probenecid
Procainamide
Quinine
Tolbutamide

Vitamins
   Ascorbic Acid
   Vitamin K

TABLE 1-7. Drugs That May Precipitate Acute Intermittent Porphyria

Barbiturates	Griseofulvin
Chlordiazepoxide	Phenytoin
Chlorpropamide	Sulfonamides
Estrogens	Tolbutamide
Glutethimide	

Prevention of Adverse Drug Reactions

Preventing or minimizing the severity of adverse drug reactions presents a perplexing problem. In spite of the desires of idealists, benefit without risk is an elusive dream. There

TABLE 1–8. Potentially Ototoxic Drugs

Aminoglycosides	Diuretics
Amikacin	Ethacrynic acid
Gentamicin	Furosemide
Kanamycin	
Neomycin	Other
Streptomycin	Ampicillin
Tobramycin	Chloramphenicol
Vancomycin	Minocycline
	Nortriptyline
Analgesics-antirheumatics	Polymyxin
Aspirin	Propranolol
Fenoprofen	Quinidine
Gold salts	Quinine
Ibuprofen	
Indomethacin	
Naproxen	
Phenylbutazone	
Tolmetin	

are, however, a number of steps that may minimize the potential of serious harm from adverse drug reactions.

A careful history of medication use and experience is essential to avoid repetition of a previous untoward experience. Patients at greatest risk, including the elderly and those with impaired renal function, should be started at conservative dosage levels, which can be increased gradually to achieve optimal therapeutic benefit without inducing significant undesired side effects. In order to monitor patients it is essential to be aware of the significant toxic reactions associated with the use of each drug. Tables 1–8, 1–9, and 1–10

TABLE 1–9. Potentially Nephrotoxic Drugs

Acetazolamide	Kanamycin*
Amikacin	Neomycin*
Amitriptyline	Nitrofurantoin
Amphotericin B	PAS
Bacitracin*	Penicillamine*
Carbonic anhydrase inhibitors	Penicillin
Cephaloridine	Phenacetin
Chlorothiazide	Phenylbutazone
Colchicine	Polymyxin B*
Cisplatin*	Probenecid
Colistimethate sodium	Salicylates
Colistin*	Streptomycin
Corticosteroids	Sulfonamides
Ethacrynic acid	Tetracyclines*
Furosemide	Thiazides
Gentamicin*	Tobramycin*
Gold compounds	Vancomycin
Hydralazine	Viomycin*
Hydrochlorothiazide	

*Designated drugs have the highest incidence of nephrotoxicity.

TABLE 1–10. Potentially Hepatotoxic Drugs

Acetaminophen	Methyldopa
Acetohexamide	Naproxen
Alcohol	Nicotinic acid
Allopurinol	Nitrofurantoin
Aminosalicylic acid	Oxyphenbutazone
Amitriptyline	Oxytetracycline
Ampicillin	Papaverine
Chloramphenicol	Penicillin
Chlordiazepoxide	Perphenazine
Chlorothiazide	Phenazopyridine
Chlorpromazine	Phenobarbital
Chlorpropamide	Phenylbutazone
Chlorthalidone	Phenytoin
Clindamycin	Probenecid
Conjugated estrogens	Procainamide
Dantrolene	Prochlorperazine
Desipramine	Propoxyphene
Diazepam	Quinidine
Erythromycin estolate	Rifampin
Ferrous sulfate	Sulfonamides
Gold salts	Sulfisoxazole
Hydralazine	Tetracycline
Hydrochlorothiazide	Thioridazine
Imipramine	Tolbutamide
Indomethacin	Tripelennamine
Isoniazid	Vitamin A
Meprobamate	

list the drugs most commonly implicated in causing ototoxic, nephrotoxic, and hepatotoxic reactions.[43–48] Periodic clinical assessment and monitoring of appropriate laboratory tests frequently make possible the detection of early manifestations of toxicity. Perhaps most significant in preventing adverse drug reactions is the avoidance of unnecessary drug exposure; prescriptions should be limited to instances in which drug therapy is clearly indicated and therapy should be discontinued when the drug is no longer necessary.

Summary

Adverse drug reactions represent real and significant risks in the use of any drug. Knowledge of the nature of adverse effects is essential to an accurate risk-benefit analysis of drug therapy. Proper drug selection and appropriate patient monitoring can minimize the risks of significant morbidity or mortality from adverse reactions. A review of most general drug information sources will provide a listing of adverse reactions that may occur with any particular drug. For more complete and detailed information relating to adverse drug reactions, the references listed in Table 1–11 are recommended.

TABLE 1–11. References on Adverse Drug Reactions

Drugs, Chemicals and Blood Dyscrasias
    Swanson, M., and Cook, R.
    Hamilton, Illinois, Drug Intelligence Publications, 1977

Meyler's Side Effects of Drugs. Ed. 9
    Dukes, M.N.G.
    Amsterdam, Excerpta Medica, 1980

Side Effects of Drugs-Annual 7
    Dukes, M.N.G.
    Amsterdam, Excerpta Medica, 1983

Textbook of Adverse Drug Reactions
    Davies D.M.
    New York, Oxford University Press, 1981

Clin-Alert (periodical)
    Louisville, Science Editors Inc.

Reactions (periodical)
    New York, ADIS Press

TABLE 1–12. References on Drug-Drug Interactions

A Guide to Drug Interactions
    James, J.D., Braunstein, M.L., Karig, A.W., and Hartshorn, E.A.
    New York, McGraw-Hill Inc., 1978

Clinical Effects of Interactions Between Drugs
    Cluff, L.E., and Petrie, J.C.
    Amsterdam, Excerpta Medica, 1978

Drug Interaction Facts
    Mangini, R.J. (Editor)
    St. Louis, Facts and Comparisons, 1984

Drug Interactions. Ed. 5
    Hansten, P.D.
    Philadelphia, Lea & Febiger, 1984

Evaluations of Drug Interactions. Ed. 2
    Washington, D.C., American Pharmaceutical Association, 1976

DRUG INTERACTIONS

Achieving an accurate diagnosis requires the evaluation and correlation of a multitude of variables that contribute to the overall assessment. Isolated factors are of little value if not considered within the context of the whole patient. Similarly, in order to insure an optimal regimen of drug therapy, consideration must be given to the potential for interactions between drugs, between drugs and laboratory test procedures, and between drugs and elements of the patient's diet.

Over the last 20 years the level of understanding of drug interactions has evolved from almost complete ignorance, through a stage of minor paranoia over multiple drug therapy. Although there is much yet to be learned, there is a wealth of information available that can serve as a guide to rational therapy with minimal risk of significant untoward effects from drug interactions.

The following discussions briefly review the areas of drug-drug, drug-laboratory test, and drug-food interactions. Emphasis is placed on a conceptual understanding of the mechanisms of drug interactions; knowledge of the mechanisms by which interactions occur can enhance anticipation of a potential interaction and suggest appropriate methods of management. Tabular compilations of drug interactions are provided as a guide to many of the more common, potentially significant drug interactions with selected drugs most commonly used by the elderly patient. For more comprehensive discussions and evaluations of drug interactions, the reference sources listed in Table 1–12 are recommended.

Drug-Drug Interactions

In the simplest terms, a drug interaction can be defined as the effect of one drug altering the usual anticipated activity of another drug. Although concern usually focuses on therapeutic failures or adverse reactions, drug interactions may also prove to be beneficial. Additive or synergistic effects that improve the efficacy of antihypertensive and antineoplastic combination regimens are common examples.

Mechanisms

There are several mechanisms by which drug interactions occur. Most interactions appear to occur by a single mechanism; however, there are many drug combinations that may interact by more than one mechanism. Drug interactions may occur by pharmacokinetic (alterations in the absorption, distribution, metabolism, or excretion) or pharmacodynamic (occurring at the drug receptor) mechanisms.

Absorption. The first parameters defining the pharmacokinetic profile of a drug relate to the rate and degree of absorption (bioavailability). Any factor that alters the rate or degree of absorption may affect the performance of the drug. Interactants that inhibit the degree or extent of absorption usually do so by physical or chemical complexation of the drug. The capacity of calcium (from milk or antacids) to complex with and inhibit the absorption of tetracycline is a common example. The physical nature of antacids, which are adsorbants as well as buffers, makes these products suspect in having the potential to alter the absorption of many drugs.

Drugs that alter gastrointestinal transit time, and therefore the time a drug is exposed to the gastrointestinal mucosa for absorption, can also affect the extent of drug absorption. Anticholinergics may therefore be expected to enhance the absorption of some drugs, whereas cathartics, which increase peristaltic activity, may decrease drug absorption. Food frequently delays the rate of drug absorption but may not alter the total amount of the drug absorbed. These interactions are of most significance with drugs having short half-lives. In such instances delayed absorption may preclude the attainment of therapeutic serum levels.

The majority of drug interactions involving impaired drug absorption can be avoided by proper timing and sequencing of drug administration. Separation of administration times by two hours is usually sufficient.

Distribution. Drugs are distributed throughout the body tissues in varying degrees. However, for the majority of drugs, both pharmacologic and toxic responses are dependent on the amount of free drug in the plasma. Any concomitant therapy that alters the distribution of the drug in tissues may significantly alter the free drug fraction and thereby affect the activity of the drug.

Interactions involving altered distribution include changes in the volume of distribution and displacement from protein binding. A large number of interactions have been reported to occur secondary to displacement from protein binding. However, many of these theoretical displacement interactions are clinically insignificant because of compensatory increases in clearance.

Metabolism. Since many drugs are inactivated by biotransformation via hepatic microsomal enzymes, alteration of the level of enzyme activity or competition for common metabolic pathways can significantly affect drug activity. Table 1–13 lists a number of drugs known to induce or stimulate the activity of hepatic microsomal enzymes.[49–51] Significant enzyme induction usually requires chronic exposure to the inducer. A common example is barbiturate-induced increased metabolism of warfarin.

Inhibition of drug metabolizing enzymes is another common occurrence; the clinical manifestations of enzyme inhibition would be expected to cause an increased pharmacologic effect and toxicity. Table 1–14 lists the most frequently encountered enzyme inhibitors. Aside from the potential for undesirable drug interactions, enzyme inhibition may be useful therapeutically. Allopurinol inhibition of xanthine oxidase, disulfiram inhibition of alcohol metabolism, and the use of monoamine oxidase inhibitors are examples of beneficial interactions of this type.

Excretion. Since most drugs and drug metabolites are excreted by renal mechanisms, any drug induced alteration in renal function

TABLE 1–13. Drugs That Induce Microsomal Enzyme Activity

Amobarbital	Meprobamate
Antihistamines	Methyprylon
Butabarbital	Nicotine
Chloral hydrate	Pentobarbital
Chlordiazepoxide (Librium)	Phenobarbital
Chlorpromazine	Phenytoin
Cortisone	Prednisolone
Diphenhydramine	Prednisone
Ethanol	Probenecid
Ethchlorvynol	Promazine
Glutethimide	Rifampin
Griseofulvin	Secobarbital
Haloperidol	Testosterone and its derivatives
Imipramine	
Insecticides, halogenated	Tolbutamide

TABLE 1–14. Drugs That Inhibit Microsomal Enzyme Activity

Acetohexamide
Allopurinol
Antipsychotic agents
Bishydroxycoumarin
Chloramphenicol
Cholinesterase inhibitors
Chlorpropamide
Cimetidine
Disulfiram
Furazolidone
Isoniazid
Methylphenidate
Metronidazole
Monoamine oxidase inhibitors
Procarbazine
Sulfonamides
D-Thyroxine
Tolbutamide

may alter drug activity. Decreases in the renal blood flow and glomerular filtration rate may lead to drug accumulation. Many drugs are secreted and at least partially reabsorbed in the renal tubules. Competition by two or more drugs for common secretory pathways can result in a decreased rate of elimination. The use of probenicid to block penicillin elimination is a beneficial application of this drug interaction mechanism. Tubular secretion and reabsorption are frequently pH dependent; alterations in urinary pH therefore can enhance or inhibit drug elimination. Basic drugs are excreted more rapidly in an acid urine and more slowly in an alkaline urine; conversely, excretion of acidic drugs can be enhanced by urinary alkalinization or inhibited by urinary acidification. Again, such interactions may be detrimental if unanticipated, yet can be used to advantage by the knowledgable therapist.

Pharmacodynamic Interactions. Drug interactions involving the receptor upon which the drug produces its pharmacologic effect are termed pharmacodynamic interactions. Such interactions may involve one or more receptors and may result in either additive or antagonistic effects. Additive pharmacologic and toxic effects occur when two drugs having similar actions are given together; such interactions are easily recognized when they are the result of the primary pharmacologic activity of the drugs, such as additive central nervous system depression from hypnotics, benzodiazepines, and narcotics. However, secondary pharmacologic effects are often forgotten or ignored, as in the case of additive anticholinergic effects of antihistamines, antidepressants, and antipsychotic drugs.

Opposing pharmacologic effects may occur with drugs acting at different receptor sites. Coadministration of an alpha-adrenergic drug (vasoconstrictor) and a beta-2-adrenergic drug (vasodilator) might result in no net effect on peripheral vascular resistance. Direct antagonism at a single receptor may occur with combinations such as a narcotic agonist and a narcotic antagonist or a cholinergic drug and an anticholinergic drug.

Management of Drug Interactions

Although there are numerous sources of information about the topic, reports of therapeutic failures and toxic reactions due to well known drug-drug interactions continue to appear in the literature. The elderly patient in particular appears to be at great risk of sustaining a drug interaction because of an increased exposure to drugs.

Knowledge of the pharmacokinetic and pharmacodynamic characteristics of medications being utilized can provide insight into the potential for drug interactions. The occurrence of an unexpected response in a patient receiving multiple drug therapy requires a careful review of the regimen for possible interactions. In such instances it is imperative to have knowledge of all the medications a patient is taking, including nonprescription products.

Few drug interactions constitute absolute contraindications to concomitant therapy. Interference with absorption can usually be avoided by separating administration of interactants by two hour intervals. Most other interactions can be compensated for by careful adjustments in drug dosages. In all cases close monitoring of the patient is essential to make appropriate adjustments in order to avoid therapeutic failure or other untoward effects. The monitoring of drug plasma levels may be extremely useful when such capabilities are available. Critical periods of observation occur when any change in therapy is instituted.

Table 1-15 summarizes many of the more common drug interactions of potential clinical significance that are most likely to occur in the geriatric patient. No attempt has been made to include all possible interactions for the drugs listed. Information in the table is presented in alphabetical order by the generic names of the drug affected. Cross references are included when interactions are listed by drug class or group.

Drug-Laboratory Test Interactions

Clinical laboratory test procedures play a significant role in contemporary health care delivery. Various tests serve as screening tools in preventive medicine and early detection programs. Many tests are invaluable as diagnostic tools to confirm clinical impressions. Monitoring the progression of disease and the response to therapeutic measures frequently requires the use of laboratory test procedures.

Proper use and interpretation of reported laboratory test values requires an appreciation of the "normal range" of reported parameters as well as the significance and probable causes of deviations from "normal." The effects of drugs on the results of various clinical laboratory test procedures must be considered in order to avoid making erroneous diagnostic or

TABLE 1–15. Potential Interactions of Drugs Used in the Elderly

Acetohexamide. See *Antidiabetics*

Allopurinol. See *Uricosurics*

Aminoglycosides
    Additive ototoxicity with
        Furosemide
        Ethacrynic acid

Amitriptyline. See *Tricyclic antidepressants*

Anticholinergics
    Additive anticholinergic effects with
        Antihistamines
        Antipsychotics
        Tricyclic antidepressants

Anticoagulants, oral
    Activity increased (hemorrhage) via *displacement* by
        Chloral hydrate
        Phenylbutazone
        Salicylates
        Sulfonamides
        Sulfonylureas
        Triclofos
    Activity increased (hemorrhage) via *enzyme inhibition* by
        Allopurinol
        Cimetidine
        Clofibrate
        Disulfiram
        Metronidazole
        Phenylbutazone
        Sulfonamides
    Activity increased (hemorrhage) via *inhibition of vitamin K* by
        Antibiotics (broad spectrum)
        Cholestyramine
        Mineral oil
    Increased bleeding tendency when given with drugs that *inhibit platelet aggregation*
        Dipyridamole
        Indomethacin
        Phenylbutazone
        Salicylates
        Sulfinpyrazone
    Activity increased (hemorrhage) by *unknown mechanism*
        Acetaminophen
        Anabolic steroids
        Thyroid products
    Activity decreased via *enzyme induction* by
        Barbiturates
        Carbamazepine
        Glutethimide
        Griseofulvin
        Rifampin
        Phenytoin
    Activity decreased via *increase in procoagulant factors* by
        Vitamin K
        Estrogens

Antidiabetics (oral)
    Activity decreased via increased blood glucose levels by
        Thiazides
    Activity increased via *displacement* by
        Sulfonamides
        Clofibrate
    Activity increased (hypoglycemia) via *unknown mechanism* by
        Monoamine oxidase inhibitors
        Corticosteroids
    Activity increased (hypoglycemia) via *inhibition of catecholamines* by
        Propranolol (beta-adrenergic blockers)
    Activity increased via *inhibition of hepatic metabolism* of sulfonylureas by
        Warfarin
        Chloramphenicol
    Activity increased via *enhancement of hypoglycemic effect* by
        Alcohol
    Activity increased (hypoglycemia) via *delayed excretion* by
        Phenylbutazone
        Oxyphenbutazone
    Activity decreased via *enzyme induction* by
        rifampin

Barbiturates
    Additive central nervous system depression with
        Alcohol
        Antipsychotics
        Narcotic analgesics
        Tricyclic antidepressants
    Activity increased via inhibition of metabolism by
        Monoamine oxidase inhibitors

Belladonna
    Activity increased via potentiation of anticholinergic effect by
        Amantadine
        Antihistamines
        Antipsychotics
        Monoamine oxidase inhibitors
        Tricyclic antidepressants

Bendroflumethiazide. See *Thiazides*

Benzodiazepines
    Activity increased via additive central nervous system depressant activity by
        Alcohol
        Antipsychotics
        Barbiturates
        Narcotics
        Nonbarbiturate sedative-hypnotics
    Activity increased via *enzyme inhibition* by
        cimetidine

Benzthiazide. See *Thiazides*

Bishydroxycoumarin. See *Anticoagulants, oral*

TABLE 1–15. *Continued*

Chlordiazepoxide. See *Benzodiazepines*

Chlorpropamide. See *Antidiabetics*

Chlorothiazide. See *Thiazides*

Codeine. See *Narcotics*

Corticosteroids
    May cause significant hypokalemia when used with
        Ethacrynic acid
        Furosemide
        Thiazide diuretics
    Activity decreased via enzyme induction by
        Barbiturates
        Phenytoin
        Rifampin

Cyclothiazide. See *Thiazides*

Desipramine. See *Tricyclic antidepressants*

Diazepam. See *Benzodiazepines*

Dicumarol. See *Anticoagulants, oral*

Digitalis glycosides
    Activity increased (toxicity) via depletion of potassium by
        Amphotericin B
        Ethacrynic acid
        Furosemide
        Corticosteroids
        Thiazide diuretics
    Activity decreased via intestinal binding by
        Antacids
        Cholestyramine
        Kaolin-pectin
    Activity increased via potentiation of pharmacological effect by
        Calcium, parenteral
        Dextrothyroxine
    Digitoxin activity decreased via enzyme induction by
        Barbiturates
    Digoxin activity increased via inhibition of clearance by
        Quinidine
        Verapamil

Doxepin. See *Tricyclic antidepressants*

Ephedrine
    Activity increased via enhancement of norepinephrine activity by
        Monoamine oxidase inhibitors
    Activity increased via unknown mechanism by
        Tricyclic antidepressants

Ethacrynic acid
    Additive ototoxicity with
        Aminoglycosides

Flumethiazide. See *Thiazides*

Furosemide
    Additive ototoxicity with aminoglycosides

Guanethidine
    Activity decreased via inhibition of uptake at adrenergic neuron by
        Amphetamines
        Phenothiazines
        Sympathomimetics
        Tricyclic antidepressants

Hydrochlorothiazide. See *Thiazides*

Hydroflumethiazide. See *Thiazides*

Imipramine. See *Tricyclic antidepressants*

Isocarboxazid. See *Monoamine oxidase inhibitors*

Levodopa
    Activity decreased via enhancement of metabolism by pyridoxine
    Activity decreased via dopamine depletion by reserpine

Meperidine. See *Narcotics*

Methenamine
    Activity decreased via alkalinization of urine by
        Acetazolamide
        Thiazides

Methyclothiazide. See *Thiazides*

Methyldopa
    Activity decreased (hypertension) by phenothiazines, mechanism unknown

Monoamine oxidase inhibitors
    Hypertensive reactions may occur with
        Amphetamine
        Levodopa
        Sympathomimetics
        Tyramine-containing foods
    Marked central nervous system depression with
        Alcohol
        Hypnotic-sedatives
        Narcotic analgesics

Morphine. See *Narcotics*

Narcotics
    Additive central nervous system depression with
        Alcohol
        Antipsychotics
        Barbiturates
        Benzodiazepines
        Nonbarbiturate sedative-hypnotics
        Tricyclic antidepressants

Nortriptyline. See *Tricyclic antidepressants*

TABLE 1–15. *Continued*

Pargyline. See *Monoamine oxidase inhibitors*

Pentobarbital. See *Barbiturates*

Phenelzine. See *Monoamine oxidase inhibitors*

Phenobarbital. See *Barbiturates*

Phenytoin
    Activity increased via inhibition of metabolism by
        Anticoagulants, oral
        Chloramphenicol
        Cimetidine
        Disulfiram
        Isoniazid (INH)
        Phenylbutazone
        Sulfonamides

Polythiazide. See *Thiazides*

Prednisone. See *Corticosteroids*

Probenecid. See *Uricosurics*

Protriptyline. See *Tricyclic antidepressants*

Quinidine
    Activity increased via alkalinization of urine by
        Acetazolamide
        Antacids
        Thiazides
    Decreased effect via enhanced metabolism by
        Phenobarbital
        Phenytoin
        Rifampin

Secobarbital. See *Barbiturates*

Sulfinpyrazone. See *Uricosurics*

Sulfonylureas. See also *Antidiabetics*

Tetracycline
    Activity decreased via impaired absorption by
        Antacids
        Iron salts
        Milk and dairy products due to calcium

Thiazides
    Activity increased (potassium loss) via potentiation by corticosteroids
    Activity increased via displacement by diazoxide

Tolazamide. See *Antidiabetics*

Tolbutamide. See *Antidiabetics*

Tranylcypromine. See *Monoamine oxidase inhibitors*

Trichlormethiazide. See *Thiazides*

Tricyclic antidepressants
    Additive anticholinergic effects with
        Anticholinergics
        Antihistamines
        Antipsychotics
    Activity increased via enhancement of renal tubular absorption by
        Acetazolamide
        Sodium bicarbonate
    Activity decreased via enhanced urinary excretion by
        Ammonium chloride
        Ascorbic acid (large doses) > 2.0 gm. per day

Uricosurics
    Antagonism of uricosuric effects by
        Salicylates
        Thiazides

Warfarin. See *Anticoagulants, oral*

---

therapeutic judgments. The large number of drugs used and the variety of laboratory parameters that may be evaluated in a given patient may lead to a multitude of possible drug–laboratory test interferences that must be considered. Medical, laboratory, and pharmacy personnel must cooperate to insure accurate evaluation of such interferences in the delivery of rational therapy.

Mechanisms of Drug–Laboratory Test Interactions

It is essential to distinguish between drug–laboratory test interactions, which may occur by two general mechanisms (i.e., methodologic interferences or biologic alterations). Methodologic interactions are the result of a drug interference with the analytical procedure used to measure the particular parameter. Such interferences result in false positive or false negative values. Biologic interactions occur when the drug causes an actual alteration in the amount of the substance being evaluated. Such alterations result in true elevations or decreases in reported values.

Methodologic Interferences. Drugs, or their metabolites, may interfere with clinical laboratory test procedures by either physical or chemical means. Physical interference occurs most commonly with drugs that impart a color to body fluids being analyzed by colorimetric or spectrophotometric means. Phenazopyridine and riboflavin are common examples of drugs that alter the color of biologic fluids.

Chemical interference may occur when the drug or its metabolites enter into a chemical reaction that is the basis for the analytical procedure. A common example is the false positive values caused by reducing agents (e.g., ascorbic acid, nalidixic acid) when urine glucose levels are determined by copper reduction methods. The interference of iodine-containing contrast media with protein bound iodine and iodine-131 uptake is another well documented laboratory interference by chemical means.

When drugs that interfere with specific test procedures are known, alternate laboratory methods are frequently available. For example, when reducing substances render copper reduction methods of glucose determination useless, glucose oxidase methods may remain accurate. It is therefore important to know the specific mechanism of drug induced interference so that appropriate alternative methods can be identified.

Biologic Alterations. In contradistinction to methodologic interferences that result in false laboratory test values, biologic alterations are true changes (elevations or decreases) in the parameter being evaluated as a result of drug administration. Such alterations may be desired and anticipated as a part of the pharmacologic response to drug therapy; other alterations may be undesirable and may occur as a result of an adverse reaction to drug therapy. Laboratory test changes that represent a therapeutic response to drug therapy are not normally considered as drug-laboratory test interactions (e.g., sulfonylureas decrease the blood glucose level, and allopurinol lowers the uric acid level).

Monitoring laboratory test values for undesired changes in physiologic parameters is an essential part of rational drug therapy for the early detection of adverse drug reactions. Toxic effects of drugs on hepatic, renal, and hematopoietic function can commonly be detected at an early stage by monitoring appropriate laboratory tests. Early detection and appropriate alterations of therapy can avoid many severe adverse drug reactions.

Summary

Tables 1–16 to 1–19 provide a brief guide to interactions between standard laboratory tests and the drugs most commonly used by elderly patients. For more extensive listings and discussions of drug–laboratory test interactions, the references in Table 1–16 are recommended.

Drug-Food Interactions

Compared to the topic of drug-drug interactions, relatively little is known concerning drug-food interactions. Few studies have been conducted documenting the mechanism or clinical significance of interactions between medications and components of the diet. This discussion reviews the types of drug-food interactions that may occur, reviews what is known concerning the mechanisms of such interactions, and identifies a number of drug-food interactions that have been reported. Drug-food interactions include both alterations in a drug's activity as a result of concurrent ingestion of food and changes in nutritional status as a result of drug use.

Mechanisms of Drug-Food Interactions

As with drug-drug interactions, drug-food interactions may occur by pharmacokinetic or pharmacologic mechanisms. Pharmacokinetic interactions result from alterations in the rate or extent of absorption, metabolism, or excretion of the drug. Pharmacologic interactions

TABLE 1–16. References on Drug–Laboratory Test Interactions

Effects of Drugs on Clinical Laboratory Tests
  Young, D.S., Pestaner, L.C., and Gibberman, V.
  Clinical Chemistry, *21*:5, 1975
  Winston-Salem, North Carolina, American Association of Clinical Chemists, Inc., 1975

Todd Sanford Davidsohn Clinical Diagnosis and Management by Laboratory Methods
  Henry, J.B. (Editor)
  Philadelphia, W.B. Saunders Company, 1979

Clinical Laboratory Medicine
  Ravel, R.
  Chicago, Year Book Medical Publishers, 1978

Drug-induced Modifications of Laboratory Test Values
  Constantino, N.V., and Kabat, H.F.
  American Journal of Hospital Pharmacy, *30*:24, 1973
  Washington, D.C., American Society of Hospital Pharmacists

Drug Interactions. Ed. 5
  Hansten, P.D.
  Philadelphia, Lea & Febiger, 1984

Handbook of Clinical Drug Data. Ed. 5
  Knoben, J.E., Anderson, P.O., and Watanabe, A.S.
  Hamilton, Illinois, Drug Intelligence Publications, Inc., 1983

TABLE 1-17. Drug Interaction with Serum Laboratory Tests

Alkaline phosphatase
    Acetohexamide — Increase
    Allopurinol — Increase
    Amitriptyline — Increase
    Anabolic-androgenic drugs — Increase
    Chlorpropamide — Increase
    Clindamycin — Increase
    Colchicine — Increase
    Erythromycin — Increase
    Estrogens — Increase
    Flurazepam — Increase
    Imipramine — Increase
    Indomethacin — Increase
    Methyldopa — Increase
    Nicotinic acid — Increase
    Nitrofurantoin — Increase
    Oxacillin — Increase
    Papaverine — Increase
    Phenothiazines — Increase
    Phenylbutazone — Increase
    Procainamide — Increase
    Propranolol — Increase
    Rifampin — Increase
    Sulfonamides — Increase
    Tetracycline — Increase
    Tolbutamide — Increase

Bilirubin
    Acetaminophen — Increase
    Acetazolamide — Increase
    Acetohexamide — Increase
    Allopurinol — Increase
    Amitriptyline — Increase
    Anabolic-androgenic steroids — Increase
    Barbiturates — Increase
    Chlordiazepoxide — Increase
    Chlorpropamide — Increase
    Clindamycin — Increase
    Desipramine — Increase
    Diazepam — Increase
    Erythromycin — Increase
    Ethacrynic acid — Increase
    Ethanol — Increase
    Flurazepam — Increase
    Gentamicin — Increase
    Imipramine — Increase
    Indomethacin — Increase
    Isoniazid — Increase
    Lincomycin — Increase
    Menadione — Increase
    Methyldopa — False positive (SMA 12/60)
    Nicotinic acid — Increase
    Nitrofurantoin — Increase
    Oxacillin — Increase
    Papaverine — Increase
    Phenazopyridine — Increase
    Phenothiazines — Increase
    Phenylbutazone — Increase
    Phenytoin — Increase
    Procainamide — Increase
    Protriptyline — Increase
    Sulfonamides — Increase/decrease
    Tetracycline — Increase
    Tolbutamide — Increase

Blood urea nitrogen (BUN)
    Acetohexamide — False positive
    Alkaline antacids — Increase
    Aminoglycosides — Increase
    Chloral hydrate — False positive (Nessler)
    Ethacrynic acid — Increase
    Furosemide — Increase
    Guanethidine — Increase and false positive
    Indomethacin — Increase
    Methyldopa — Increase
    Nalidixic acid — Increase
    Nitrofurantoin — Increase
    Phenothiazines — Decrease
    Polymyxin B — Increase
    Propranolol — Increase
    Radiopaque contrast media — Increase
    Salicylates — Increase
    Tetracyclines — Increase
    Thiazide diuretics — Increase
    Vancomycin — Increase

Calcium
    Acetazolamide — Decrease
    Alkaline antacids — Increase
    Anabolic-androgenic steroids — Increase
    Corticosteroids — Decrease
    Estrogens — Increase
    Ethacrynic acid — Decrease
    Furosemide — Decrease
    Insulin — Decrease
    Iron — False positive (EDTA titration)
    Laxatives (excessive use) — Decrease
    Potassium — False positive (flame photometry)
    Sodium — False positive (flame photometry)
    Thiazide diuretics — Increase
    Vitamin D — Increase

Chloride
    Acetazolamide — Increase
    ACTH-corticosteroids — Increase/decrease
    Androgenic steroids — Increase
    Bicarbonate — Decrease
    Ethacrynic acid — Decrease
    Furosemide — Decrease
    Oxyphenbutazone — Increase
    Phenylbutazone — Increase
    Thiazide diuretics — Decrease

Cholesterol
    ACTH-corticosteroids — Increase and false positive (ferric chloride)
    Anabolic steroids — Increase
    Androgenic steroids — Decrease
    Antidiabetic drugs — Decrease
    Chlortetracycline — Decrease
    Cholestyramine resin — Decrease
    Clofibrate — Increase/decrease
    Colchicine — Decrease
    Cortisone — Increase
    Dextrothyroxine — Decrease
    Estrogens — Decrease
    Haloperidol — Decrease
    Neomycin — Decrease
    Nicotinic acid — Decrease
    Nitrates — False negative (Zlatkis-Zak)
    Phenothiazines — Increase
    Phenytoin — Increase
    Salicylates — Decrease
    Thyroid — Decrease

Creatine phosphokinase (CPK)
    Ampicillin (intramuscular administration) — Increase
    Carbenicillin (intramuscular administration) — Increase
    Chlorpromazine (intramuscular administration) — Increase
    Clindamycin — Increase
    Clofibrate — Increase

TABLE 1–17. *Continued*

Creatinine		Phosphate (inorganic)	
Aminoglycosides	Increase	Alkaline antacids	Decrease
Ascorbic acid	False positive (Heinegarb and direct methods)	Aluminum hydroxide	Decrease
		Epinephrine	Decrease
Barbiturates	Increase	Insulin	Decrease
Clofibrate	Increase	Tetracycline	Increase/decrease
Gentamicin	Increase		
Glucose	False positive (Heinegarb and Jaffe reaction)	Potassium	
		Acetazolamide	Decrease
Kanamycin	Increase	Cephaloridine	Increase
Methyldopa	False positive (Fuller's earth and alkaline picrate)	Chlorthalidone	Decrease
		Corticosteroids	Decrease
		Diuretics (oral)	Decrease
Triamterene	Increase	Insulin	Decrease
		Isoniazid	Increase
Glucose		Laxatives (excessive)	Decrease
Acetaminophen	Decrease/false positive (SMA 12/60)	Lithium carbonate	Increase/decrease
		Salicylates	Decrease
Acetazolamide	Increase	Spironolactone	Increase/decrease
Acetohexamide	Decrease	Tetracyclines	Increase/decrease
Anabolic steroids	Decrease	Triamterene	Increase/decrease
Ascorbic acid	False positive (SMA 12/60)		
Ascorbic acid	False negative (glucose oxidase)	Protein (total)	
		Anabolic steroids	Increase
		Androgenic steroids	Increase
Caffeine	Increase	Clofibrate	Increase
Chlorpropamide	Decrease	Corticosteroids	Increase
Chlorthalidone	Increase	Insulin	Increase
Clofibrate	Decrease	Radiographic contrast media	False positive (turbidity)
Corticosteroids	Increase		
Dextrothyroxine	Increase	Thyroid preparations	Increase
Diazoxide	Increase		
Estrogens	Increase		
Ethacrynic acid	Increase/decrease	Serum glutamic oxaloacetic transaminase (SGOT)	
Ethanol	Increase/decrease		
Fructose	False positive (SMA 12/60)	Acetaminophen	Increase
Fructose	False negative (hexokinase)	Acetaminophen	False positive (Morgenstern, SMA 12/60)
Furosemide	Increase		
Guanethidine	Decrease	Ampicillin	Increase
Haloperidol	Increase/decrease	Anabolic-androgenic drugs	Increase
Imipramine	Increase/decrease	Carbenicillin	Increase
Insulin	Decrease	Cephalothin	Increase
Isoniazid	Increase/false negative (glucose oxidase)	Clindamycin	Increase
		Clofibrate	Increase
Lithium carbonate	Increase	Colchicine	Increase
Monoamine oxidase inhibitors	Decrease	Desipramine	Increase
		Erythromycin	Increase/false positive (colorimetric)
Nalidixic acid	False positive (copper reduction)		
		Flurazepam	Increase
Nicotinic acid	Increase	Gentamicin	Increase/false positive (Babson)
Nitrofurantoin	Increase		
Phenytoin	Increase	Indomethacin	Increase
Propoxyphene	Decrease	Isoniazid	Increase/false positive (SMA 12/60)
Propranolol	Decrease		
Reserpine	Increase	Lincomycin	Increase
Salicylates	Increase/decrease	Meperidine	Increase
Thiazide diuretics	Increase	Methyldopa	Increase/false positive (SMA 12/60, Babson)
Thyroid preparations	Increase		
Tolazamide	Decrease/false negative (glucose oxidase)	Nalidixic acid	Increase
		Nitrofurantoin	Increase
Tolbutamide	Decrease	Phenothiazines	Increase
Tolbutamide	False positive (glucose oxidase)	Phenytoin	Increase
		Procainamide	Increase
Tolbutamide	False negative	Propranolol	Increase
		Rifampin	Increase
Lactic dehydrogenase		Salicylates	Increase
Ascorbic acid	False negative (SMA 12/60)	Sulfamethazole	Increase
		Tetracycline	Increase
Clofibrate	Increase/decrease		
Meperidine	Increase	Sodium	
		Ammonium chloride	Decrease
Lipids (total)		Anabolic agents	Increase
Cholestyramine resin	Decrease	Corticosteroids	Increase
Coffee	Increase	Diuretics, oral	Decrease
Estrogens	Increase	Laxatives	Decrease

THERAPEUTIC DILEMMAS IN THE ELDERLY/27

TABLE 1-17. Continued

Sodium *continued*		Ascorbic acid	False positive (Cu-chelate, Klein, Nishi)
Methyldopa	Increase		
Oxyphenbutazone	Increase	Bishydroxycoumarin	Decrease
Phenylbutazone	Increase	Chlorthalidone	Increase
Potassium	False positive (flame photometry)	Clofibrate	Decrease
		Coffee	False positive (Bittner)
Rauwolfia alkaloids	Increase	Corticosteroids	Decrease
Spironolactone	Decrease	Diazoxide	Increase
Thiazide diuretics	Decrease	Diuretics	Increase
		Ethacrynic acid	Increase/decrease
Triiodothyronine [(T₃) uptake]		Ethanol	Increase
Anabolic-androgenic drugs	Increase	Furosemide	Increase
Anticoagulants, oral	Increase	Gentamicin	Increase
Antithyroid drugs	Decrease	Levodopa	Increase and false positive (Cu-chelate, Nishi, phosphotungstate)
Chlordiazepoxide	Decrease		
Corticosteroids	Increase/decrease		
Dextrothyroxine	Increase	Lithium carbonate	Decrease
Estrogens	Decrease, false positive (Thyopac)	Methotrexate	Increase/decrease
		Methyldopa	False positive (phosphotungstate)
Phenylbutazone	Increase		
Phenytoin	Increase	Nicotinic acid	Increase
Salicylates	Increase	Nitrogen mustards	Increase/decrease
Sulfonylureas	Increase	Oxyphenbutazone	Decrease
Thiazides	Decrease	Phenothiazines	Increase/decrease
Thyroid therapy	Increase	Phenylbutazone	Increase/decrease
		Probenecid	Decrease
Uric acid		Rifampin	Increase
Acetazolamide	Increase	Salicylates	Increase (low dose)
Acetohexamide	Decrease	Salicylates	Decrease (high dose)
Adrenocortical steroids	Increase/decrease	Spironolactone	Increase
Allopurinol	Decrease	Sulfinpyrazone	Decrease
Aminophylline	False positive (Bittner)	Thiazide diuretics	Increase
Anticoagulants	Increase	Triamterene	Increase

TABLE 1-18. Drug Interactions with Hematology Values

Erythrocyte count or hemoglobin		Leukocytes	
Acetaminophen	Decrease	Acetohexamide	Decrease
Chloramphenicol	Decrease	Acetominophen	Decrease
Chloroquine	Decrease	Allopurinol	Increase/decrease
Diiodohydroxyquin	Decrease	Ampicillin	Increase (eosinophilia)/decrease
Ethosuximide	Decrease		
Hydralazine	Decrease	Barbiturates	Decrease
Indomethacin	Decrease	Cardiotonic glycosides	Increase (eosinophilia)/decrease
Isoniazid	Decrease		
Monoamine oxidase inhibitors	Decrease	Cephalothin	Increase (eosinophilia)/decrease
Mercurial diuretics	Decrease	Chloramphenicol	Increase/decrease
Methyldopa	Decrease	Chlordiazepoxide	Decrease
Nitrites	Decrease	Chlorpropamide	Increase/decrease (increase eosinophilia)
Nitrofurantoin	Decrease		
Oxyphenbutazone	Decrease		
Penicillin	Decrease	Clindamycin	Increase/decrease (increase eosinophilia)
Phenobarbital	Decrease		
Phenylbutazone	Decrease		
Primaquine	Decrease	Clofibrate	Decrease
Rifampin	Decrease	Corticosteroids	Decrease
Spectinomycin	Decrease	Diazepam	Decrease
Sulfonylureas	Decrease	Desipramine, imipramine	Increase/decrease (increase eosinophilia)
Tetracycline	Decrease		
Thiazide diuretics	Decrease		

TABLE 1–18. Continued

Digitalis	Increase (eosinophilia)/decrease	Streptomycin	Decrease
Erythromycin	Increase/decrease	Sulfonamides	Increase/decrease
Ethacrynic acid	Decrease	Sulfonamides, long acting	Increase
Furosemide	Decrease	Sulfonylureas	Decrease
Gold compounds	Increase/decrease (increase eosinophilia)	Tetracyclines	Increase/decrease
		Thiazide diuretics	Decrease
		Triamterene	Increase (eosinophilia)
Haloperidol	Decrease		
Hydantoins	Increase/decrease (increase eosinophilia)	Thrombocytes (platelets)	
		Acetazolamide	Decrease
Hydralazine	Decrease	Acetohexamide	Decrease
Indomethacin	Decrease	Cardiotonic glycosides	Decrease
Isoniazid	Increase (eosinophilia)/decrease	Chloramphenicol	Decrease
		Colchicine	Decrease
Kanamycin	Increase (eosinophilia)	Ethacrynic acid	Decrease
Meprobamate	Decrease	Gold salts	Decrease
Methyldopa	Increase/decrease (increase eosinophilia)	Oxyphenbutazone	Decrease
		Penicillins	Decrease
		Phenothiazines	Decrease
Methyprylon	Decrease	Phenylbutazone	Decrease
Nalidixic acid	Increase (eosinophilia)	Procainamide	Decrease
Nitrofurantoin	Decrease	Propranolol	Decrease
Oxyphenbutazone	Increase/decrease	Quinidine sulfate	Decrease
Penicillins	Decrease	Quinine	Decrease
Phenothiazines	Increase/decrease	Rifampin	Decrease
Phenylbutazone	Increase/decrease	Salicylates	Decrease
Procainamide	Decrease	Sulfonamides	Decrease
Quinine	Increase/decrease	Sulfonylureas	Decrease
Rifampin	Decrease	Thiazide diuretics	Decrease

TABLE 1–19. Drug Interactions with Urine Laboratory Tests

Acetone		Isoniazid	False positive (copper reduction)
Insulin	Increase		
Isoniazid	Increase	Levodopa	False positive (Clinitest)
Levodopa	False positive (nitroprusside)	Levodopa	False negative (glucose oxidase)
		Lithium carbonate	Increase
Bilirubin		Methyldopa	False positive (Clinitest)
Mefenamic acid	False positive (Diazo)	Nalidixic acid	False positive (copper reduction, Fehlings)
Phenothiazines	Increase		
		Nicotinic acid	Increase
Glucose		Nitrofurantoin	False positive (Benedict's)
Abscorbic acid	False negative (glucose oxidase)	Penicillin	False positive (copper reduction)
Cephaloridine	False positive (copper reduction)	Phenacetin	False positive (Benedict's)
Cephaloridine	False positive (Clinitest)	Phenothiazines	Increase
Chloral hydrate	False positive (Benedict's)	Probenecid	False positive (copper reduction)
Chloral hydrate	False negative (Clinistix, Diastix)	Salicylates	Increase/decrease
Chloramphenicol	False positive (copper reduction)	Salicylates	False positive (Benedict's)
Corticosteroids	Increase	Salicylates	False negative (glucose oxidase)
Ephedrine	Increase		
Ethacrynic acid	Increase	Streptomycin	False positive (Benedict's)
Isoniazid	Increase		

TABLE 1–19. Continued

Glucose *continued*		Ethacrynic acid	Decrease/increase (intravenous)
Sulfonamides	False negative (Benedict's)	Methyldopa	False positive (phosphotungstate)
Tetracycline	Increase		
Tetracycline	False positive (copper reduction)	Probenecid	Increase/decrease
		Salicylates	Increase/decrease
Tetracycline	False negative (glucose oxidase)	Salicylates	False positive (nonspecific)
Thiazide diuretics	Increase	Thiazide diuretics	Decrease
Vaginal powders	False positive (contamination)	Triamterene	Increase
		Urine color change	
Protein (as albumin)		Amitriptyline	blue-green
Chlorpropamide	Increase	Cascara	brown (acid), yellow-pink (alkaline), black on standing
Corticosteroids	Increase		
Gentamicin	Increase		
Gold salts	Increase	Ethanol	lighter color
Isoniazid	Increase	Indomethacin	green
Kanamycin	Increase	Levodopa	red tinged, blackens on standing
Lithium carbonate	Increase		
Neomycin	Increase	Methyldopa	red, brown-black on standing
Penicillin	False positive (sulfosalicylic acid)		
		Nitrofurantoin	brown or rust yellow
Phenylbutazone	Increase	Phenolphthalein	orange rust (acid), pink, red, purple (alkaline)
Radiopaque contrast media	Increase and false positive (acid, Doetsch)		
Sulfonamides	False positive (sulfosalicylic acid)	Phenothiazines	pink, purple, orange, rust
		Phenytoin	pink, red, red-brown
Tetracyclines	Increase	Primaquine	rust yellow, brown
Tolbutamide	False positive (sulfosalicylic acid)	Quinine	brown
		Riboflavin	yellow
		Rifampin	red-orange
		Senna	yellow-brown (acid), yellow-pink (alkaline)
Uric acid			
Allopurinol	Decrease		
Caffeine	False positive (phosphotungstate)	Sulfonamides	rust yellow or brown
Corticosteroids	Increase	Triamterene	bluish color, green

occur when the interactant enhances or antagonizes the effects of the drug at the effector site.

Absorption. By far the most common type of drug-food interactions involve alteration of the bioavailability of the drug. Concurrent ingestion of food with drugs may alter both the extent and the rate of drug absorption. There are many instances in which consumption with food delays absorption of the drug but does not affect the total amount of drug absorbed. Such interactions are not clinically significant for most drugs; however, for drugs that must rapidly achieve high serum levels to produce the desired response, a delay in the rate of absorption may be significant. Interactions in which the extent of absorption is affected are more likely to be clinically significant, especially for drugs with a narrow therapeutic index.

Alterations in drug bioavailability can occur by a variety of mechanisms. The physical mass of food may restrict contact of the drug with the absorbing surface of the gastrointestinal mucosa, thus inhibiting or delaying absorption. Chemical complexation, as with the effects of calcium from milk on tetracyclines, may also inhibit absorption. Food may alter the amount of secretion of gastric acid, digestive enzymes, and bile. Subsequent alterations in gastric pH may affect the degree of ionization of weakly acidic or basic drugs and therefore affect their absorption.

Changes in gastrointestinal motility, particularly gastric emptying time, will affect the time a drug is exposed to the gastrointestinal mucosa for absorption and may also alter the dissolution rate of some drugs. Changes in hepatic blood flow in response to a meal have been reported to decrease the extent of first pass metabolism of propranolol, thus enhancing the oral bioavailability of the drug. Table

TABLE 1-20. Drugs Whose Absorption Is Decreased When Given with Food

Ampicillin	Penicillins
Isoniazid	Rifampin
Levodopa	Tetracyclines
Lincomycin	

1-20 lists a number of drugs whose absorption is inhibited by food, and Table 1-21 lists drugs that are known to have improved bioavailability when given with food.

Metabolism. A potentially significant drug-food interaction involving altered drug metabolism is the effect of charcoal broiled meat on phenacetin and theophylline kinetics. Enzyme induction by polycyclic hydrocarbon compounds present in charcoal broiled foods significantly enhances the rate of elimination of theophylline in man.[52] Similarly, cabbage and brussels sprouts have been found to induce the metabolic clearance of antipyrine and to enhance the metabolism of phenacetin. The effect on phenacetin is believed to occur either in the gastrointestinal tract or as a first pass hepatic effect. Although few interactions of this type have been documented, it is likely that other dietary components may similarly affect the metabolic fate of drugs.

In contrast to foods altering drug metabolism, drugs may significantly alter the metabolic fate of dietary constituents. The most remarkable of these interactions is the hypertensive response to dietary tyramine in patients taking monoamine oxidase inhibitors. Tyramine is a potent pressor, which is normally inactivated by monoamine oxidase enzymes. Reactions may range from headache to potentially fatal hypertensive crisis in patients taking monoamine oxidase inhibitors as antidepressants or antihypertensive drugs. Table 1-22 lists the commercially available monoamine oxidase inhibitors and a number of foods known to contain significant amounts of tyramine.

TABLE 1-21. Drugs Whose Absorption Is Enhanced When Given with Food

Carbamazepine	Methoxsalen
Dicumarol	Metoprolol
Erythromycin stearate	Nitrofurantoin
Griseofulvin (fatty foods)	Phenytoin
Hydralazine	Propranolol
Hydrochlorothiazide	Riboflavin
Lithium	Spironolactone

TABLE 1-22. Monoamine Oxidase Inhibitors and Foods Containing Tyramine

Monoamine Oxidase Inhibitors	Tyramine Containing Foods
Isocarboxazid (Marplan)	Aged cheeses
Pargyline (Eutonyl)	Beer
Phenelzine (Nardil)	Broad beans
Tranylcypromine (Parnate)	Caffeine (excessive)
	Chocolate (excessive)
	Pickled herring
	Wine (chianti)
	Yeast extract
	Yogurt

Excretion. Excessive intake of dietary constituents that alter the pH of the urine could affect the urinary excretion of weakly acidic or basic drugs that are subject to pH dependent excretion and reabsorption. Acidic drugs are excreted more rapidly in a basic urine and more slowly in an acid urine; conversely the excretion of basic drugs is enhanced in an acid urine and delayed in a basic urine. Alteration of urinary pH may also present a problem with methenamine or aminoglycosides, which are most active in an acid urine. Conversely, an alkaline urine is desirable to maximize the solubility of sulfonamides. Dietary constituents that are capable of altering urinary pH are listed in Table 1-23.

Another potentially significant dietary interaction involves lithium. The excretion of lithium is decreased in sodium depletion states. Low sodium intake therefore may predispose the patient to lithium toxicity. Patients who are taking lithium should be encouraged to maintain an adequate sodium intake.

Pharmacologic Interactions. Antagonism of the hypoprothrombinemic effects of orally administered anticoagulants may occur if a

TABLE 1-23. Foods That Can Alter Urinary pH

Alkalinizers	Acidifiers
Almonds	Bacon
Chestnuts	Breads
Coconuts	Cheese
Citrus fruits	Corn
Milk	Cranberries
Vegetables	Eggs
	Fish
	Fowl
	Lentils
	Meat
	Pasta
	Plums

patient ingests excessive quantities of foods containing vitamin K. Cabbage, green tea, turnip greens, broccoli, and brussels sprouts all contain significant amounts of vitamin K. The efficacy of the thiazide diuretics is enhanced by dietary sodium restriction; conversely, excessive sodium intake decreases the efficacy of thiazide therapy.

Summary

Alterations in the anticipated effects of drugs may occur as a result of concomitant administration with food. Although a number of these interactions have been documented, relatively little is known concerning the mechanisms, incidence, or clinical significance of these interactions. Known interactions should be avoided if they have the potential for untoward effects. Conversely, beneficial interactions may be used to advantage. The potential of unknown drug-food interactions represents another factor that must be considered if unexpected results occur with drug therapy.

RATIONAL PRESCRIBING

The path to an ideal therapeutic regimen for any given patient includes a variety of obstacles that can lead to undesirable consequences. To avoid therapeutic misadventures, practitioners must make a concerted effort to tailor therapy to the unique characteristics of each patient. The complexity of interrelationships between the patient, the conditions being treated, and the therapeutic modalities being utilized preclude the use of cookbook approaches to rational prescribing.

The discussions of therapeutic dilemmas have been directed at increasing the reader's awareness of these potential hazards associated with drug therapy. Although these problems exist in treating patients of all ages, the elderly patient is at greater risk of suffering clinically significant complications of a therapeutic misadventure. On the basis of previous discussions, the following is a brief summary of the principles essential to the pursuit of a safe and effective therapeutic regimen.

Taking a Medication History

No patient's medical history is complete without a complete medication history. In addition to current prescriptions, specific inquiry should be made regarding previous drug experience. Nonprescription drugs or home remedy use should be noted as well as alcohol consumption patterns.

Striving for an Accurate Diagnosis

Drug therapy cannot be properly planned in the absence of an accurate diagnosis. Prescribing without a clear indication for therapy exposes the patient to unnecessary risks of untoward effects and expense, without a reasonable expectation of therapeutic benefit. In any patient currently taking medication of any type, evaluation of new complaints should rule out drug therapy as a contributing factor to the problem.

Prescribing the Right Drug

Proper drug selection requires consideration of factors beyond an indication of efficacy for the condition being treated. Has one chosen the *best* drug for *this patient*? Consideration must be given to drug-disease interactions (contraindications) and drug-drug interactions with any other medication the patient may require. Obviously knowledge of the drug is paramount to a full assessment of these factors. In this regard, all health professionals must acknowledge the limitations of the human memory and must not hesitate to take the brief moment occasionally required to consult a reliable source of information to confirm and reinforce their drug knowledge.

Simplifying the Regimen

Complicated regimens enhance the probability that the patient will be unable or unwilling to comply. Avoidance of any nonessential medication will simplify the regimen, decrease the potential for an adverse response, and save money. The selection of pharmacokinetically long acting agents or the use of sustained release dosage forms will limit the number of repetitive doses required. Similarly, the use of fixed dosage combination products is appropriate when compatible with the patient's dosage requirements for all components of the formulation. Administration times that are compatible with the patient's daily routine may also minimize noncompliance.

Educating the Patient

Informing the patient of the nature of the drug and emphasizing the importance of properly following directions should be viewed as a responsibility rather than an imposition. Patients should be encouraged to ask questions and deserve an informative response. Full and clear directions for use as well as the name and purpose of the medication should be included on the prescription label. Although verbal instructions are important to clarify instructions and to verify the patient's understanding, written instructions are important for future reference. Because of the patient's limitations of memory, any essential or important instruction or information should be communicated in written form.

Monitoring Therapy

Drug therapy in the elderly patient usually should be initiated at low dosage levels. Periodic monitoring at appropriate intervals guides the dosage adjustments necessary to optimize therapy. Failure to achieve a therapeutic response following a reasonable time is an indication to re-evaluate the diagnosis and the drug selection. Knowledge of drug effects and observation for evidence of adverse reactions permit early detection and possibly avoidance of a severe drug reaction.

Discontinuing Therapy

When therapeutic benefits are no longer being realized, therapy should be discontinued. Periodic re-evaluation should be made of all drug therapy. When a substitute medication is prescribed, it is important to inform the patient to discontinue the previous prescription. Limitations on and cautious monitoring of prescription refills is helpful to prevent inappropriate continuation of a prescription.

Summary

Contemporary drug therapy is one of the greatest achievements in improved health care delivery. Proper application of pharmacotherapeutic principles can alleviate unnecessary suffering and significantly prolong life. Yet in spite of the benefits, there remain numerous hazards that can produce effects more deleterious than the benefits to be derived. The elderly patient presents a particular challenge as a unique patient who has been largely neglected. Practitioners must make concerted efforts to gain an understanding of geriatric drug therapy. With increased recognition of the necessity for specialization in this area, the future promises to provide a greater level of understanding and an improved level of patient care.

REFERENCES

1. Gibson, R.M., Mueller, M.S., and Fisher, C.R.: Age difference in health care spending. Fiscal year 1976. Soc. Sec. Bull., *40*:3–14, 1977.
2. Kasper, J.A., et al.: Expenditures for personal health services: findings from the 1977 national medical care expenditures survey. Presented at Annual Meeting, American Public Health Association, Detroit, October 21, 1980.
3. Covington, T.R., and Pfeiffer, F.G.: The pharmacist-acquired medication history. Am. J. Hosp. Pharm., *29*:692, 1972.
4. Milliren, J.W.: Some contingencies affecting the utilization of tranquilizers in long-term care of the elderly. J. Health Soc. Behav., *18*:206, 1977.
5. Adamson, K.A., and Smith, D.L.: Nonprescription drugs and the elderly patient. Can. Pharm. J., *111*:80, 1978.
6. Caranasos, G.J., Stewart, R.B., and Cluff, L.E.: Drug-induced illness leading to hospitalization. J.A.M.A., *228*:713, 1974.
7. Smith, F.A., et al.: Health information during a week of television. N. Eng. J. Med., *286*:516, 1972.
8. Law, R., and Chalmers, C.: Medicines and elderly people: a general practice survey. Br. Med. J., *1*:565, 1976.
9. Newmann, K.: Why patients seek unorthodox health care. Am. Druggist, *182*:52, 1980.
10. Ellison, N.M.: Unproven methods of cancer therapy. Drug Ther., *10*:73, 1980.
11. Hecht, A.: Hocus-pocus as applied to arthritis. FDA Consumer, 24–30, September 1980.
12. Isler, C.: The fatal choice cancer quackery. RN Magazine, September 1974.
13. Medical Letter, May 5, 1981.
14. Consumer Reports, 1979.
15. Eisele, J.W., and Reay, D.T.: Deaths related to coffee enemas. J.A.M.A., *244*:1608.
16. Ostfeld, A., et al.: The systemic use of procaine in the treatment of the elderly: a review. J. Am. Geriat. Soc., *25*:1, 1977.
17. FDA, HHS News, 80–61, December 15, 1980.
18. Haynes, R.B., Taylor, D.W., and Sackett, D.L.: Compliance in Health Care. Baltimore, Johns Hopkins University Press, 1979.
19. Boyd, J.R., et al.: Drug defaulting, Part II: Analysis of noncompliance patterns. Am. J. Hosp. Pharm., *31*:485, 1974.
20. Gilbert, J.R., et al.: Predicting compliance with a regimen of digoxin therapy in family practice. Can. Med. Assoc. J. *123*:119, 1980.
21. Mushlin, A., et al.: Diagnosing potential noncompliance. Arch. Int. Med., *137*:318, 1977.
22. Fed. Reg., *45*:60754.

23. Weintraub, M.: Reducing medication costs: a common sense approach. Drug Ther., 9:48, 1979.
24. Capel, W.C., and Stewart, G.T.: The management of drug abuse in aging populations: New Orleans findings. J. Drug Issues, 1:114, 1971.
25. Pascarelli, E.F., and Fischer, W.: Drug dependence in the elderly. Int. J. Aging Hum. Dev., 5:347, 1974.
26. Winick, C.: Maturing out of narcotic addiction. Bull. Narc., 14:1, 1962.
27. Zimberg, S.: The elderly alcoholic. Gerontologist, 14:221, 1974.
28. Cahalan, D., and Cisin, I.H.: Drinking behavior and drinking problems in the United States. In Kissin, B., and Begleiter, H. (Editors): The Biology of Alcoholism. New York, Plenum Press, 1976, Vol. 4.
29. Wood, W.G.: The elderly alcoholic: some diagnostic problems and considerations. In Storandt et al. (Editors), Clinical Psychology of Aging. New York, Plenum Press, 1978.
30. Gaitz, C.M., and Baer, P.E.: Characteristics of elderly patients with alcoholism. Arch. Gen. Psychiatry, 24:372, 1971.
31. Karch, F.E., and Lasagna, L.: Adverse drug reactions: a critical review. J.A.M.A., 234:1236, 1975.
32. Irey, N.S.: Diagnostic problems and methods in drug-induced diseases. Washington, D.C., American Registry of Pathology, Armed Forces Institute of Pathology, Part I (1966), Part II (1967), Part III (1968).
33. Wang, R.I.H., and Terry, L.C.: Adverse drug reactions in a Veterans Administration hospital. J. Clin. Pharmacol., 11:14, 1971.
34. Borda, I.T., et al.: Assessment of adverse reactions within a surveillance program. J.A.M.A., 205:645, 1978.
35. Domecq, C., et al.: Int. J. Clin. Pharmacol. Ther. Toxicol., 18:362, 1980.
36. Hurwitz, N.: Predisposing factors in adverse reactions to drugs. Br. Med. J., 1:536, 1969.
37. Swanson, M.: Drugs, chemicals and hemolysis. Drug Intell. Clin. Pharmacol., 7:6, 1973.
38. Chan, T.K., Todd, D., and Tso, S.C.: Drug-induced hemolysis in glucose-6-phosphate dehydrogenase deficiency. Br. Med. J., 2:1227, 1976.
39. Beutler, E.: Drug-induced hemolytic anemia. Pharmacol. Rev., 21:73, 1969.
40. Visconti, J.A., Dasta, J.F., and Grotting, M.A.: Drug information forum. U.S. Pharmacist, 3:10, 1978.
41. Eales, L.: Acute porphyria: the precipitating and aggravating factors. S. Afr. J. Lab. Clin. Med., 17:120, 1971.
42. deMatteis, F.: Disturbances of liver porphyrin metabolism caused by drugs. Pharmacol. Rev., 19:529, 1967.
43. Sheffield, P.A., and Turner, J.S.: Ototoxic drugs: a review of clinical aspects, histopathologic changes and mechanisms of action. South. Med. J., 64:359, 1971.
44. Ajodhia, J.M., and Dix, M.R.: Drug-induced deafness and its treatment. Practitioner, 216:561, 1976.
45. Dukes, M.N.G.: Meyler's Side Effects of Drugs. Amsterdam, Excerpta Medica, 1980.
46. Rosenstein, S., and Lamy, P.P.: Drug-induced diseases; the kidney. Hosp. Form. Manag., 5:34, 1970.
47. Mangini, R.J., and Gambertoglio, J.G.: Adverse effects of drugs on the kidney. In Koda-Kimble, M.A., Katcher, B.S., and Young, L.Y. (Editors): Applied Therapeutics for Clinical Pharmacists. Ed. 2. San Francisco, Applied Therapeutics, Inc., 1978, pp 384–409.
48. Koda-Kimble M.A., Katcher B.S., and Young L.Y.: Applied Therapeutics for Clinical Pharmacists. Ed. 2. San Francisco, Applied Therapeutics, Inc., 1978.
49. Kuntzman, R.: Drugs and enzyme induction. Am. Rev. Pharmacol., 9:21, 1969.
50. Conney, A.H.: Pharmacological implications of microsomal enzyme induction. Pharmacol. Rev., 19: 317, 1967.
51. Conney, A.H., et al.: Adaptive increases in drug-metabolizing enzymes induced by phenobarbital and other drugs. J. Pharmacol. Exp. Ther., 130:1, 1960.
52. Kappas, A., et al.: Effect of charcoal-broiled beef on antipyrine and theophylline metabolism. Clin. Pharm. Ther., 23:445, 1978.

# CHAPTER 2

MODIFYING DRUG DOSAGE IN ELDERLY PATIENTS

Peter P. Lamy

Geriatric drug therapy, a most difficult undertaking, has been the subject of many literature reviews.[1-11] In general, these reviews reflect the fact that there is still much uncertainty about the use of drugs for older adults. The difficulty is in matching the right drug and dose to the right disease in the right patient. Yet in the absence of explicit rules or appropriate tools, the decision making process (clinical judgment) is still predominantly used, and the management of uncertainty remains one of the major tasks of the provider caring for elderly patients. Improper dosages have probably become a far greater cause of error in therapy than is the use of an inappropriate drug, and often it is not recognized that different dosages are needed for different conditions and different patients.[12,13] All currently available knowledge has been gained from cross sectional studies, which yield information about age differences. Longitudinal studies are needed to provide more definitive knowledge about biological changes that occur with aging.[14]

It is well known that responses to some drugs are altered in the elderly.[15] These changes are often ascribed to the aging process and its effects, but they may well be due to other factors that might vary with age. Some of the increased sensitivity to drug action in the elderly can be related to changed pharmacokinetic parameters, but others, particularly those reported for drugs acting on the central nervous system, are most likely due to an increase in intrinsic sensitivity.[16]

The increased incidence of adverse effects in the elderly supports the assumption that complex changes in the physiology and biochemistry in humans with advancing age affect responsiveness to drugs by changing the processes of drug disposition or drug-receptor relationships.[17] For example, the responsiveness to beta-adrenoreceptor agonists is decreased in old age.[18] This chapter presents the effect of aging on numerous characteristics relative to the pharmacokinetics of drugs and discusses how one might more effectively apply pharmacokinetic principles in dosage adjustment.

SOME REASONS FOR PRESCRIBING DIFFICULTIES

A number of factors combine to make prescribing for older adults difficult. Among them should be listed atrophy of disuse, differences in drug responses between the sexes, malnutrition, chronic use of drugs, the multimorbidity often faced by the elderly, and difficulties in the diagnostic process.

Atrophy of Disuse. Many elderly people prefer or are forced into a sedentary, inactive life. Atrophy of disuse decreases functional ability. Although even large tissue and organ losses do not necessarily jeopardize life itself, they can and do influence drug action.

Sex Differences. More than 70 per cent of all residents in nursing homes are females, and the disproportional ratio between males and

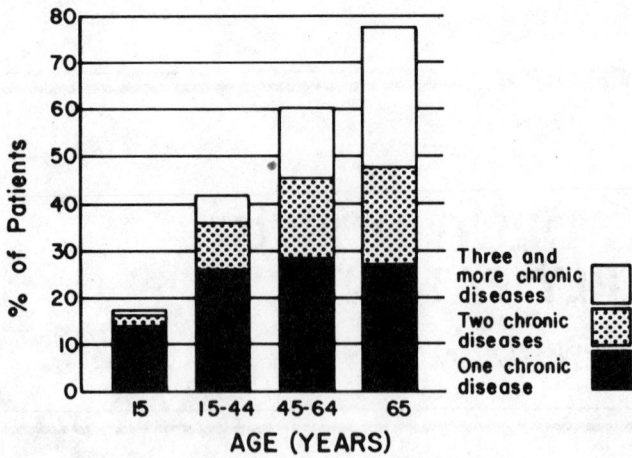

Figure 2–1. Incidence of chronic disease with advancing age.

females is increasing. It is well known that females often react to drugs in ways that are different from those in males. This holds true for such drugs as diazepam and chlordiazepoxide, among many others.[19–21]

Malnutrition. Altered dietary habits make drug therapy more difficult in the elderly, in whom malnutrition is an often encountered problem.[22,23]

Chronic Drug Use. Little is known about the long range effect of chronic drug use. Certain cautions ought to be exercised when chronic drug use is anticipated, particularly in view of the fact that many chronically used drugs may interfere with a patient's nutritional status.[24] Generally the chronic use of a drug is justified only if the drug decreases the overall morbidity and mortality of the disease process, there is no substantial drug induced toxicity, and the benefit to risk ratio of the drugs used is favorable.

Multimorbidity. Health in the elderly is viewed somewhat differently from that in younger persons, or as complete physical, mental, and social well-being, not just the absence of disease or infirmity. With advancing age, patients are faced with an increasing number of diseases, predominantly chronic diseases and disabilities (Figs. 2–1, 2–2). Many elderly patients suffer from four or more different conditions, with as many as nine different pathologic conditions frequently identified in persons 70 years and older.[25,26] It is also not uncommon for a patient to be seen by several different physicians and to patronize multiple pharmacies. The problem may be compounded by the fact that many disabilities remain unknown to the primary provider. The consequence of this situation is that one physician may be unaware of what another has prescribed and may thus duplicate drug orders or increase the interaction potential between

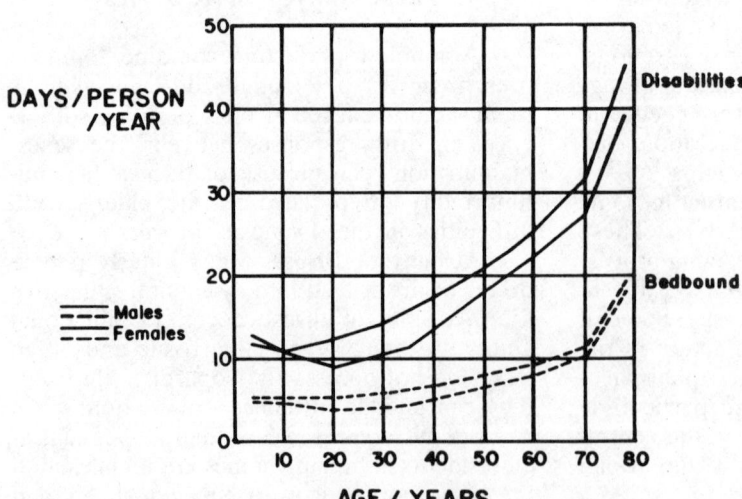

Figure 2–2. Incidence of disability with advancing age.

drugs. Additionally, failure of the patient to patronize a single pharmacy precludes the maintenance of a comprehensive patient drug profile, thus prohibiting effective drug utilization review by the pharmacist. Finally, the action of drugs can be seriously and markedly affected by intercurrent diseases.

Diagnostic Difficulties. Rational prescribing must start with a rational diagnostic process, particularly in elderly patients. This practice, however, is at times extremely difficult because of patient characteristics, changing diagnostic parameters, the frequent atypical presentation in the elderly patient, and the fact that some diagnostic criteria apparently change with age (Table 2–1). In a study of 53 different blood tests, 15 per cent of the findings were outside the accepted normal ranges in elderly patients; thus ranges for "normal" references probably need to be expanded.[28] Some of the changes in laboratory test values have now been documented, but it is likely that more need to be recognized.[29]

KEY CONSIDERATIONS IN GERIATRIC MEDICINE AND PRESCRIBING

The prescriber should be aware of the following points when managing diseases in the elderly with drug therapy:

1. First one considers the illness and only then the patient's chronologic age and its possible effect on the course of the illness and its management.

2. The therapeutic goal in treating chronic illness in the elderly is often not to cure but rather to successfully manage the disease. The goal of drug therapy should be to stabilize the patient, maintain as much functional and intellectual capability as possible, and maintain the patient's quality of life at the highest level possible.

3. One must carefully evaluate all organ systems.

4. Diagnostic findings should be separated by the degree of severity and priorities in treatment should be based on findings.

5. Before initiating drug therapy, all alternate methods of treatment should be considered (e.g., diet, physical therapy, occupational therapy).

6. If drug treatment cannot be avoided, the number of drugs used should be kept to an absolute minimum.

7. Elderly patients may be expected to have a reduced capacity to detoxify and excrete drugs.

8. Many drugs used in geriatric medicine have a narrow therapeutic index.

9. For many drugs used in geriatric medicine there is no readily measurable therapeutic endpoint.

10. Among the elderly there is a wide fluctuation between standard dosages and therapeutic responses.

11. Multiple drug therapy compounds the difficulty in predicting the patient's response.

12. Interactions (drug-drug, drug-disease, and drug-food) may occur. They may be difficult to detect and evaluate in complex clinical cases.

13. The incidence of adverse drug reactions increases with advancing age.

14. The effects of adverse drug reactions are more severe in the elderly than in younger populations.

TABLE 2–1. Possible Diagnostic Difficulties with Elderly Patients

Type of Difficulty	Example
Hoarding of illness	Elderly accept physical limitations as normal concomitant of aging
	Elderly are poor in self-referral
	Elderly may present only the chief complaint
Diagnostic parameters	Some relatively unreliable (e.g., fever, pain, thirst)
	May indicate serious disease, although often ascribed to old age (e.g., confusion, falls, fatigue)
Atypical presentation	Myocardial infarction; there may be no significant chest pain but radiation of pain into abdomen
	Sepsis without fever
	Nonbreathless pulmonary edema
	Pneumonia may present as confusion
	In angina there may be dyspnea instead of chest pain
	Pain and discomfort may be due to stress equivalent and not organic disease
	Chest pain may indicate angina pectoris, arthritis, heart disease, hiatal hernia, peptic ulcer, or pneumonia
	Cough and wheezing are frequent in elderly patients with heart disease

There are numerous reasons, other than physiologic ones, why the elderly experience drug induced adverse effects. Frequently cited reasons for these adverse reactions for which the prescriber bears direct responsibility are an excessive dose, an excessively long duration of therapy, a wrong drug (e.g., antibiotics in viral infections), an incorrect dosage form (e.g., an oral dosage form when a parenteral dosage form is indicated), and failure to use an equally or more effective drug having less toxicity.

It has been suggested almost universally that drug dosages be adjusted downward in order to protect the elderly patient from adverse drug reactions. For example, the dose of psychoactive drugs, in general, should be reduced by half in patients over 65 years of age, and by another half in those patients who also suffer from organic brain syndrome.[30] Experience has shown that some physicians seldom adjust dosages.[13] However, it is more than questionable that even a universal downward adjustment of dosages will absolutely accomplish the goal of less hazardous drug therapy for the elderly.[31] What is needed, and what will bring that goal closer to accomplishment, is a realization of the dynamics of drug action with advancing age. First, it must be realized that senescent function acts on drug action and that drug action, in turn, influences senescent function. Further, it is clear that several factors combine to yield an unpredictable drug effect in the elderly patient. Changes in enzyme and organ function (primary aging) interact with multipathologic disorders (secondary aging) and changes in income, dietary habits, and dentition (sociogenic aging), for example, to produce unpredictable drug effects (Fig. 2–3). Drug therapy itself can then create even more unpredictability. Clearly, more intense efforts are needed to understand drug action in the elderly and to provide guidelines and tools for more rational geriatric drug therapy. Much of this can be provided by a clearer understanding of the changes in pharmacodynamics and pharmacokinetics with age.

THE THERAPEUTIC GOAL

In the past, trial and error were the primary tools of the clinician who wanted to establish the appropriate dose for a particular patient. Very simply, the optimal dose was established by administering a fixed dose and, on the basis of observation of the patient, adjusting the dose whenever necessary.

Recently optimal therapeutic plasma drug concentration ranges have been established for many drugs (Table 2–2). It is important to note that some patients (the elderly, for example) may well exhibit the desired therapeutic effect at a lower than optimal level, whereas others may need higher than "optimal levels."

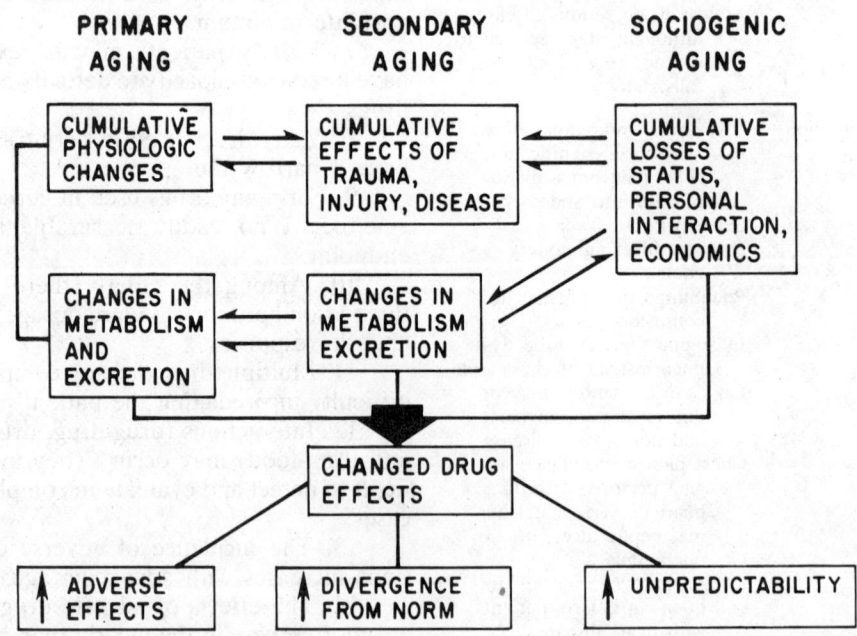

Figure 2–3. Selected factors combining to produce unpredictable drug effects in the elderly.

TABLE 2–2. Optimal Therapeutic Plasma Concentration Ranges

Drug	Therapeutic Plasma Range
Amitriptyline (amitriptyline plus nortriptyline)	> 100 ng./ml.*
Carbamazepine	8–12 mcg./ml.
Chlorpromazine	150–300 ng./ml.
Clonazepam	0.012–0.072 mcg./ml.
Clorazepate	0.075 mcg./ml.*
Desipramine	> 125 ng./ml.*
Digitoxin	10–30 ng./ml.
Digoxin	0.6–2.0 ng./ml.
Doxepin (doxepin plus desmethyldoxepin)	>100 ng./ml.*
Ethosuximide	50–100 mcg./ml.
Flurazepam	0.05 mcg./ml.
Imipramine (imipramine plus desipramine)	> 200 ng./ml.*
Lidocaine	1.2–5.0 mcg./ml.
Lithium	0.8–1.5 mEq./L. (for acute manic episodes)
	0.6–1.2 mEq./L. (for maintenance therapy)
Maprotiline	200–300 ng./ml.
Nortriptyline	75–140 ng./ml.
Phenobarbital	10–40 mcg./ml.
Phenytoin	10–20 mcg./ml.
Primidone	5–12 mcg./ml.
Procainamide	4–8 mcg./ml.
Propranolol	50–100 ng./ml.
Protriptyline	> 100 ng./ml.*
Quinidine	2–7 mcg./ml.
Salicylate	15–30 mg./100 ml.
Theophylline	10–20 mcg./ml.
Valproate	50–100 mcg./ml.

*Minimal effective plasma levels.

It is now the primary goal of the provider utilizing drug therapy to insure that a minimal effective concentration of drug is reached while avoiding a maximal level, at which toxicity tends to appear (Fig. 2–4). The minimal effective concentration is that concentration of a drug needed to produce the desired clinical effect, when the drug concentration in plasma is equilibrated with that in tissues. After the dosage form (orally administered) has undergone dissolution and the drug has reached the systemic circulation, it is distributed to all tissues. Concurrently the elimination process takes place, by excretion, metabolism, or both mechanisms. An increase in the dosage of a drug exhibiting a minimal effective plasma concentration will increase its effectiveness (within limits, indicating that a higher number of receptors is occupied), but an indiscriminate increase in dosage will result in toxic levels, particularly in elderly patients. In geriatric medicine, therefore, it is important to achieve a trough level above the minimal effective concentration but below the maximal level at which toxic reactions will be manifest.

Other drugs, mainly the antibiotics, exhibit a minimal inhibitory concentration. Theoretically, at least, an increase beyond that concentration will not increase the effectiveness of the drug. Again a maximal level can be reached at which toxicity occurs. However, two thoughts merit some consideration. First, a considerable body of literature seems to indicate that the effectiveness of some antibiotics increases at concentrations higher than the minimal inhibitory concentration and as the duration of the concentration above the minimal inhibitory concentration lengthens.[32-37] Furthermore, when bacteriostatic drugs are used in the elderly, who are more likely to be immunosuppressed, it is possible that their effectiveness is decreased, because bacteriostatic drugs depend on the patient's immune system, at least in part, for their effectiveness. Finally, many elderly suffer from urinary tract infections, and the minimal inhibitory concentration would most likely not be applicable. It is the drug's concentration in the urine that is important, and the plasma concentration most likely should be below the minimal inhibitory concentration for systemic infections.

CLINICAL PHARMACOKINETICS

Pharmacokinetics involves the application of kinetics to drugs. It is the science involving a quantitative analysis of the relation between

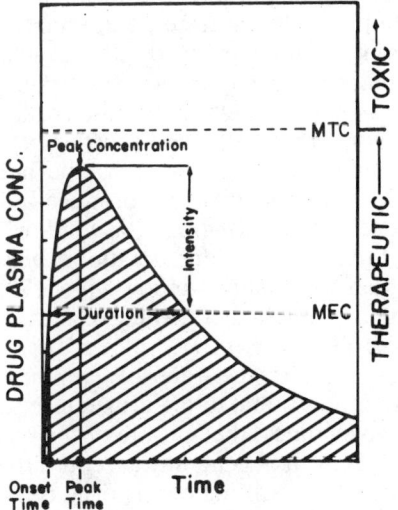

Figure 2–4. Drug plasma level–time curve following oral administration. MEC, minimal effective concentration. MTC, minimal toxic concentration.

organism and drug, not just simply the study of absorption, distribution, metabolism, and excretion of drugs.[38] The biologic rate processes control the onset, intensity, and duration of action of any drug by determining the concentration of the drug, its active metabolites, or both at the receptor site.[39] Thus, clinical pharmacokinetics can provide a valuable tool for understanding and interpreting the response of an individual patient to a given drug regimen. If used correctly, clinical pharmacokinetics can be used to calculate the expected plasma concentration of a given drug that will be achieved over a fixed time interval following a given dose.

If one accepts that the drug response in the elderly is often uncertain and unpredictable, knowledge of kinetic parameters should prove more than useful in attaining optimal drug use for individual patients. This is true particularly for drugs that have a narrow therapeutic index (often used for the elderly) and for patients who have diseases affecting drug disposition (also often true for the elderly).

The pharmacokinetic properties of a drug can be described in terms of three variables: the serum half-life ($T_{1/2}$), the elimination constant (K_e), and the apparent volume of distribution (V_d).[40,41] Each of these three factors must be taken into consideration when one wants to determine or predict the steady state level of a drug. After administration of a drug, body and plasma concentrations increase exponentially, following first the initial distribution phase (alpha phase) and then the elimination phase (beta phase). A drug continues to accumulate until the rate of accumulation is equilibrated with the rate of elimination. At that point a plateau or steady state is achieved. The ability to predict steady state concentrations assumes particular importance with drugs that follow other than the expected behavior. Some drugs, for example, must be administered in a fashion that will produce a steady state level within a "therapeutic window" (Fig. 2-5). Steady state concentrations below or above that therapeutic window will yield no, or less than optimal, therapeutic results.

Half-life. If a drug follows first order kinetics (i.e., if the rate of elimination is directly proportional to the drug concentration at any given time), the half-life of the drug can be calculated. It is generally accepted that five to six times the half-life of any drug is the time required to achieve steady state plasma levels. Table 2-3 indicates the rate of elimination after a drug has been discontinued.

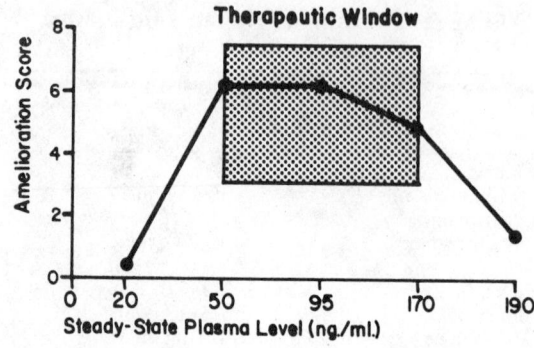

Figure 2-5. Demonstration of therapeutic window concept indicating that steady state blood levels of drug below or above the therapeutic window will have a less than optimal effect.

The half-life of a drug represents the elimination half-time. In general, 97 per cent of a drug will be eliminated within five half-lives regardless of the route of elimination, whether by metabolism, renal, or nonrenal elimination. The half-life therefore can be used to calculate the time it will take to achieve steady state levels, i.e., the drug concentration that will be optimal for a particular patient:

Time to achieve steady state = half-life × 5

It is important to understand the many parameters that can affect the half-life. For example, the half-life depends on the rate of drug metabolism and excretion:

Half-life = rate of elimination

but

Rate of elimination = elimination + metabolism

Metabolism can convert a drug from a pharmacologically active substance to an inactive metabolite, and the pharmacologic activity may be eliminated although the metabolite is not. Therefore, the elimination rate does not

TABLE 2-3. Rate of Drug Elimination After Drug Has Been Discontinued

Drug in Body (%)	Time
100	0
50	1 half-life
25	2 half-lives
12.5	3 half-lives

necessarily refer to the actual elimination of the drug from the body.

Some other precautions deserve discussion. First, any factor that alters a drug's half-life will also alter that drug's steady state concentration. Furthermore, even though the steady state concentration (serum drug concentration) appears to provide good guidance for dosage selection, there are drugs that exhibit a poor correlation between serum level and clinical activity. Therefore, the half-life may well not be representative of a particular drug's action.[42] Moreover, the exact meaning of "half-life" is not always clear. For example, for heparin, half-lives have been reported to vary between 23 minutes and 2.48 hours. This variation probably reflects the fact that various authors report the half-life of a bioassayed heparin concentration, the half-life of the extension of the clotting time, or the half-life of the clotting time itself.[43]

Elimination Constant. Drug clearance represents the volume of plasma in the vascular compartment that is cleared of drug per unit time. Clearly the mechanisms or process of clearance is not taken into consideration in this statement. The total clearance of a drug relates the rate of elimination under steady state conditions to the concentration in the serum. Alternatively stated, total body clearance is the pharmacokinetic parameter that determines the plasma concentration of a drug at steady state during administration of the drug at a fixed dose and dosing interval.

The elimination constant represents the fraction of the total amount of active drug eliminated in a given time interval for a given patient. The constant is inversely proportional to the half-life of a drug:

$$K_e = 0.693/\text{half-life}$$

Such factors as renal clearance, tissue and protein binding, lipid solubility, and metabolism of a drug enter into the determination of this constant. Renal clearance represents all clearance by the kidney, whereas nonrenal clearance represents all other types of clearance. Because the liver is the most important organ of metabolism as well as biliary excretion, nonrenal clearance is often equated to hepatic clearance. For many drugs, the elimination rate constant has been presented as:

$$K_e = K_{NR} + \alpha\, C_{cr}$$

where K_{NR} is the nonrenal elimination rate constant and alpha C_{cr} is a constant relating renal elimination to glomerular filtration rate as measured by creatinine clearance.

Since the elimination rate constant is inversely related to the half-life, one would expect that decreasing values of creatinine clearance would markedly lengthen the half-life, while the half-life would decrease with higher creatinine clearance values.

The nonrenal elimination process also can markedly influence total clearance. Variations from person to person must be expected for drugs that are primarily metabolized by the liver, for microsomal enzyme activity varies markedly from person to person. Clearance is also decreased when the metabolic process is saturable, but increases (with higher dosage rates) when serum protein binding is saturated.[44]

Apparent Volume of Distribution. Upon administration, a drug is distributed throughout the body. Because of various physiologic factors such as body size and body composition, as well as certain properties of the drug, such as solubility, individual tissues attain different concentrations of a drug depending on that drug's affinity for the particular tissue. Thus, in pharmacokinetics the apparent volume of distribution is used. This is the volume into which the drug appears to be distributed in a concentration equal to that of plasma or blood. The apparent volume of distribution, then, does not correspond to a true anatomic body compartment. Rather it is a theoretical space only. Its value varies with variations in the serum protein binding of a drug, tissue binding, and the relative water or lipid solubility of a drug. The apparent volume of distribution is the pharmacokinetic parameter that determines the initial plasma concentration following a loading dose. The apparent volume of distribution includes total body fluids, extracellular fluids, and intracellular fluid, as well as the tissues into which the drug is distributed (Table 2–4). A drug exclusively distributed throughout the total body water would have an apparent volume of distribution of 41 L.

Most often, however, drugs do not follow that pattern of distribution, but rather concen-

TABLE 2–4. Major Fluid Compartments

Compartment	Volume (L.)	Percentage of Body Weight
Intracellular	3–4	4
Extracellular	12	17–20
Total body water	41	58

trate in specific tissues. Lipid soluble drugs are attracted mainly to fatty tissues. These, as well as drugs that are avidly bound to tissue sites and those not highly protein bound, will have relatively high apparent volumes of distribution. A high volume of distribution would generally indicate that a low plasma level can be expected. On the other hand, highly protein bound drugs will stay primarily within the vascular space and these will exhibit a relatively low apparent volume of distribution. To achieve maximal therapeutic benefit and to eliminate, as much as possible, the uncertainty of geriatric drug therapy, it is important to determine whether a drug is distributed into fatty tissue so that the loading dose can be calculated on the basis of the correct body weight.

The apparent volume of distribution is a proportionality constant. It can be calculated from data obtained after intravenous administration of a drug (incomplete absorption and the first pass effect do not permit calculation after oral administration of a drug) and, in general, for drugs following first-order kinetics:

$$V_d = \frac{\text{Total amount of drug in body at time T}}{\text{Plasma concentration at time T}}$$

when both are in equilibrium. It can also be represented as:

$$V_d = \text{dose administered}/C_0$$

where C_0 is the calculated initial concentration derived from a half-life plot of the drug.

The apparent volume of distribution therefore yields information about the amount of drug in fluids that are in equilibrium with the plasma. If the amount of dose absorbed, the half-life of the drug, and the dose administration interval are kept constant, the steady state level is inversely proportional to the apparent volume of distribution.

PHARMACOKINETIC VARIATIONS WITH AGE

Many factors can interfere with achieving and maintaining the optimal blood levels desired for an individual patient. These factors are often present in elderly patients in multiple form, accounting for some of the difficulties of geriatric medicine. Among these factors are bed rest, dietary changes, multiple drug therapy, dehydration, fever, malnutrition, stress, and altered body temperature. Of particular importance are the effects of primary and secondary aging on drug dynamics.

The availability of a drug and thus its clinical effect depend on the biologic rate processes controlling the movement of the drug through the body. This movement in turn depends on the drug's absorption, distribution, metabolism, and excretion. Combined, these factors form a complex process that in the elderly can be and often is changed by the effects of primary aging (physiologic changes with age), secondary aging (pathophysiologic changes and, in particular, multiple disease processes with advancing age), and other factors, such as multiple drug administration (Fig. 2–6). There is no question that increasing age has many variable and clinically important effects on drug actions and that the pharmacokinetics of a drug may be influenced and changed by a host of factors, such as those produced by primary aging and secondary aging.[45] For example, changes in protein binding and variation in the volume of distribution can and should be expected, as should the influence of cardiac failure, hypothermia, hypo- or hyperthyroidism, hyperbilirubinemia, inflammatory diseases, and respiratory failure, among others.

Absorption. Little is known about the effects of aging on the human gastrointestinal system. The systemic absorption of a drug from the gastrointestinal tract depends on the dosage form (which can be controlled) and the anatomy and physiology of the absorption site. Gastrointestinal absorption involves several processes that occur simultaneously and sequentially.

Extensive changes take place in the gastrointestinal system with advancing age, but its general anatomic and physiologic integrity is maintained at an adequate level.[46–48] The effects of primary aging on the gastrointestinal system and the prescribing process for elderly patients are poorly elucidated, although there are several points of concern.

Major changes occur in the oral cavity with aging. The most obvious and frequent change is loss of teeth and, disturbingly, a frequent lack of replacements. (This loss is actually not an aging effect but is due to disease processes stemming from poor dental care.) This loss is paralleled by a reduction in salivary flow, and in very advanced old age there may be a complete lack of salivary flow.[49] There is

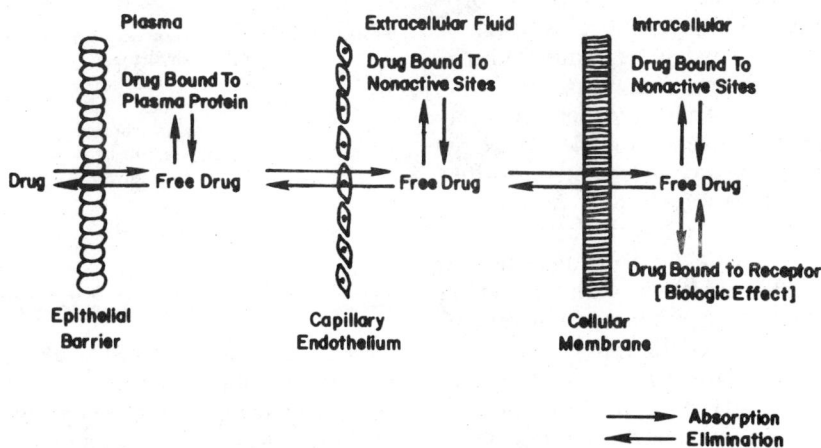

Figure 2–6. Normal movement of drug from absorption to receptor. (From Pippenger, C.E.: Syva Monitor, August 1978.)

also a marked decrease in the ptyalin content of the saliva.[50] The reduction in salivary flow may be exacerbated further by disease processes. Depression, frequently encountered among the elderly, is a strong salivary depressant and so are antidepressants with a significant anticholinergic component. Lack of salivary flow may lead to difficulties in swallowing, perhaps of solid dosage forms. A reduced salivary flow, coupled with loss of dentition, a considerable decrease in the number and sensitivity of taste buds, and a reduction in the sensitivity of the olfactory cells may cause a drastic alteration in the dietary intake of elderly persons, who are likely to switch to more easily chewable and more "gratifying" foods.[10] This, in turn, could lead to a reduction in the level of plasma proteins and altered drug action. The oral mucosa also changes with age, and these changes may be responsible for occasional treatment failure when buccal or sublingual tablets are used.[51]

In the aging esophagus one may encounter defects in deglutition, relaxation of the lower esophageal sphincter, delayed esophageal emptying, dilation of the esophagus, and an increase in nonpropulsive contractions. Reflux esophagitis is probably present in 75 per cent of all people between the ages of 50 and 80 years but is rarely symptomatic.[52]

The passage of oral solid dosage forms may be delayed by the effects of primary and secondary aging on the esophagus, leading to ulceration. Ulceration has been reported with potassium chloride tablets, and doxycycline and tetracycline capsules and tablets have been retained as long as 10 minutes and sometimes much longer.[53–56] Therefore, many oral solid dosage forms prescribed for elderly patients should be taken with meals or with large volumes of fluid. Overall, the decrease in peristaltic activity in the esophagus with advancing age may contribute to less consistent and slower absorption of drugs and, thus, to a less predictable drug effect. Once a drug reaches the stomach, the absorptive process may begin.

Most drugs are absorbed by passive diffusion, but some are absorbed by active transport. Absorption is described in terms of both rate and extent of absorption, and aging processes might interfere with one or both of these. In long term drug administration, the most frequent mode of drug administration for the elderly, the rate of absorption is less important than the fraction of drug absorbed, because accumulation will occur as long as administration intervals are selected correctly.

It has been suggested that there may be diminished absorption because of the theoretical consideration that with aging the enzyme systems involved may be less efficient. It has also been suggested that for the majority of drugs absorbed by passive diffusion there would not be a discernible effect on the absorptive process owing to aging effects. Investigations involving acetaminophen, aspirin, indomethacin, phenylbutazone, propicillin, quinine, and sulfamethiazole indicate that absorption does not seem to be influenced.

Passive diffusion of a drug depends on its solubility, which in turn depends on its degree of ionization. Gastric acidity, or more precisely the pH encountered by a drug in the stomach, may therefore influence solubility and absorption. With advancing age there is often a decrease in basal and histamine stimulated acid secretion in the stomach, resulting in an increase in gastric pH. Anacidity (achlorhydria) or hypochlorhydria occurs much more frequently in older than in younger persons (often accompanied by hyposecretion of pepsin and intrinsic factor), and it has therefore been deduced that weakly acidic drugs may not be well absorbed in the elderly.[10,57] This change in the gastric milieu is accompanied by a general decrease in the volume of fluids in the gastrointestinal tract. Therefore, because of both the change in gastric pH and the reduction in fluids, it is thought that poorly soluble drugs, such as ampicillin, digoxin, and griseofulvin, may not be as well absorbed in older people, but studies to document this possibility are still lacking. It is believed that an elevated pH only plays a role in the bioavailability of a drug with either marginal bioavailability or a potential for pH induced physicochemical problems in vivo; there is no real evidence that changes in gastric acidity impede drug absorption.[48,58]

Once a dosage form has been deaggregated and the drug has been dissolved in the intraluminal fluid, the drug is partitioned between the intestinal wall and the intraluminal contents according to the pKa and the lipid-water solubility characteristics of the drug. Previously it was thought that acidic drugs would be absorbed from the stomach and weak bases from the alkaline environment of the intestine. However, this concept is no longer rigidly applied. The gastric mucosa has only limited absorptive capability, whereas the small intestine, particularly the duodenal mucosa, provides a large area for drug absorption. It is therefore now believed that most absorptive processes take place there.

It has been postulated that two additional factors might interfere with drug absorption in the elderly. Gastric motility may be adversely affected by such diseases as atrophic gastritis, which occurs in the elderly more frequently than in the young. Again this change may account for drug absorption that is less consistent and slower in older adults. Also, if one accepts the fact that most of a drug will be absorbed from the duodenum, gastric emptying becomes a rate limiting factor, and changes in gastric emptying may be responsible for altering the rate with which a drug is absorbed and, consequently, enters the circulation.[59] Delayed gastric emptying also can decrease the bioavailability of a drug significantly.[60] This principle applies particularly to drugs such as chlorpromazine, which are tightly bound to the intestinal wall and are metabolized in the intestine. Factors that may delay gastric emptying include meals high in fat (likely in elderly, urban poor), drugs, and diseases (Tables 2–5, 2–6).

Emotional stress, not infrequent among the elderly, can also inhibit gastric emptying and, presumably, change the absorption of drugs.[61] Finally, if pyloric opening is impaired, the drug will be only slowly released to the duodenum. Therefore, the drug will be exposed to the "first pass" effect for a longer period of time, and losses due to that effect (metabolic inactivation) could be greater than usual.[62] Thus, the rate at which a drug is transferred from the stomach to the duodenum is an important determinant of the overall absorption rate for most drugs, and the rate may be slowed with advancing age because of nutritional factors, disease factors, or multiple drug therapy.

Once a drug is expelled from the stomach, it reaches the duodenum. The upper small intestine is very important in the absorptive process because it has an exceedingly large absorptive surface, which with advancing age may show a decrease in absorptive cells and, thus, the absorbing mucosal surface.[46,50] Theoretically, normal peristaltic movements of the duodenum are helpful in absorption by bringing drug particles into close contact with the

TABLE 2–5. Drugs That May Delay Gastric Emptying Time

Aluminum hydroxide
Analgesics (narcotic)
Anticholinergics
Drugs with anticholinergic activity
Antihistamines
Phenothiazines
Tricyclics
Ganglionic blockers
Isoniazid
Lithium

TABLE 2–6. Diseases That May Delay Gastric Emptying Time

"Acute abdomen"	Myocardial infarction
Gastric ulcer	Myxedema
Hepatic coma	Pain
Intestinal obstruction	Paralytic ileus
Migraine	Trauma

intestinal mucosa. There are few data relating to the role of intestinal motility on drug absorption, but it is assumed that decreased motility may increase the rate of absorption, particularly of poorly soluble drugs, because they tend to stay in contact with the absorbing surfaces longer.[62,63] It has been suggested that peristaltic activity in the intestinal tract decreases with age, reflecting an age related decrease in the control exercised by the central nervous system. Amylase, trypsin, and phosphorylation activity is also thought to be decreased in the aging intestine.[64] Diseases can affect the functional state of the upper small intestine. Among them are lactose intolerance (apparently increasing among elderly persons), small bowel diverticulosis, and duodenal diverticula, which afflict the elderly more frequently than younger adults.

An interesting thesis has been advanced recently.[65] The following metabolic processes may take place in the gastrointestinal tract: hydrolysis, dehydroxylation, decarboxylation, dealkylation, dehalogenation, deamination, and reduction. The rate of absorption of the drug (particularly compounds with an azo bond or a glycine conjugate) determines whether metabolism will take place and its extent. If absorption from the upper gastrointestinal tract is delayed, metabolism by microorganisms will take place, potentially influencing or altering drug activity. However, if a compound is rapidly absorbed, microbial metabolism will probably not take place. Thus, if peristaltic activity is reduced and drugs remain longer before being absorbed, it is again possible that unexpected results will occur.

Relaxation of the colonic musculature may be responsible, in part at least, for constipation about which the elderly complain frequently. The general loss of elastic tissue leads to the formation of diverticula of the large bowel, and it has been suggested that up to 40 per cent of all elderly people over the age of 70 years may be affected.[10] Symptomatic diverticular disease is accompanied by constipation in over one-third of all patients. Constipation can alternate with diarrhea and periods of normal bowel behavior.[66]

Drugs such as the opiates and tricyclics are also often responsible for constipation in the elderly, as is a reduction in fluid intake and decreased exercise. Minor pain from anal fissures may lead to a voluntary suppression of the urge to defecate, and constipation in the elderly may also be caused by an enlarged prostate, or it may accompany diabetes mellitus or hypothyroidism. Constipation is often treated with drugs, most often with self-selected and self-administered drugs, resulting in a cycle of slowed and quickened gastrointestinal motility, which can be responsible for erratic therapeutic results with concurrently administered drugs.

The intestine is perfused by the mesenteric blood vessels, which carry the absorbed drug to the liver via the hepatic portal vein, then to the general circulation, and finally to the target organ. Thus, it has been postulated that any decrease in the mesenteric blood flow would decrease the rate of removal of drug, reducing the bioavailability of the drug. With advancing age there is a pronounced decrease in splanchnic blood flow, possibly by as much as 50 per cent once a person reaches age 65.[10,46,50,57] It has been speculated, but not proven, that this could reduce or delay drug absorption. Emotional stress also decreases intestinal blood flow, causing drug absorption to become slow and erratic.[61] In patients with congestive heart failure, there is also a diminished intestinal blood flow and slower and more erratic drug absorption. Low blood pressure may exert a similar effect, and decreased or erratic absorption of drugs should also be expected as a result of diminished perfusion following shock or hypothermia.

The elderly are known to be recipients of an extraordinarily high number of drugs.[67] Multiple drug therapy can lead to drug interactions and to altered absorption of drugs. The elderly frequently are given antacids containing magnesium or calcium. These can reduce drug dissolution or bind drugs in the gastrointestinal tract, inhibiting absorption of such drugs as chlordiazepoxide, chlorpromazine, digoxin, or tetracycline.[68] Of particular interest for the elderly who may suffer from an unrecognized subclinical vitamin deficiency is the fact that absorption of vitamins and trace elements can be adversely affected by antacid therapy. For example, absorption of vitamin A, calcium, iron salts, and phosphorus may be impaired in the elderly.[68] On the other hand, antacids containing magnesium and aluminum hydroxide can enhance levodopa absorption.[10] Antacids also seem to decrease the absorption of digitoxin, indomethacin, isoniazid, pentobarbital sodium, propranolol, and quinine, while enhancing the absorption of aspirin, bishydroxycoumarin, nalidixic acid, naproxen, and pseudoephedrine.[69]

Amitriptyline and nortriptyline increase the absorption of dicumarol, and propantheline can be responsible for increased absorption of digoxin. On the other hand, such drugs as cholestyramine and kaolin-pectin are responsible for decreased absorption of a host of drugs.[70] Factors that may affect drug absorption are summarized in Table 2–7.

After a drug reaches the fluids of distribution, the disposition phase begins, involving distribution, metabolism, and excretion. Physiologic factors such as body weight as well as nutritional and disease factors may alter drug disposition.[71] Cardiac output decreases considerably with age and the blood volume is also redistributed.[10,46] Even in the absence of disease, the cerebral tissue and coronary and skeletal muscles receive proportionally more of the diminished cardiac output than do the liver and the kidneys, the main metabolic and excretory organs. The normal disposition of drugs may also change owing to changes in peripheral resistance, which increases at a rate corresponding to the rate of change in cardiac output. Furthermore, aging is characterized by a reduction in adaptive capacity in many organs.[72] One of the systems working less efficiently is the aged homeostatic mechanism, which responds less quickly in the elderly, and therefore the elderly are particularly sensitive to excessive doses of various drugs. Delivery to and removal from target organs may become more unpredictable with age, leading to less predictable drug effects. There may be alterations in plasma and tissue binding. The apparent volume of distribution may change for some drugs, as may the processes of metabolism and excretion.[1,2]

Distribution. Impaired drug distribution can alter or even seriously affect a specific therapeutic outcome. Among other factors, decreased and redistributed cardiac output, increased circulation time, and cardiovascular diseases can impair drug distribution in the elderly.[10] Drug action, as a result, could be delayed or in some instances even prolonged because removal to the site of metabolism may also be delayed.

Body Weight and Composition. Both body weight and body composition change with advancing age, and these changes can (and have been documented to) affect drug action (Table 2–8).[73,74] In general, the elderly lose weight with advancing age, particularly when they are very old. Loss of weight may influence the therapeutic plasma level of drugs directly or indirectly. At a given dose plasma and tissue levels will most likely be higher than

TABLE 2–7. Summary of Various Effects on Drug Absorption in the Elderly*

Changes	Effect
Oral cavity	Mucosal changes, perhaps leading to erratic absorption of buccal and sublingual tablets Dietary and nutritional changes, perhaps leading to reduced albumin levels or changes in rate of gastric emptying
Esophagus	Possible ulceration Changed peristaltic movement, perhaps causing erratic drug effect
Stomach	Anacidity or hydrochlorhydria; no significant drug effect documented as yet Delayed gastric emptying; could lead to reduced rate of absorption Delayed gastric emptying may lead to longer exposure to first pass effect and accelerated metabolic inactivation
Duodenum	Reduced peristalsis may cause erratic absorption Reduced peristalsis may cause increased metabolism of certain drugs Reduced absorptive surface; no significant effect proven as yet
Colon	Changes lead to constipation; both constipation and its treatment can lead to erratic drug action
Mesenteric blood flow	Postulated, but not proven, that reduction affects drug action
Diseases	Many diseases can and do affect drug absorption
Drugs	Drugs can both increase and decrease absorption of other drugs

*From Kalow, W., et al.: A method for studying drug metabolism in populations. Clin. Pharmacol. Ther., 26:766, 1979.

TABLE 2–8. Changes in Body Composition with Age

Compound Change	Approximate Change Between Ages 25 and 65
Total body water	15–20% decrease
Extracellular fluid	35–40% decrease
Body fat/body weight	25–45% increase
Body fat	
Males	18–36% increase
Females	33–48% increase

desired. The body weight of females is generally considerably lower than that of males, and females (who predominate among the elderly) would receive larger relative doses than males if both were given the same absolute doses.[75] Many dosage recommendations do not take this weight variation into account.[30,76]

In the elderly the ratio between lean body mass and fatty tissue changes. There is a reduction in the proportion of lean body mass to total body weight. This can have several effects. If drugs are primarily distributed in body water, higher plasma levels can be expected because their volume of distribution is reduced. On the other hand, adipose tissue is metabolically inert tissue. With an increase in fatty tissue, the volume of distribution of lipid soluble drugs increases, and there is the potential for prolongation of drug action. The apparent half-life of lipid soluble drugs will probably be increased, but clearance may not be affected because most lipid soluble drugs are cleared mainly by metabolism.

In order to overcome the effect of the changes in body composition, it has been suggested that drugs be prescribed on the basis of the ideal body weight. Current dosing recommendations are usually based on total body weight, but for drugs with a low therapeutic index, the difference in the dose calculated on the basis of either total or ideal body weight may be substantial and result in significantly changed clinical effects. Consideration should be given to utilizing standardized calculation schedules for dosing drugs such as digoxin, gentamicin, and theophylline.[77-79] The currently held belief that lean body mass is replaced by increased amounts of adipose tissue is being challenged. It has been proposed that lean body mass remains constant and does not decline with age, while adipocyte numbers actually increase very late in life, suggesting that old age is accompanied by relative obesity, probably caused by hyperplasia of adipose stores.[80]

The pronounced changes in total body water that take place with advancing age affect the action of polar, water soluble drugs. Their volume of distribution decreases as the total body water decreases, and this could result in a prolonged drug half-life.[1,2] Significant changes in the apparent volume of distribution have been documented for ethanol, lidocaine, and propicillin.

Elderly persons may exhibit a diminished thirst mechanism. The elderly are therefore particularly sensitive to dehydration, because of either reduced fluid intake or drug action such as that of diuretics. Dehydration, and possibly changed drug action, should be considered in elderly patients who are unconscious, confused, or severely depressed, those who receive tube feedings or intravenous infusions, patients with poor appetites or inability to feed themselves, chair- or bedbound patients, and those who receive diuretics or use laxatives frequently. In those patients the hematocrit, hemoglobin, serum sodium, and serum protein levels will most likely be elevated. Dehydration is, as a matter of fact, one of the most common reasons for the appearance of an elevated blood urea nitrogen level. The elderly clearly are at great risk of dehydration, and this should be taken into consideration when changes in drug distribution and drug action due to the changed distribution are suspected.

Plasma Protein Binding. Many factors can exert a crucial influence on the transport of a drug to and from the target organ. Therefore, these factors can influence, and in some instances change in important ways, the pharmacokinetics of drugs. Drug protein binding is such a factor, and it can be an important determinant of pharmacokinetics and renal disposition of a drug. The duration of action of a drug and the intensity of its effect may therefore also be influenced by the binding or displacement of a drug to or from serum protein.

The major plasma and tissue protein responsible for binding of most drugs is albumin.[81,82] Sixty per cent of the total albumin is in the extravascular space. The skin contains 18 per cent of the total exchangeable albumin, and muscle accounts for approximately 15 per cent. Albumin moving out of plasma is returned via the lymphatic circulation. Other serum protein components that may be involved in protein binding are the globulins, lipoproteins, and glycoproteins.

Weakly acidic drugs are generally highly bound to plasma albumin (Table 2-9). Basic drugs such as quinidine exhibit a high degree of affinity for albumin as well as lipoproteins, and alpha$_1$ acid glycoprotein. Hormones, vitamins, and steroids usually bind to serum globulins. Drug protein binding can be influenced by species differences, interindividual differences, electrolytes, pH, endogenous substances, drug concentration, protein concentration, and other drugs. The plasma protein concentration, in turn, is controlled by protein synthesis, protein catabolism, distribution of albumin

TABLE 2–9. Selected Drugs More Than 80 Per Cent Bound to Plasma Protein

Acetazolamide	Imipramine
Acetylsalicylic acid	Metolazone
Amitriptyline	Nafcillin
Amphotericin B	Nalidixic acid
Bishydroxycoumarin	Nortriptyline
Cefazolin	Phenindione
Chlordiazepoxide	Phenylbutazone
Chlorpromazine	Phenytoin
Chlorthalidone	Prazosin
Cloxacillin	Propranolol
Desmethylimipramine	Protriptyline
Dicloxacillin	Quinidine
Digitoxin	Rifampin
Doxepin	Spironolactone
Doxycycline	Sulfisoxazole
Furosemide	Trimipramine
Hydralazine	Warfarin sodium

between the intravascular and extravascular spaces, and excessive elimination of plasma protein, particularly albumin.

The adsorption of a drug on the surface of plasma proteins is called protein binding. Protein binding is a reversible interaction between a drug (a relatively small molecule) and a protein (a macromolecule). At any given time a certain percentage of the drug in the serum is bound to protein molecules which, because of their size, cannot diffuse through capillary walls to reach the site of intended drug action. The bound drug is therefore not subject to metabolism or elimination. The bound drug is in reversible equilibrium with the free (unbound) drug. Some of the drug-protein complex continuously dissociates as free drug diffuses out of the blood through capillary membranes. Only the free drug, and not the bound drug, is in equilibrium with body tissues, and it is therefore only the free drug that is therapeutically active. Binding therefore influences drug activity by determining the proportion of the dose available to the site of action. For drugs that are less than 80 per cent protein bound, binding is not likely to be clinically important.[83] However, this theory should be used only as a guide, not a dictum. When a drug with a narrow therapeutic index is used, a 200 or 300 per cent variation in the free drug fraction is likely to be clinically significant, particularly in the elderly, who are very sensitive to adverse drug actions, even with drugs that are not that highly bound.

Primary aging brings about a fall in mean serum albumin levels, from about 4.0 gm. per 100 ml. at age 40 or less to approximately 3.58 gm. per 100 ml. in those 80 or older.[84] Others have indicated a 15 to 25 per cent reduction in the serum albumin level in persons over 60 years of age as compared to those under 40 years.[85,86] Theoretically, then, one might anticipate accelerated elimination of drugs in the elderly, because of the fact that a reduced albumin level will lead to higher levels of free drug (there are fewer binding sites available) and these higher levels are, of course, subject to metabolism and elimination. In practice, however, the elimination rates for several highly bound drugs are unchanged or even reduced, not increased, indicating the influence of other factors.[64] However, if the plasma albumin level is decreased, then for any given dose of a drug, the concentration of the free moiety may well be higher than anticipated, leading to a more intense and possibly undesirable effect. Indeed reduced plasma albumin levels have been shown to be responsible for greater unbound drug fractions in the elderly. Diflunisal, phenytoin, and warfarin have been involved. With warfarin (97 per cent bound), reduced protein binding leads to a more intense drug effect.[87] On the other hand, reduced binding of phenytoin leads to faster clearance and possibly to a less intense effect and a shorter duration of action.[85] Adverse reactions to phenytoin occurred in more than 11 per cent of patients with a serum albumin concentration of less than 3 gm. per 100 ml. but only in 3.8 per cent of the patients with normal albumin levels.[88] Serum albumin levels have also been correlated with the clearance of antipyrine, diazepam, and propranolol. Secondary aging effects (e.g., diseases) are known to affect protein concentrations and, thus, drug action. Diseases may be accompanied by both hypoalbuminemia and changes in the molecular structure of the albumin molecule, and either or both could be responsible for reduced binding. Bed rest and immobilization also lower the plasma albumin concentration. In renal disease many drugs may accumulate that can occupy drug binding sites on the albumin molecule and therefore cause less protein binding. Bilirubin, uric acids, and thyroxine may be responsible for less drug binding.

Hypoalbuminemia should be expected in chronic liver disease and chronic kidney disease (when both glomeruli and tubules are affected). Acute infections, myocardial infarction, and pneumonia also can be responsible for lowered albumin levels. In addition, decreased protein synthesis (liver disease), increased protein catabolism (surgery, trauma), and excessive elimination of protein (renal disease) produce hypoalbuminemia.

With renal disease a change in the molecular structure of the albumin molecule has been suggested, resulting in a decreased binding of acidic drugs, such as aspirin, phenylbutazone, phenytoin, sulfadiazine, and thiopental. Even such neutral molecules as digitoxin apparently bind less in renal disease.[89-91] In contrast, anxiety or agitation can cause an increase in albumin concentrations.

Other plasma components deserve mention because they may also bind drugs, and their concentrations may change with age or disease. Myocardial infarction, pneumonia, and febrile illnesses usually cause increased gamma globulin levels,[89] and it might be speculated that this could alter the kinetics and action of hormones, vitamins, and steroids.

Many drugs bind to lipoproteins. Among them are chlorpromazine, quinidine, reserpine, various steroids, and tetracycline. It is not unreasonable to assume that increased plasma lipoprotein levels may affect the concentration of the unbound active fraction of a drug. More of reserpine is associated with lipoproteins in hyperlipoproteinemic patients than in normal individuals. Imipramine probably binds to lipoproteins more avidly and with greater capacity than to albumin.[92,93]

Normal free fatty acid concentrations in plasma range from 200 to 500 micromoles. Fasting, bacterial infection, diabetes mellitus, and hyperthyroidism can cause concentrations of more than 2500 micromoles.[94] Plasma concentrations of free fatty acid increase with renal failure owing to mobilization of adipose tissue. Heparin, used in the treatment of pulmonary embolism, deep vein thrombosis, and other conditions, increases the concentration of free fatty acid, inhibiting the binding capacity of serum albumin with such drugs as bishydroxycoumarin, phenylbutazone, phenytoin, salicylates, sulfadiazine, and thiopental, thus possibly changing their kinetic behavior. Alpha$_1$ acid glycoprotein is an acute-phase plasma protein, which increases in response to certain diseases, such as infections, inflammatory rheumatoid arthritis, chronic renal failure, cancer, and trauma. One should expect higher levels of alpha$_1$ acid glycoprotein in those diseases as well as with stress, and possibly lower levels in diseases such as the nephrotic syndrome, or malnutrition.[83,95-97] Binding to alpha$_1$ acid glycoprotein seems to be most intensive in rheumatoid arthritis and inflammatory complications in renal failure. Thus, although a reduction in albumin levels may take place, and one would expect higher levels of free drug, more drug may be bound to alpha$_1$ acid glycoprotein, leading in fact to lower levels of unbound drug. The cationic drugs probably bind most frequently to alpha$_1$ acid glycoprotein. Alprenolol, chlorpromazine, imipramine, quinidine, and propranolol have been identified as drugs that bind to alpha$_1$ acid glycoprotein and that may exhibit marked differences in action with plasma increases in alpha$_1$ acid glycoprotein.

Concurrent administration of two drugs, both protein bound, can be a strong determinant of drug interactions, and it is likely that this type of interaction occurs frequently in the elderly. Phenytoin, for example, is displaced by salicylic acid and phenylbutazone, increasing the unbound fraction of the drug up to threefold. The magnitude of the interaction depends on the avidity with which each drug binds to the protein molecule. The more avidly bound drug will displace a less avidly bound drug already in place. On the other hand, a concurrently administered drug may increase the percentage bound of another drug. For example, approximately 9 per cent of gentamicin is normally bound, but in the presence of heparin, 55 per cent of gentamicin is bound, most likely because of a complex interaction between heparin, serum proteins, divalent cations, and gentamicin.[98] It has also been shown that such substances as plasticizers from intravenously administered materials can displace basic drugs bound to alpha$_1$ acid glycoprotein.[99] Thus, altered drug action is most likely to be expected in multiple drug therapy because of this type of interaction, making drug therapy uncertain in elderly patients, who almost by definition receive multiple drug therapy. These interactions, with their potentially serious adverse clinical effects, in the elderly are of particular importance because the magnitude of interactions affecting displacement from albumin of one drug by another is greater in older than in younger people.[100]

Finally, binding to red blood cells can change with age.[101] Meperidine binds less to red blood cells with advancing age, leading to higher plasma concentrations with a given dose in elderly patients. Other drugs that are bound to red blood cells are acetazolamide and chlorthalidone.[102]

Elimination. Drugs are removed from the body primarily by either one or both of two major routes. The first of these involves the metabolism of the drug by the liver. Less active or inactive metabolites are formed, which in turn are most often excreted by the kidney. The kidneys provide the second major route of elimination of drugs. In that case it is usually the unaltered drug that is excreted. Both these functions may be, and indeed often are, altered in elderly persons. The impaired ability of the elderly to eliminate drugs may account in part for the often reported increased incidence of adverse drug reactions in that population.

Hepatic Metabolism. The liver, the largest single organ in the body, probably continues to function well in elderly, reasonably fit individuals without liver disease. Liver and body weights correlate with one another, both starting to decline in the fifth or sixth decade of life.[46] A majority of elderly persons may well have even more than one abnormality in liver function, but serious deterioration of liver function is not consistent with the effects of primary aging and is induced only by a large loss of functioning liver cells.

Carbohydrates, fats, and proteins are metabolized by the liver, which also acts as a storage depot for certain nutrients. Part of the 5000 (or more) known biochemical reactions taking place in the liver are also involved in drug metabolism. A satisfactory index to use in predicting a person's capacity to metabolize drugs is not yet available. Although liver weight and the number of functioning hepatic cells decrease with increasing age, there is no convincing evidence that this decline impairs drug metabolism in the elderly.[103] In general, bile salt production, necessary for fat absorption, is not affected by the processes of primary aging either. However, questions have been raised about other factors that may be important in hepatic metabolism. Among those are liver blood flow and the activity of the drug metabolizing systems, particularly the inducible microsomal enzymes involved in oxidation and reduction mechanisms. Changes in either or both of these, singly or combined, may have important effects on the overall elimination rate of lipophilic drugs from the body and may contribute to the increased incidence of adverse drug effects in the elderly.[104]

Some drugs—those under polymorphic control—are metabolized via a nonmicrosomal enzyme pathway. These include hydralazine, isoniazid, procainamide, and many sulfonamides. These drugs undergo hepatic acetylation. The acetylator phenotype can influence the therapeutic effects and toxicity of these drugs.[105] Mongoloid populations are primarily rapid acetylators, while among American Indians, 79 per cent are likely to be rapid acetylators, and among American blacks and whites, 45 to 48 per cent are rapid acetylators.

Slow acetylators are more apt to develop higher and longer lasting blood levels with the drugs mentioned, even when they receive the "usual" dose and consequently develop signs of toxicity. Other drugs that demonstrate acetylation polymorphism are dapsone, phenelzine, and nitrazepam, and, depending on the phenotype, the drugs may be more active or cause more toxicity. Thus, although the specific phenotype is not susceptible to change with aging, in the elderly, in whom it is often important to reduce drug hazards to a minimum, it might be advisable to determine the patient's phenotype. A simple method for determining the acetylator phenotype is available. Only one serum and one urine specimen are needed, neither requiring special handling.[107,108]

Metabolite patterns can also vary with racial characteristics of a patient. Figure 2–7 clearly shows differences in the metabolite patterns of Oriental and Caucasian subjects to whom amobarbital was administered. The Caucasians excreted, on the average, about

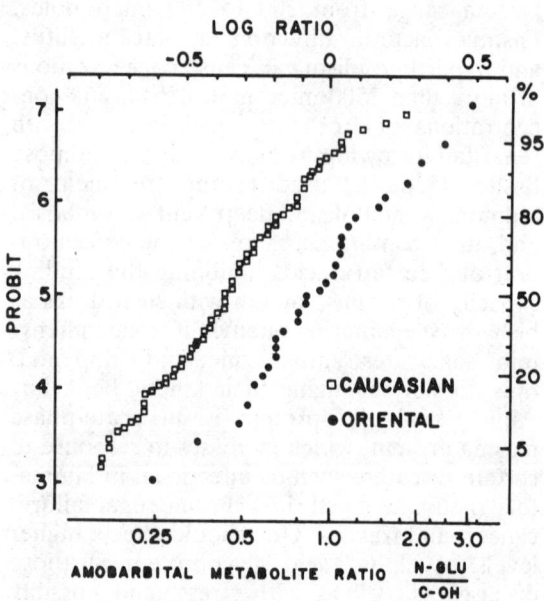

Figure 2–7. Distribution of urinary metabolites of amobarbital in populations of 139 Caucasian and 30 Oriental subjects. Scales of the abscissas are logarithmic; ordinates indicate cumulative frequencies in the form of probits.

50/MODIFYING DRUG DOSAGE IN ELDERLY PATIENTS

TABLE 2–10. Drugs Frequently Prescribed for the Elderly Susceptible to Microsomal Enzyme Metabolism

Barbiturates	Phenylbutazone
Chlorpromazine	Phenytoin
Corticosteroids	Thyroxine
Coumarin derivatives	Tolbutamide
Digitoxin	Vitamin D
Estrogens	Warfarin sodium
Oxyphenbutazone	

two-thirds of the two major amobarbital metabolites as C-OH and one-third as N-glu.[106]

Most drugs, however, are under polygenic control and are metabolized by microsomal enzymes. Selected drugs that frequently induce enzyme activity and those that can inhibit enzyme activity are found in Tables 1–14 and 1–15 of Chapter 1. Drugs that are susceptible to microsomal metabolism and that frequently are used to treat elderly patients are listed in Table 2–10. A comparison of the drugs listed in this table shows clearly that some drugs are capable of inducing their own metabolism.

Metabolic conversion of drugs (usually from a fat soluble to a water soluble and, therefore, excretable form) occurs most often in two phases. The purpose of phase I metabolism is to introduce an anion into the drug molecule, which can then react with a conjugating agent in phase II of metabolism. In phase I, oxidation, reduction, or hydrolytic reactions take place most commonly. These reactions take place mostly in the endoplasmic reticulum of the cell.

A common oxidizing system involving cytochrome P-450 has been proposed for most xenobiotics. Reduction reactions are catalyzed by cytochrome reductase. Most often, the transformation step (phase I) is followed by a synthesis step (phase II), which usually abolishes the action of the drug undergoing metabolism. If the activity of the substance resides in the original molecule, the metabolic process will eliminate its activity. Metabolism, though, can also result in the formation of one or more active metabolites, as in the case of some tricyclics or benzodiazepines, and the overall effect then depends on the activity of the metabolite(s). An important concept to realize is that the chief site for liver metabolism of drugs is in the lipid membranes surrounding the liver microsomes. Thus, liver metabolism is an enzyme mediated, probably saturable process.

Drugs absorbed from the stomach or intestine are delivered via the hepatic portal vein to the liver before reaching the general circulation. Because metabolism is enzyme mediated and is therefore a saturable process, the metabolism of a drug will depend, in part at least, on the rate at which a drug enters the liver. If a drug enters quickly, the system will be partially (or even totally) saturated, permitting more of the unmetabolized drug to reach the general circulation. If, on the other hand, a drug enters the liver slowly, saturation will most likely not be reached, and more of the drug will be metabolized. Thus, the effect (or action) of a drug may well depend on liver perfusion.

Little is known about liver blood flow. A decline over years similar to the decline in cardiac output has been suggested. It is also known that because of the reduced cardiac output due to age, less blood flow goes to the liver than before. When liver blood flow is quantitatively important in the hepatic clearance of a drug, aging can impair this process and lead to prolongation of the terminal half-life of a drug, provided other disposition factors are not affected.[109,110] Liver perfusion also can be affected by a number of physiologic, pathologic, or pharmacologic factors (Table 2–11). A reduction in hepatic blood flow, the consequence of prolonged administration of beta-blockers or other factors, can reduce the extent of hepatic drug clearance. Higher blood levels and longer plasma half-lives of drugs with high hepatic clearance may result.

The degree of liver metabolism that takes place following absorption is called the first pass effect or presystemic elimination. The bioavailability of a drug varies with the capacity of the hepatic-portal system to metabolize the drug during the initial transport from the gastrointestinal tract into the general circulation. Drugs that are highly metabolized by the

TABLE 2–11. Factors Affecting Variations in Liver Perfusion

Factor	Increase	Decrease
Physiologic	Bedbound Ingestion of food	Hyperthermia Dehydration
Pathologic	—	Cardiac and circulatory failure
Pharmacologic	Isoproterenol Phenobarbital	Propranolol

liver demonstrate poor systemic availability when given orally. Theoretically this can be overcome by increasing the dose of the drug, but another result of a strong first pass effect is greater individual variation in plasma levels and drug response. Sometimes, to overcome the first pass effect, the dosage form is changed to a more rapidly absorbed dosage form. One can also change the route of administration to sublingual, topical, or rectal if such dosage forms exist.

A word of caution should be added. An increment in dosage, designed to overcome a strong first pass effect, may lead to saturation of the enzymatic hepatic metabolic mechanism. Thus, two factors would combine to cause higher than anticipated plasma drug levels. First, would be the increased dose and, second, the decreased metabolism. Whether the metabolism of a drug will be affected by age related decreases in hepatic enzyme activity depends on the fraction of the drug dose removed during the first pass effect. The amount of drug so removed is characterized by the hepatic extraction ratio (Table 2–12). An extraction ratio may be expressed as the percentage of drug entering the liver minus the relative concentration of drug removed by the liver. The extraction ratio may vary from zero to 1.0. An extraction ratio of 0.25 means that 25 per cent of the drug is removed during the first pass of the drug. If both the hepatic extraction ratio and the blood flow to the liver are known, the hepatic clearance may be calculated.

For example, if 50 per cent of a drug is removed during the first pass through the liver, the drug's hepatic extraction ratio is 0.5. Normal liver blood flow is approximately 1.5 liters per minute. The product of these two factors is then 0.75 liters per minute. This is the hepatic clearance. The lower the extraction ratio, the more drug is available to produce the anticipated systemic effect. The metabolism of drugs with low extraction ratios is influenced by the decline in the activity of drug metabolizing enzymes. Thus, even in apparently healthy elderly persons, the metabolism of many drugs may be slowed.

For some drugs the extraction ratio is high (greater than 0.7). Those drugs are removed by the liver almost as rapidly as the liver is perfused by the blood containing the drugs. Among those drugs can be listed isoproterenol, lidocaine, and nitroglycerin. For those drugs, changes in hepatic blood flow can change the rate of their metabolism, an increase causing an increase in the rate of drug removal. So-called high clearance drugs are highly tissue localized and exhibit avid hepatic elimination (chlorpromazine, for example). For them one can expect a decrease in volume of distribution and a shortening of half-life if plasma binding increases. Some drugs such as the beta blockers inherently decrease hepatic blood flow by decreasing cardiac output, thus decreasing their own clearance.

Drugs with low extraction ratios (e.g., phenylbutazone, procainamide, theophylline) are less affected by hepatic blood flow. These drugs are more affected by the intrinsic activity of the mixed function oxidases (enzyme metabolism). Other drugs that have an inherently low extraction ratio, like diazepam or digitoxin, may be affected by an age related reduction in hepatic extraction. Note should be taken of the fact that an extraction ratio is not constant but can change with blood flow and the intrinsic clearance of a drug. The intrinsic clearance describes the inherent activities of the microsomal enzymes indirectly by describing the capacity of the liver to remove a drug in the absence of flow limitations.

The rate of liver drug metabolism is related to the free or nonprotein bound plasma concentration of a drug. Drugs that are protein bound fail to reach the site of enzyme activity, whereas the unbound part will. For drugs with a high extraction ratio, the percentage of drug that is protein bound will not significantly affect the rate of metabolism, since the drug is removed from the plasma binding sites during circulation through the liver. For drugs with low extraction ratios and low plasma binding, the concentration of drug at the enzyme site will not be changed significantly when the drug is displaced from binding.

TABLE 2–12. Hepatic Extraction Ratios of Selected Drugs

High	Intermediate	Low
Isoproterenol	Aspirin	Amobarbital
Lidocaine	Desipramine	Diazepam
Meperidine	Nortriptyline	Digitoxin
Morphine	Quinidine	Isoniazid
Nitroglycerin		Phenobarbital
Pentazocine		Phenylbutazone
Propoxyphene		Phenytoin
Propranolol		Procainamide
		Salicylic acid
		Theophylline
		Tolbutamide
		Warfarin

Drug metabolizing enzymes are apparently more easily stimulated in younger than in older persons, and therefore the possibility of a reduced induction response and a more intense or longer duration of drug action exists in the elderly.[111] Drug metabolism also may be changed by other factors in the elderly.[112] As previously discussed, drug oxidation is performed primarily by inducible microsomal enzyme systems for which multiple cytochrome P-450 enzymes serve as the terminal oxygenases. The rates of oxidative metabolism of drugs in man can be substantially altered by nutritional factors and by liver disease, as well as by long term drug ingestion, which predominates among the elderly.[113,114] Levels of hepatic cytochrome P-450 and activities of aryl hydrocarbon hydroxylase and ethylmorphine demethylase are increased by drugs in patients without liver disease, with mild to moderate hepatitis, and in patients with inactive cirrhosis. It has also been suggested that age related change originating at the brain-pituitary level may delay the induction of liver enzymes.[115] Finally, there may be, in the elderly, a diminished rate of albumin liver synthesis secondary to progressive, age related deficits in liver function, which may lead to altered protein binding of drugs.

Drug induced hepatitis and hepatic necrosis occur more frequently in older patients, and this can affect drug metabolism.[116] Penicillamine therapy can cause liver abnormalities, including increased levels of lactic dehydrogenase and alkaline phosphatase.[117] In patients with liver disease, sedatives and narcotic analgesics may cause coma, possibly as a result of altered oxidative biotransformation of these drugs.[118,119] Hepatic extraction and clearance can change with age, depending on the effects of primary and secondary aging and drug administration. Plasma half-life and clearance are changed with age for a number of drugs, lowered plasma clearance indicating a lower rate of metabolism. However, there is no uniform change in the plasma clearance of drugs with age. Sometimes prolonged plasma half-lives in the elderly may be offset by increased distribution volumes. Thus, although significant age related increases in plasma steady state levels may be anticipated for drugs extensively metabolized by the liver, and age and plasma drug concentrations are well correlated in some cases, no across the board statement can be made at this time for all drugs.[120-122] Since, however, metabolic processes change with age, a knowledge of physiologic, pathologic, or pharmacologic factors and their effects in the elderly can help eliminate variability in drug response and prevent drug interactions.

Renal Excretion. Many changes in renal structure and function take place with advancing age, and it is well established that renal function declines with age, even in the absence of disease.[123] Altered renal function is probably the single most important factor and the factor most responsible for altered drug levels and, therefore, altered drug action, in the elderly (Table 2-13).

Changes in Kidney Structure. In normal adults the combined weight of the kidneys is less than 1 per cent of total body weight. Yet the normal kidneys receive approximately 20 per cent of the cardiac output. The normal nephrons process more than 170 liters of glomerular filtrate daily. Structural age related changes are manifested by a weight loss of the kidneys. Between the fourth and eighth decades the kidneys lose approximately one-fifth of their weight, more weight being lost from the cortex than from the medulla.[124] Stated differently, with advancing age, the kidney loses mass, which declines from about 270 gm. during the third and fourth decades to 185 gm. in the ninth decade.[123] The absolute volume of the renal cortex reaches its peak during the third to fifth decades and then declines. The number of nephrons declines by 50 per cent, but the surviving units seem to contribute increasingly toward maintenance of homeostasis.[125]

Kidney size and the number of glomeruli and tubule cells decrease with age,[46] although there is wide interindividual variation in the decrease in the number of glomeruli. Fibrotic changes also may take place in the glomeruli. Degenerative tubular changes take place, particularly in the proximal convoluted tubule where interstitial fibrosis can be pronounced after the seventh decade. Vascular changes also take place, even in the absence of hypertension. Vascular changes in normotensive patients over the age of 70 years are similar to those observed in younger hypertensive patients.[10]

Functional Kidney Changes. Both of the broad excretory functions of the kidney—to preserve the volume of body fluids and to maintain composition of these fluids—are affected by aging.[10] Even in apparently healthy older adults, functional changes in the kidney are the rule rather than the exception. After the fourth decade there is a progressive decline

TABLE 2–13. Renal Factors Affecting Excretion and Reabsorption of Drugs

Process	Comments
Glomerular filtration	Probably all drugs of low molecular weight that are water soluble and their metabolites are excreted by glomerular filtration. The amount excreted is directly related to the concentration of nonprotein bound drug in plasma. In the elderly both the amount of drug available to the glomeruli and the amount that can be filtered may be altered. For drugs excreted only by this process, the elimination half-life may change markedly with changes in protein binding.
Tubular secretion	This process, which occurs in renal tubules, appears to be linear under most clinical conditions. The rate of renal tubular secretion may be proportional to the concentration of free or total drug in plasma and may or may not be affected by blood flow. The slight reduction due to primary aging is usually not a problem in drug therapy. However, this may not be true in dehydrated patients or in those with heart failure or extensive or chronic renal failure (examples: organic acids and antibiotic metabolites).
Tubular reabsorption	May be active or passive. Follows glomerular filtration from renal tubular lumen. Many drugs (both weak acids and weak bases) and a large number of electrolytes are reabsorbed into the blood. The rate of reabsorption is proportional to the concentration gradient of diffusible (free and nonionized) drug. Urinary pH is the primary factor influencing tubular reabsorption. Normal urinary pH may fluctuate between 4.5 and 8.0, depending on the diet, pathophysiology, and drug intake; may also be affected by changes in urine flow rate.

of about 10 per cent per decade in the total renal blood flow and a progressive reduction in mean blood flow per unit mass.[123] If renal blood flow is 600 ml. per minute at age 40, it would be about 300 ml. per minute four decades later. Reduced glomerular flow results in part from reduced cardiac output and the redistribution of that output, the renal fraction being further reduced with age. The decreased renal perfusion associated with aging is most pronounced in the renal cortex.

Formation of glomerular filtrate and tubular excretory capacity both decline about 40 per cent between the ages of 20 and 90 years. Because glomerular and tubular functions decline in a similar fashion, the balance between the two functions remains virtually unaltered. The glomerular filtration rate is reduced as a function of normal aging, showing a progressive decline as a function of increasing age, from 100 to 120 ml. per minute at age 40 to about 60 to 70 ml. per minute at age 85. Failure to modify dosage schedules for drugs eliminated primarily by renal mechanisms can lead to significant dosage errors.

Renal function is best measured by the glomerular filtration rate. The "normal" standards available to estimate the glomerular filtration rate must be age adjusted if one attempts to estimate renal function in older persons. Renal function can be estimated by first measuring the urinary creatinine level and then the serum creatinine level. One then can calculate creatinine clearance. However, normal serum creatinine values for an elderly patient do not provide proof of a normal glomerular filtration rate, because decreased production in many elderly will result in normal values despite decreased glomerular filtration. The reduction in creatinine clearance is paralleled by a reduction in the daily urinary creatinine excretion, reflecting a decreased muscle mass. There may also be a constancy of serum creatinine concentration when the glomerular filtration rate and the creatinine clearance decline. A serum creatinine level of 1.0 mg. per 100 ml. may indicate a creatinine clearance of 120 ml. per min. at age 20, but only 60 ml. per min. at age 80. A nomogram has been developed to aid in the determination of creatinine clearance changes with age.[126]

With advancing age there is also likely to be a reduction in the number of functioning tubules. This would mean that both the maximal rate of urine flow and the diluting capacity of the kidney would diminish with age. Renal tubular transport of anions depends on the number of nephrons, the activity of the transport mechanism, and the availability of free drug, and it is clear that with advancing age that process may change as a result of changes in one or more of these factors.[127]

Tubular reabsorption of some drugs follows pH dependent kinetics. Increases in urinary pH would cause increased elimination of weakly acidic drugs but decreased elimination of weak bases. In the elderly, nutritional factors may well affect urinary pH to a greater extent than in younger persons. Many elderly people apparently switch to low protein diets with advancing age, often because of economic considerations, and low protein diets support an alkaline urinary pH. Vegetable diets or diets rich in carbohydrates result in a higher urinary pH, whereas high protein diets will result in a lower urinary pH.

Urinary pH also can be affected by drugs, both prescription and nonprescription. Vitamin C, for example, may be responsible for an acid urinary pH, whereas diuretics and antacids often produce an alkaline urinary pH. However, one must not assume that administration of these drugs will automatically change the urinary pH. For example, administration of vitamin C for the purpose of acidifying the urine may have variable effects.[128]

Secondary Aging Effects on Kidneys. A number of diseases are responsible for altered renal function, diseases, and conditions that occur frequently among elderly patients. Among them are diabetes mellitus, hypovolemia, and pyelonephritis. Acute glomerulonephritis can develop at a very late age, possibly following nonstreptococcal infections such as pneumococcal pneumonia.[129] Arteriosclerosis often may be responsible for decreased functional ability, as may hypertension. The kidney is most severely affected by hypertension. The more pronounced the blood pressure elevation, the more severe the damage. Thus, renal senescence, cumulative effects of kidney infections, and impaired vascular and humoral responses may combine to alter kidney function and, therefore, drug action.

Effects of Drugs. The renal system is very susceptible to drug toxicity. Various drugs can produce nephrotoxic reactions, leading possibly to acute or chronic renal failure, nephrotic syndrome, renal tubular syndromes, and other disorders. Drugs of course are also known to disturb the fluid and electrolyte balance.[130] The nephrotoxic effects of drugs may be responsible for arteritis, glomerular changes, acute tubular necrosis, and interstitial nephritis. The elderly male is further at risk to the cumulative effect of drugs that can cause acute urinary retention, such as decongestants found in many nonprescription drugs and anticholinergic medication.

Clinical and Pharmacokinetic Effects of Impaired Renal Function. Even in patients with normal renal function, a wide variation in drug response is to be expected. In one study the recommended dose of gentamicin would have been too low for 47 per cent of the patients and too high in 17 per cent of the patients studied—all patients with normal renal function.[131] Therefore, even more caution must be exercised when drugs are prescribed that depend primarily on renal excretion, because they may accumulate in patients with renal impairment, leading to toxic reactions.[132]

Clinical effects of renal impairment may have a variety of causes and presentations.[7] Reduced renal perfusion may well be responsible. Reduction of the blood supply to any organ reduces that organ's capacity to respond to stress, and drugs, as foreign substances, produce stress. Thus, reduction of the reserve capacity of the kidney can have serious consequences if the kidney is overloaded with drugs. In particular, cationic electrolyte overload is not too infrequent in elderly patients. It can cause major clinical problems. Most often mentioned are the penicillins, which can induce a sodium overload, leading to congestive heart failure or decompensation of stabilized congestive heart failure. Reduced renal function, and therefore increased drug hazard, should be considered in prescribing such water soluble drugs as digoxin, the aminoglycosides (their serum levels may also be altered by changed body temperature and lean body mass), the long acting sulfonamides, the penicillins and tetracyclines, phenobarbital, procainamide, and most antihypertensive agents.

The clinical effect of poor renal function on the elimination of lipid soluble drugs is not easily predictable. It would be reasonable to assume that no adverse effects resulting from poor renal function would occur when metabolism of such drugs leads to the formation of inactive metabolites that cause no toxic effects. However, the importance of the prescriber's knowledge of a drug's metabolism is highlighted by such drugs as phenytoin. This drug is extensively metabolized, and one therefore would not expect decreased elimination of it in renal insufficiency. However, metabolism of this drug leads to the formation of a metabolite that is excreted by the kidney, and therefore renal status must be taken into consideration when prescribing this drug.[133]

The clinical effect of reduced glomerular

TABLE 2–14. Selected Clinical Effects of Reduced Glomerular Filtration Rate

Drug	Effect of Change in Glomerular Filtration Rate (ml./min.)
	Ineffective in urinary infection when glomerular filtration rate is:
Carbenicillin	< 20
Cephalothin	< 20
Cephapirin	< 10
Chloramphenicol	< 40
Tetracyclines	< 20
	Hyperkalemia common when glomerular filtration rate is:
Spironolactone	< 25
Triamterene	< 25
	Ineffective when glomerular filtration rate is:
Thiazides	< 25

function for some drugs is shown in Table 2–14. In other cases the clinical effect may be more subtle. Apparently one should expect increased patient sensitivity to narcotic analgesics and sedatives in renal failure. It has been speculated that this may be due to an altered permeability to the blood-brain barrier or tissue receptor sites.[134]

Reduced renal function may lead to edema, which in turn could lead to changes in the absorption of drugs administered intramuscularly or subcutaneously. Edema may also occur in the gastrointestinal tract, leading to altered bioavailability of some drugs. This has been documented for furosemide.[135,136] Edema can decrease the bioavailability of furosemide from approximately 74 per cent to 17 per cent in addition to having numerous other effects (Table 2–15).

TABLE 2–15. Effect of Edema on Kinetics of Orally Administered Furosemide*

	No Edema	Edema
Plasma half-life (hr.)	1.52	1.15
Area under plasma conc. time curve (ng./mg./hr.)	6179	1930
Apparent volume of distribution (L.)	21.3	12.0
Plasma clearance (ml./min.)	162	120
Bioavailability	74.7	17.3

*Adapted from Odlind, B.G., and Beerman, B.: Diuretic resistance: reduced bioavailability and effect of oral furosemide. Br. Med. J., 280:1577, 1980.

Renal impairment can lead to disturbances in electrolyte and fluid balance, which in turn can lead to changes in the volume of distribution. There may also be changes in the intravascular volume that can affect the processing of drugs by the proximal tubules. Thiazides can cause lithium to be reabsorbed in a volume contracted state, leading to lithium toxicity. On the other hand, administration of saline solutions can bring about volume expansion, and thereby subtherapeutic drug levels.

As previously discussed, the disposition of drugs can be importantly influenced by binding of drugs to both plasma and tissue constituents. Renal impairment may disturb binding, leading to alterations in drug distribution and elimination.[137–141] Most affected are the weakly acidic drugs; the weakly basic drugs are less affected.

A number of reasons for reduced binding in renal impairment have been advanced. These patients may well be hypoproteinemic, and, given the usual dose, the free amount of drug will change, leading to toxicity even if serum levels do not change. Impaired or reduced glomerular filtration may result in the accumulation of fluid and blood nitrogenous substances. The presence of both irreversible and competitive inhibitors may then be responsible for reduced protein binding. Finally, in renal impairment the composition of albumin may be altered also. A decrease in drug-protein binding results in an increase in the volume of distribution, possibly facilitating biotransformation and excretion of a drug. However, because the effect of reduced glomerular filtration often dominates, the net elimination of a drug is rarely increased.

Kidney disease may also adversely affect drug metabolism. Apparently drug oxidation and glucuronide conjugation are not affected, but reduction to inactive metabolites appears to be slower and acetylation metabolism, more variable. Low molecular weight proteins, such as insulin, tend to accumulate in renal failure. There has also been the suggestion that the processes leading to the formation of active metabolites may be impaired in renal failure.[142]

It seems clear, therefore, that any renal impairment mandates a cautious approach to drug therapy. Many drugs are eliminated through a combined effect of extrarenal and renal elimination. When extrarenal elimination predominates, blood flow and metabolic capacity should be evaluated. If renal clearance predominates, drugs eliminated primarily by the kidney should be used with caution, particularly drugs with a low margin of safety. In the elderly the combined effects of primary and secondary aging in addition to the effects of multiple drug therapy may and often do cause unexpected drug effects and increase the hazard of drug therapy.

BIOAVAILABILITY

The term "bioavailability" is often used interchangeably with the term "bioequivalence." Either term denotes the amount of active ingredient available for absorption into the circulation and action. An understanding of the concept of bioavailability can contribute greatly to safe drug therapy for the elderly.

The possible influence of various dosage forms on serum levels (and thereby the intensity and duration of drug action) is shown in Figure 2-8. When this information is translated to a real drug, one that poses considerable hazard to elderly patients, it shows that when digoxin is administered in tablet form, 65 per cent of the dose will be absorbed. However, if an elixir dosage form is used, the fraction of the dose absorbed is increased to 80 per cent; intravenous administration yields 100 per cent absorption.[143]

For the elderly, the bioequivalent concept is particularly important when viewed in economic terms. Often generic products may be less costly than trade named products. However, a patient well stabilized on a particular drug should not necessarily change. For example, available data suggest that various marketed brands of the same orally administered tricyclic antidepressants may not have the same comparable therapeutic effects.[144,145] Other differences in bioequivalence have been reported.[146] Bioequivalence, and an appreciation for its possible influence on drug action, may assume particular importance when a different dosage form is selected to overcome the first pass effect.

The concepts just discussed are well established and, one would assume, well known. Yet reality seems to offer a slightly different and disturbing picture. One need only recall the many patients who were switched from 300 mg. phenytoin capsules to the oral, liquid dosage form (also 300 mg. per dose) and the resultant and apparently unexpected change in drug action and patient response.

A similar disturbing factor is the continued incorrect use of some antibiotics. For example, an elderly patient was found to have a Pseudomonas infection in a surgical incision in the left thigh. The laboratory reported Pseudomonas to be sensitive to carbenicillin, and the physician prescribed oral doses of carbenicillin, unaware of the fact that the parenteral dosage form would have to be used if therapeutic blood levels were to be achieved. (Incidentally, the danger of cationic electrolyte overload mentioned previously was also over-

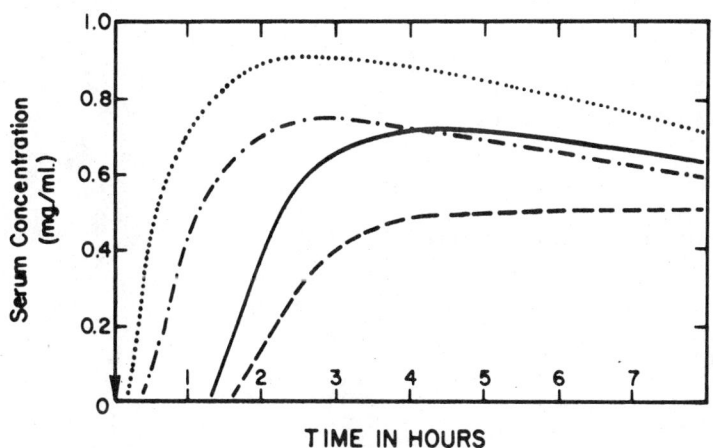

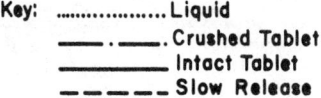

Figure 2-8. Graph demonstrating the influence of the dosage form on the rate of absorption, serum concentration, and duration of action.

looked.) This particular elderly patient was being treated for congestive heart failure, and the sodium overload produced by the oral dosage form of carbenicillin caused decompensation. Thus, the goal of geriatric medicine to use drugs in a manner that would optimize benefit while decreasing, to the largest degree possible, their hazard often mandates a careful evaluation of bioequivalence factors.

MODIFYING DOSAGES IN THE ELDERLY

There is no question that advancing age changes the pharmacokinetics of many drugs. Many of these changes have recently been summarized (Table 2–16). Others have shown that the biologic half-life of theophylline varies from 5.4 to 9 hours in elderly patients, that steady state levels of cimetidine are higher and persist longer in older adults, and that elimination processes, of salicylate, for example, may be very complicated and, if not taken into consideration, can lead to toxic reactions in the elderly, in whom desired serum concentrations may be very close to toxic concentrations.[148–150]

These changes in pharmacokinetic parameters of drugs can lead to drug toxicities that the elderly are ill equipped to overcome. Additionally, drug therapy in the elderly can be incredibly complicated, with results depending on many different factors. For example,

TABLE 2–16. Effects of Age on Drug Disposition*

Drug	Elimination Rate		aVd	Apparent Mechanism for Age Related Change
	Young Adult	*Geriatric*		
Acetanilide	$t\frac{1}{2} = 1.45$ hr.	$t\frac{1}{2} = 2.07$ hr.	—	Decreased metabolism
Aminopyrine	$t\frac{1}{2} = 3.0$ hr.	$t\frac{1}{2} = 10.0$ hr.	—	
Ampicillin	$t\frac{1}{2} = 1.0$ hr.	$t\frac{1}{2} = 1.2$ hr.	—	
Amylobarbitone	Urinary metabolite excretion = 14.2%	Urinary metabolite excretion = 4.3%	—	Decreased metabolism
	Plasma drug level = 1.3 µg./ml.	Plasma drug level = 1.0 µg./ml.		
Antipyrine	1st study: $t\frac{1}{2} = 12$ hr.	$t\frac{1}{2} = 17.4$ hr.	—	
	2nd study: no change in MCR of nonsmokers; MCR decreased with age in smokers		—	
Chlordiazepoxide	Clearance = 26.6 ml./min.	Clearance = 46.3 ml./min.	↑ in elderly	
Diazepam	$t\frac{1}{2} = 20$ hr.	$t\frac{1}{2} = 80$ hr.	↑ 3× in elderly	
Digoxin	$t\frac{1}{2} = 51$ hr.	$t\frac{1}{2} = 73$ hr.	—	Decreased renal function
Dihydrostreptomycin	$t\frac{1}{2} = 5.2$ hr.	$t\frac{1}{2} = 8.4$ hr.	—	Decreased renal function
Doxycycline	$t\frac{1}{2} = 11.95$ hr.	$t\frac{1}{2} = 17.74$ hr.	—	Decreased renal function
Flurazepam	Incidence of flurazepam toxicity increased with age		—	
Indocyanine green	MCR decreased with age		—	Decreased liver blood flow
Isoniazid	$t\frac{1}{2} = 2.5$ hr.	$t\frac{1}{2} = 2.9$ hr.	—	
Kanamycin	$t\frac{1}{2} = 107$ min.	$t\frac{1}{2} = 282$ min.	—	Decreased renal function
Lithium	Clearance = 41.5 ml./min.	Clearance = 7.7 ml./min.	—	
Lorazepam	Clearance = 0.99 ml./min./kg.	Clearance = 0.77 ml./min./kg.	↑ 2.5× in elderly	
Nitrazepam	Clearance = 4.1 l./hr.	Clearance = 4.7 l./hr.	↑ 2.0× in elderly	
Penicillin	$t\frac{1}{2} = 0.55$ hr. (penicillin G)	$t\frac{1}{2} = 1.0$ hr. (penicillin G)	—	
	$t\frac{1}{2} = 10$ hr. (procaine penicillin)	$t\frac{1}{2} = 18$ hr. (procaine penicillin)		
Pethidine (meperidine)	Plasma levels twice as high in elderly		—	
Phenobarbital	$t\frac{1}{2} = 71$ hr.	$t\frac{1}{2} = 107$ hr.	—	Decreased metabolism
Phenylbutazone	1st study: $t\frac{1}{2} = 81$ hr.	$t\frac{1}{2} = 105$ hr.	—	
	2nd study: $t\frac{1}{2} = 87$ hr.	$t\frac{1}{2} = 110$ hr.		
Phenytoin	Clearance = 26 ml./kg./hr.	Clearance = 42 ml./kg./hr.	—	
Practolol	$t\frac{1}{2} = 7.1$ hr.	$t\frac{1}{2} = 8.6$ hr.	—	Decreased renal function
Propicillin	Serum levels are twice as high in elderly		↓ in elderly	Decreased distribution volume
Propranolol	Clearance decreases with age only in smokers		—	
Quinidine	Clearance = 4.04	Clearance = 2.64	No change	Decreased metabolism and renal function
Tetracycline	$t\frac{1}{2} = 3.5$ hr.	$t\frac{1}{2} = 4.5$ hr.	—	

*Reproduced with permission from Vesell, E.S.: The influence of host factors on drug response. II. Age. Ration. Drug Ther., *14*(4):1–7, 1980. A publication of the American Society for Pharmacology and Experimental Therapeutics. Published by W.B. Saunders Company, Philadelphia, Pennsylvania.

more than 37 per cent of the elderly receive diuretics. They are likely to develop hypokalemia because their dietary intake of potassium tends to be reduced, the gastrointestinal absorption of potassium may be decreased, and reduced muscle mass may further diminish total body potassium reserves. Yet even if the challenge of the use of a diuretic that can increase urinary potassium loss is recognized and a potassium sparing diuretic is used, hypokalemia can still develop.[151] The provider then must consider not only the possible clinical effects of hypokalemia but also the effects on the patient's quality of life, which may be considerably reduced by apathy, lethargy, and fatigue.

Incidentally, fatigue is apparently a common side effect of many drugs (particularly beta-blockers), but it has been given relatively little attention and its effect on the quality of life in elderly patients has probably not yet been well evaluated.[152] One might speculate that it is most often overlooked and ascribed to "growing old."

Without doubt, then, drug therapy for elderly patients demands a much more sophisticated approach than may have been practiced in the past. However, one must still note the absence of a comprehensive body of knowledge about drugs and aging, and this lack poses a serious problem, to both the provider and the patient.

It is relatively simple to state that drugs should be administered to older adults according to the principle that enough drug is given to achieve the desired therapeutic response with a minimal number of adverse effects. To achieve that, the impaired capacity of the elderly patient to tolerate complex drug regimens (or even a single potent drug) should be kept in mind. Failure to quantitate the reactive capacities of the aging body should be avoided, and the prescriber must be familiar with confirmed pharmacologic and pharmacokinetic data with respect to the elderly.[10]

A rational prescribing process and a modification of dosages might start with acceptance of the fact that this is a shared responsibility of provider and patient. Some problems are attributable to the provider at the very start of the process of rational drug therapy.[159] These include lack of appreciation of the effects of primary and secondary aging, inaccuracies in drug treatment, unnecessary multiple drug administration, and deliberate overmedication.

Safer drug therapy may also result when there is a better understanding of the continuum of care of the elderly. In one survey only 21 per cent of the physicians interviewed believed that they continued to be in charge of their patient after the patient had become a resident in a nursing home.[154] Drug therapy for the elderly may also become safer when it is recognized that the young-old die mostly from arteriosclerotic disease and the old-old from infection, pulmonary emboli, and cancer. One can then become intimately familiar with these disease processes and the drugs used to manage them. A more comprehensive knowledge is needed about the drugs that most often cause adverse effects in the elderly (e.g., the diuretics) and those that pose the highest risk to elderly patients (e.g., antihypertensives, antiparkinson drugs, psychotropics, and digoxin). One recent study documented a surprising lack of knowledge of the pharmacology, pharmacokinetics, and toxicology of drugs used for the elderly by those who prescribe them.[155]

One must hasten to add that some of this type of knowledge is not yet readily available and in some instances may be difficult to compile. For example, quinidine is excreted by a combination of renal excretion of intact drug (15 to 40 per cent of the total clearance) and hepatic biotransformation of a variety of metabolites (60 to 85 per cent of the total clearance). Many of the metabolites apparently are active. Quinidine clearance is reduced with age and is also reduced in patients with cirrhosis of the liver and congestive heart failure. To predict the action of quinidine, it must further be noted that it is 70 to 95 per cent protein bound, primarily to albumin but also to other plasma constituents. Since elderly patients often are thought to suffer from unrecognized drug-drug interactions, it would also be necessary to be familiar with its particular metabolic pathways, for interactions may occur with drugs that share quinidine's metabolic pathways.

Further complicating the prescribing process is the fact that in the elderly the response to a given dose may vary widely and unpredictably. This has been shown to be true for phenylbutazone, for example.[156] When patients in one study received 0.25 gm. of chloroquine daily, serum concentrations ranged from less than 0.2 to more than 0.8 mcg. per ml.[157]

Because of the limited knowledge of drug effects in the elderly, the admonition "Start low, go slow" is a commonly heard direction. Theoretically, then, the dose would be adjusted, on the basis of the patient's response (Fig. 2–9). Although this is an appealing

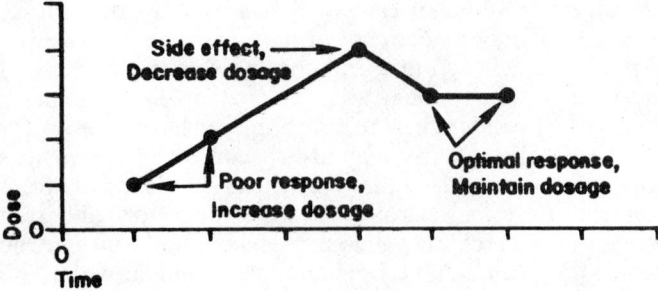

Figure 2–9. Illustration of the importance of individualizing therapy and adjusting dosages to optimize the therapeutic response while minimizing toxicity.

concept, it requires close supervision of the elderly patient, which often cannot or does not take place; secondly, a reduction in the dose might still lead to unexpected results. As Figure 2–10 indicates, normal subjects received a dose of 5 mg. of prazosin and patients with congestive heart failure a dose of 2 mg., but even though higher prazosin peak levels were seen in the normal subjects, the area under the curve for the patients with congestive heart failure is substantially greater.[158]

DOSE ADJUSTMENT BASED ON RENAL FUNCTION

Pharmacokinetic principles enable the provider to arrive at dosage regimens based on the quantity of drug administered. For drugs with first order kinetics, calculations are based on the direct relationship between the total daily dose and the steady state plasma concentration:

Dose response ratio = drug plasma concentration (mcg. per ml.) × total daily dose (mg. per kg.)

Obviously each milligram of drug administered contributes a certain amount (mcg. per ml.) to the steady state plasma level, and therefore:

Expected plasma concentration = dose response ratio (mcg. per ml. per mg. per kg.) × total daily dose (mg. per kg.)

Use of this formula can yield a valuable first indication of the dose that must be used to attain a certain steady state concentration, the desired optimal therapeutic concentration. Application of these principles also enables the provider to select the dosage and the dosing interval so that an optimal plasma concentration can be reached and maintained below the level at which toxic effects may occur.

In many instances physiologic factors (e.g., weight) and pathologic factors (e.g., dehydration) have to be considered because they too may mandate adjustment of both the dose and the dosing interval. For example, in diabetes mellitus, the anticipated response to an antibiotic will likely be changed, especially if the antibiotic is administered intramuscularly, probably as a result of microangiopathic changes.

From a clinical point of view it is important to modify drug dosages and dosage intervals, particularly for elderly persons with impaired renal function. As previously documented, most elderly patients probably do present with functional impairment of the kidney, a factor still all too often overlooked and not considered in prescribing for the elderly.

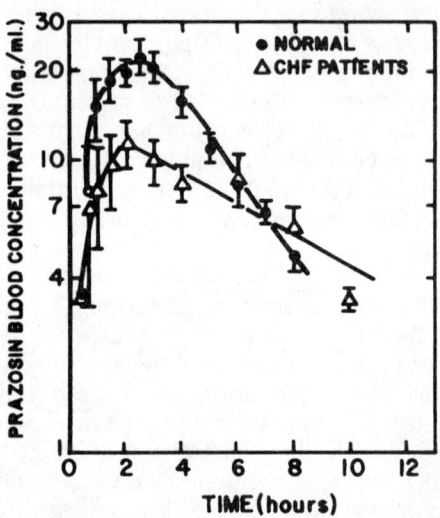

Figure 2–10. Blood prazosin concentration in normal subjects and patients with congestive heart failure after administration of the first dose. Normal subjects received a 5 mg. dose and patients with congestive heart failure, a 2 mg. dose. Although normal subjects received higher concentrations, the area under the curve is greater in patients with congestive heart failure.

A combination of factors determines which drugs should be considered especially for dose adjustment in the elderly. The use of antibiotics, in particular, is difficult in elderly patients. The elderly, for example, are increasingly susceptible to allergic reactions when treated with antibiotics.[159] Tetracyclines may cause azotemia in patients with renal impairment by increasing catabolism; therefore, except for doxycycline and minocycline, they should be avoided.[159] The aminoglycosides are themselves nephrotoxic, and their use can lead to even more serious kidney impairment. Others, such as nitrofurantoin and nalidixic acid, are not effective in renal failure.[160] Mental disturbances with some antibiotics occur in the elderly, even when reduced doses are used. The possibility of a sodium overload must not be overlooked. Routine doses of carbenicillin and ticarcillin act as nonreabsorbable anions, possibly leading to an efflux of hydrogen and potassium ions and producing hypokalemic alkalosis. Other antibiotics may exhibit other peculiarities that must be taken into consideration. After multiple dosing of gentamicin, for example, there is tissue accumulation of the drug.[161]

Other considerations enter into the selection of the proper dose. For example, there may be an interaction between two drugs, such as occurs between lidocaine and propranolol.[162] Sometimes it may be important to know the exact mechanism of renal clearance. With digoxin, for example, both glomerular filtration and tubular secretion take place, and when its plasma concentration is elevated, the amount of digoxin excreted by glomerular filtration increases proportionally.[163] Tubular secretion also increases with increasing plasma concentration but reaches a maximum at which this mechanism is saturated; it is during this active process (tubular secretion) that interactions can occur.

Clearly, then, a number of factors need to be considered before a particular antibiotic (or any other drug) is selected for use. Following the selection based on all other considerations, two factors generally determine whether a dose or dosage interval will have to be adjusted. If the amount of drug excreted unchanged by the kidney is great, one must expect a clinically significant adverse effect when renal function is impaired. This principle usually applies with all drugs with a narrow therapeutic index. The drugs listed in Table 2-17 are examples of drugs with a relatively narrow therapeutic index that would require a dosage adjustment in case of renal impairment. However, some drugs exhibit a very wide therapeutic margin of safety. If that is the case, as happens with the cephalosporins, dosage adjustment based on impaired renal status is most likely not needed.

TABLE 2-17. Dosage Adjustment Needed if Renal Impairment Exists

Aminoglycosides	Digoxin
Amikacin	Lithium
Gentamicin	Procainamide
Kanamycin	Theophylline
Tobramycin	

HOW TO ADJUST THE DOSE

Two basic methods are available to achieve an optimal drug effect while minimizing drug toxicity in elderly patients with renal impairment. In principle, a dosage regimen may be adjusted either by lowering the maintenance dose or by prolonging the dosage interval. It should be the specific goal of the treatment regimen to achieve the desired therapeutic plasma concentration, which, once achieved, is maintained by multiple dosing. During the course of treatment the drug concentration will fluctuate between a maximal and a minimal level. Selection of the particular method of administration or dose adjustment should proceed according to particular characteristics of the drug to be administered.

Variable Dose Regimen. When it is important to achieve an effective dose level, but when higher doses would not produce a corresponding therapeutic effect, the variable dose method is usually selected. The dosage reduction method, in which dosage intervals are maintained as usual, has been recommended for drugs for which a relatively constant blood level is desired, such as the anticoagulants, the antidiabetics, and the corticosteroids. It has also been suggested that this method be used for drugs that are relatively slowly excreted.

Variable Frequency Regimen. This method, also referred to as the interval extension method, has been recommended for the administration of many analgesics, cardiovascular drugs, and antibacterial drugs. In general, this method of dosage adjustment is used for drugs with short half-lives. Use of this method may lead to higher peak and lower trough levels. Since the half-life of many drugs in renal failure is greatly prolonged, it often takes too long to reach the steady state level, the desired, optimal level. Therefore, in critical cases, as with the use of antibiotics, for example, a loading dose may be necessary. After the loading dose has been administered, the standard dose of the drug is given at the standard intervals. Often the exact timing is determined by renal function or such pharmacokinetic variables as the serum half-life or excretion constant.

Combination of Variable Dose and Variable Frequency Methods. In selecting the specific method, one can use recommendations as listed in the literature.[164] The major factors to be considered are the peak-trough differences and possible toxic reactions at peak levels, the maintenance of the minimal level required, and the half-life of the drug.

Not too infrequently either or both methods will still result in wide swings in serum levels, alternating between subtherapeutic and toxic levels. This must be expected, particularly in the elderly, in whom drug responses are very unpredictable and responses are often more scattered than in a normal population. These swings can be hazardous to the elderly. Therefore, a combination of the variable dose and variable frequency methods is often necessary.

DOSE ADJUSTMENT METHODS

Many dose adjustment methods have been proposed. That so many exist speaks to the fact that there is probably as yet no one method for any one drug that can be considered "best." Most must be preceded by an assessment of the kidney status.

Assessment of Kidney Status. Two factors are mainly responsible for serum creatinine levels, i.e., the rate of production of muscle mass and the glomerular filtration, which is assumed to reflect the rate of excretion. It is further assumed that when the serum creatinine concentration doubles, the glomerular filtration rate decreases by one-half. Small changes in the serum creatinine level therefore can reflect marked changes in the glomerular filtration rate. However, still often not sufficiently appreciated in the prescribing process is the dependency of the serum creatinine concentration on muscle mass, and that "normal" values do not exclude significant changes in elderly patients, in whom muscle production may be reduced. Creatinine clearance reflects the volume of serum completely cleared of creatinine in a given time interval (ml. per min.). It is a more accurate reflection than serum creatinine of the glomerular filtration rate and renal function.

To assess renal function correctly, the steady state of renal function must be determined. Unless an elderly patient suffers from abnormal liver function or muscle disease, two rapid methods have been suggested to evaluate renal function. The first takes into account lean body weights and differences in sex; the second, utilizing a nomogram, takes into consideration weight and age, as well as sex.[165,166] Once the kidney status has been assessed, a particular method of dose adjustment can be chosen.[167]

Welling and Craig have suggested a method that utilizes a nomogram.[168] The changes in the percentage of normal elimination rate constants and the consequent increase in elimination half-life are described as a function of creatinine clearance. The method provides a convenient means for estimating the ratio of the uremic elimination rate constant to the normal elimination rate constant on the basis of creatinine clearance. Wagner's method takes advantage of the fact that the elimination constant can be obtained from the creatinine clearance.[169]

The method advanced by Giusti and Hayton assumes that the effect of reduced kidney function on the renal portion of the elimination constant can be estimated from the ratio of the uremic creatinine clearance.[170] Kampmann and Hansen have suggested a practical way to adjust dosage regimens for elderly patients.[171] Using this method, one first determines the normal adult dose, based on normal creatinine clearance. Second, the amount of unchanged drug and active metabolites excreted by the kidneys is determined. Finally, the endogenous creatinine clearance yields the kidney status. Next one determines the half-life of the drug to be administered for the particular patient, which is compared with the half-life of the drug for the person with a normal creatinine clearance. The former is divided by the latter, yielding a ratio value. If the variable dose method is chosen, the "normal dose" is divided by that dosage adjustment factor (the ratio value). If the variable frequency method is chosen, the "normal interval" is multiplied by this factor, yielding the new interval tailored to the specific patient with renal impairment.

PRECAUTIONS IN USING DOSAGE ADJUSTMENT METHODS

Certain assumptions are made in all dosage adjustment methods:
1. The drug in question follows dose independent kinetics.
2. The volume of distribution remains relatively constant.
3. The original molecule is the active part.
4. The pharmacologic response to the drug in the uremic patient remains the same.

Therefore—and this is an important point to remember—dosage adjustment is only a preliminary step, a step that must necessarily be followed by further dosage adjustment based on observation of the clinical response. One additional word of caution is necessary: A significant error could be introduced by calculating drug clearance using the one compartment formula for drugs whose disposition follows multicompartment kinetics.[172] Errors ranging from 12 to 196 per cent can be introduced. It is noteworthy that in some instances, the error was reduced because of the patient's disease state. Those drugs for which one compartment calculations are apparently sufficient are listed in Table 2–18.

It has been suggested that a classification of drugs into three categories based on creatinine clearance may be helpful in predicting possible effects of renal impairment.[173] Three types of drugs have been designated, types A, B, and C (Table 2–19). Type A drugs are water soluble and are normally eliminated almost entirely by the kidneys. The half-life of a type A drug increases slightly with decreasing values of creatinine clearance, until a critical clearance value has been reached. Beyond that critical value (clearance of 10 to 20 ml. per min.), the half-life increases dramatically. In

TABLE 2–18. Drugs Whose Clearance Can Apparently Be Calculated Using One-Compartment Kinetics

Ascorbic acid	Propranolol*
Amobarbital	Quinidine*
Chlordiazepoxide	Salicylic acid
Clonazepam	Sulfisoxazole
Diazepam*	Theophylline
Meperidine*	Tobramycin
Nortriptyline	Tolbutamide
Pentobarbital	Warfarin
Phenytoin	

*In hypertension or hepatic cirrhosis.

TABLE 2–19. Relationship Between the Elimination Rate of Some Antimicrobials and Their Endogenous Creatinine Clearance*

Drug	Type A, B, or C†
Antituberculars	
Aminosalicylic acid	C
Ethambutol	A
Isoniazid	C
Rifampin	B
Aminoglycosides	
Amikacin	A
Gentamicin	A
Kanamycin	A
Neomycin	A
Streptomycin	A
Cephalosporins	
Cefamandole	A
Cefazolin	A
Cephalexin	A
Cephalothin	C
Cephapirin	C
Cephradin	A
Penicillins	
Amoxicillin	A
Ampicillin	C
Carbenicillin	C
Cloxacillin	C
Dicloxacillin	C
Methicillin	C
Nafcillin	B
Oxacillin	C
Penicillin G	C
Ticarcillin	A
Tetracyclines	
Doxycycline	C
Minocycline	B
Tetracycline	C
Others	
Chloramphenicol	C
Clindamycin	C
Erythromycin	B
Nalidixic acid	A
Vancomycin	A

*Polar drugs are usually eliminated by the renal route, whereas lipophilic drugs are preferentially metabolized.

†Type A: half-life increases with decreasing renal clearance. Type B: half-life unchanged by decrease in renal clearance. Type C: half-life variably affected by decrease in renal clearance.

elderly patients, type A drugs should be used cautiously, particularly if the drugs exhibit a low margin of safety. Type B drugs are almost entirely eliminated by extrarenal mechanisms. Decreasing renal clearance values would not significantly affect their half-lives. Those drugs with both renal and extrarenal clearance (type C) would be variably affected by decreased renal clearance, and a very precise understanding of their pharmacokinetics is necessary

TABLE 2-20. Digoxin Dosing*

Parameters entered†		Parameters entered	
Weight	110	Weight	110
CCR	25	CCR	25
ITBC	0	ITBC	0
T1	0	T1	0
DTBC	13	DTBC	13
DI	1	DI	1
Route	Oral	Route	Oral
Loading dose	0.7629718554 mg	Loading dose	0.7629718554 mg
Maintenance dose	0.1516631387 mg	Maintenance dose	0.1516631387 mg
Enter mg to be used	0.125 mg	Enter mg to be used	0.1875 mg
Estimated glycoside TBC		Estimated glycoside TBC	
Peak	10.71453495	Peak	16.07180242
End	8.584705403	End	12.8770581

*Reprinted with permission from Gregory, A.: Programmed pharmacokinetic dosing regimens. Hosp. Pharm., 15:31, 1980.

†CCR = creatinine clearance. ITBC = initial total body concentration. T1 = time between estimation of initial concentration and time at which next dose is given. DTBC = desired total body concentration. DI = dosing interval.

when they need to be prescribed for elderly patients with renal impairment.

THE USE OF COMPUTER PROGRAMS IN DOSAGE ADJUSTMENT

More and more the recent literature describes the use of programmable calculators or computer programs to assist the provider in dosage adjustment calculations. Two are included in Table 2-20.

Programmed Pharmacokinetic Dosing Regimens*

Digoxin Dosing

The patient illustrated in Table 2-20 weighs 110 lb. (lean body weight) with a creatinine clearance of 25 ml. per min. per 1.73 sq. m. The initial total body concentration is 0, and the desired total body concentration is approximately 13 mcg. per kg. of lean body weight. The patient is being dosed on a daily basis and the drug is to be given orally. The loading dose (as calculated) is 0.75 mg.; the maintenance dose is 0.15 mg. daily. In one case the operator indicates that a 0.125 mg. daily dose would be given, and the estimated peak and trough levels were calculated. In the second case a dose of 0.1875 mg. daily is indicated, and again peak and trough estimations are printed out.

Antimicrobial Dosing

Antimicrobial dosages have also been calculated using a computer, according to the following formulas:*

Adjustments to antimicrobial doses are directly related to the elimination rate fraction, which describes the elimination rate of the drug in a patient as a fraction of its "normal" elimination rate constant.

The following abbreviations are used in the equations for calculation of the dose regimens:

Q	= Elimination rate fraction.
K(f)	= Fraction of the drug eliminated per hour in the patient with renal failure.
K(n)	= Fraction of the drug eliminated per hour in "normal" subjects.
CCr(f)	= Creatinine clearance in the patient with renal failure (ml./min./1.73 m.²).
CCr(n)	= Age-related creatinine clearance in "normal" subjects. If age is > 6

---

*This system is composed of a Texas Instruments programmable calculator (TI-59) attached to a printer unit. The calculator is preprogrammed with equations derived from the pharmacokinetic literature.

*Copyright 1980, American Society of Hospital Pharmacists. All rights reserved. Reprinted with permission from Wraith Bennett, S., and Scott, A.C.: Computer-assisted customized antimicrobial dosages. Am. J. Hosp. Pharm., 37:523, 1980.

months old, value is 100 ml./min./1.73 m.^{2}; 1 week < age < 6 months, 80 ml./min./1.73 m.^{2}; 1 day < age < 1 week, 45 ml./min./1.73 m.^{2}.

- a = Fraction of the drug eliminated per hour by nonrenal means.
- b = Slope of K vs. CCr line.
- fe = Fraction excreted unchanged in the urine.
- D(f) = Maintenance dose of the drug for the patient in renal failure.
- D(n) = Maintenance dose of the drug in "normal" subjects.
- LD = Loading dose.
- τ(f) = Dosing interval for the patient in renal failure.
- τ(n) = Dosing interval in patients with normal renal function.
- τ(s) = Selected dosing interval.

The elimination rate of the drug is linearly related to the endogenous creatinine clearance as shown in the following formula:

$$Q = K(f)/K(n) = (a + b\ CCr(f))/(a + b\ CCr(n))$$

The pharmacokinetic variables used in the formula above were extracted from literature references. For some antimicrobials, it was necessary to estimate the values of variables a, b, and K(n) from half-life information. This was done using the relationship that exists between K and the creatinine clearance, based upon normal and anuric half-life values.

The following formula is used to determine Q for drugs for which the values of a or b could not be determined:

$$Q = K(f)/K(n) = 1 - fe[1 - (CCr(f)/CCr(n))]$$

Using the elimination rate fraction, the dosage regimen is adjusted in three ways:

(1) The dose (D) can be decreased while the dosing interval (τ) remains the same

$$D(f) = D(n) \times Q;$$

(2) The dosing interval can increase while the dose remains the same

$$\tau(f) = \tau(n)/Q;\ or$$

(3) The user can select a more convenient dosing interval

$$D(f) = D(n) \times Q \times (\tau(s)/\tau(n))$$

Finally, the loading dose is calculated depending on the dose regimen, in the following ways:

(1) If the dose is changed,

$$LD = D(f)/(1 - e^{-K(f)\tau(n)})$$

(2) If the dosing interval is changed,

$$LD = D(n)/(1 - e^{-K(f)\tau(f)})$$

(3) If both the dose and the interval are changed,

$$LD = D(f)/(1 - e^{-K(f)\tau(f)})$$

SOME FINAL CONSIDERATIONS

Whenever available data or experience permits, one should try to forecast the therapeutic dosage range that will most likely be obtained by regulating the drug dosage.[174] Although the concept of a "therapeutic range," i.e., the optimal plasma concentration range of a particular drug for a particular patient, is not synonymous with a "nontoxic" range, regulation of a dosage to achieve that optimal range seems to be the most reasonable approach for most, but not all, drugs.[175] Forecasting must link dosage, time, observable patient features, disease states, sex, age, weight, and functional capacity of organs of elimination. It may be difficult and at times even hazardous to generalize about the drug dose and plasma concentration. Ultimately an individualized dosage regimen must evolve.

Even though it seems simple to state that the cumulation characteristics, which possibly pose the greatest danger to the elderly, depend only on two factors, i.e., the elimination rate constant and the dosing interval, many other factors must be considered if an individualized dosage regimen is to be achieved. This decision making process should start with a serious consideration as to the drug selected. Has the right drug been selected? Apparently it is still not being recognized that the majority of patients with a history of heart disease and heart failure, not including those with rapid atrial fibrillation, do not need long term digitalis therapy.[176] Furthermore, is the drug to be used for an emergency or for a prolonged period? It is known that any factor that alters a drug's half-life will alter its steady state concentration. Multiple drug therapy, often the result

TABLE 2–21. Influence of Some Drugs on Digoxin Plasma Concentration Levels

Drug	Effect
Antacids	Decrease
Kaolin-pectin	Decrease
Penicillamine	Decrease
Quinidine	
If added	Increase
If withdrawn	Decrease
Spironolactone	Increase
Sulfasalazine	Decrease

of long term therapy, may cause changes in metabolism because drugs may compete for the same metabolic sites. If a drug is displaced from that site, its half-life may be prolonged. This in turn will lead to a higher steady state level of that drug. Interactions can interfere with many drugs. Table 2–21 uses digoxin as one example. Another example of changed drug action with time is provided by propranolol, whose systemic availability differs for short and long term dosing.[177] The influence of various pathologic conditions on the serum digoxin plasma concentration is revealed in Table 2–22.[175,178]

The prescriber using drug therapy for elderly patients should expect extended half-lives. The causative factors may range from impaired kidney function and decreased ability of the liver microsomal enzymes to metabolize a drug to changes in the volume of distribution. Often, particularly in long term drug therapy, it is not enough to know that the half-life changes; the reason must be elucidated.[179] For example, in order to minimize toxic reactions to digoxin, it is not enough to know that digoxin excretion is reduced commensurate with decreased renal function.[180] Other possible variables must be considered.

TABLE 2–22. Effects of Disease on Variations in Serum Digoxin Levels and Action

Disease	Effect
Advanced renal failure	Half-life increased from 1.5 to 3.5–5 days
Atrial fibrillation	Altered sensitivity at "normal" levels
Cor pulmonale	Expect toxicity at lower serum levels
Hyperthyroidism	Expect lower serum levels
Hypothyroidism	Expect elevated serum levels
Hypoxia	Expect increased sensitivity at "normal" levels

Serum Levels. The ability to monitor plasma levels of drugs holds promise for a safer, more rational approach toward drug therapy. However, caution must be exercised so that the process of blood level monitoring does not create unjustified expectations.[181] Standardization of analytical techniques still is needed, for the particular technique selected by a particular laboratory can cause wide variations in reported kinetic variables.[182]

When one considers the dose-effect relationship, it is not too difficult to conclude that measurement of plasma concentration yields a much better correlation with the desired clinical effect than does the total daily dose. The probability of attaining a given blood level from a given dose is much less than that of obtaining a specific effect from a given plasma concentration. Yet in some instances, as with digoxin, the relationship between the total daily dose, steady state, and toxic reactions is very poor, and unless one can reasonably expect a usable result, blood level monitoring should possibly not be used.[183,184] For example, a digoxin level determination costs approximately $28.00, whereas medical assistance reimbursement per day for a patient may be only $31.00. Furthermore, a determination of a blood level may not be quick enough in an emergency, and, again in the case of digoxin, an electrocardiogram may be much more applicable in a case of suspected toxicity.[185] Thus, the purpose and the result expected often should determine whether a blood level estimation is performed.

For most drugs there is a linear relationship between the dose of the drug and the plasma concentration achieved. However, it would be fallacious to assume that as the dosage is increased, a concomitant increase in the plasma level directly proportional to the increase in dose would occur. Often a linear dose-concentration relationship occurs only over a given range. A marked increase in the plasma level may indeed occur with a very small increase in the dose, as can happen with amitriptyline or phenytoin, reflecting saturation kinetics. In other instances it may not be the serum level that should be used for predictive or monitoring purposes.

For example, red cell levels are more closely related to lithium side effects than plasma levels and may be better predictors of lithium brain concentration as well.[186,187] Extrapyramidal symptoms due to chlorpromazine are possibly better related to the drug's concentration in the cerebrospinal fluid, and it is

TABLE 2-23. Signs of Digoxin Psychotoxicity in the Elderly

Anxiety	Impairment of memory
Confusion	Lack of motivation
Depression	Lethargy
Emotional instability	Loss of capacity for self-care
Hyperventilation	

not at all clear whether data obtained from plasma levels can be applied to patients given long term chlorpromazine therapy.[188,189] As another example, the antihypertensive dose-response curve of chlorothiazide, hydrochlorothiazide, furosemide, and possibly chlorthalidone may be better related to their urinary recovery than to plasma levels.[190]

Finally, the clinician cannot and must not depend only or entirely on the monitoring of serum drug levels. At best, these levels can only complement personal observation. For example, the elderly patient taking digoxin should be continuously observed for subtle noncardiac symptoms of toxicity, which often occur much earlier than the traditional signs of digoxin toxicity found in younger persons. Possible signs of digoxin psychotoxicity in the elderly are documented in Table 2-23.[191]

SUMMARY

On the basis of all the considerations discussed, the characteristics of the ideal drug for the elderly are listed in Table 2-24. Dosage adjustment for most drugs used in disease management of the elderly, particularly in long term management, is almost mandatory. The kidney status of the patient is probably the prime factor determining the need for dose adjustment. Pharmacokinetics can be of immense help in providing drug therapy to the elderly on a level of sophistication that will serve to increase the benefit of drug therapy and decrease the hazards. This demands an intimate and complete knowledge of a drug's kinetics and possible side effects as well as characteristics of the patient and the disease that may complicate therapy. In any case, pharmacokinetics can only complement but cannot and should not take the place of patient observation.

TABLE 2-24. Characteristics of the Ideal Drug for Elderly Patients

Characteristic	Therapeutic Advantage
Complete absorption	Less scatter in drug response
	Low oral dose
High bioavailability	Low daily dose
Low first pass effect	Little effect of hepatic extraction and hemodynamics
	Low daily dose; no saturation effect
Low protein binding	Small variations in plasma levels and drug effects due to multiple drug therapy, disease, malnutrition
Balanced clearance by kidney and liver	No accumulation in patients with renal or hepatic impairment

REFERENCES

1. Triggs, E.J., and Nation, R.L.: Pharmacokinetics in the aged: a review. J. Pharmacokinet. Biopharm., 3:387, 1975.
2. Triggs, E.J., Nation, R.L., Long, A., and Ashley, J.J.: Pharmacokinetics in the elderly. Eur. J. Clin. Pharmacol., 8:55, 1975.
3. Crooks, J., O'Malley, K., and Stevenson, I.H.: Pharmacokinetics in the elderly, Clin. Pharmacokinet., 1:280, 1976.
4. Judge, T.G., and Caird, F.I.: Drug Treatment of the Elderly Patient. Turnbridge Wells, England, Pitman Medical Publishing, 1978.
5. Vestal, R.E.: Drug use in the elderly: a review of problems and special considerations, Drugs, 16:358, 1978.
6. Lamy, P.P., and Vestal, R.E.: Drug prescribing for the elderly. In Reichel, W. (Editor): The Geriatric Patient. New York, H.P. Publishing Co., Inc., pp. 1-8.
7. Lamy, P.P.: Modifying drug dosage in elderly patients. Therapeutics, 28:1, 1978.
8. Lamy, P.P.: Considerations in drug therapy of the elderly. J. Drug Issues, 9:27, 1979.
9. Schumacher, G.E.: Using pharmacokinetics in drug therapy. VII. Pharmacokinetic factors influencing drug therapy in the aged, Am. J. Hosp. Pharm., 37:559, 1980.
10. Lamy, P.P.: Prescribing for the Elderly. Littleton, Massachusetts, Publishing Sciences Group, Inc., 1980.
11. Lamy, P.P.: Misuse and abuse of drugs by the elderly: another view, Am. Pharm., NS20:14, 1980.
12. Sice, J.: How much is enough? Clin. Pharmacol. Ther., 26:537, 1979.
13. Editorial: Digoxin, more problems than solutions, Lancet, 2:1288, 1978.
14. Rowe, J.W.: Clinical research on aging: straegies and directions. N. Engl. J. Med., 297:1332, 1977.
15. O'Malley, K., Judge, T.G., and Crooks, S.J.: Geriatric clinical pharmacology and therapeutics. In Avery, G.S. (Editor). Drug Treatment. Sidney, Australia, ADIS Press, 1976, pp. 123-142.
16. Reidenberg, M.M., Levy, M., Warner, H., Coutinho, C.B., Schwartz, M.A., Yu, C., and Chripko, J.: Relationship between diazepam dose, plasma level, age, and central nervous system depression. Clin. Pharmacol. Ther., 23:371, 1978.

17. Hurwitz, N.: Predisposing factors in adverse reactions to drugs. Br. Med. J., *1*:536, 1969.
18. Vestal, R.E., Wood, A.J.J., and Shand, D.G.: Reduced beta-adrenoreceptor sensitivity in the elderly. Clin. Pharmacol. Ther., *26*:181, 1979.
19. Greenblatt, D.J., Allen, M.D., Harmatz, J.S., and Shader, R.I.: Diazepam disposition determinants. Clin. Pharmacol. Ther., *27*:301, 1980.
20. Roberts, R.K., Desmond, P.V., Wilkinson, G.R., and Schenker, S.: Disposition of chlordiazepoxide: sex differences and effects of oral contraceptives. Clin. Pharmacol. Ther., *25*:826, 1979.
21. Proksch, R.A., and Lamy, P.P.: Sex variation and drug therapy. Drug Intell. Clin. Pharm., *11*:398, 1977.
22. Dans, P.E., and Kerr, M.R.: Gerontology and geriatrics in medical education. N. Engl. J. Med., *300*:228, 1979.
23. Zilli, A.: Multimorbiditaet und alter. *In* Platt, D. (Editor): Forum Medici: Der Arzt Spricht zum Arzt. Nyon, Switzerland, Zyma, 1979, pp. 36–48.
24. Winick, M.: Nutrition in the elderly: Practical recommendations. *In* Practical Guide to Geriatric Medication. Oradell, New Jersey, Medical Economics Co., 1980, pp. 139–153.
25. Zilli, A., Sdraffa, L., Germano, G., Bogliolo, C., and del Soldato, G.: Misplacement of the old in a psychiatric ward. J. Gerontol., *17*:735, 1969.
26. Franke, H.: Das wesen der polypathie bei hundertjaehrigen. *In* Schubert, R., and Stoermer, A.: Multimorbiditaet. Muenchen-Graefelfing, Werk-Verlag Dr. E. Banaschewskim, 1973, pp. 50–75.
27. Williamson, J., Stokoe, I.H., Gray, S., Smith, A., McGhee, A., and Stephenson, E.: Old people at home: their unreported needs. Lancet, *1*:1117, 1964.
28. Jernigan, J.A., Gudat, J.C., Blake, J.L., Bowen, L., and Lezotte, D.C.: Reference values for blood findings in relatively fit elderly persons. J. Am. Geriatr. Soc., *28*:308, 1980.
29. Ravel, R.: Clinical Laboratory Medicine. Chicago, Year Book Medical Publishers, Inc., 1978, pp. 232, 253, 300, 318, 304, 341.
30. Dorsey, R., Ayd, F.J., Cole, J., Klein, D., Simpson, G., Tupin, J., and DiMascio, A.: Psychopharmacological screening criteria development project. J.A.M.A., *241*:1021, 1979.
31. Lamy, P.P.: Operation common sense. Contemp. Pharm. Pract. (In press.)
32. Schumacher, G.E.: Paper presented, Baltimore, 1979.
33. Eagles, H., Fleischman, R., and Levy, M.: "Continuous" vs. "discontinuous" therapy with penicillin. N. Engl. J. Med., *248*:481, 1953.
34. Jaffe, H.W., Schroeter, A.L., Reynolds, G.H., Zaidi, A.A., Martin, J.E., and Thayer, J.D.: Pharmacokinetic determinants of penicillin cure of gonococcal urethritis. Antimicrob. Agents Chemother., *15*:587, 1979.
35. Klastersky, J., Daneau, D., Swings, G., and Weerts, D.: Antibacterial activity in serum and urine as a therapeutic guide in bacterial infections. J. Infect. Dis., *129*:187, 1974.
36. Grasso, S., Meinardi, G., De Carneri, I., and Tammasia, V.: New in vitro model to study the effect of antibiotic concentration and rate of elimination on antibacterial activity. Antimicrob. Agents Chemother., *13*:570, 1978.
37. Zagar, A.: Kinetics of antibacterial inhibition power of ampicillin, cloxacillin, carbenicillin and gentamicin at changing concentration similar to that in the body fluids. Adv. Antimicrob. Antineoplastic Chemother., I/2, 715, 1972.
38. Wagner, J.G.: Fundamentals of Clinical Pharmacokinetics. Hamilton, Illinois, Drug Intelligence Publishers, Inc., 1975.
39. Azarnoff, D.L.: Use of pharmacokinetic principles in therapy. N. Engl. J. Med., *289*:635, 1973.
40. Dettli, L.: Individualization of drug dosage in patients with renal disease. Med. Clin. N. Am., *58*:977, 1974.
41. Greenblatt, D.J., and Koch-Weser, J.: Drug therapy—clinical pharmacokinetics. N. Engl. J. Med., *293*:702, 1973.
42. Koch-Weser, J.: Drug therapy—serum drug concentrations as therapeutic guide. N. Engl. J. Med., *287*:227, 1972.
43. McAvoy, T.J.: The biological half-life of heparin. Clin. Pharmacol. Ther., *25*:372, 1979.
44. Furst, D.E., Tozer, T.N., and Melmon, K.L.: Salicylate clearance, the resultant of protein binding and metabolism. Clin. Pharmacol. Ther., *26*:380, 1979.
45. Ouslander, J.: Theophylline dosage in the elderly. N. Engl. J. Med., *301*:435, 1979.
46. Lamy, P.P.: Aging: how human physiology responds. *In* Busse, E.W. (Editor): Theory and Therapeutics of Aging. New York, MEDCOM, Inc., 1973, pp. 12–29.
47. Berman, P.M., and Kirsner, J.B.: The aging gut. II. Diseases of the colon, pancreas, liver, and gallbladder, functional bowel disease and iatrogenic disease. Geriatrics, *27*:117, 1972.
48. Richey, D.P., and Bender, A.D.: Effects of human aging on drug absorption and metabolism. *In* Goldman, R., and Rockstein, M. (Editors): The Physiology and Pathology of Human Aging. New York, Academic Press, Inc., 1975, pp. 59–93.
49. Stare, P.J.: Three score and ten plus more. J. Am. Geriatr. Soc., *25*:529, 1977.
50. Bayless, T.M.: Malabsorption in the elderly. Hosp. Pract. *14*:57, 1979.
51. Shklar, G.: The effects of aging upon the oral mucosa. J. Invest. Dermatol., *47*:115, 1966.
52. Berman, P.M., and Kirsner, J.B.: Recognizing and avoiding adverse gastrointestinal effects of drugs. Geriatrics, *29*:59, 1974.
53. Bokey, L., and Hugh, T.B.: Oesophageal ulceration associated with doxycyclin therapy. Med. J. Aust., *1*:236, 1975.
54. Crowson, T.D., Head, L.H., and Ferrante, W.A.: Esophageal ulcers associated with tetracycline therapy. J.A.M.A., *235*:2747, 1976.
55. Evans, K.I., and Roberts, G.M.: Where do all the tablets go? Lancet, *2*:1237, 1976.
56. Pemberton, J.: Oesophageal obstruction and ulceration caused by oral potassium therapy. Br. Heart J., *32*:267, 1970.
57. Stevenson, I.H., Salem, S.A.M., and Shepherd, A.M.M.: Studies on drug absorption and metabolism in the elderly. *In* Crooks, J., and Stevenson, I.H. (Editors): Drugs and the Elderly. Baltimore, University Park Press, 1979, pp. 51–63.
58. Kramer, P.A., Chapron, D.J., Benson, J., and Mercik, A.S.: Tetracycline absorption in elderly patients with achlorhydria. Clin. Pharmacol. Ther., *23*:467, 1978.
59. Bianchine, J.R., Calimlim, L.R., Morgan, J.P., Dujovne, C.A., and Lasagna, L.: Metabolism and absorption of L-3,4-dihydroxyphenylalanine in patients with Parkinson's disease. Ann. N.Y. Acad. Sci., *179*:126, 1971.

60. Rivera-Calimlim, L., Kerzner, B., and Karch, F.E.: Effect of lithium on plasma chlorpromazine levels. Clin. Pharmacol. Ther., 23:451, 1978.
61. Johnson, G., Sjogren, J., and Solvell, L.: Beta-blocking effect of alprenolol in man after administration of ordinary and sustained release tablets. Eur. J. Clin. Pharmacol., 3:74, 1971.
62. Matilla, M.J., and Venho, V.M.K.: Drug absorption from abnormal gastrointestinal tract. Progr. Pharmacol., 2:58, 1979.
63. Romankiewicz, J.A., and Reidenberg, M.M.: Factors that modify drug absorption. Ration. Drug Ther., 12(10):1, 1978.
64. Vesell, E.S.: The influence of host factors on drug response. II. Age. Ration. Drug Ther., 14(4):1, 1980.
65. Boxenbaum, H.G., Bekersky, I., Jack, M.L., and Kaplan, S.A.: Influence of gut microflora on bioavailability. Drug Metab. Rev., 9:259, 1979.
66. Steinheber, F.U.: Interpretation of gastrointestinal symptoms in the elderly. Med. Clin. N. Am., 6:1141, 1976.
67. Grindstaff, G.F., Hirsch, B., and Silverman, H.A.: Use of prescription drugs by aged persons enrolled for supplementary medical insurance, 1967–1977. Baltimore, Health Care Financing Administration. (In preparation.)
68. Hurwitz, A.: Antacid therapy and drug kinetics. Clin. Pharmacokinet., 2:269, 1977.
69. Romankiewicz, J.A.: Effects of antacids on gastrointestinal absorption of drugs. Primary Care, 3:537, 1976.
70. Parsons, R.L.: Drug absorption in gastrointestinal disease with particular reference to malabsorption syndromes. Clin. Pharmacokinet., 2:50, 1977.
71. Wagner, J.G.: An overview of determinants of drug activity. *In* McMahon, F.G. (Editor): Pharmacokinetics, Drug Metabolism, and Drug Interactions. Principles and Techniques of Human Research and Therapeutics. New York, Futura Publishing Co., Inc., 1974, Vol. 3.
72. Shock, N.W.: Systems physiology and aging: introduction. Fed. Proc. 38:161, 1979.
73. Edelman, L.S., and Leibman, J.: Anatomy of body water and electrolytes. Am. J. Med., 27:256, 1959.
74. Novak, L.P.: Ageing, total body potassium, fat free mass and cell mass in males and females between the ages of 18 and 85 years. J. Gerontol., 27:438, 1972.
75. International Comm. Radiol. Protection: Report of the Task Group on Reference Man. New York, Pergamon Press Inc., 1974, Ch. 1.
76. Levy, G., and Giacomini, K.M.: Rational aspirin dosage regimens. Clin. Pharmacol. Ther., 23:247, 1978.
77. Gal, P., Jusko, W.J., Yurchak, A.M., and Franklin, B.A.: Theophylline disposition in obesity. Clin. Pharmacol. Ther., 23:438, 1978.
78. Ewy, G.A., Groves, B.M., Ball, M.F., Nimmo, L., Jackson, B., and Marcos, F.: Digoxin metabolism in obesity. Circulation, 44:810, 1971.
79. Hull, J.H., and Sarubbi, F.A.: Gentamicin serum concentrations: pharmacokinetic predictions. Ann. Intern. Med., 85:183, 1976.
80. Masoro, F.J.: Physiologic changes with aging. *In* Winnickm, M. (Editor): Nutrition and Aging. New York, John Wiley & Sons, Inc., 1976, Ch. 4.
81. Jusko, W.J., and Gretch, M.: Plasma and tissue protein binding of drugs in pharmacokinetics. Drug Metab. Rev., 5:43, 1976.
82. Yacobi, A.: Clinical implications of protein binding of drugs, Ration. Drug Ther., 12(11):1, 1978.
83. Routledge, P.A., Barchowsky, A., Bjornson, T.D., Kitchell, B.B., and Shand, D.G.: Lidocaine plasma protein binding. Clin. Pharmacol. Ther., 27:347, 1980.
84. Greenblatt, D.J.: Reduced serum albumin concentration in the elderly: a report from the Boston Collaborative Drug Surveillance Program. J. Am. Geriatr. Soc., 27:20, 1979.
85. Hayes, M.J., Langman, M.J.S., and Short, A.H.: Changes in drug metabolism with increasing age: phenytoin clearance and protein binding. Br. J. Clin. Pharmacol., 2:73, 1975.
86. Wallace, S., Whiting, B., and Runcie, J.: Factors affecting drug binding in plasma of elderly patients. Br. J. Clin. Pharmacol., 3:327, 1976.
87. Hayes, M.J., Langman, M.J.S., and Short, A.H.: Changes in drug metabolism with increasing age. 1. Warfarin binding and plasma proteins. Br. J. Clin. Pharmacol., 2:73, 1975.
88. Boston Collaborative Drug Surveillance Program: Diphenylhydantoin side effects and serum albumin levels. Clin. Pharmacol. Ther., 14:529, 1973.
89. Casey, A.E., Gilbert, F.E., Copeland, H., Downey, E.L., and Casey, J.G.: Albumin, alpha-1,2, beta and gamma globulin in cancer and other diseases. South. Med. J., 66:179, 1973.
90. Erill, S., Calvo, R., and Carlos, R.: Plasma protein carbamylation and decreased acidic drug protein binding in uremia. Clin. Pharmacol. Ther., 27:612, 1980.
91. Ecanow, B., Gold, B.H., and Tunkunas, P.: Serum albumin and urea during states of anxiety and depression. J.A.M.A., 226:356, 1973.
92. Danon, A., and Chen, Z.: Binding of imipramine to plasma proteins: effect of hyperlipoproteinemia. Clin. Pharmacol. Ther., 25:316, 1979.
93. Bickel, M.H.: Binding of chlorpromazine and imipramine to red cells, albumin, lipoproteins and other blood components. J. Pharm. Pharmacol., 27:733, 1975.
94. Verbeek, R.K., and De Schepper, P.J.: Influence of chronic renal failure and hemodialysis on diflunisal plasma protein binding. Clin. Pharmacol. Ther., 27:628, 1980.
95. Piafsky, K.M., and Borga, O.: Plasma protein binding of basic drugs. II. Importance of alpha$_1$-acid glycoprotein for interindividual variation. Clin. Pharmacol. Ther., 22:545, 1977.
96. Piafsky, K.M., Borga, O., Odar-Cederloef, I., Johansson, C., and Sjoeqvist, F.: Increased plasma protein binding of propranolol and chlorpromazine mediated by disease-induced elevation of plasma alpha$_1$-acid glycoprotein. N. Engl. J. Med., 299:1435, 1978.
97. Vermeij, P., and Van Zwieten, P.A.: Monitoring of free plasma propranolol. Pharmaceut. Weekbld. (Sc. Ed.), 1:105, 1979.
98. Myers, D.R., DeFehr, J., Bennett, W.M., Porter, G.A., and Olsen, G.D.: Gentamicin binding to serum and plasma proteins. Clin. Pharmacol. Ther., 23:356, 1978.
99. Wiegand, U.W., Hintze, K.L., Slattery, J.T., and Levy, G.: Protein binding of several drugs in serum and plasma of healthy subjects. Clin. Pharmacol. Ther., 27:297, 1980.
100. Wallace, S., Whiting, B., and Runcie, J.: Factors

affecting drug binding in plasma of elderly patients. Br. J. Clin. Pharmacol., *3*:327, 1976.
101. Chan, K., Kendell, M.J., Mitchard, M., Wells, W.D.E., and Vickers, M.D.: The effect of aging on plasma pethidine concentration. Br. J. Clin. Pharmacol., *2*:297, 1975.
102. Beerman, B., Hellstroem, K., Lindstroem, B., and Rosen, A.: Binding site interaction of chlorthalidone and acetazolamide, two drugs transported by red blood cells. Clin. Pharmacol. Ther., *17*:424, 1975.
103. Sata, T., Miwa, T., and Tauchi, H.: Age changes in the human liver of different races. Gerontologia, *16*:368, 1970.
104. Zilly, W., Breimer, D.D., and Richter, E.: Hexobarbital disposition in compensated and decompensated cirrhosis of the liver. Clin. Pharmacol. Ther., *23*:525, 1978.
105. Drayer, D.E., and Reidenberg, M.M.: Clinical consequences of polymorphic acetylation of basic drugs. Clin. Pharmacol. Ther., *22*:251, 1977.
106. Kalow, W., Tang, B.K., Kadar, D., Endrenyi, L., and Chan, F.-Y.: A method for studying drug metabolism in populations: racial differences in amobarbital metabolism. Clin. Pharmacol. Ther., *26*:766, 1979.
107. Price Evans, D.A.: An improved and simplified method of detecting the acetylator phenotype. J. Med. Genet., *6*:405, 1969.
108. Varley, H.: Practical Clinical Biochemistry. London, William Heinemann Medical Books, Ltd., 1967, p. 744.
109. Sherlock, S., Bearn, A.G., Billing, B.H., and Paterson, J.C.S.: Splanchnic blood flow in man by the bromsulfalein method: the relation of peripheral plasma bromsulfalein level to the calculated flow. J. Lab. Clin. Med., *35*:923, 1950.
110. Wood, A.J.J., Vestal, R.E., Wilkinson, G.R., Branch, R.A., and Shand, D.G.: Effect of aging and cigarette smoking on antipyrine and indocyanine green elimination. Clin. Pharmacol. Ther., *26*:16, 1979.
111. Salem, S.A.M., Rajjayabun, P., Shepherd, A.M.M., and Stevenson, I.H.: Reduced induction of drug metabolism in the elderly. Age Ageing, *7*:68, 1978.
112. Gorrod, J.W.: Absorption, metabolism and excretion of drugs in geriatric subjects. Gerontol. Clin., *16*:30, 1974.
113. Anderson, K.E., Conney, A.H., and Kappas, A.: Nutrition and oxidative drug metabolism in man: relative influence of dietary lipids, carbohydrate and protein. Clin. Pharmacol. Ther., *26*:493, 1979.
114. Farrell, G.C., Cooksley, W.G.E., and Powell, L.W.: Drug metabolism in liver disease: activity of hepatic microsomal metabolizing enzymes. Clin. Pharmacol. Ther., *26*:483, 1979.
115. Finch, C.E.: Neuroendocrine mechanisms and aging. Fed. Proc., *38*:178, 1979.
116. Drugs in the elderly. Med. Lett. Drugs Ther., *21* (10):43, 1979.
117. Wollheim, F.A., and Lindstrom, C.G.: Liver abnormalities in penicillamine treated rheumatoid arthritis. Scand. J. Rheum., Suppl. 28, 100, 1979.
118. Kraus, J.W., Desmond, P.V., Marshall, J.P., Johnson, R.F., Schenker, S., and Wilkinson, G.R.: Effects of aging and liver disease on disposition of lorazepam. Clin. Pharmacol. Ther., *24*:411, 1978.
119. Fessell, J.M., and Conn, H.O.: An analysis of the causes and prevention of hepatic coma. Gastroenterology, *62*:191, 1972.
120. Wilkinson, G.R., and Shand, D.G.: A physiological approach to hepatic drug clearance. Clin. Pharmacol. Ther., *18*:377, 1975.
121. O'Malley, K., Crooks, J., Duke, E., and Stevenson, I.H.: Effect of age and sex on human drug metabolism. Br. Med. J., *3*:607, 1971.
122. Nies, A., Robinson, D.S., Friedman, M.J., Green, R., Cooper, T.B., Ravaris, C.L., and Ives, J.O.: Relationship between age and tricyclic antidepressant levels. Am. J. Psychiatry, *134*:790, 1977.
123. Epstein, M.: Effects of aging on the kidney. Fed. Proc., *38*:168, 1979.
124. McLachlan, M.S.F.: The ageing kidney. Lancet, *2*:143, 1978.
125. Bricker, N.S.: On the pathogenesis of the uremic state. N. Engl. J. Med., *286*:1093, 1972.
126. Rowe, J.W., et al.: Age-adjusted standards for creatinine clearance. Ann. Intern. Med., *84*:567, 1976.
127. Bowman, R.H.: Renal secretion of ^{35}S furosemide and its depression by albumin binding. Am. J. Physiol., *229*:93, 1975.
128. Naccarto, D., Bell, C., and Lamy, P.P.: Appraisal of ascorbic acid for acidifying the urine of methenamine-treated geriatric patients. J. Am. Geriatr. Soc., *27*:34, 1979.
129. Montoliu, J., Darnell, A., Torras, A., and Revert, L.: Primary acute glomerular disorders in the elderly. Arch. Intern. Med., *140*:755, 1980.
130. Roxe, D.M.: Toxic nephropathy due to drugs. Ration. Drug Ther., *9*(12):1, 1975.
131. Zaske, D.E., Cipolle, R.J., and Strate, R.J.: Gentamicin dosage requirements: wide interpatient variations in 242 surgery patients with normal renal function. Surgery, *87*:164, 1980.
132. Vestal, R.E.: Drugs and the elderly, *In* Drugs and the Elderly. Publ. No. 720–295/4058–31. Washington, D.C., U.S. Government Printing Office, 1978.
133. Borga, O., Hoppel, C., Odar-Cederlof, I., and Garle, M.: Plasma levels and renal excretion of phenytoin and its metabolites in patients with renal failure. Clin. Pharmacol. Ther., *26*:306, 1979.
134. Lowenthal, D.T.: Tissue sensitivity to drugs in disease states. Med. Clin. N. Am., *58*:1111, 1974.
135. Benet, L.Z.: Pharmacokinetics/pharmacodynamics of frusemide in man: a review. J. Pharmacokinet. Biopharm., *7*:1, 1979.
136. Odlind, B.G., and Beerman, B.: Diuretic resistance: reduced bioavailability and effect of oral frusemide. Br. Med. J., *280*:1577, 1980.
137. Rane, A., Villeneuve, J.P., Stone, W.J., Nies, A.S., Wilkinson, G.R., and Branch, R.A.: Plasma binding and disposition of furosemide in the nephrotic syndrome and in uremia. Clin. Pharmacol. Ther., *24*:199, 1978.
138. Anton, A.H., and Solomon, H.M.: Drug protein binding. Ann. N.Y. Acad. Sci., *226*:1–362, 1973.
139. Reidenberg, M.M.: The binding of drugs to plasma proteins from patients with poor renal function. Clin. Pharmacokinet., *1*:121, 1976.
140. Reidenberg, M.M.: Effect of disease states on plasma protein binding of drugs. Med. Clin. N. Am., *58*:1103, 1974.
141. Koch-Weser, J., and Sellers, E.M.: Drug therapy—binding of drugs to serum albumin. N. Engl. J. Med., *294*:311, 1976.
142. Reidenberg, M.M.: Kidney disease and drug metabolism. Med. Clin. N. Am., *58*:1059, 1974.
143. Johnson, B.F., and Bye, C.: Maximal intestinal

absorption of digoxin and its relation to steady state plasma concentration. Br. Heart J., *37*:203, 1975.
144. Ostroff, R.B., and Docherty, J.P.: Tricyclics, bioequivalence, and clinical response. Am. J. Psychiatry, *135*:1560, 1978.
145. Crout, J.R.: Tricyclic antidepressants: proposed bioequivalence requirement. Fed Reg., *43*:3965, 1978.
146. Meyer, M.C., Gollamudi, R., and Straughn, A.B.: The influence of dosage form on papaverine bioavailability. J. Clin. Pharmacol., *19*:435, 1979.
147. Vesell, E.S.: The influence of host factors on drug response. II. Age. Ration. Drug Ther., *14*(4):1, 1980.
148. Nielsen-Kudsk, F., Magnussen, I., and Jacobsen, P.: Pharmacokinetics of theophylline in ten elderly patients. Acta Pharmacol. Toxicol., *42*:226, 1978.
149. Gugler, R., and Somogyi, A.: Reduced cimetidine clearance with age. N. Engl. J. Med., *301*:435, 1979.
150. Levy, G., and Tshuchiya, T.: Salicylate accumulation kinetics in man. N. Engl. J. Med., *287*:430, 1972.
151. Hamdy, R.C., Tovey, J., and Petera, N.: Hypokalemia and diuretics. Br. Med. J., *280*:1187, 1980.
152. Editorial. Lancet, *1*:1285, 1980.
153. Gollub, J.: Psychoactive drug misuse among the elderly: a review of prevention and treatment programs. *In* The Aging Process and Psychoactive Drug Use. DHEW Publ. No. (ADM) 79–813. Rockville, Maryland. U.S. Drug Abuse and Mental Health Administration, 1979.
154. Miller, D.B., Lowenstein, R., and Winston, R.: Physician's attitudes toward the ill aged and nursing homes: J. Am. Geriatr. Soc., *24*:498, 1976.
155. Gottlieb, R.M., Nappi, T., and Strain, J.J.: The physician's knowledge of psychotropic drugs: preliminary results. Am. J. Psychiatry, *135*:29, 1978.
156. O'Malley, K., Cusack, B., Kelly, J., and Stevenson, I.H.: Drugs in the elderly: pharmacokinetics and effects of some metabolized drugs. *In* Kitani, K. (Editor): Liver and Aging. New York, Elsevier North-Holland, Inc., 1978.
157. Frisk-Holmberg, M., Bergkvist, Y., Domeij-Nyberg, B., Hellstroem, L., and Jansson, F.: Chloroquine serum concentration and side effects: evidence of dose-dependent kinetics. Clin. Pharmacol. Ther., *25*:345, 1979.
158. Jaillon, P., Rubin, P., Yee, Y.-G., Ball, R., Kates, R., Harrison, D., and Blaschke, T.: Influence of congestive heart failure on prazosin kinetics. Clin. Pharmacol. Ther., *25*:790, 1979.
159. Lutwick, L.I.: Principles of antibiotic use in the elderly. Geriatrics, *35*(2):54, 1980.
160. Appel, G.B., and Neu, H.C.: The nephrotoxicity of antimicrobial agents. N. Engl. J. Med., *296*:663, 1977.
161. Schentag, J.J., Jusko, W.J., Plaut, M.E., Cumbo, T.J., Vance, J.W., and Abrutyn, E.: Tissue persistence of gentamicin in man. J.A.M.A., *238*:327, 1977.
162. Ochs, H.R., Carstens, G., and Greenblatt, D.J.: Reduction in lidocaine clearance during continuous infusion and by coadministration of propranolol. N. Engl. J. Med., *303*:373, 1980.
163. Waldorff, S., Andersen, J.D., Heebøll-Nielsen, O.G., Moltke, E., Sørensen, U., and Steiness, E.: Spironolactone-induced changes in digoxin kinetics. Clin. Pharmacol. Ther., *24*:162, 1978.
164. Bennett, W.M., Singer, I., Golper, T., Feig, P., and Coggins, C.J.: Guidelines for drug therapy in renal failure. Ann. Intern. Med., *86*:754, 1977.
165. Jeliffe, R.W.: Estimation of creatinine clearance when urine cannot be collected. Lancet, *1*:975, 1971.
166. Kampmann, J., and Siersback-Nielsen, J.M.: Rapid evaluation of creatinine clearance. Acta Med. Scand., *196*:517, 1974.
167. Dettli, L.: Elimination kinetics and dosage adjustment of drugs in patients with kidney disease. *In* Grobecker, H., et al. (Editors): Progress in Pharmacology. New York, Gustav Fischer Verlag, 1977.
168. Welling, P.G., and Craig, W.E.: Pharmacokinetics in disease states modifying renal function. *In* Benet, L.Z. (Editor): The Effects of Disease States on Drug Pharmacokinetics. Washington, D.C., American Pharmaceutical Association, 1976.
169. Wagner, J.G.: Fundamentals of Clinical Pharmacokinetics. Hamilton, Illinois, Drug Intelligence Publishers, Inc., 1975, p. 161.
170. Giusti, D.L., and Hayton, W.L.: Dosage regimen adjustments in renal impairment. Drug Intell. Clin. Pharm., *7*:382, 1973.
171. Kampmann, J.P., and Mølholm Hansen, J.E.: Renal excretion of drugs. *In* Crooks, J., and Stevenson, I.H. (Editors): Drugs and the Elderly. Baltimore, University Park Press, 1979, p. 77.
172. Dvorchik, B.H., and Vesell, E.S.: Significance of error associated with use of one-compartment formula to calculate renal clearance of thirty-eight drugs. Clin. Pharmacol. Ther., *23*:617, 1978.
173. Kunin, C.M., and Finland, M.: Persistence of antibiotics in blood of patients with acute renal failure. III. Penicillin, streptomycin, erythromycin, kanamycin. J. Clin. Invest., *38*:1509, 1959.
174. Sheiner, L.B., Beal, S., Rosenberg, B., and Marathe, V.V.: Forecasting individual pharmacokinetics. Clin. Pharmacol. Ther., *26*:294, 1979.
175. Carlstedt, B.C.: Blood levels: digoxin and digitoxin, U.S. Pharm., *4*(10):26, 1979.
176. Spector, R.: Digitalis therapy in heart failure: a rational approach. J. Clin. Pharmacol., *19*:992, 1979.
177. Vestal, R.E., Wood, A.J.J., Branch, R.A., Shand, D.G., and Wilkinson, G.R.: Effects of age and cigarette smoking on propranolol disposition. Clin. Pharmacol. Ther., *26*:8, 1979.
178. Weintraub, M.: Interpretation of the serum digoxin concentration. Clin. Pharmacokinet., *2*:205, 1977.
179. Gilette, J.R.: Biotransformation of drugs during aging. Fed. Proc., *38*:1900, 1979.
180. Cusack, B., Kelly, J., O'Malley, K., Noel, J., Lsvan, J., and Horgan, J.: Digoxin in the elderly: pharmacokinetic consequences of old age. Clin. Pharmacol. Ther., *25*:772, 1979.
181. Latini, R., Bonati, M., and Tognoni, G.: Clinical role of blood levels. Ther. Drug Monit., *2*:3, 1980.
182. Tilstone, W.J., and Fine, A.: Furosemide kinetics in renal failure. Clin. Pharmacol. Ther., *23*:644, 1978.
183. Duhme, D.W., Greenblatt, D.J., and Koch-Weser, J.: Reduction of digoxin toxicity associated with measurement of serum levels: a report from the Boston Collaborative Drug Surveillance Program. Ann. Intern. Med., *80*:516, 1974.
184. Ochs, H.R., Greenblatt, D.J., Harmatz, J.S., and Bodem, G.: Serum digoxin concentrations and subjective manifestations of toxicity. Pharmacology (Basel), *20*:149, 1980.
185. Erbel, R., Kraemer, R., Kleesiek, K., Schweizer, P., Pop, T., and Effert, S.: Suizidale digitalisintoxikation: beziehung zwischen der digitalis serumkonzentration und den elektrokardiographischen befunden. Z. Kardiol., *68*:590, 1979.

186. Elizur, A., Graff, E., Steiner, M., and Davidson, S.: Intra/extra red blood cell lithium and electrolyte distributions as correlates of neurotoxic reactions during lithium therapy. *In* Gershon, E.S., et al. (Editors): The Impact of Biology on Modern Psychiatry. New York, Plenum Publishing Corp., 1977, pp. 55–64.
187. Frazer, A., Mendels, J., Secunda, S.K., Cochrane, C.M., and Bianchi, C.P.: The prediction of brain lithium concentrations from plasma or erythrocyte measures. J. Psychiatr. Res., *10:*1, 1973.
188. Wode-Helgodt, B., Borg, S., Fyro, B., and Sedvall, G.: Clinical effects and drug concentrations in plasma and cerebrospinal fluid in psychotic patients treated with fixed doses of chlorpromazine. Acta Psychiatr. Scand., *58:*149, 1978.
189. Sakalis, G., Curry, S.H., Mould, G.P., and Lader, M.H.: Physiologic and clinical effects of chlorpromazine and their relationship to plasma level. Clin. Pharmacol. Ther., *13:*931, 1972.
190. Fleuren, H.L.J., Verwey-van Wissen, C., and Van Rossum, J.M.: Dose-dependent urinary excretion of chlorthalidone. Clin. Pharmacol. Ther., *25:*806, 1979.
191. Portnoi, V.A.: Digitalis delirium in elderly patients. J. Clin. Pharmacol., *19:*747, 1979.

PART TWO

PHARMACOLOGICAL MANAGEMENT OF COMMON DISORDERS IN THE ELDERLY

CHAPTER 3

PSYCHIATRIC DISORDERS

J. Ingram Walker and Timothy R. Covington

An estimated one-third of United States citizens over 60 years of age receive at least one psychotropic medication over the course of one year.[1] A survey at Duke University Medical Center indicated that approximately 28 per cent of elderly citizens living in Durham County were receiving psychoactive medications.[2] For elderly patients residing in long term care facilities this figure is frequently in excess of 50 per cent. In a study by Prien et al. involving patients over 60 years of age at 12 Veterans Administration hospitals, it was revealed that 70 per cent of the patients with a diagnosed mental disorder received a psychoactive drug, while 23 per cent with no diagnosed mental disorder received one or more psychoactive drugs.[3] The most commonly prescribed psychoactive medications in this study were thioridazine (21 per cent of the orders), chlorpromazine (16 per cent of the orders), diazepam (7 per cent of the orders), dihydroergotoxine (7 per cent of the orders), amitriptyline (5 per cent of the orders), and trifluoperazine (5 per cent of the orders). United States Department of Health, Education, and Welfare statistics from 1974 indicate that in a random analysis of 288 long term care facilities, 46.9 per cent of the patients over the age of 65 received tranquilizers, with 26 per cent of the population receiving thioridazine.[4]

There is a profound paucity of psychopharmacologic studies involving the elderly.[5] All too often the choice of drug appears to be based on conjecture and habit rather than on informed decision making and sound therapeutic judgment. This chapter addresses the appropriate use of specific psychotropic drugs in the elderly and provides some guidelines for monitoring both drug induced toxicity and therapeutic effectiveness.

THE EFFECT OF AGING ON THE ACTIVITY OF PSYCHOTROPIC MEDICATION

Physiologic changes associated with aging alter the activity of psychotropic medication considerably (see Chapter 2).[5] A reduction in digestive enzymes, a decrease in gastric acidity, a smaller intestinal absorbing surface, impaired epithelial transport systems, and reduced mesenteric blood flow result in decreased absorption of drugs in the elderly.[6] Decreased cardiac output contributes to slower transportation of drugs. Bender found that cardiac output declines approximately 1 per cent a year from age 19 to 86, with a proportionately larger blood flow to the brain and coronary vasculature than to the liver and kidneys.[7] This redistribution of blood flow causes an increase in drug activity in the brain and heart with a decrease in drug elimination. A decreased cardiac output, vasoconstriction of the renal vasculature, and a decrease in the renal tubular mass cause a 55 per cent reduction in renal clearance from age 40 to 89.[6] Protein decreases while body fat increases with age. Thus, highly lipid soluble drugs remain in the circulation longer. The duration of action of highly lipid soluble drugs is prolonged in the elderly because of increased total body fat; decreased enzyme activity and increased liver disease in the elderly result in slower drug metabolism. The decreased concentration of the active drug may be due in part to a decrease in protein binding capacity.[8]

A decrease in the number of receptors and the concentrations of neurotransmitters as well as structural changes in the responsive tissues may alter drug activity in the elderly despite normal psychoactive blood levels.[5] Dopamine, norepinephrine, and serotonin concentrations and the activity of cholinesterase and tyrosine hydroxylase in the brain all decrease with age.[9] The activity of monoamine oxidase, which metabolizes norepinephrine, serotonin, and dopamine, increases with age, particularly in the fifth, sixth, and seventh decades.[10]

In view of the altered physiology in the elderly, the dosage determination of psychotropic drugs requires special attention and careful titration. Strict monitoring for drug toxicity is essential owing to the unpredictability of drug responses in the elderly and the narrow therapeutic range of some psychotropic drugs. If the initial dose is too large, the therapeutic range can be passed rapidly, drug toxicity will be induced, and no objective judgment of the effectiveness of therapy can be made. In treating the elderly it is strongly recommended that the physician initiate therapy with low doses and increase dosage levels at appropriate intervals.[11]

TREATMENT OF SCHIZOPHRENIA AND FUNCTIONAL PARANOID DISORDERS

Blazer, in summarizing three epidemiologic studies, reported that the incidence of schizophrenia and paranoid psychosis in the elderly was 1 to 3.5 per cent.[12] Schizophrenia in the elderly nearly always is associated with delusions and auditory hallucinations.[13] The delusions, varying from persecutory to grandiose, frequently involve neighbors, landlords, relatives, or nursing home staff. Elderly schizophrenic patients frequently report thought intrusions, experiences of influence, and voices discussing the patient in the third person.[14] In addition, elderly schizophrenics demonstrate marked personal and social deterioration.[13]

Kay and Roth found that 10 per cent of all psychiatric admissions in patients over 60 years of age could be classified as paraphrenic (or to use the criteria of the third edition of the *Diagnostic and Statistical Manual of Mental Disorders*—paranoiac).[15,16] These patients had paranoid delusions and hallucinations without the personal, affective, and social deterioration found in schizophrenics; the persecutory symptomatology was not related to organic or depressive illness.

Antipsychotic Drugs

The antipsychotic medications can be used to help control the primary symptoms of schizophrenia and the agitation and hallucinations associated with paranoid disorders. There are five major classes of antipsychotic medications, all of which are believed to act to block the dopamine receptor sites in the central nervous system (Table 3–1).

The selection of an antipsychotic drug depends not only on the drug's pharmacologic properties and the patient's previous response to medication, but also on the drug's potential for producing side effects (Table 3–2).

The high potency drugs, powerful blockers of dopamine receptors, require a lower dose to produce the same effects as the low potency antipsychotic drugs, which are weaker blockers of dopamine receptors. The low potency antipsychotic drugs most frequently used in the elderly, chlorpromazine and thioridazine, have strong sedative effects (due to alpha-adrenergic blocking properties), marked anticholinergic effects, and a low incidence of extrapyramidal reactions. The high potency compounds most frequently used in the elderly—acetophenazine, fluphenazine, perphenazine, trifluoperazine, and haloperidol—have fewer sedative and anticholinergic effects, but a greater tendency to produce extrapyramidal side effects.[5]

Antipsychotic drugs are absorbed into the blood five to 10 minutes after intramuscular injection and 30 to 60 minutes after oral administration. They readily cross the blood-brain barrier, are highly lipid soluble, and are slowly metabolized because of tissue binding. The hepatic microsomal enzymes (decreased in the elderly) break down the antipsychotic drugs into inactive water soluble products that are excreted primarily in the urine and bile.[17]

In initiating antipsychotic medication in the elderly, a small test dose should be administered. If no major side effects develop, the dose may be increased in steps until therapeutic benefit or toxicity develops. Occa-

TABLE 3–1. Equivalent Dosages and Daily Dosage Ranges of Commonly Used Antipsychotic Drugs by Chemical Type*

Generic Name	Trade Name	Approximate Equivalent Daily Dosage (mg.)	Approximate Daily Dosage Range (mg.)
Phenothiazines			
Aliphatic			
Chlorpromazine	Thorazine	50.0	50–1000
Promazine	Sparine	100.0	50–1000
Triflupromazine	Vesprin	12.5	60–150
Piperidines			
Thioridazine	Mellaril	50.0	150–800
Mesoridazine	Serentil	25.0	30–400
Piperacetazine	Quide	5.0	20–160
Piperazines			
Acetophenazine	Tindal	10.0	60–120
Fluphenazine	Prolixin, Permitil	1.0	2.5–20
Perphenazine	Trilafon	4.0	6–64
Trifluoperazine	Stelazine	2.0	2–40
Prochlorperazine	Compazine	5.0	15–150
Carphenazine	Proketazine	12.5	25–400
Butaperazine	Repoise	5.0	15–100
Thioxanthenes			
Aliphatic			
Chlorprothixene	Taractan	50.0	30–600
Piperazine			
Thiothixene	Navane	2.0	6–60
Butyrophenone			
Haloperidol	Haldol	1.0	1–15
Dibenzoxazepine			
Loxapine	Loxitane	5.0	20–250
Indol derivative			
Molindone	Moban, Lidone	5.0	15–225

*Reprinted with permission from Facts and Comparisons, 1981, p. 265.

sionally after an adequate trial of two to three weeks, a patient fails to respond to a particular antipsychotic drug. If this occurs, the drug should be switched to one of a different class. There is no apparent advantage to adding another antipsychotic medication to a regimen that has not been effective alone. The most common cause of drug failure is patient noncompliance.

Owing to their long half-life, it takes four to seven days for antipsychotic drugs to reach steady state plasma levels; therefore dosage adjustments should not be made more often than every week with maintenance therapy. The maintenance dose should be the lowest possible that can sustain the patient at an acceptable level of improvement. Because of the long half-life of the antipsychotic drugs, the medication can be given in single night-time doses if this does not result in orthostatic hypotension. In the normal adult the half-life of the antipsychotic drugs ranges from 20 to 24 hours, although extremes in half-life from eight to 44 hours have been reported.[18] In the elderly the half-life of antipsychotic drugs is approximately 20 per cent longer than in the younger population.[5]

Drug free holidays can lessen the chance of long term side effects, including tardive dyskinesia.[19] Because of the long half-life of the antipsychotic drugs, most elderly patients can skip antipsychotic medications for two or three days weekly without an increase in symptomatology. Gardos and Cole suggested that patients who have been taking low doses of antipsychotic drugs for many years without

TABLE 3–2. Potential of Antipsychotic Medications for Producing Selected Adverse Effects*

Drug	Sedation	Adverse Effects Extrapyramidal Symptoms	Anticholinergic Symptoms	Orthostatic Hypotension
Phenothiazines				
Aliphatic				
Chlorpromazine (Thorazine)	+ +	+	+ +	+
Promazine (Sparine)	+	+	+ +	+
Triflupromazine (Vesprin)	+ +	+	+ +	+
Piperidines				
Thioridazine (Mellaril)	+ +	±	+ +	+
Piperacetazine (Quide)	+	+	+	±
Mesoridazine (Serentil)	+ +	±	+	+
Piperazines				
Acetophenazine (Tindal)	+	+ +	±	±
Perphenazine (Trilafon)	±	+ +	±	±
Carphenazine (Proketazine)	+	+ +	±	±
Butaperazine (Repoise)	+	+ +	±	±
Prochlorperazine (Compazine)	+	+ +	±	±
Fluphenazine (Prolixin)	±	+ +	±	±
Trifluoperazine (Stelazine)	±	+ +	±	±
Thioxanthines				
Chlorprothixene (Taractan)	+ +	±	+	+ +
Thiothixene (Navane)	±	+ +	±	±
Butyrophenone				
Haloperidol (Haldol)	±	+ +	±	±
Indole derivative				
Molindone (Moban)	+	+	+	+
Dibenzoxazepine				
Loxapine (Loxitane)	+	+ +	±	±

*Reprinted with permission from Facts and Comparisons, 1981, p. 265.

fluctuation in clinical course probably can be withdrawn from their medications; in a review of outpatient drug withdrawal studies, they concluded that as many as 50 per cent of chronic schizophrenic patients may not need antipsychotic medication at all.[20] Prien and his associates reported that elderly schizophrenic patients receiving dosages equivalent to less than 250 mg. of chlorpromazine per day can tolerate discontinuation of the drug without an exacerbation of symptoms.[21]

Thioridazine, the most commonly used antipsychotic drug in the elderly, has anticholinergic properties that can protect against extrapyramidal side effects, minimizing the tendency for drug induced movement disorders.[17] Unfortunately the same anticholinergic properties contribute to the development of cardiac arrhythmias and toxic delirium. Branchey and associates reported electrocardiographic changes, decreased blood pressure, and weight gain in 27 of 30 elderly schizophrenic patients treated with thioridazine.[22] The alpha-adrenergic blocking properties of thioridazine result in sedation that is more profound than that found with such high potency antipsychotic drugs as haloperidol and trifluoperazine. Thioridazine may cause inhibition of ejaculation, a side effect that could have serious psychologic consequences in an elderly individual already concerned about his deteriorating physical condition. Pigmentary retinopathy may develop in patients who are maintained on dosages of thioridazine greater than 800 mg. daily.[17]

In a survey of 12 Veterans Administration hospitals, chlorpromazine was the second most frequently used antipsychotic drug—employed in 22 per cent of the elderly schizophrenic patients.[21] Stotsky reviewed studies of the use of chlorpromazine in treating elderly psychotic patients and found dosages to range from 50 to 300 mg. daily.[23] Because chlorpromazine can cause hypotensive crises, especially in debilitated patients, supine and standing blood pressure measurements should be done in the elderly patient before and after a test dose of chlorpromazine prior to routine administration of the drug.

The piperazine drug trifluoperazine (Stelazine) was used in 8 per cent of elderly schizophrenics in the 12 hospital Veterans Administration study.[21] The effective dose for trifluoperazine in the elderly ranges from 2 to 20 mg.[23] Trifluoperazine, a high potency antipsychotic drug, can produce acute dystonic muscle spasms, Parkinson-like side effects, and motor restlessness. In a crossover study Branchey and associates compared fluphenazine hydrochloride (dosage range, 1.5 to 5.0 mg. daily) with thioridazine (dosage range, 84 to 285 mg. daily) in 30 elderly patients.[22] From this study they concluded that although the clinical efficacy of the two antipsychotic drugs was similar, the side effects of fluphenazine were less severe.

If the patient is not reliable enough to take his oral medication or if it is suspected that the medication is poorly absorbed when given orally, the long acting parenterally administered (intramuscularly) piperazine drugs fluphenazine decanoate (with a duration of action of 14 to 21 days) and fluphenazine enanthate (with a duration of action of 10 to 14 days) can be used. Approximately 25 mg. of enanthate or decanoate given every other week is equal to 5 mg. of fluphenazine administered orally once daily.[24]

The butyrophenone, haloperidol, has minimal alpha-adrenergic blocking properties and few anticholinergic side effects; therefore fewer sedative, electrocardiographic, and hypotensive effects are produced. Haloperidol, however, induces a high frequency of extrapyramidal side effects. To lessen the chance of extrapyramidal side effects, the elderly patient should receive 0.5 mg. of haloperidol initially, and the dosage should be increased gradually to control agitation, grandiosity, and hallucinations; the average dosage in the elderly is 2 mg. daily.[23]

Side Effects

The prevalence of side effects is difficult to estimate. Because side effects are relatively rare, it is necessary to observe a large number of patients over an extended period of time to obtain accurate data. Most information about side effects reflects differences in definitions. Schizophrenic patients, when not taking medicine, often complain of symptoms similar to drug induced side effects. Furthermore, subjective information is difficult to quantitate. For example, chlorpromazine induced drowsiness occurs in 2 to 92 per cent of the patients.[25]

Acute Extrapyramidal Disorders. An estimated 50 per cent of all patients taking antipsychotic drugs between the ages of 60 and 80 have extrapyramidal symptoms at some time during the course of treatment; 90 per cent of these reactions occur during the first two months of therapy.[8] The elderly have a greater likelihood of developing a Parkinson-like syndrome, whereas younger patients tend toward dyskinesia, and patients between age 40 and 50 are more susceptible to akathisia. The extrapyramidal symptoms appear to be related to dopamine blockage: the antipsychotic drugs with strong dopamine blocking properties have a tendency to produce extrapyramidal symptoms. In regard to the three dopamine pathways in the central nervous system—the nigrostriatal, the mesolimbic, and the tuboinfundibular—dopamine blockage in the mesolimbic terminals is believed to reverse psychotic thought, whereas dopamine blockage in the nigrostriatal pathway results in extrapyramidal symptoms.

Acute dystonic reactions, characterized by acute spasms of the truncal, nuchal, buccal, and oculomotor muscle groups, usually occur within the first hour to five days of the onset of treatment with antipsychotic drugs. Benztropine (Cogentin), 0.5 to 2.0 mg. intravenously, or diphenhydramine (Benadryl), 25 to 50 mg. intravenously, can dramatically reverse acute dystonia.[24]

Akathisia (motor restlessness with an inability to sit still) usually develops within the first few weeks of treatment. Akathisia can be misdiagnosed as agitation, causing the physician to erroneously increase the dose of antipsychotic medication. This increased dosage will result in more restlessness or lead to sedation and rigidity. Amphetamines, coffee (more than three cups daily), and ingestion of alcohol exacerbate akathisia. Benztropine or trihexphenadyl (Artane) generally reduces the symptoms of akathisia.[24] Switching to another antipsychotic drug is usually also effective.[25]

A Parkinson-like syndrome, more common in the elderly than dyskinesia or akathisia, is characterized by bradykinesia, a shuffling gait, resting tremor, masked facies, muscle rigidity, and occasional drooling. These symptoms may cause the patient to appear depressed. Instead of adding an antidepressant, the physician should prescribe an anticholinergic medication. Either benztropine (Cogentin), 0.5 to 2.0 mg. orally daily, or trihexphenadyl (Artane), 2 to 8 mg. orally, given in daily divided doses is effective in managing Parkinson-like side effects; both restore the cholinergic-dopaminergic balance in the caudate nucleus. When antipsychotic drugs block dopaminergic activity, cholinergic activity dominates, resulting in extrapyramidal symptoms. An anticholinergic medication reduces cholinergic activity, restoring the cholinergic-dopaminergic balance and thus relieving the extrapyramidal symptoms.[27]

Anticholinergic medications should be given only when extrapyramidal symptoms develop, for the following reasons:[5]

1. Anticholinergic medications decrease antipsychotic blood levels.

2. Anticholinergic drugs slow intestinal motility and decrease the absorption of antipsychotic drugs.

3. Anticholinergic medications exacerbate tardive dyskinesia, presumably by antagonizing the dopamine system.

4. The anticholinergic drugs may produce side effects such as toxic delirium, constipation, urinary retention, blurred vision, prostatic hypertrophy, cardiac arrhythmias, or aggravation of glaucoma. In patients who are given anticholinergic medications to control extrapyramidal symptoms, the anticholinergic drugs may be discontinued after two or three months because extrapyramidal symptoms tend to dissipate after a few months of antipsychotic therapy (probably as a result of tolerance to the dopaminergic blockage in the caudate nucleus).[17,28]

Tardive Dyskinesia. A neurologic condition consisting of abnormal motor movements of the face, tardive dyskinesia is sometimes referred to as the buccolingual masticatory syndrome. The typical facial movements include grimacing, involuntary protrusion of the tongue, pushing out of the cheeks, chewing movements, and licking of the lips. Less commonly choreoathetoid movements of the extremities and ballistic movements of the arms are involved.[25]

Tardive dyskinesia should be carefully looked for, because, unlike many other toxic effects, it is sometimes irreversible. Because the syndrome can be volitionally suppressed, the physician should observe the patient unawares—when the patient is talking to a family member or another patient.[25] Any abnormal rhythmic movement should be considered an early manifestation of tardive dyskinesia until proven otherwise. Early signs may include rhythmical vermiform movements of the tongue and the inability to protrude the tongue for more than a few seconds.[29] Slight involuntary movements of the fingers (digital dyskinesia) may also be an early sign.[17]

The prevalence of tardive dyskinesia varies tremendously, from 0 to 40 per cent of the patients surveyed.[25] The syndrome is most common in individuals who have been taking antipsychotic medication for a long period of time (hence the term "tardive") and is also most frequently found in the elderly and in women.[30]

Whether the total dosage of an antipsychotic drug taken over time is responsible and whether a particular drug is more implicated than others have not been ascertained,[25] but studies done by Borison indicate that the development of tardive dyskinesia depends on the capacity of a particular drug to block dopamine receptors in the extrapyramidal system.[31] Borison found that haloperidol has a greater likelihood of blocking dopamine receptors in the extrapyramidal system than does thioridazine.[31] Thioridazine, on the other hand, has a higher propensity for blocking dopamine receptors in the limbic system, the area believed to be responsible for antipsychotic effects of medications.

The pathophysiology of tardive dyskinesia is unknown, although several theories have been advanced.[25] Prange and associates proposed that tardive dyskinesia is caused by a dopaminergic overactivity in the extrapyramidal system (nigrostriatum), thereby disrupting the normal dopamine-acetylcholine ratio.[32] With tardive dyskinesia there is overactivity of dopamine; with Parkinson's disease there is overactivity of acetylcholine. The anticholinergic drugs are believed to exacerbate tardive dyskinesia, since they increase the acetylcholine-dopamine imbalance by lowering the effective acetylcholine concentration.[33] Klawans suggested that antipsychotic drugs cause hypersensitivity of the dopamine receptors in the nigrostriatal area.[34] Eventually the dopamine that escapes blockade by the antipsychotic drug stimulates the receptors, producing the symptoms of tardive dyskinesia.

There are two types of central dopamine receptors—those inhibitory and those facilitatory to motor movements.[25] Hypersensitivity of the facilitatory receptors may produce tardive dyskinesia, whereas blockade of the inhibitory receptors may produce drug induced parkinsonism.[34] The observation that tardive dyskinesia develops most frequently in patients with extrapyramidal side effects seems to contradict the denervation hypersensitivity theory.[35]

Since there is no effective treatment for tardive dyskinesia, every effort should be made to achieve therapeutic benefits with the least dosage of an antipsychotic drug administered for the shortest period of time. The condition can be suppressed temporarily by increasing the dose of the antipsychotic drug, but there soon will be an "escape" and the medication will be necessary in ever increasing doses, eventually failing completely.[5] In an extensive review of the literature, Klein and associates reported some moderately encouraging findings in the use of a variety of drugs to treat tardive dyskinesia.[25] Reserpine, physostigmine, lecithin, deanol, lithium carbonate, l-tryptophan, and apomorphine have all proved to be somewhat effective in small uncontrolled studies. A critical review of these studies, however, leads to the conclusion that the only practical treatment is to stop the antipsychotic medication as soon as dyskinesia is detected. Unfortunately it is impossible to withhold antipsychotic medications in some patients for an extended period of time; in these situations the patient and his family should be fully informed and included in the decision making process.

Central Anticholinergic Syndrome. Another common problem in the elderly is a central anticholinergic syndrome. This condition is especially common in patients treated with thioridazine and chlorpromazine (as well as those treated with tricyclic antidepressants) because of the strong anticholinergic side effects of these drugs. The frequency varies from 16 to 35 per cent of elderly patients receiving psychoactive medication.[5] Symptoms include agitation, anxiety, delirium, restlessness, disorientation, impaired memory, hallucinations, and slurred speech. Peripheral signs include cardiac arrhythmias, dilated pupils, which react slowly to light, erythema, and warm dry skin. Treatment consists of 1 to 2 mg. of physostigmine given slowly intravenously and repeated as needed every 15 to 30 minutes. The clinician should be cautious about inducing a physostigmine toxicity marked by the opposite peripheral signs of atropine toxicity in addition to confusion, seizures, nausea, and hallucinations. The treatment of physostigmine induced cholinergic excess is to give atropine subcutaneously, 0.5 mg. for every milligram of physostigmine previously given.[17]

Peripheral Anticholinergic Effects. Elderly patients are particularly susceptible to the peripheral anticholinergic effects of the antipsychotic drugs, such as blurred vision, urinary retention, dry mouth, paralytic ileus, constipation, and orthostatic hypotension. Orthostatic hypotension commonly causes weakness and dizziness in the elderly, particularly those treated with chlorpromazine and thioridazine. Patients taking these drugs should be warned to avoid sudden shifts in posture. The use of surgical stockings to prevent venous pooling in the extremities is helpful. Tolerance to orthostatic hypotension usually develops, and the side effect is seldom a long term problem.[25]

Dry mouth can be particularly distressing to the elderly. Oral lesions and parotid infections secondary to dry mouth can occur.[5] Good oral hygiene, adequate hydration, and the chewing of sugarless gum can be helpful. A saliva substitute (VA/Oral Lube) has recently been found effective, as has bethanecol, 25 mg. orally three times a day.[25,36] Bethanecol also can be used to treat urinary retention and other anticholinergic side effects of the antipsychotic drugs.

Approximately 2 per cent of the population over age 40 have undiagnosed glaucoma.[8] The atropine-like effects of the antipsychotic drugs can precipitate an acute attack of previously undetected glaucoma, an event that requires immediate ophthalmologic consultation. Patients maintained on cholinomimetic eyedrops for chronic glaucoma can receive antipsychotic medications.[17]

The sedative effects of the antipsychotic drugs, especially chlorpromazine, may lead to an unacceptable degree of lethargy, loss of motor coordination, and delayed reaction time.[25] In some patients who have trouble arising in the morning, the key point is to get these individuals out of bed, for once they are up and moving, the drowsiness clears. The clinician should be alert concerning interactions between antipsychotics and other drugs that also produce sedation (the anticholinergics, antihistamines, alcohol, and minor tranquilizers, to name a few); medications should be limited only to those that are absolutely necessary.

Electrocardiographic Changes. The phenothiazines, especially thioridazine, can produce electrocardiographic changes resembling those in hypokalemia.[25] Branchey and associates reported electrocardiographic changes in 90 per cent of the elderly patients treated with thioridazine.[22] The combination of thioridazine and tricyclic antidepressants may be particularly dangerous.[37]

Other Side Effects. Agranulocytosis, a life threatening complication of antipsychotic drug administration, usually occurs in the first two months of treatment and is accompanied by a sore throat, ulcerations, and high fever.[25] If the antipsychotic medication is discontinued quickly enough, the leukocyte count returns to normal within seven to 10 days. Agranulocytosis has been reported in one in 200 elderly patients, compared to one in 6000 of the general population.[8] Seventy-five per cent of all cases of drug induced agranulocytosis occur in patients over 50 years of age.[8]

Chlorpromazine induced jaundice, believed to be a hypersensitivity reaction resulting in small bile duct obstruction, occurs in approximately 1 per cent of the patients. The disorder is preceded by fever, malaise, and nausea, followed by liver enlargement and jaundice.[25] Most patients recover spontaneously after discontinuation of the antipsychotic drug. The frequency of chlorpromazine induced jaundice appears to be decreasing, possibly because of better quality control in drug manufacture.[25]

The antipsychotic drugs produce a variety of effects involving the skin and eyes. An estimated 4 per cent of the elderly have photosensitivity reactions secondary to antipsychotic medication.[38] A chronic blue-gray discoloration over areas exposed to sunlight can result from long term antipsychotic drug administration.[25] The low potency antipsychotic drugs can bring about the formation of pigment deposits in the lens, cornea, and retina. Patients who are receiving more than 800 mg. of thioridazine daily are particularly vulnerable to pigmentary retinopathy.[17]

Low potency antipsychotic drugs can produce seizures, particularly with high dosages or rapid increases in dosage level. There is no evidence that adding an anticonvulsant drug protects against seizures; the one effective treatment is to decrease the dosage slightly.[25] Patients with pre-existing seizure disorders are least likely to have drug induced seizures with the high potency piperazines or haloperidol.[17]

All antipsychotic drugs cause an elevation of plasma prolactin due to receptor blockade of the tuberoinfundibular dopaminergic neurons.[25] Klein and associates in an extensive review of the literature concluded that there was no evidence linking antipsychotic drugs to breast cancer.[25] Because breast cancer is the leading cause of cancer death in women, periodic breast examination in the female is advised, particularly in patients with a family history of breast cancer.

Numerous other adverse effects have been reported with use of the antipsychotic drugs, but their incidence and dose-response relationship are poorly defined.[5] These include lactation and breast engorgement in the female, gynecomastia in the male, false positive pregnancy test results, hypoglycemia, glycosuria, and amenorrhea. Antipsychotic drugs have been reported to aggravate pre-existing peptic ulcer, suppress the cough reflex, and suppress the thirst reflex. Because of the potential for numerous side effects, the implications of all the foregoing are obvious, and patients should be monitored closely over long periods of therapy.

The ratio of toxic dose to effective dose (the therapeutic index) is very high with antipsychotic drugs.[5] Respiratory depression, coma, and sudden death are extremely uncommon. The potential for suicide by an overdose should not be overlooked, however. Unfortunately the antipsychotic drugs are not easily dialyzable because of their lipid and protein binding properties.[17]

AFFECTIVE DISORDERS

The third edition of the *Diagnostic and Statistical Manual of Mental Disorders* divides the affective disorders (primary mood disturbances) into three types:[16]

1. Major affective disorders—a full affective syndrome, either bipolar or depressive.

2. Other specific affective disorders—a partial affective syndrome of at least two years' duration.

3. Atypical affective disorders—a category for affective conditions that cannot be classified as episodic, chronic, or adjustment disorders.

Table 3–3 further subdivides these three groups.

Bipolar disorders are further divided into two types—conditions in which episodes of mania alternate with periods of normal mood and affective disorders characterized by depressive and manic episodes separated by essentially normal mental functioning. Mania is characterized by the triad of hyperactivity, pressured speech, and elated mood; major

TABLE 3–3. Types of Affective Disorders

Classification	Characteristics
Major affective disorders	Severe depression or mania
Bipolar disorder	Includes unipolar mania and manic episodes alternating with depressive episodes
Major depression, single episode or recurrent	Biological signs of depression with severe dysphoria
Other specific affective disorders	Partial affective syndrome
Cyclothymic disorder	Chronic mood disturbance involving episodes of depression and elation not sufficiently severe to be classified as a major affective disorder
Dysthymic disorder (depressive neurosis)	Lifelong pattern of depressive symptoms
Atypical affective disorders	Unusual affective features
Atypical bipolar disorder	A major depressive episode followed by a hypomanic episode ("bipolar II")
Atypical depression	Depression that fits none of the foregoing categories

depression consists of a dysphoric mood combined with sleep disturbance, weight fluctuation, decreased sexual drive, and diminished energy. A patient with mild fluctuations in mood would be classified as having a cyclothymic disorder; one with a lifelong pattern of depression would be diagnosed as having a dysthymic disorder.

Lithium in the Treatment of Mania and Bipolar Disorders

Lithium is indicated for the treatment of bipolar disorders. The use of lithium can prevent the recurrence of manic attacks and modify mood swings. Tricyclic antidepressants are the drugs of choice for depressive episodes in bipolar patients. Lithium should be given concurrently to prevent a swing into a manic episode. Although acute episodes of mania or hypomania occur infrequently for the first time in the elderly, many patients who have begun taking lithium earlier in life need to be maintained on the medication to prevent recurrent attacks.

Lithium offers advantages in the management of bipolar affective disorders owing to its specificity, few adverse effects at stable therapeutic dosage levels, prophylactic value, insignificant sedative properties, high patient acceptability, and the availability of objective blood level measurements for monitoring therapy. The prescriber must be aware, however, that there is a narrow margin between therapeutic and toxic doses of lithium, and if toxicity does occur, it can be life threatening. Since the use of lithium is associated with numerous side effects, the physician should use clinical judgment as to whether the patient's abnormal mood swings are significant enough to merit continued long term treatment risk. Because of the danger of lithium overdosage, suicidal or impulsive patients are poor candidates for therapy.

Once the decision is made to begin lithium therapy, certain laboratory studies should be performed. A baseline serum creatinine determination is necessary to evaluate renal function. Because lithium may induce leukocytosis, a complete blood count is required. A urinalysis will give a baseline specific gravity value, which may be altered if a diabetes insipidus-like syndrome develops. Thyroid function tests are necessary because lithium may induce thyroid enlargement and contribute to hypothyroidism. Physical examination and the taking of a history should be directed toward detection of cardiovascular, renal, or organic brain disease. Periodic evaluation of the foregoing parameters in patients given long term lithium therapy is advised.

A desirable blood level for the treatment of an acute manic episode is 0.8 to 1.5 mEq. per liter. The achievement of this blood level normally requires a daily dosage of 1500 to 2400 mg. of lithium carbonate. The desirable blood level for maintenance therapy is 0.6 to 1.2 mEq. per liter, which for most patients is achieved within a 900 to 1500 mg. daily dosage range of lithium carbonate. To provide a reliable measure of the lithium level, the blood sample should be drawn approximately 12 hours after the last lithium dose, when absorption is complete and excretion less erratic.[39]

It takes four to 10 days for lithium to become effective; therefore it may be necessary to use an antipsychotic medication such as haloperidol or chlorpromazine concomitantly to control acute manic episodes. Once therapeutic serum lithium levels are achieved, the dosages of the neuroleptic drugs may be tapered and then discontinued and lithium alone continued. Approximately 80 per cent of the patients having acute manic episodes respond to lithium in one to two weeks.[40]

Over 99 per cent of a single oral dose of lithium is absorbed within eight hours. Serum levels reach a peak in one to three hours. Lithium is not bound to plasma proteins, and most is excreted unchanged in the urine at the rate of approximately half the ingested dose within 24 hours after administration in the person with normal renal function. Excretion varies considerably with age, the elimination half-life ranging from 18 hours in young adults to 36 hours in the elderly.[39] Elderly patients therefore require less lithium to achieve a therapeutic serum level.

Since sodium and lithium compete for reabsorption at the proximal renal tubule, a deficit in sodium results in an increase in lithium reabsorption. A fall in the total body sodium level resulting from salt restriction, fasting, crash diets, dehydration, increasing perspiration, or diuretic medication leads to lithium retention and an increased risk of toxicity. In addition to diuretics, numerous other drugs may affect renal excretion of lithium (Table 3–4).

The initial dose of lithium depends on the severity of the illness and the patient's age, weight, physical condition, and kidney function. Since elderly patients excrete lithium slowly, they require less medication in order for therapeutic blood levels to be obtained. Although a younger manic patient may require 1500 to 2400 mg. daily initially in management of the acute phase and 900 to 1500 mg. daily in long term management to reach a lithium level in the therapeutic range, an elderly manic patient may require only 600 to 900 mg. daily to maintain a therapeutic serum level. Blood levels should be determined every second or third day after initiation of therapy and until the manic episode subsides.

After the patient has been discharged from the hospital, it is judicious to monitor serum levels once a week for four weeks and then once a month for 12 months. Once a satisfactory dose has been established, it can often be maintained in a particular patient for many years; however, serum levels should be determined frequently (every one to two months) to insure compliance and safety. Signs of a manic or depressive episode, an intercurrent disease, a significant change in salt intake, or the institution of symptoms of intoxication requires more frequent monitoring of the lithium level.

Although much has been printed about the value of prophylactic lithium therapy, a single attack of mania or a rare attack of mania is not sufficient reason for initiating lithium prophylaxis. In individuals experiencing their first manic episode, lithium should be gradually withdrawn after three months of therapy. Patients in whom there is a recurrence of manic behavior more frequently than every year or two are candidates for lithium prophylaxis. Good compliance and patient reliability are essential, because a constant therapeutic blood level must be maintained.

Lithium Toxicity

Mild symptoms of lithium toxicity generally begin at a blood level of 1.5 mEq. per liter or less. At 1.5 to 2.0 mEq. per liter, symptoms of toxicity become serious; lithium levels greater than 3.0 mEq. per liter are life threatening (Table 3–5). Elderly patients are susceptable to severe toxic symptoms despite a serum lithium level in the therapeutic range; thus, clinical judgment should be the final determining factor in evaluating a patient with possible lithium toxicity. The earliest toxic signs include nausea, vomiting, diarrhea, thirst, polyuria, lethargy, slurred speech, and an exaggerated tremor of the hands. Electrocardiographic changes may include flattening

TABLE 3–4. Potential Drug Interactions with Lithium

Drug	Effect on Renal Clearance of Lithium	Effect on Serum Lithium Level
Diuretics		
Thiazides	↓	↑↑
Furosemide	↓	↑
Ethacrynic acid	↓	↑
Spironolactone	None	None
Triamterine	?	?
Aminophylline	↑	↓
Mannitol	↑	↓
Urea	↑	↓
Acetazolamide	↑	↓

TABLE 3–5. Adverse Effects Induced by Lithium at Various Blood Levels

Lithium Blood Level	Adverse Effect
1.5 mEq./l. or less	Nausea Vomiting Diarrhea Thirst Polyuria Lethargy Slurred speech Fine hand tremor Muscle weakness
1.5–2.0 mEq./l.	Coarse hand tremor Persistent gastrointestinal effects Mental confusion Hyperirritability of muscles Electrocardiographic changes
>2.0 mEq./l.	Electrocardiographic changes (possible flattening and inversion of T wave) Fasciculations Tinnitus Blurred vision Clonic movements Seizures Electroencephalographic changes Stupor Coma Hypotension Death

and inversion of the T wave. As intoxication increases, neurologic symptoms become prominent, with tinnitus, fasciculations, blurred vision, clonic movements, electroencephalographic changes, seizures, stupor, and finally coma. Fatalities are usually secondary to pulmonary complications resulting from coma.[5]

If lithium toxicity develops, the drug should be stopped immediately and the patient monitored with daily or more frequent lithium levels, electrolyte determinations, and electrocardiograms. Electrolytes should be replaced as needed. Lithium excretion is enhanced by increasing the fluid intake to 5 to 6 liters a day.

When lithium elimination must be hastened, 20 grams of urea given intravenously two to five times daily (or mannitol, 50 to 100 grams intravenously daily in the nonrenally impaired patient) also increases lithium diuresis. Aminophylline, 500 mg., given by slow intravenous push every six hours, suppresses tubular reabsorption of lithium in addition to increasing blood flow through the tubules, thus enhancing lithium clearance.

Hemodialysis should be considered for refractory lithium toxicity.[5]

Chronic Side Effects

Patients maintained on lithium may develop side effects unrelated to blood levels. These chronic side effects are reversible when lithium is discontinued. An initial sodium diuresis, common during the first few weeks of lithium treatment, may persist as chronic polyuria in some patients. Rarely polyuria develops into a nephrogenic diabetes insipidus-like syndrome secondary to lithium interference with the action of antidiuretic hormone. This syndrome is characterized by an excessive intake of fluids, constant thirst, and a large output of very dilute urine (3 or more liters per day).

Prolonged exposure to lithium has been correlated with nonspecific renal lesions in a small percentage of patients.[41] With prolonged therapy, routine monitoring of the serum creatinine level should be carried out every three to six months. Some clinicians advocate a creatinine clearance every six to 12 months.[25] This approach may be overly cautious, particularly in patients with no increase in the serum creatinine value. If the serum creatinine value increases 50 per cent over baseline values, more intensive monitoring is indicated.

Benign diffuse enlargement of the thyroid gland secondary to an impaired thyroid response to thyroid stimulating hormone occurs in approximately 3 per cent of the patients given long term lithium therapy. In patients who develop thyroid dysfunction, a decision as to whether to continue lithium depends on the severity of the affective illness and the degree of thyroid impairment. Rarely, localized edema or folliculitis may develop, but the condition is usually only a minor cosmetic problem. Some patients develop a fine hand tremor, which is usually of no functional significance.[25] An insignificant leukocytosis (10,000 to 14,000) without a left shift found in infection may develop in patients given lithium treatment.[5]

Treatment of Depression

Approximately 20 per cent of elderly adults suffer from significant symptoms of depression.[42] Affective disorders are present in somewhat more than 50 per cent of hospitalized geropsychiatric patients aged 60 to 70, and in somewhat less than 50 per cent of the patients ages 70 to 80.[43] Currently less than one-fourth of the patients with depression receive any treatment.[44]

Manifestations of the depressive syndrome include emotional, cognitive, physiologic, and behavioral aspects. Emotional aspects include the symptoms of sadness, apathy, irritability, anxiety, or anger. Cognitive symptoms of depression include loss of self-esteem, a negative attitude, guilt, and a sense of worthlessness. Physiologic symptoms, which may mimic organic disease, most commonly involve the gastrointestinal, cardiac, and musculoskeletal systems. Behavioral symptoms of depression include reduced interest in social, familial, and occupational activities. Additionally, some elderly patients develop depressive illnesses that appear to mimic dementias, and symptoms may include an impaired ability to concentrate, decreased attention to personal tidiness, anorexia, and sleep disturbance.

When attempting to diagnose depressive illness in the elderly patient, one must consider the possibility that the depression may be drug induced or that it may be a manifestation of a pre-existing disease that has been improperly managed.[45] Drugs known to precipitate depression in some patients are included in Table 3–6. The sympatholytic antihypertensive drugs are particularly notorious in producing symptoms of depression, reserpine being the primary offender. Table 3–7 presents physical illnesses that are frequently associated with depressive symptoms. The approach first is to identify the physical illness in question and to treat it properly. If depressive illness persists, specific antidepressant therapy may be indicated. A definitive diagnosis of depression, beyond ruling out the possibility that the depression may be drug induced or induced by a pre-existing disease, requires numerous diagnostic steps. These include the clinical interview, a self-report inventory, physical examination, and laboratory work (including a complete blood count; urinalysis; thyroid function, blood urea nitrogen, serum electrolyte, and fasting blood sugar determinations; electrocardiography; and liver function tests).

Perhaps the most difficult task in the differential diagnosis of depression is its distinction from dementia.[46] Failure to distinguish depression from organicity can result in the depressed patient's placement in a long term care facility where he may be neglected. A thorough mental status examination with detailed evaluation of cognitive functioning (orientation, the ability to name objects and remember them, knowledge of current events, and memory for important dates) can help in distinguishing between depression and organicity.

Drug therapy management of depressive disorders in the elderly is very much like the management of depressive illness in younger age groups except that strict attention must be directed toward the appropriateness of the dose, the frequency of drug administration, and the potential for antidepressant drugs to interact with numerous other drugs the patient may be consuming to manage a myriad of chronic or acute diseases. The drugs most

TABLE 3–7. Illnesses Frequently Associated with Depression

Anemia (pernicious)
Addison's disease
Cancer of the pancreas
Cerebral arteriosclerosis
Cushing's disease
Diabetes
Disabling diseases of any type
Hepatitis
Hyperparathyroidism
Hyperthyroidism
Hypoglycemia
Hypothyroidism
Malignant disease
Parkinson's disease
Senile dementia
Systemic lupus erythematosus

TABLE 3–6. Drugs That May Precipitate Depression

Drug Class and Generic Names	
Antihypertensives	Anticonvulsants
Clonidine	Succinimide derivatives
Guanethidine	Carbamazepine
Hydralazine	
Methyldopa	Antineoplastics
Propranolol	Vincristine
Reserpine	Vinblastine
Antiarthritic drugs	Corticosteroids
Indomethacin	Entire class
Phenylbutazone	
	Hormones
Antiparkinson drugs	Estrogen
L-dopa	Progesterone
Amantadine	
Anti-infectives	
Sulfonamides	
Cycloserine	

useful in treating depression in the elderly include the tricyclic antidepressants; the tetracyclic antidepressant, maprotiline; monoamine oxidase inhibitors; and, for recurrent depressions with mania, lithium. The antipsychotic drugs are useful in delusional depressions.[5] Central nervous system stimulants, barbiturates, the nonbarbiturate sedative-hypnotics, and the benzodiazepines are of no value in managing depressive disorders.[5]

Tricyclic Antidepressants

Bielski and Friedel have reported that predictors of a positive response to tricyclic antidepressants include upper socioeconomic class, an insidious onset, anorexia, weight loss, middle and late insomnia, and psychomotor disturbance.[47] They also reported that predictors of poor response to tricyclic drugs include hypochondriasis, hysterical traits, multiple prior episodes, and delusions.

It has been suggested that depression may exist as two biochemical subtypes characterized by either a norepinephrine or a serotonin deficiency.[48] As Table 3–8 indicates, individuals with norepinephrine deficiency, as determined by low urinary excretion of the norepinephrine metabolite 3-methoxy-4-hydroxyphenylglycol, are more likely to respond to secondary amine tricyclic antidepressants (amoxapine, desipramine, nortriptyline, and protriptyline) and to the tertiary amine, imipramine, which is partially metabolized to desipramine. Conversely, individuals with normal 3-methoxy-4-hydroxyphenylglycol levels may have low levels of the major metabolite of serotonin, 5-hydroxyindoleacetic acid, and should respond best to the tertiary amines (amitriptyline, doxepin, and trimipramine).

The eight tricyclic compounds have a common structure, consisting of two benzene rings between a seven member central ring containing a side chain.[5] Minor changes in the central ring and the side chain result in differences in their clinical effects. Thus amitriptyline has the most anticholinergic and sedative properties, whereas desipramine, nortriptyline, and protriptyline are the least sedative tricyclic compounds (Table 3–8).

The tricyclic antidepressants are rapidly absorbed after oral administration. In middle aged adults approximately 10 per cent of the drug is found in the blood in the active unbound form; in the elderly, who have less plasma protein, higher levels of unbound tricyclic compounds circulate in the blood, resulting in a potentially higher incidence of side effects than in the population under age 60 if appropiate dosage adjustments are not made.[7]

The rate of metabolism for the tricyclic antidepressants decreases in the elderly, probably because of a loss of liver mass and a gradual decrease in liver enzyme concentrations. Nies and associates, studying the plasma levels of imipramine, desipramine, and amitriptyline in older depressed patients, found that patients over 65 years of age had higher plasma levels than those in a group of younger patients, even though the older patients re-

TABLE 3–8. Summary of the Relative Anticholinergic, Sedative and Amine Uptake Blocking Activity of the Tricyclic Antidepressants*

Drug	Major Side Effects		Amine Uptake Blocking Activity	
	Anticholinergic	*Sedative*	*Norepinephrine*	*Serotonin*
Tertiary amines				
Amitriptyline (Elavil)	+++	+++	0	++
Doxepin (Sinequan)	++	+++	0^2	$+^?$
Imipramine (Tofranil)	++	++	$++^1$	+
Trimipramine (Surmontil)	++	+++	$-^2$	$-^2$
Secondary amines				
Amoxapine (Asendin)	++	++	++	±
Desipramine (Norpramin, Pertofrane)		+	+++	0
Nortriptyline (Aventyl)	+	+	++	±
Protriptyline (Vivactil)	++	0^2	$+^2$	0^2

*Adapted with permission from Facts and Comparisons, 1982, p. 263.
[1]Via desipramine, the major metabolite.
[2]Studies are lacking to produce definitive information.

ceived lower daily doses of the tricyclic compounds.[49] In addition, although the steady state in the average adult was achieved in five to 10 days, elderly patients did not achieve a steady state plasma level for two to three weeks. Elimination of the tricyclic antidepressants took twice as long in the older group as in the younger age group.

Because of the higher plasma levels found in the elderly, amitriptyline, desipramine, and imipramine should be started at a dosage of 25 mg. daily; this dosage can be increased gradually every four to seven days to a maximal limit of 100 mg. daily, or until troublesome side effects develop. For other tricyclic drugs a good rule of thumb in initiating therapy in the elderly, if there are no extenuating precautions, is to begin with a dosage estimated to be one-quarter to one-third the expected therapeutic dosage, increasing every four to seven days until the desired response is achieved (Table 3–9). Because there is a lag period before the onset of an antidepressant effect, the therapeutic trial period for antidepressant drugs in the elderly may be as long as six weeks, as opposed to three weeks in the normal adult. The onset of action of amoxapine (which may prove to be the least cardiotoxic of the tricyclic drugs) appears to be somewhat faster, a clinical response being seen in some patients after four to seven days of therapy.[50] Trimipramine can be used safely in the elderly but requires a decrease in dosage and increased monitoring.[51]

Friedel and Raskin[52] studied the plasma levels of doxepin in 15 elderly depressed patients treated with dosages ranging from 50 to 300 mg. daily. Seven patients who responded had a mean steady state plasma concentration of doxepin and its metabolite desmethyldoxepin of 111 ng. per ml.; those who failed to respond had a mean plasma concentration of 60 ng. per ml. Patients who responded were treated with an average daily dosage of 164 mg. without adverse effects. This small sample may indicate that the elderly can tolerate higher dosages of doxepin than of the other tricyclic antidepressants (i.e., approximately 150 mg. daily).

Regardless of the tricyclic drug chosen, once there has been a complete remission of symptoms, the dosage may be reduced gradually every 14 days to approximately half the therapeutic dosage.[5] Since episodes of depression usually last longer in aged persons— sometimes up to two years—low dose maintenance therapy should be considered for longer than one year in the elderly.[53]

Plasma Levels. Because there are individual differences in absorption and metabolism, the determination of tricyclic plasma levels can aid in evaluating therapeutic dosage ranges, especially in the elderly in whom a small change in dosage might lead to toxicity. Plasma level determinations should be ordered whenever there appears to be a lack of response to therapy, unexpected or serious side effects occur, or there is a suspicion of noncompliance.[5] Because there is a lag of steady state plasma tricyclic antidepressant drug levels of up to two to three weeks in the elderly, the assay should not be carried out earlier than the fourteenth day of treatment.[49] The sample is usually collected from the fasting patient before the morning dose in Venojet tubes or syringes, since Vacutainer tubes contain a substance that causes tricyclic drugs to shift from the plasma to the red blood cells, causing falsely low plasma levels.[54] The range of effective plasma levels of selected tricyclic antidepressants is illustrated in Table 3–10.[55]

Side Effects. The most common side effects of tricyclic antidepressants, resulting from their anticholinergic properties, include dry mouth, sweating, blurred vision, constipation, urinary retention, tachycardia, palpitations, ar-

TABLE 3–9. Tricyclic Antidepressant Dosing Information for the Elderly

Drug	Adult Starting Dose (Mg./Day)	Usual Adult Maintenance Dose (Mg./Day)	Adult Therapeutic Dosage Range (Mg./Day)	Plasma Half Life (Hours)
Amitriptyline	25–75	100–150	50–300	10–50
Amoxapine	75–150	150–250	150–600	—
Desipramine	25–50	100	75–300	13–23
Doxepin	25–50	75–100	75–300	8–23
Imipramine	25–75	100–125	50–300	8–16
Nortriptyline	20–40	50–75	40–100	16–45
Protriptyline	10	10–30	10–40	54–198
Trimipramine	50–75	100–200	100–300	—

TABLE 3–10. Range of Effective Plasma Levels of Selected Tricyclic Antidepressants

Amitriptyline > 100 ng./ml. (amitriptyline plus nortriptyline)

Imipramine > 200 ng./ml. (imipramine plus desipramine)

Doxepin > 100 ng./ml. (doxepin plus desmethyldoxepin)

Desipramine > 125 ng./ml.

Nortriptyline > 75 ng./ml.

Protriptyline > 100 ng./ml.

rhythmias, hypertension, and paralytic ileus.[17] Confusional episodes resembling those with atropine poisoning have been reported in 35 per cent of the patients over 40 years of age receiving such drugs.[56] Amitriptyline has the greatest potential for producing adverse anticholinergic effects.

Various skin reactions, such as rash, pruritus, urticaria, and photosensitization, as well as drug fever, have been reported with the tricyclic drugs. An allergic obstructive type of jaundice has also been reported.[17] Although agranulocytosis is rare, the incidence increases with age.[5] The seizure threshold is lowered by the tricyclic drugs.[17]

Tricyclic antidepressants directly suppress the contractility of the myocardium, increasing the risk of left ventricular hypertrophy, cardiac arrhythmias, and congestive heart failure.[17] They exacerbate tardive dyskinesia and other choreas and also can precipitate manic attacks in patients with bipolar disorders.[57]

A major side effect from tricyclic antidepressants that deserves special attention is their capacity for producing episodes of orthostatic hypotension. Many elderly individuals suffer from idiopathic orthostatic hypotension secondary to cardiovascular impairment; in others orthostatic hypotension is secondary to medication they are using to control symptoms of other diseases. To superimpose still another drug onto a regimen that has a known potential for producing orthostatic episodes increases the risk of stroke, myocardial infarction, and other syndromes resulting from low perfusion pressure. Additionally, if the orthostatic episode produces significant dizziness when the patient rises from a lying to a standing position, falls and subsequent fractures are major risks in the elderly. The dizziness may also contribute to a general loss of confidence or to fear regarding mobility.

If a patient experiences a pressure drop of 25 mm. Hg systolic and 10 mm. Hg diastolic when changing from a lying to a standing position, a reduction in dosage is indicated.[45] Moreover, tricyclic drugs are best administered in divided doses rather than as a single dose in the elderly, since side effects, particularly orthostatic hypotension, are associated with blood level peaks.

Because the elderly take large numbers of medications, the clinician should be aware of drug-drug interactions between tricyclic antidepressants and other drugs consumed by the elderly (Table 3–11). Tricyclics prolong central nervous system depression associated with alcohol, the barbiturates, sedative-hypnotics, antianxiety drugs, and antipsychotic drugs. The anticholinergic and orthostatic hypotensive activity of tricyclics also can be increased by antipsychotic drugs. The tricyclic antidepressants interfere with the antihypertensive effects of guanethidine (Ismelin) and other sympatholytic antihypertensives by blocking their uptake in the postganglionic adrenergic receptor sites.[17] The antihypertensives alpha-methyldopa (Aldomet) and reserpine can exacerbate depression, probably secondary to their central adrenergic properties.[17] Diuretics are effective and safe when used with the tricyclic antidepressants for the treatment of hypertension. Propranolol (Inderal) in combination with hydralazine (Apresoline) may be used in more refractory hypertensive patients, although high doses of propranolol may cause enough sedation to exacerbate depressive symptomatology.[17]

Toxicity. Intentional tricyclic overdosage is a major clinical problem. Overdosage and subsequent toxicity may be significantly curtailed by limiting prescriptions to 1.25 grams of amitriptyline or its equivalent. Acute overdosage produces extreme anticholinergic toxicity, which may be manifested as hyperpyrexia, respiratory depression, cardiac depression, cardiac arrhythmias, delirium, seizures, coma, or death.[58]

Treatment of overdosage is based on removal of the ingested drug via emesis or gastric lavage and supportive measures. Forced diuresis, hemodialysis, and peritoneal dialysis are of little value.[59] Supportive measures include correction of acidosis and support of body functions. Physostigmine may be useful in managing neurologic and cardiac symptoms. One to 3 mg. of physostigmine should be given

TABLE 3–11. Tricyclic Antidepressant Drug Interactions

Drug	Effect
Anticholinergics	Potentiation of anticholinergic (atropine-like) side effects
Anticoagulants Dicoumarol	Bioavailability increased, probably secondary to displacement from plasma protein
Antihistamines	Potentiation of anticholinergic (atropine-like) side effects
Antihypertensives Guanethidine Clonidine Reserpine Methyldopa	Partially block the antihypertensive effects of these drugs; additionally, reserpine and methyldopa alone may produce depression with chronic use
Antiparkinson drugs	Increase risk of anticholinergic (atropine-like) side effects and episodes of orthostatic hypotension
Central nervous system depressants Alcohol Barbiturates Nonbarbiturates Sedative-hypnotics Minor tranquilizers Major tranquilizers	Potentiation of sedative properties; additionally, with chronic use, barbiturates may induce hepatic microsomal enzymes, which will enhance the metabolism of tricyclic antidepressants, thus decreasing the plasma level of tricyclic antidepressants
Monoamine oxidase inhibitors	Hyperpyretic crises, severe convulsions, hypertensive episodes, and deaths have resulted from combined therapy
Phenothiazines	Increase risk of anticholinergic and orthostatic hypotensive episodes; inhibit metabolism of tricyclic antidepressants and may lead to increased tricyclic antidepressant plasma levels
Sympathomimetics	Potentiation of the effects of endogenous catecholamines; methylphenidate appears to inhibit the metabolism of tricyclic antidepressants, thus increasing plasma levels
Thyroid replacement drugs	Improve the clinical response to tricyclic antidepressants but may predispose to untoward cardiac effects such as tachycardia and cardiac arrhythmias

slowly by the intravenous route in increments of 0.5 mg. Because the duration of action of physostigmine is only one to two hours, the dose should be repeated as necessary.

Tetracyclic Antidepressants

Maprotiline (Ludiomil) was the first tetracyclic antidepressant to receive FDA approval.[60] It is indicated for use in the treatment of all types of mental depression or depressive mood disorders but does not appear to offer any compelling advantage over the tricyclic antidepressants.

The four ring composition of the tetracyclic structure produces a more rigid molecular arrangement alleged to have greater specificity and selectivity than tricyclic drugs. It has been postulated that maprotiline exerts its antidepressant and anxiolytic effects by preventing the re-uptake of norepinephrine at synaptic nerve junctions.

Maprotiline, available in 25 and 50 mg. tablets, is slowly and completely absorbed following oral administration. Its serum half-life is approximately two days. Maprotiline is slowly eliminated, principally as the glucuronide metabolite, about two-thirds of the dose appearing in the urine and one-third in the feces.

Except for a higher incidence of skin rashes, maprotiline causes adverse effects similar to those induced by the tricyclic drugs, such as psychiatric (e.g., nervousness, anxiety, insomnia, and agitation), neurologic (e.g., drowsiness, dizziness, tremor, headache, weakness, and fatigue), anticholinergic (e.g., dry mouth, constipation, nasal congestion, and blurred vision), and gastrointestinal symptoms (e.g., nausea). An optimal therapeutic response with a minimum of drug induced toxicity appears to occur when maprotiline blood levels reach 200 to 300 ng. per ml. Higher blood levels produce more pronounced and frequently occurring adverse effects, although nonlinear relationships between the blood levels of maprotiline, the clinical response, and drug induced toxicity have been reported.

Maprotiline is well tolerated by elderly patients.[61] Several controlled trials have failed to distinguish between the antidepressant efficacy and the side effects of maprotiline and amitriptyline or imipramine.

Maprotiline should not be administered within two weeks of treatment with monoamine oxidase inhibitors, for the drug-drug interaction may lead to serious hypertensive sequelae. Maprotiline may interfere with blood pressure control in hypertensive patients receiving treatment with adrenergic blocking drugs such as guanethidine.

Maprotiline should be used with caution in patients with hepatic or renal damage, glaucoma, prostatic hypertrophy, coronary artery disease, cardiac arrhythmias, and obstructive disorders of the urinary tract. A rare complication of maprotiline therapy, the development of grand mal seizures at normal therapeutic doses in patients with or without a history of seizure disorders, necessitates caution when the drug is given to individuals with known seizure disorders. Maprotiline, like other drugs having effects on the central nervous system, may impair the patient's coordination, reaction time, and ability to perform motor functions optimally. The drug may diminish alcohol tolerance.

The usual starting dosage for outpatients with mild to moderate depression is 75 mg. daily given as a single dose at night, or three 25 mg. divided doses. Two to three weeks of therapy is usually necessary before clinical improvement is seen. In more severe or resistant episodes of depression, an initial daily dosage of 150 mg. may be indicated. If a satisfactory response is not seen after three weeks of therapy, the dosage may be increased incrementally based on the needs and tolerance of the individual patient. Most patients respond to a dosage of 150 mg. per day. The recommended maintenance dosage is 75 to 150 mg. per day.

Trazodone Hydrochloride

Trazodone (Desyrel) represents a unique addition to management of depression. The precise mechanism by which the drug exerts its antidepressant action in humans has not been defined. In animals trazodone selectively inhibits serotonin uptake by brain synaptosomes and potentiates the behavioral changes induced by the precursor of serotonin, 5-hydroxytryptophan. Efficacy in managing depressed inpatients and outpatients with and without anxiety has been demonstrated. Approximately one-third of the inpatients and one-half of the outpatients treated with trazodone have a significant therapeutic response by the end of the first week of treatment. Three-fourths of all responders demonstrate a significant therapeutic effect by the end of the second week. In one-fourth of the responders two to four weeks is required to demonstrate a significant therapeutic response.

Trazodone is well absorbed orally. The drug is extensively metabolized in the liver, with less than 1 per cent excreted unchanged. Elimination is biphasic, with a half-life of three to six hours and five to nine hours respectively.

Trazodone is not recommended for use during the initial recovery phase of myocardial infarction. Numerous reports indicate that trazodone may induce cardiac arrhythmias in patients with pre-existing cardiac disease. If the drug is utilized in such patients, close cardiac monitoring is necessary. Trazodone may cause drowsiness, dizziness, or blurred vision, and outpatients should be cautioned about driving or performing other tasks requiring alertness, coordination, and dexterity. Patients with significant hepatic disease may require substantial dosage reductions because of impaired capacity to metabolize the drug.

Numerous interactions are possible between trazodone and other drugs. Central nervous system depression may be magnified substantially when trazodone is administered with alcohol, barbiturates, tranquilizers, and other depressants. Alcohol should be avoided and other depressant drugs administered with caution. Trazodone has been reported to increase serum levels of digoxin and phenytoin, but the clinical significance of these interactions has not been determined. Trazodone given alone may induce hypotension, and therefore, concurrent administration with antihypertensive drugs may necessitate a dosage reduction of antihypertensive medication.

Trazodone may cause dry mouth, blurred vision, dizziness, lightheadedness, drowsiness, irregular heart rhythm, shortness of breath, nausea, and vomiting. If these adverse effects occur, the physician should be notified. Other adverse effects, which occur rarely, include allergic skin disorders, syncope, hostility, nightmares, confusion, disorientation, headache, insomnia, decreased libido, anemia, decreased appetite, and various blood dyscrasias.

The manufacturer does not provide specific dosage guidelines for the elderly. The usual initial adult dosage is 150 mg. per day in divided doses taken shortly after meals or a light snack. This dosage may be increased by 50 mg. per day every three to four days. The maximal dosage for outpatients is 400 mg. per day in divided doses. Inpatients may receive up to 600 mg. per day. Such a dosage schedule may not be appropriate in the elderly. The physician may wish to initiate therapy at a daily dosage less than 150 mg. per day. The occurrence of drowsiness may require the administration of a major portion of the dosage at bedtime. Once an adequate response has been achieved the dosage may be gradually reduced, with subsequent adjustment based on clinical response.

Monoamine Oxidase Inhibitors

Monoamine oxidase is a complex enzyme system widely distributed throughout the body and is responsible for the metabolic decomposition of biogenic amines, thus terminating their activity. Drugs that inhibit this enzyme system, specifically monoamine oxidase inhibitors, cause an increase in the concentration of endogenous epinephrine, norepinephrine, and serotonin in storage sites throughout the nervous system.[5] It is believed that the increase in the concentration of monoamines in the central nervous system is the basis for their antidepressant activity.

The indications for treatment with monoamine oxidase inhibitors include atypical depression (patients with pananxiety, phobias, hypersomnolence, and hypochondriacal complaints associated with depression), failure to respond to tricyclic drugs, and a history of a response to monoamine oxidase inhibitors.[25] The monoamine oxidase inhibitors lack the cardiotoxic effects of the tricyclic drugs and offer a relative advantage in patients with heart disease and hypertension, provided these patients can be closely monitored (Table 3–12).

There are two classes of monoamine oxidase inhibitors available in the United States, the hydrazines—phenelzine (Nardil) and isocarboxazide (Marplan), and the nonhydrazine—tranylcypromine (Parnate). Another nonhydrazine, pargyline (Eutonyl), has been approved only as an antihypertensive. Because phenelzine has been more extensively studied and appears to be safer and more effective than the other monoamine oxidase inhibitors, it is considered the drug of choice in that class for the elderly.

In an extensive review of the literature, Klein and associates[25] found phenelzine to be superior to placebo in 10 of 11 studies. Ravaris and coworkers studied the inhibition of platelet monoamine oxidase as an index of brain monoamine oxidase inhibition.[62] They found that approximately 85 per cent inhibition of brain monoamine oxidase is needed before increases in platelet monoamines occur. They suggested that at least 60 mg. of phenelzine a day is required to achieve 85 per cent monoamine oxidase inhibition. In the elderly the starting dosage of phenelzine is 15 mg. three times daily, gradually increased to 60 mg. per day. Many patients may not show a response until four weeks after the initiation of treatment.

Side Effects. Both minor and serious side effects can be encountered with monoamine oxidase therapy. Common adverse reactions include orthostatic hypotension, disturbances in cardiac rhythm, dizziness, vertigo, constipation, headache, hyper-reflexia, tremors and muscle twitching, mania, hypomania, jitteriness, confusion and memory impairment, insomnia, edema, weakness, fatigue, drowsiness, dry mouth, blurred vision, hyperhidrosis, anorexia, and minor dermatologic reactions. Infrequent adverse effects include glaucoma, akathisia, ataxia, coma, dysuria, euphoria, hematologic changes, incontinence, neuritis, photosensitivity, sexual disturbances, urinary retention, nystagmus, hypernatremia, tachycardia, palpitations, chills, respiratory depression, leukopenia, reversible jaundice, hepatitis, acute anxiety reaction, and convulsions.

Most monoamine oxidase inhibitors reduce the amounts of intestinal monoamine oxidase, thus allowing increased concentrations of tyramine and other sympathomimetics to be absorbed. This mechanism is believed to contribute to the pathogenesis of the hypertensive crisis.[25] Patients taking monoamine oxidase inhibitors should avoid tyramine containing foods, such as cheese, wine, beer, yogurt, broad beans, unfresh meats, yeast, and pickled products. All sympathomimetic drugs, including nonprescription "cold" preparations containing decongestants, should be avoided. It is estimated that only 2 per cent of the patients being treated with monoamine oxidase inhibitors will develop headaches and 0.3 to 0.5 per cent hypertensive crises; death will occur in fewer than 0.001 per cent.[25] The death rate in monoamine oxidase treated patients is approximately one per 100,000, compared to one in 2000 cases treated with electroconvulsive therapy.[25]

If a patient is being switched from a tricyclic antidepressant, there should be a delay of at least seven to 10 days before beginning monoamine oxidase therapy in order to prevent severe interactions.[5] Combined tricyclic and monoamine oxidase therapy requires further investigation before it can be recommended for use in the elderly.[5]

Lithium. Although several studies have suggested that lithium can be used to treat

TABLE 3-12. General Characteristics of Monoamine Oxidase Inhibitors*

Precautions	Contraindications	Drug Interactions
Warn patient to:	Patients over 60 years of age	Alcohol: inhibits monoamine oxidase inhibitor (possible hypertensive crisis if beverage contains tyramine)
Report headache, dizziness or unusual symptoms immediately	Tricyclic drugs (concurrent use) Stop monoamine oxidase inhibitor a minimum of 14 days before beginning tricyclic antidepressants	
Avoid self-medication (including over-the-counter drugs like cold and sinus drugs and analgesics)	Amphetamines Sympathomimetic amines Hypertension	Sympathomimetic amine—potentiate amines, risk of hypertensive crisis
Avoid tyramine-containing foods—cheese, wine (especially sherry and Chianti), beer, pickled herring, yeast extracts, chicken liver, cream, chocolate, fava beans	Cardiovascular disease Cerebrovascular disease Headaches Pheochromocytoma Liver or advanced renal disease Quiescent schizophrenia	Anesthetics—increase central nervous system depression Anticholinergics—effect increased Antiparkinson drugs—potentiated Barbiturates—potentiated
Avoid excess amount of caffeine	Avoid combinations with dopa, amphetamines, hypoglycemics, alcohol, narcotics, diuretics, levodopa, meperidine, methyldopa, barbiturates, antiparkinson drugs, insulin, guanethidine, sympathomimetic amines, reserpine, anticholinergics, antihypertensives, antihistamines, hypnotics, other monoamine oxidase inhibitors, anesthetics, phenothiazines	Caffeine—hypertension
Also avoid Marmite, Bovril, yogurt, bee stings		Chloral hydrate—potentiated
Use analgesics in lower doses if needed		Chocolate—hypertension
Taper off when stopping		Cocaine—potentiated, hypertensive crisis
Safe use in pregnancy not yet established		Curare—effect increased
		Foods with tyramine†—hypertensive crisis
		Meperidine—hypotension potentiated, may inhibit monoamine oxidase inhibitor
Avoid drugs and foods that may interact with monoamine oxidase inhibitors for at least two weeks after discontinuation of monoamine oxidase inhibitors		Methyldopa (Aldomet)—hypertension, excitation; minor tranquilizers—potentiated
		Other monoamine oxidase inhibitors—additive
Possibility of lowered convulsive threshold in seizure disorders		Phenothiazines—potentiated, may inhibit monoamine oxidase inhibitors
		Thiazide diuretics—hypotension, potentiate monoamine oxidase inhibitors
		Tricyclic antidepressants—potentiate both, hyperpyretic crisis, convulsions, hypertensive episodes

*Adapted from Goldstein, B. J.: Drug therapy for the depressed patient. Hospital Formulary, December 1977.
†Foods high in tyramine content include aged cheeses, wines, beers, pickled herring, broad bean pods, chicken liver, and yeast extract.

acute depression and prevent recurrent attacks of depression, the Food and Drug Administration has yet to approve it for this use.[5,39] Kupfer and associates found that lithium responsive patients with unipolar depression had relatively normal premorbid personalities, whereas unipolar tricyclic responders showed every evidence of chronic anxiety and obsessiveness.[63] Depressed patients with a bipolar disorder (a history of mania) are more likely than those with unipolar depression to show an antidepressant response to lithium. Depressed lithium responders have a tendency to eat and sleep more under stress, have labile moods, and are more likely to have a family history of mania.[64]

Antipsychotic Drugs. In agitated depressed patients, especially those with paranoid ideation and somatic delusions, antipsychotic medications are the drugs of choice.[25] In an extensive review of the literature, Bielski and Friedel concluded that depressed patients with delusions fail to respond to tricyclic antidepressants.[65] Because high potency antipsychotic drugs produce less sedation and have fewer cardiovascular side effects, they may be the treatment of choice for delusionally depressed patients with serious medical illnesses.[5] On the other hand, Klein and associates suggested that the low potency antipsychotic drugs thioridazine and chlorpromazine (because of their sedative effects), are the treatment of choice for agitated depressed patients, with or without delusions.[25] The choice of an antipsychotic drug depends on clinical judgment and the needs of the individual patient.

Stimulant Drugs. The stimulant drugs amphetamine, methamphetamine, and methylphenidate are ineffective as antidepressants.[17] The stimulants carry a high risk of abuse and can induce paranoid psychosis, agitation, and confusion. Prolonged use can produce depression on withdrawal. Short term use of a stimulant medication might be helpful as a psychomotor activator in patients with mild anergy, but they should never be used to treat major depression in the elderly.[66]

Benzodiazepines. There is little evidence to support the usefulness of the benzodiazepines in the treatment of depressive symptoms. In studies comparing tricyclics and benzodiazepines, the benzodiazepines were never found to be superior.[25] Furthermore, the benzodiazepines have the potential for producing oversedation, confusion, concentration difficulties, and paradoxical angry outbursts.[17]

Electroconvulsive Therapy. Electroconvulsive therapy is a safe and effective treatment for depression, with marked improvement occurring in 80 to 90 per cent of the patients.[67] Electroconvulsive therapy is effective with many depressed patients who fail to respond to psychopharmacologic drugs, especially those with somatic delusions. However, because of recent legal issues and the possibility of increased confusion with electroconvulsive therapy in the elderly, the latter is recommended only if the patient is so severely depressed that food intake is inadequate to maintain life or the suicide risk is high and the use of drug therapy will take an unacceptably long period for a therapeutic response.[68]

The mortality associated with electroconvulsive therapy is approximately one per 100,000 patients treated, death generally being secondary to cardiac complications. Electroconvulsive therapy may be used following a myocardial infarction once electrocardiographic changes and cardiac enzyme levels have stabilized.[69] Patients with peptic ulcer, substernal hematoma, aortic aneurysm, and other conditions that might lead to hemorrhage tolerate electroconvulsive therapy when muscle relaxation is used.[70] Increased intracranial pressure is the only definite contraindication.[71]

The standard medical work-up includes the following laboratory procedures: electrocardiography, chest x-ray examination, electroencephalography, spinal x-ray studies (to assess the degree of osteoporosis), a complete blood count, and routine blood chemistry determinations.[67] Since there is some evidence that psychotropic drugs increase the cardiovascular complications of electroconvulsive therapy, these medications should be discontinued for one to three days prior to convulsive therapy, if possible.[69]

Technique. Approximately 15 minutes prior to electroconvulsive therapy the patient is given 0.6 to 1.0 mg. of atropine intramuscularly to decrease morbidity due to cardiac arrhythmias and aspiration. Just prior to electroconvulsive therapy the patient is sedated with an intravenous dose of 30 to 100 mg. of sodium methohexital (Brevital). To modify the motor aspects of a cerebral seizure, 30 to 80 mg. of succinylcholine (0.75 to 1.5 mg. per kg.) is given rapidly intravenously immediately after the onset of anesthesia. A few seconds later, muscle fasciculation will begin in the rostral portion of the body and move caudally. During this time it is recommended that the patient receive 100 per cent oxygen by bag inhalation. Once fasciculations in the feet diminish, a mouthpiece is inserted, the neck is extended, and the electrical stimulus is given. Generally the elderly have a higher seizure threshold than younger patients, and 130 volts of current for 0.1 to 0.5 second may be necessary. Oxygenation should be resumed following passage of the current and continued until the patient is able to breathe unassisted.[67]

A complete course of electroconvulsive therapy generally consists of six to eight seizures induced twice weekly. To decrease the possibility of memory impairment, treatments should be kept to a minimum, and with the first signs of improvement, the older patient can be switched to an antidepressant drug. Unilateral electroconvulsive therapy with the electrodes placed over the nondominant hemisphere reduces memory loss without significantly diminishing the efficacy of the treatment.[72]

Patients with a recent history of cardiac arrhythmias or myocardial infarction should be monitored with an electrocardiogram during treatment. In hypertensive patients, 5 mg. of diazepam given slowly intravenously may be used to replace pretreatment atropine. To prevent prolonged sleep following electroconvulsive therapy, elderly patients may require less barbiturate anesthesia. In elderly patients who are susceptible to pulmonary and cardiovascular complications, a subconvulsive stimulus to render the patient unconscious can be given instead of barbiturates just prior to the time the patient begins to experience respiratory distress from the succinylcholine.[70]

In patients with an increased susceptibility to fractures, doses up to 150 mg. of succinylcholine can be given without prolonged respiratory depression as long as the patient does not have a deficiency of pseudocholinesterase (which metabolizes succinylcholine). A genetic abnormality, liver disease, or cholinesterase inhibitors such as echothiophate (used to treat glaucoma) can produce a deficiency of pseudocholinesterase. In addition, the half-life of succinylcholine may be greatly increased by a number of medications, including quinidine, some antibiotics, phenelzine, and lithium carbonate.[67] Variations in succinylcholine metabolism may produce prolonged apneic states.

TREATMENT OF DEMENTIA

Dementia, characterized by a decrease in intellectual ability, memory loss, disorientation, and impaired judgment, is found in approximately 20 per cent of mental hospital first admissions and in 40 per cent of chronically hospitalized psychiatric patients.[73] In a review of the diagnoses in six studies of 417 patients fully evaluated for dementia, Wells postulated that 10 to 15 per cent of the patients with dementia have reversible illnesses.[74] For example, patients with normal pressure hydrocephalus, thyroid disease, benign intracranial masses, pernicious anemia, drug toxicity, and hepatic disease will respond to appropriate surgical or medical treatments. Another 25 to 30 per cent of demented patients have disorders that call for specific therapy. For example, patients with multi-infarct dementia respond, at least partially, to the reduction of hypertension. Patients with alcoholic deterioration benefit from abstinence from alcohol and improved nutrition. Those with neurosyphilis can be improved with adequate dosages of penicillin. Demented patients with secondary depression benefit from antidepressant medication. Indeed, many patients with depression characterized by social withdrawal, loss of energy, and apparent impairment of cognitive functioning are misdiagnosed as having dementia. Whenever depression is suspected, a therapeutic trial of antidepressants is indicated.[75]

In the study conducted by Wells, almost half the patients were found to have progressive idiopathic dementia (senile dementia).[74] Among the most important pharmacologic agents investigated for the treatment of senile dementia are the cerebral vasodilators, procaine solution, psychostimulants, the "nootropics," neuropeptides, and neurotransmitter precursors or agonists.[76]

Vasodilators

The original justification for the use of vasodilators in dementia was the assumption that arteriosclerotic narrowing was the primary cause of senile dementia. However, more recent findings indicate that senile dementia is a degenerative disease unrelated to cerebral blood flow. Many of the vasodilators are now postulated to exert their primary effects through metabolic enhancement or through their anxiolytic or antidepressant effects.[76]

Hyperbaric oxygen was suggested by Jacobs and associates for the treatment of dementia in 1969.[77] Since then a definitive double blind study of the procedure with 82 elderly outpatients who had senile dementia showed no significant difference in patients treated with hyperbaric oxygen when compared with patients placed in the chamber under normobaric conditions.[78]

Hydergine, consisting of three hydrogenated alkaloids of ergot, has been postulated to have a primary effect on ganglion cell metabolism. In experimental animals given hydergine, changes in the lactate-pyruvate ratio have been found, indicating improved oxygenation in the cells. This improved oxygenation in turn is believed to lead to a decrease in local edema with secondary improvement in the microcirculation. Placebo controlled studies have demonstrated improvement in mood, unsociability, confusion, recent memory, anxiety, initiative, dizziness, and levels of performance of self-care in the elderly treated with hydergine.[79] The usual dosage is a single 1 mg. oral tablet three times daily, although the dosage can range from 3.0 to 4.5 mg. daily. Hydergine should be given for at least three months before being deemed ineffective. Sinus bradycardia, nausea, and vomiting are rare complications.

Papaverine (Pavabid), 150 mg. twice daily, cyclandelate (Cyclospasmol), 800 to 1200 mg. daily, and isoxsuprine (Vasodilan), 10 to 20 mg. three to four times daily, have all been found superior to placebo in alleviating at least some symptoms in patients with senile dementia.[76] Side effects include nausea, rash, dizziness, headaches, flushing, and hypotension.[5] Carbonic anhydrase inhibitors, another group of substances that increase cerebral blood flow, may prove useful in treating senile dementia.[76]

Anticoagulants

In a review of the literature, Reisberg and associates found no well controlled studies demonstrating the usefulness of anticoagulants in the treatment of senile dementia.[76] The obvious hazards of long term anticoagulant therapy limit the utility of this treatment.

Procaine Solution

Gerovital H3, a procaine solution developed by Aslan in Romania, has been reported to improve memory, mobility, attention span, concentration, skin texture, and hair color, but the results have been inconsistent and the studies poorly controlled.[80] The clinical effect of procaine is believed to be secondary to its mild monoamine oxidase inhibiting properties.[81] Although procaine solution may be an effective antidepressant, there is no good evidence regarding its cognitive effects in senile dementia.[76]

Psychostimulants

Most adequately controlled studies of the stimulants dextroamphetamine, methylphenidate (Ritalin), and pentylenetetrazol (Metrazol) fail to substantiate the rationale for their use in the treatment of senile dementia.[76] The risk of drug dependency, paranoid reactions, accelerated heart rate, hypertension, anorexia, and irritability supersedes the possible benefits of these medications.

Nootropics

Piracetam (2-oxo-1-pyrrolidine acetamide), a cyclic derivative of gamma-aminobutyric acid, is an intriguing new compound with unique central nervous system effects, hence the term "nootropic." Piracetam is believed to enhance learning by improving the interhemispheric transfer of information.[76] Although Piracetam has definite effects on central nervous system activity, it does not possess any analgesic, sedative, antihistaminic, anticholinergic, antiserotonergic, or tranquilizing properties. Piracetam does not appear to have any effect on regional cerebral blood flow, and no peripheral effects have been demonstrated.[76]

Dimond and Brouwers found that students receiving Piracetam performed significantly better in learning measures than did control subjects.[82] Mindus and associates, in a double blind, intraindividual, crossover design study, found that individuals with subjective memory impairment who received Piracetam performed significantly better than control subjects in terms of a variety of cognitive variables.[83] Stegink found that elderly individuals with mild to moderate cognitive impairment had significant positive benefit in cognitive functioning when given Piracetam.[84] Individuals with severe dementia failed to respond to Piracetam. Piracetam may be the forerunner of a new pharmacologic class of compounds that may be useful in improving functioning in patients with mild to moderate senile dementia.[76]

Neuropeptides

The neuropeptides, ACTH, vasopressin, and enkephalins, have been shown to enhance learning.[76] Although animal studies have demonstrated that the heptapeptide $ACTH_{4-10}$ enhances conditioned avoidance behavior, current evidence does not indicate clinical utility in humans.[76] Legros and associates in a double blind study found that patients receiving vasopressin performed better on memory and nonmemory cognitive tasks.[85] The enkephalins, postulated neurotransmitters in certain central pathways, have been found to affect learning in rats.[86] Clearly, more studies of the cognitive effects of the neuropeptides are needed.

Neurotransmitters

Pathologic studies have revealed a widespread deficiency of the enzyme choline acetyltransferase in the brains of patients with senile dementia.[87-89] The possibility of a cholinergic deficit in senile dementia suggests that a diet rich in choline and lecithin may prove to be of benefit in patients with senile dementia, but as yet no long term dietary studies have been reported. Ferris and associates investigated the cholinomimetic drug, Deanol, in an open trial involving 14 patients with mild to moderate cognitive functioning: none of the patients showed improvement in cognitive functioning.[90] In another study no improvement in cognitive function was found in patients taking up to 20 grams of choline chloride daily.[91]

Antipsychotic Drugs

Acute episodes of agitation and restlessness associated with senile dementia can be controlled with the judicious use of antipsychotic drugs.[5] Haloperidol, with the fewest anticholinergic side effects, is probably the antipsychotic drug of choice in senile patients with agitation. The starting dose of 0.5 mg. once or twice daily can be gradually increased until symptoms are controlled.

TREATMENT OF ALCOHOL WITHDRAWAL

Alcoholism accounts for 12 per cent of elderly male and 4 per cent of elderly female admissions to inpatient psychiatric facilities.[5] The treatment of alcohol withdrawal in the elderly is essentially the same as that in the normal aged population. In all patients immediate administration of thiamine, 100 to 200 mg. intramuscularly or intravenously, should be undertaken to prevent irreversible brain damage. Doses of 100 mg. of thiamine are repeated, orally or parenterally, for at least the next three consecutive days.[92] In addition, all patients should receive folic acid, 1 to 5 mg. daily, orally or intramuscularly. Finally, a daily multivitamin supplement should be given. Five to 10 mg. of vitamin K can be given in a single parenteral dose if the prothrombin time is prolonged more than three seconds beyond the control value.[92] Diazepam, 5 to 10 mg. two to three times daily, or chlordiazepoxide, 10 to 25 mg. two to three times daily, can be used for sedation and to prevent delirium tremens. Therapy must be carefully individualized and titrated; the cumulative effects and long duration of action of diazepam and chlordiazepoxide must be kept in mind. Fluid and electrolyte deficits should be corrected as indicated, with no more than 50 per cent of the initial deficit replaced in the first 24 hours. Because elderly patients tolerate a mild degree of volume depletion much better than overhydration, the physician should use extreme caution when administering parenteral fluid.[92]

Because most alcoholic patients are magnesium depleted regardless of serum concentrations, withdrawing alcoholics should receive 2 to 4 ml. of 50 per cent magnesium sulfate intramuscularly every eight hours for at least three doses.[92] Patients who are known to have grand mal seizures with alcohol withdrawal can be given anticonvulsants prophylactically. A patient known to have had seizures who has not been given maintenance therapy with anticonvulsants for five days prior to admission requires a loading dose of phenytoin (Dilantin). One gram of Dilantin should be added to 500 ml. of 5 per cent dextrose in water and given by continuous intravenous infusion over a four hour period. After the loading dose, most patients require 300 to 400 mg. of Dilantin per day in divided oral doses to maintain daily effective serum concentrations of 10 to 20 mcg. per ml.[92] Antipsychotic drugs should be used with extreme caution and given only if necessary to control hallucinations, frightening delusions, or agitation.[5]

TREATMENT OF ANXIETY

Anxiety, one of the most frequent diagnoses made in general medical practice, is a complicating factor in the illnesses of at least 30 to 40 per cent of all patients.[93] Anxiety is characterized by tremulousness, fatigue, inability to relax, sweating, dizziness, palpitations, and apprehensive expectation marked by rumination or worry. Numerous medical conditions can mimic anxiety, including cardiovascular disorders, respiratory disorders, metabolic and hormonal disorders, nutritional disorders, and drug or alcohol intoxication. The most difficult differential is between anxiety and depression. A patient who complains of anxiety but who has biologic signs of depression (for example, anorexia with a change in weight, sleep disturbance, decreased sex drive, and decreased energy) should undergo a therapeutic trial of antidepressants.

The treatment of anxiety involves a wide range of procedures, including behavioral therapy, goal directed psychotherapy, psychodynamic psychotherapy, and drug therapy. Medications should be used only as adjuncts to psychotherapy, and the duration of drug therapy should be limited to one to two weeks. When prescribing antianxiety medications, the clinician should be mindful that moderate levels of anxiety stimulate adaptive functions necessary to cope successfully with problems. Extreme caution should be taken to avoid hindering these adaptive forces with medications.

Benzodiazepines

Benzodiazepines are the most frequently prescribed medications in the United States. Approximately 100 million prescriptions are written each year in the United States for chlordiazepoxide (Librium) and diazepam (Valium), at a cost approaching $500 million annually.[17]

The benzodiazepines selectively depress the limbic system, sparing the cerebral cortex and the reticular activating system so that sedative side effects are much less than those with the barbiturates. Table 3–13 summarizes

TABLE 3–13. Selected Pharmacokinetic Characteristics of Benzodiazepines*

Drug	Equivalent Dose (Mg.)[1]	Peak Plasma Level (Hours)[2]	Elimination t½ (Hours)	Metabolites
Oxazepam (Serax)	15.0	2–4	5–20	Inactive glucuronide
Lorazepam (Ativan)	1.0	2.5	10–15	Inactive glucuronide
Chlordiazepoxide (Librium)	10.0	1–4	5–30	Desmethylchlodiazepoxide (M) Demoxepam Desmethyldiazepam
Diazepam (Valium)	5.0	1–2	20–50	Desmethyldiazepam (M) Temazepam
Prazepam (Centrax)	10.0	6	30–100[1]	Desmethyldiazepam
Clorazepate (Tranxene)			30–100[3]	Desmethyldiazepam
Dipotassium	7.5	—		
Alprazolam (Xanax)	0.5	1–2	12–15	Alphahydroxyalprazolam Benzophenone
Halazepam (Paxipam)	40	1–3	14	Desmethyldiazepam (M) 3-Hydroxyhalazepam

*Reprinted with permission from Facts and Comparisons, 1982, p. 261.
[1]Estimated values; patient response is variable.
[2]Oral administration.
[3]Half-life of desmethyldiazepam, the active metabolite of the drug.
M = major metabolite.

the major pharmacokinetic variables of the benzodiazepines. The benzodiazepines are rapidly absorbed after oral administration. With the exception of oxazepam and lorazepam, they are converted to active metabolites in the liver. Intramuscular absorption of the benzodiazepines can be slow and unpredictable because of the tendency of these medications to accumulate in the tissues.[94] Diazepam, with a marked tendency to accumulate in the fat tissue, has an elimination half-life of 20 to 50 hours. In the general population chlordiazepoxide has a half-life of five to 30 hours, but preliminary studies indicate that its half-life may be much longer in the elderly. Clorazepate has a half-life of 30 to 100 hours in the general population.[95] Because oxazepam has no active metabolites or tendency to accumulate in the tissues, this drug may be safer for use in the elderly, although few patients over age 65 have been studied. Shader and Greenblatt report the half-life of oxazepam to be five to 20 hours.[95] Reidenberg reported that plasma levels of diazepam were inversely correlated with age and that the elderly were more sensitive to the sedative and depressant effects of diazepam.[96]

Because of the extremely long half-life of chlordiazepoxide, diazepam, and clorazepate, the medications need not be taken any more often than once or twice daily. Oxazepam can be given three times daily because of its shorter period of activity. A reasonable starting dose of diazepam in the elderly would be 2 mg. at bedtime. Alternatively 3.75 mg. of clorazepate given at bedtime or 5 mg. of chlordiazepoxide at bedtime can be given. The elderly generally tolerate 10 mg. of oxazepam twice daily.[5]

The major side effects of the benzodiazepines are drowsiness, ataxia, headache, and lethargy. The sedative effects of the benzodiazepines can easily produce confusion in elderly individuals. Paradoxical reactions, common in the elderly, include hallucinations, agitation, insomnia, and rage.[5] In addition, the sedative-hypnotics, alcohol, narcotics, antipsychotics, and antidepressants mutually potentiate the benzodiazepines.[5] In rare cases, overdoses of a benzodiazepine equivalent to a two week supply have resulted in death, especially when they have been combined with some other medication.[17] Withdrawal from large doses of benzodiazepines can produce shakiness, anxiety, insomnia, nightmares, and, if the benzodiazepines have been taken in large doses for a prolonged period of time, seizures.[17]

Propranolol

Propranolol (Inderal) is a beta-adrenergic blocking drug that can effectively control the somatic symptoms of anxiety, although it has not been approved by the Food and Drug Administration for this use. Suzman studied 725 patients with anxiety marked by tremor, palpitations, headache, hyperventilation, and muscular weakness.[97] Therapy was initiated with 40 to 80 mg. of propranolol daily in four divided doses, and the dosage was gradually increased to control symptoms. Generally 80 to 320 mg. of propranolol was needed to control the somatic symptoms of anxiety.

Contraindications to the use of propranolol include obstructive pulmonary disease, asthma, congestive heart failure, heart block, and allergic rhinitis. Depression is a common psychiatric complication of propranolol treatment.[98]

Tricyclic Antidepressants

Two recent studies reviewed the treatment of panic and phobic disorders: the tricyclic antidepressant, imipramine, was compared with placebo and behavioral therapy.[99,100] Imipramine, in initial doses of 25 mg. before bedtime gradually increased to 150 mg. at bedtime, was found to be significantly more effective than the other treatment methods. In the elderly, dosages of imipramine greater than 100 mg. daily should be carefully monitored with plasma levels.[5]

Other Medications

The barbiturates, because of their potential for producing mental confusion and oversedation, are not recommended in elderly patients. In addition, the barbiturates have a high abuse potential and a propensity to produce paradoxical agitation in the elderly.[5] Lethal overdosage is not uncommon. The barbiturates increase liver enzyme activity, resulting in increased metabolism of steroids, the tricyclic antidepressants, and warfarin.[17]

The propanediols (meprobamate-like drugs) have no place in modern drug treatment of anxiety disorders. The propanediols produce psychologic and physical dependence, as well as inducing hepatic enzymes.[5] The addicting dose of meprobamate overlaps the therapeutic dose.[17] As with the barbiturates, the propanediols are not recommended in the elderly.

TREATMENT OF SLEEP DISORDERS

Between 12 and 15 per cent of the population in the United States—approximately 30,000,000 people—have sleep complaints.[101] The average sleep time in young adults is seven hours and 45 minutes, while the minimal sleep requirement appears to be about four to five hours at night.[102] Sleep efficiency, total sleep time, and the amount of REM sleep decrease as people age.[102]

Many elderly individuals are convinced that they have insomnia because they feel they should be sleeping as much as in former years. Normal aging is associated with decreased sleep time, an increased number of awakenings during the night, decreased deep sleep, and a decrease in REM sleep. In some elderly patients merely informing them that the expected sleep quantity and quality decrease with age may help them adjust to their misperception of sleep requirement.

Because there are a wide variety of causes of sleep disturbance, including drug dependency insomnia, conditioned sleep disturbance, phase lag syndrome, stimulation overload, nocturnal myoclonus, sleep apnea, depression, and dream disturbances, the clinician should perform a thorough diagnostic examination prior to prescribing medication. The treatment of sleep disorders consists of more than prescribing a mild sedative, and a discussion of the numerous therapeutic modalities is beyond the scope of this chapter. Suffice it to say that sedatives should be used only for the short term treatment of situational insomnia.

Flurazepam (Dalmane), temazepam (Restoril), and triazolam (Halcion) are the drugs of choice. In the elderly an initial dose of 15 mg. of flurazepam or temazepam at bedtime increased to 30 mg. if necessary is appropriate. In the elderly triazolam should be administered at a dose of 0.125 mg. before retiring and adjusted up to 0.25 mg. at bedtime if necessary. According to most studies, REM sleep is relatively unimpaired in dosages recommended by the manufacturers and approved by the Food and Drug Administration. These three drugs do possess the potential for producing the side effects of the other benzodiazepines.[5] The antihistamines, diphenhydramine (Benadryl), 25 to 50 mg. at bedtime, and hydroxyzine (Atarax), 10 to 25 mg. at bedtime, have sedative properties; these drugs, however, can cause acute toxic delusions secondary to their anticholinergic properties. Chloral hydrate, in doses of 500 mg. to 1 gram, has sedative effects but can produce gastric irritation. Chloral hydrate also potentiates the effects of Coumadin, and some studies suggest that it depresses REM sleep.[5] The hypnotics, glutethimide (Doriden), ethchlorvynol (Placidyl), and methaqualone (Quaalude), and the barbiturates are contraindicated as long term sleep aids in the elderly. In addition to having the potential for habituation and abuse, these drugs can cause confusional reactions and depress cardiac and respiratory functions.

Withdrawal from sedative-hypnotics should be done gradually to prevent REM rebound, nightmares, agitation, and seizures. The medication can be reduced in increments of one-tenth the daily dosage until the drug is completely withdrawn.[5]

CONCLUSION

The clinician who prudently applies his general knowledge of psychopharmacology can avoid most of the therapeutic dilemmas associated with overmedication, subtherapeutic treatment, drug toxicity, and polypharmaceutical use. Knowledge of drug therapy will enable the clinician to better assist the elderly patient's adjustment to the psychiatric problems of older life with optimal therapeutic outcomes and minimal drug induced morbidity.

REFERENCES

1. Eisdorfer, C., and Fann, W. (Editors): Psychopharmacology and Aging. New York, Plenum Press, 1973.
2. Maddox, G., et al.: Report to the Community on Durham's Elderly by the Older Americans Resources and Science Program. (Unpublished material.)
3. Prien, R.F.: A survey of psychoactive drug use in the aged at Veterans Administration hospitals. In Gershon, S., and Raskin, D. (Editors): Aging. New York, Raven Press, 1975, pp. 143–154.
4. Physician's drug prescribing patterns in the skilled nursing facilities: Long-term facility campaign. Monograph No. 2. DHEW Publication No. 76–50050. Washington, D.C., U.S. Government Printing Office, 1976.
5. Walker, J.I., and Brodie, H.K.H.: Neuropharmacology of aging. In Busse, E.W., and Blazer, D.G. (Editors): Handbook of Geriatric Psychiatry. New York, Van Nostrand Reinhold Co., 1980, pp. 102–124.

6. Verwoerdt, A.: Clinical Geropsychiatry. Baltimore, The Williams & Wilkins, Co., 1976.
7. Bender, D.: The effect of increasing age on the distribution of peripheral blood flow in man. J. Am. Geriatr. Soc., *13:*192–198, 1965.
8. Holloway D.: Drug problems in the geriatric patient. Drug Intell. Clin. Pharm., *8:*632–642, 1974.
9. Meier-Ruge W., et al.: Experimental pathology in the aging brain. *In* Gershon, S., and Raskin, M. (Editors): Aging. New York, Raven Press, 1975, pp. 55–126.
10. Nies A., et al: Changes in monoamine oxidase with aging. *In* Eisdorfer, C., and Fann, W. (Editors): Psychopharmacology and Aging. New York, Plenum Press, 1973, pp. 41–54.
11. Fann, W.: Pharmacotherapy in older depressed patients. J. Gerontol., *31:*304, 1976.
12. Blazer, D.: The epidemiology of mental illness in late life. *In* Busse, E.W., and Blazer, D.G. (Editors): Handbook of Geriatric Psychiatry. New York, Van Nostrand Reinhold Co., 1980, pp. 249–271.
13. Eisdorfer, C.: Paranoid and schizophrenia disorders in later life. *In* Busse, E.W., and Blazer, D.G. (Editors): Handbook of Geriatric Psychiatry. New York, Van Nostrand Reinhold Co., 1980, pp. 329–337.
14. Post, F.: Paranoid disorders in the elderly. Postgrad. Med., *53:*52, 1973.
15. Kay, D.W.K., and Roth, M.: Environmental and hereditary factors in the schizophrenia of old age late paraphrenia and their bearing on the general problem of causation in schizophrenia. J. Ment. Sci., *107:*649–686, 1961.
16. American Psychiatric Association: Diagnostic and Statistical Manual of Mental Disorders, Ed. 3. Washington, D.C., American Psychiatric Association, 1980.
17. Baldessarini, R.J.: Chemotherapy in Psychiatry. Cambridge, Harvard University Press, 1977.
18. Kastrup, E.K., and Boyd, J.R. (Editors): Antipsychotic agents. Facts Comparisons, p. 265a, March, 1981.
19. Crane, G.E.: Prevention and management of tardive dyskinesia. Am. J. Psychiatry, *129:*126–127, 1972.
20. Gardos, G., and Cole, J.O.: Maintenance antipsychotic therapy: is the treatment worse than the disease? Am. J. Psychiatry, *133:*32–36, 1976.
21. Prien, R.F., Haber, P.A., and Caffey, E.M.: The use of psychoactive drugs in elderly patients with psychiatric disorders: survey conducted in 12 Veterans Administration hospitals. J. Am. Geriatr. Soc., *23:*104–112, 1975.
22. Branchey, M.H., et al.: High and low potency neuroleptics in elderly psychiatric patients. J.A.M.A., *239:*1860–1867, 1978.
23. Stotsky, B.: Psychoactive drugs for geriatric patients with psychiatric disorders. *In* Gershon, S., and Raskin, D. (Editors): Aging. New York, Raven Press, 1975, Vol. 2, pp. 229–253.
24. Shader, R., and Jackson, A.: Approaches to schizophrenia. *In* Shader, R. (Editor): Manual of Psychiatric Therapeutics. Boston, Little, Brown and Company, 1975, pp. 63–101.
25. Klein, D.F., Gittelman, R., Quitkin, F., and Rifkin, A.: Diagnosis and Drug Treatment of Psychiatric Disorders: Adults and Children. Ed. 2. Baltimore, The Williams & Wilkins Co., 1980.
26. Friedel, R.: Norepinephrine, dopamine and serotonin: CNS distribution biosynthesis and metabolism. *In* Eisdorfer, C., and Fann, W. (Editors): Psychopharmacology and Aging. New York, Plenum Press, 1973, pp. 11–16.
27. Eadie, M.J.: Tardive Dyskinesia. Med. J. Australia, *1:*682–683, 1977.
28. Kobarjashi, R.M.: Drug therapy of tardive dyskinesia. N. Engl. J. Med., *296:*257–260, 1977.
29. American College of Neuropsychopharmacology—Food and Drug Administration Task Force: Drug therapy; neurological syndromes associated with antipsychotic drug use. N. Engl. J. Med., *289:*20–23, 1973.
30. Malletta, G.J.: The use of psychotropic drugs in the older patient, with particular emphasis on the antipsychotics. *In* Malletta G., and Pirozzola, F. (Editors): The Aging Nervous System. New York, Praeger Publishers, 1980.
31. Borison, R.L.: Thioridazine and extrapyramidal syndrome evidence for site specificity. Lecture presented to the Duke University Department of Psychiatry, Durham, North Carolina, September 18, 1980.
32. Prange, A.J., Lipton, M., and Wilson, I.: Clinical intimations of amine balance and permission. Psychopharmacol. Bull., *10:*53–54, 1974.
33. Klawans, H.L., and Rubovits, R.: Effects of cholinergic and anticholinergic agents on tardive dyskinesia. J. Neurol. Neurosurg. Psychiatry, *37:*941–947, 1974.
34. Klawans, H.L.: The pharmacology of tardive dyskinesia. Am. J. Psychiatry, *120:*82–86, 1973.
35. Crane, G.E.: Pseudoparkinsonism and tardive dyskinesia. Arch. Neurol., *27:*426–430, 1972.
36. Fann, W., and Shannon, I.: A treatment for dry mouth in psychiatric patients. Am. J. Psychiatry, *135:*251–252, 1978.
37. Heisman, E.M.: Cardiac toxicity with thioridazine-tricyclic antidepressant combination. J. Nerv. Ment. Dis., *165:*139–143, 1977.
38. Leroyd, B.: Psychotropic drugs in the aging population. Med. J. Australia, *11:*1131, 1973.
39. Walker, J.I., and Brodie, H.K.H.: Current concepts of lithium treatment and prophylaxis. J. Cont. Ed. Psychiatry, *39:*19–30, 1978.
40. Gershon, S.: Lithium. *In* Arieti, S. (Editor): American Handbook of Psychiatry. Ed. 2. New York, Basic Books, 1975, Vol. 1, pp. 490–513.
41. Hestbeck, J., Hansen, I.T., Amdisen, A., and Olsen, S.: Chronic renal lesions following long-term treatment with lithium. Kidney Int., *12:*205–213, 1977.
42. Weissman, M.M., and Myers, J.K.: Affective disorders in a U.S. community: the use of research diagnostic criteria in an epidemiological survey. Arch. Gen. Psychiatry, *35:*1304–1311, 1978.
43. Ban, T.A.: Treatment of depressed geriatric patients. Am. J. Psychother., *27:*93–104, 1978.
44. Hirschfeld, R.M.A., and Klerman, G.L.: Treatment of depression in the elderly. Geriatrics, *34:*51–57, 1979.
45. Blumenthal, M.D.: Depressive illness in old age: getting behind the mask. Geriatrics, *35:*34–43, 1980.
46. Roth, M.: The psychiatric disorders of later life. Psychiatr. Ann., *6:*417–445, 1976.
47. Bielski, R.J., and Friedel, R.O.: Prediction of tricyclic antidepressant response: a critical review. Arch. Gen. Psychiatry, *33:*1479–1489, 1976.
48. Maas, J.W.: Biogenic amines and depression: biochemical and pharmacological separation of two types of depression. Arch. Gen. Psychiatry, *32:*1357–1361, 1975.
49. Nies, A.: Relationship between age and tricyclic antidepressant plasma levels. Am. J. Psychiatry, *134:*790–793, 1977.

50. Ayd, F.J.: Amoxapine: a new tricyclic antidepressant. Int. Drug Ther. News., *10*, November/December 1980.
51. Settle, E.C., and Ayd, F.J.: Trimipramine: twenty years' worldwide clinical experience. J. Clin. Psychiatry, *41*:266–274, 1980.
52. Friedel, R., and Raskin, D.: Relationship of blood levels of Sinequan to clinical effects in the treatment of depression in the aged patients. *In* Mendels (Editor): Sinequan: A Monograph of Recent Clinical Studies. pp. 51–53.
53. Klerman, G.L.: Long-term treatment of affective disorders. *In* Lipton, M.A., DiMascio, A., and Killam, K.F. (Editors): Psychopharmacology: A Generation of Progress. New York, Raven Press, 1978, pp. 1303–1312.
54. Brunswick, O.J., and Mendels, J.: Reduced levels of tricyclic antidepressants in plasma from vacutainers. Commun. Psychopharmacol., *1*:131–134, 1977.
55. Kastrup, E.K., and Boyd, J.R.: Facts and Comparisons. St. Louis, Facts and Comparisons Inc., 1981, p. 263a.
56. Davies, R.K.: Confusional episodes and antidepressant medication. Am. J. Psychiatry, *128*:95–99, 1971.
57. Salzman, C., Shader, R., and Van der Kolk, B.: Clinical psychopharmacology in the elderly patient. N.Y. State J. Med., *76*:71–77, 1976.
58. Hollister, L.E.: Tricyclic antidepressants. N. Engl. J. Med., *299*:1101–1108, 1978.
59. Fischer, J.M., and Kroboth, P.D.: Update: tricyclic antidepressant therapy. U.S. Pharmacist, *4*:42, 1980.
60. New Drugs/Drug News. Drug Ther., *2*:40, 1981.
61. Kastrup, E.K., and Boyd, J.R.: Facts and Comparisons. St. Louis, Facts and Comparisons, Inc., 1981, p. 263d.
62. Ravaris, C.L., Nies, A., Robinson, D.S., Ives, J.O., Lamborn, K.R., and Korson, L.: A multiple-dose controlled study of phenelzine in depression-anxiety states. Arch. Gen. Psychiatry, *33*:347–350, 1976.
63. Kupfer, D.J., et al.: Are there two major types of unipolar depression? Arch. Gen. Psychiatry, *32*:866–871, 1975.
64. Stern, S.L., Rush, J.A., and Mendels, J.: Toward a rational pharmacotherapy of depression. Am. J. Psychiatry, *137*:545–552, 1980.
65. Bielski, R.J., and Friedel, R.D.: Predictions of tricyclic antidepressant response. Arch. Gen. Psychiatry, *33*:1479–1489, 1976.
66. Fann, W., and Wheless, J.: Depression in elderly patients. South. Med. J., *68*:468–473, 1975.
67. Weiner, R.D.: The psychiatric use of electrically induced seizures. Am. J. Psychiatry, *136*:1507–1517, 1979.
68. American Psychiatric Association: Task Force Report 14. Electroconvulsive Therapy. Washington, D.C., American Psychiatric Association, 1978.
69. Salzman, C.: Electroconvulsive therapy. *In* Shader, R. (Editor): Manual of Psychiatric Therapeutics. Boston, Little, Brown and Company, 1975, pp. 115–124.
70. Kalinowsky, L.B.: The convulsive therapies. *In* Freedman, Kaplan, and Sadock (Editors): Comprehensive Textbook of Psychiatry, Ed. 2. Baltimore, The Williams & Wilkins Co., 1975, Vol. 3, pp. 1969–1976.
71. Dressler, D., and Folk, J.: The treatment of depression with ECT in the presence of brain tumor. Am. J. Psychiatry, *132*:1320–1321, 1975.
72. Squire, L.: ECT and memory loss. Am. J. Psychiatry, *134*:997–1001, 1977.
73. National Institutes of Mental Health: Patients in Mental Institutions. Washington, D.C., U.S. Government Printing Office, 1964, Vol. 2.
74. Wells, C.E.: Diagnosis of dementia. Psychosomatics, *20*:517–522, 1979.
75. Walker, J.I.: Clinical Psychiatry in Primary Care. Menlo Park, California, Addison-Wesley Publishing Co., Inc., 1981.
76. Reisberg, B., Ferris, S.H., and Gershon, S.: An overview of pharmacologic treatment of cognitive decline in the aged. Am. J. Psychiatry, *138*:593–600, 1981.
77. Jacobs, E.A., et al.: Hyperoxygenation effects on cognitive functioning in the aged. N. Engl. J. Med., *281*:753–757, 1969.
78. Raskin, A.S., et al.: The effects of hyperbaric and normobaric oxygen on cognitive impairment in the elderly. Arch. Gen. Psychiatry, *35*:50–56, 1978.
79. Gaitz, C.M., Varner, R.V., and Overall, J.E.: Pharmacotherapy for organic brain syndrome in later life. Arch. Gen. Psychiatry, *34*:839–845, 1977.
80. Aslan, A.: Theoretical and practical aspects of chemotherapeutic techniques in the retardation of the aging process. *In* Rockstein, M. (Editor): Theoretical Aspects of Aging. New York, Academic Press, Inc., 1974.
81. Jarvik, L.F., and Milne, J.F.: Gerovital H3: a review of the literature. *In* Gershon, S., Raskin, D. (Editors): Aging. New York, Raven Press, 1975, Vol. 2, pp. 203–223.
82. Dimond, S.J., and Brouwers, E.Y.M.: Increase in the power of human memory in normal man through the use of drugs. Psychopharmacology (Berlin), *49*:307–309, 1976.
83. Mindus, P., et al.: Piracetam induced improvement of mental performance: a controlled study on normally aging individuals. Acta Psychiatr. Scand., *54*:150–160, 1976.
84. Stegink, A.J.: The clinical use of Piracetam, a new nootropic drug: the treatment of symptoms of senile involution. Arzneimittelforsch., *22*:975–977, 1972.
85. Legros, J.J., et al.: Influence of vasopressin on learning and memory. (Letter to the Editor.) Lancet *1*:41–42, 1978.
86. Rigter, H.: Attenuation of amnesia in rats by systemically administered enkephalin. Science, *200*:83–85, 1978.
87. Bowen, D.M., et al.: Neurotransmitter related enzymes and indices of hypoxia in senile dementia and other abiotrophies. Brain, *99*:459–496, 1976.
88. Davies, P., and Maloney, A.J.F.: Selective loss of central cholinergic neurons in Alzheimer's disease. Lancet, *2*:1403, 1976.
89. Perry, E.K., et al.: Neurotransmitter enzyme abnormality in senile dementia: cholineacetyltransferase and glutamic and decarboxylase activities in necropsy brain tissue. J. Neurol. Sci., *34*:347–365, 1977.
90. Ferris, S.H., et al.: Senile dementia: treatment with Deanol. J. Am. Geriatr. Soc., *25*:241–244, 1977.
91. Ferris, S.H., et al.: Long-term choline treatment of memory impaired elderly patients. Science *205*:1039–1040, 1979.
92. Greenblatt, D., and Shader, R.: Treatment of alcohol withdrawal syndrome. *In* Shader, R. (Editor): Manual of Psychiatric Therapeutics. Boston, Little, Brown and Company, 1975, pp. 211–236.

93. Kolb, L.C.: Modern Clinical Psychiatry. Ed. 9. Philadelphia, W.B. Saunders Company, 1977.
94. Greenblatt, D.J.: Slow absorption of intramuscular chlorodiazepoxide. N. Engl. J. Med., *291*:1116–1118, 1974.
95. Shader, R., and Greenblatt, D.J.: Clinical implications of benzodiazepine pharmacokinetics. Am. J. Psychiatry, *134*:652–656, 1977.
96. Reidenberg, M.M.: Relationship between diazepam dose, plasma level, age, and central nervous system depression. Clin. Pharmacol. Ther., *23*:371–374, 1978.
97. Suzman, N.M.: Propranolol in the treatment of anxiety. Postgrad. Med., J., *52*:168–174, 1976.
98. Waal, H.J.: Propranolol induced depression. Br. Med. J., *2*:50, 1967.
99. Zitrin, C.M., Klein, D.F., and Woerner, M.G.: Behavioral therapy, supportive psychotherapy, imipramine and phobias. Arch. Gen. Psychiatry, *35*:307–316, 1978.
100. Sheehen, D.V., Ballenger, J., and Jacobson, G.: Treatment of endogenous anxiety with phobic, hysterical, and hypochondriacal symptoms. Arch. Gen. Psychiatry, *37*:51–59, 1980.
101. Dement, W.L.: Normal sleep and sleep disorders. *In* Usdin, G., and Lewis, J.M. (Editors): Psychiatry in General Practice. New York, McGraw-Hill, Inc., 1979.
102. Walker, J.I., and Cavenar, J.O.: Sleep disorders. *In* Cavenar, J.O., and Brodie, H.K.H. (Editors): Signs and Symptoms in Psychiatry. Philadelphia, J.B. Lippincott Company, 1982.

CHAPTER 4

PULMONARY DISEASES AND DISORDERS OF RESPIRATION

Carl B. Sherter, Charles C. Depew, and Richard A. Matthay

Elderly patients are subject to the entire spectrum of respiratory diseases, and secondary factors related to the aging process and coexisting disorders make this population even more susceptible to respiratory disorders, particularly respiratory infections and chronic obstructive lung disease. Several factors may contribute to an increased susceptibility to respiratory diseases. These include age related physiologic alteration in the lung, a decrease in mucociliary clearance, probable decline in immune function, and the frequent presence of other pulmonary diseases. These factors should be kept in mind as the physician evaluates respiratory disease in elderly patients.

OBSTRUCTIVE AIRWAY DISEASES

The elderly population is subject to many chronic ailments. Obstructive airway diseases account for a significant number of these chronic disabilities. The elderly patient who has mild asthma and is otherwise healthy can be treated like any other patient with mild asthma regardless of age. The patient with moderate to severe obstructive airway disease who also has cardiac disease, liver disease, or other major illnesses must be given special therapeutic considerations. These diseases can alter drug disposition and response and increase the risk of adverse drug reactions. These special considerations include not only the foregoing but also the choice of drug, ease of drug administration, drug cost, and nondrug treatment.

The obstructive airway diseases include asthma, chronic bronchitis, and pulmonary emphysema. The usual patient presents with a mixed disorder, e.g., chronic bronchitis accompanied by acute exacerbations of asthma. Although the diseases are characterized by separate pathologic and epidemiologic conditions, the drug treatment plans have many similar components.

Unfortunately, controlled drug studies examining the choice of drug, the therapeutic response, and combination therapy are lacking in the elderly population with asthma or chronic bronchitis. Thus therapeutic management is based on controlled studies in the population at large, evidence of subjective and objective improvement, and knowledge of airway disease reversibility and the potential for adverse effects.

Although the purpose of this chapter is to emphasize the pharmacologic management of patients with obstructive airway disorders, this should not be the only approach to treatment. There is extensive overlap among separate entities of the obstructive airway diseases, necessitating an accurate diagnosis and a comprehensive treatment plan. The treatment plan must consider physical therapy, preventative therapy, psychologic support, patient and family education, home oxygen therapy, management of heart failure, breaking the cigarette habit, removal of noxious occupational agents, control of infection, and removal of secretions.

Asthma

The clinical manifestations of asthma include episodic cough, wheezing, and dyspnea stemming from bronchial airway narrowing and increased air flow resistance. Blood and sputum eosinophilia may be associated with the episodic nature of the disease. The diagnosis is further supported by a 15 per cent or greater increase in the forced expiratory volume in one second (FEV_1) after administration of an aerosolized bronchodilator.

Asthma is often divided into extrinsic asthma and intrinsic asthma. People with extrinsic asthma are usually young, have a personal or family history of atopy, and often can gain bronchospastic relief by removal of environmental factors such as smoke, dust, and hairs. The term intrinsic asthma is used to describe persons who develop airway disease after age 35 that is not associated with any identifiable allergies. Both types are reversible with bronchodilator therapy. (The reader is referred to other sources for detailed descriptions of the pathogenesis, epidemiology, and chemical mediation of asthma.[4,6])

It is estimated that 10 per cent of asthmatic patients develop the disease after age 65.[1] Lee and Stretton studied 15 patients who developed asthma after the age of 60.[2] Dominant features included cough, paroxysmal nocturnal dyspnea, wheezing, and blood and sputum eosinophilia. Conrad described six patients (16 to 40 years of age) in whom a chronic cough without a history of episodic wheezing was the sole presenting feature of bronchial asthma.[3] All responded to bronchodilator therapy. Thus, the characteristic wheezing may not always be present.

The most common precipitating factors that bring on asthma include environmental agents, cigarette smoke, bacterial and viral upper respiratory tract infections, exertion, cold dry air, and stressful situations. Episodes of wheezing may last minutes to hours or days. The chest often becomes hyperinflated and hyper-resonant to percussion during the attack. If the attack persists and is refractory to standard bronchodilators, the patient is in status asthmaticus. The patient usually shows signs of cyanosis, is exhausted from labored breathing and lack of sleep, is often dehydrated, and may be approaching respiratory failure if not properly treated.

Pulmonary function testing may be quite helpful in quantitating the amount of airflow obstruction in any patient and determining its reversibility.[4] Static lung volumes can show an increased total lung capacity (TLC) and increased residual volume (RV). The RV/TLC ratio can increase. Dynamic lung volumes can show a forced expiratory volume (FEV) in one second—a forced vital capacity (FVC) ratio (FEV_1/FVC) of less than 75 per cent. After inhalation of a bronchodilator the FEV_1/FVC value usually improves, although a lack of response to the bronchodilator does not mean that the patient's disease is irreversible. Many patients with reversible disease do not achieve good topical deposition of sympathomimetic aerosol and may require more prolonged systemic therapy for a response.

In severe asthma, as mucous plugging worsens, the ventilation/perfusion ratio (V/Q) abnormalities worsen and arterial hypoxemia may develop. Hypercapnia can develop as a result of decreased alveolar ventilation in an asthmatic patient with fatigue or severe airway obstruction.

Chronic Bronchitis

Chronic bronchitis is defined as a production of excess sputum associated with chronic cough. The disease is characterized by cough and sputum on most days for at least three months of the year during two successive years. The symptoms range from morning cough and sputum expectoration to air flow obstruction, hypoxia, and hypercapnia. The excessive mucus accumulation in the tracheobronchial tree may predispose the patient to numerous respiratory infections, occasionally resulting in an asthmatic attack. Arterial blood gas levels may be abnormal, showing hypoxemia and carbon dioxide retention. Advanced disease is characterized by cyanosis, breathlessness, a blunted respiratory drive, and wheezing. Cor pulmonale and respiratory failure mark the end stage process in severe disease.[13-15]

Chronic bronchitis is most often associated with smoking or air pollution.[5] It often occurs with emphysema and occasionally with asthma. Breaking the cigarette habit is essential to therapy.

Emphysema

Emphysema is classified by anatomic terms rather than the clinical history. There is a destruction or loss of structure of alveoli or respiratory bronchioles. Cigarette smoking is a major etiologic factor.[6] Although emphysema is much more common in the elderly, there is no evidence to suggest that it is part of the normal aging process.[7] Breathlessness, prolonged expiration, and decreased breath sounds most often bring the patient to the physician.

In general, most patients do not have pure emphysema but rather a combination of both emphysema and chronic bronchitis. Some patients often have evidence of asthma as well. The astute physician should use his pulmonary function laboratory to help determine whether the patient with mixed respiratory disease has a reversible component.

Management with Drug Therapy

There are five categories of drugs available for the treatment of obstructive airway disease. These include theophylline and its derivatives, sympathomimetics, cromolyn sodium, anticholinergics, and corticosteroids. With the exception of cromolyn, these drugs can be administered by several different routes. The drug and route of choice depend on the severity of the patient's symptoms, the underlying disease states, and whether the patient is to be treated as an outpatient, in the emergency room, or in the hospital.

Mechanism of Action of Bronchodilators

Bronchial smooth muscle cell contraction and relaxation appear to be regulated by a balance of cyclic nucleotides within the bronchial smooth muscle fiber, chemical mediators released from mast cells, and parasympathetic nervous system alteration. Acetylcholine released from vagal efferent fibers in the bronchial tree causes bronchoconstriction.[8-12]

The balance between intracellular levels of adenosine $3',5'$-monophosphate (c-AMP) and guanosine $3',5'$-monophosphate (c-GMP) regulates bronchial smooth muscle contraction. An increase in c-AMP or a decrease in c-GMP tends to cause bronchial smooth muscle relaxation, whereas a decrease in c-AMP or an increase in c-GMP tends to cause contraction.

In vitro studies of the allergic reaction have shown that the IgE activated release of mediators from mast cells is modulated by the same cyclic nucleotides. The IgE becomes fixed to mast cells upon re-exposure to an antigen, which in turn leads to the formation and release of histamine, eosinophil chemotactic factor, and slow reacting substance of anaphylaxis. These mediators can directly promote bronchoconstriction. Increasing the intracellular c-AMP or decreasing c-GMP is thought to have a membrane stabilizing effect on the mast cell, thus preventing mediator release.

Theophylline and its derivatives elevate the intracellular c-AMP level and decrease the c-GMP level by phosphodiesterase inhibition. Most authorities agree that the phosphodiesterase inhibition is the major mechanism of action. There is some evidence that a change in cell membrane permeability to calcium may also play a role.[30]

The sympathomimetics increase intracellular c-AMP levels by stimulating $beta_2$ receptors in bronchial smooth muscle and mast cells. Activation of $beta_2$ receptors stimulates the enzyme adenyl cyclase to increase conversion of ATP to c-AMP. This effect can be blocked by beta adrenergic antagonists.

A synergistic effect from theophylline and sympathomimetics would be expected, since the molecular mechanisms of action share a final common pathway. Hanna and Eyre reviewed the literature and in summary stated that although the combination of theophylline and sympathomimetics interacts synergistically to increase intracellular c-AMP levels in bronchial smooth muscle, they do not act synergistically to inhibit smooth muscle contraction and alleviate various types of human asthma.[16] However, the clinical occurrence of an additive effect is well documented.

The anticholinergic drugs atropine and ipratropium bromide (SCH-1000) block exaggerated parasympathetic bronchial smooth muscle tone, mucus secretion, and mediator release from sensitized mast cells. This blockade decreases acetylcholine induced elevations of c-GMP.

Multiple mechanisms of action have been proposed for corticosteroids. Which is of the most significance is not yet known. Such mechanisms include an inhibition of mediator release from mast cells, a reduction of the threshold for beta adrenergic stimulation of bronchial smooth muscle relaxation, a decrease in mucosal edema, enhancement of adrenal gland synthesis of epinephrine, and suppression of immune reactions. (For a more detailed review of the biochemical actions of corticosteroids, the reader is referred to other sources.[123–125]) Although the molecular mechanisms of actions are not completely understood for any of the bronchodilators, this fact does not often alter the clinical use of the drugs.

Theophylline

In addition to its clinical use as a bronchodilator, theophylline is effective in producing sustained improvement in both right and left heart performance in chronic obstructive pulmonary disease.[18,19] Intravenous infusion of aminophylline and oral administration of a sustained release theophylline preparation significantly enhanced both right and left ventricular ejection fraction in normal control subjects and patients with chronic obstructive lung disease. This improved cardiac performance was evident after a follow-up period as long as 32 weeks. Thus, in patients with obstructive airway disease and heart failure, theophylline is useful for its cardiac actions in addition to its bronchodilatory effects.

Theophylline also has a mild diuretic action, although this is not sustained with prolonged use. The other extrapulmonary physiologic effect is on the central nervous system. The stimulant action on the central nervous system produces an increase in ventilation that occasionally may be beneficial. When therapeutic levels are exceeded, toxic effects including seizures resulting in death may occur.[17,20]

Pharmacokinetics. The proliferation in recent years of articles on theophylline pharmacokinetics is a result of an increase in reports of theophylline toxicity. Guidelines have been developed that, when used in conjunction with serum levels, can lead to much safer and efficient use of this drug. Interpatient variability with respect to theophylline disposition guarantees that not all patients will follow the same simple kinetic model, however.

Theophylline is well absorbed after oral administration.[21] There is little difference in total bioavailability between aminophylline uncoated tablets (theophylline ethylene diamine) and liquid preparations, although liquids are absorbed faster. Some liquid products (Elixophyllin, Theophyl-225, Choledyl, Quibron) do contain alcohol. The enteric coated preparation, oxtriphylline (Choledyl), is absorbed completely, although the onset of absorption is delayed for several hours.[22]

Until recently the use of sustained release preparation has been discouraged because of erratic and incomplete absorption. Manufacturing techniques have largely eliminated this problem in some of the products available (Theo-dur, Elixophyllin SR, Theobid Duracaps, Theolair SR, Slo-Phyllin Gyrocaps). Studies in adults with obstructive lung disease show that a steady serum theophylline level can be maintained with an every 12-hour regimen, and once the optimal dose is determined, levels within the therapeutic range can be sustained.[22–25] The authors report similar experiences when a product is chosen with 100 per cent bioavailability and demonstrates a constant rate of absorption. This can be especially helpful in patients with nocturnal asthma or compliance problems. The clinician must screen the sustained release products carefully, however, because there are still a number of them available that do not have the desired qualities.

Depending on the type of meal consumed, food can slightly delay the absorption of theophylline.[26] A meal high in fat content tends to yield lower serum levels, although the clinical significance of this interaction is unknown.

There are a number of changes in the gastrointestinal tract in the elderly that might be expected to alter the absorption of a drug. For example, the pH rises with advancing age and intestinal blood flow decreases. There is also a reduction in the number of absorbing cells, a delay in gastric emptying time, and a decrease in gastric motility in the elderly.[27] Whether these changes ultimately affect the rate or extent of theophylline absorption in the elderly has never been conclusively demonstrated.

The absorption of aminophylline suppositories is slow and erratic; this seems to be a function of formulation rather than the site of administration because rectal solutions are well absorbed.[28,29] Severe toxicity and deaths in children have occurred after repeated rectal use in cases of progressively worsening symptoms because early signs of theophylline toxicity were not recognized. When there is a lack of patient supervision and monitoring, use of aminophylline suppositories is a poor choice. In patients on nothing-by-mouth orders, the rectal route represents an obviously easy form of administration. If this is the case, a rectal retention enema or rectal aminophylline solution, when retained, is a reasonable alternative because absorption is reliable and complete.[29] With this form of therapy, the efficacy of an aminophylline enema is similar to that of an intravenous injection if a delay of 15 to 30 minutes is allowed for absorption. Close monitoring is advised, with frequent use of serum theophylline levels as a guide. Intramuscular administration is painful and is not recommended because of questionable absorption.[31]

Theophylline is eliminated in the body by biotransformation in the liver.[30-33] Less than 10 per cent is excreted unchanged by the kidney. Although the 3-methylxanthine metabolites accumulate in the serum in concentrations up to 2 to 3 mcg. per ml., the activity of this metabolite as well as the others is unknown.[34] This information may be important in renal failure. In rats the conversion of 1-methylxanthine to 1-methyluric acid is xanthine oxidase dependent.[35] Whether this is true in humans is unknown, although a case has been reported that suggested that allopurinol, a xanthine oxidase inhibitor, might have limited this metabolic pathway, resulting in theophylline toxicity.[36] Vozeh et al. measured the effect of allopurinol on theophylline clearance in healthy adults and found no significant changes in disposition.[37]

Striking interpatient differences in theophylline blood levels are seen with equivalent doses of the drug. This variability in theophylline serum levels is explained by differing rates of hepatic metabolism among individuals.[38] Several studies have confirmed that the mean elimination half-life is four to eight hours, with a two- to threefold variation in normal adult patients.[38-40] There are several factors, including age, disease state, smoking habit, and the use of other drugs that influence theophylline disposition. These considerations should have great impact when choosing a dosage regimen (Table 4–1).

The clearance of theophylline in children is significantly greater than in adults, and increased dosage requirements in children have been observed.[41-44] Theophylline disposition has not been well described in nonsmoking patients over 60 years of age. A study by Powell et al. showed no significant difference in theophylline elimination between three control patients 65 to 70 years of age and other control patients less than 65 years of age.[45] Cusack et al. studied theophylline clearance in five young adults (21 to 30 years of age) and six elderly adults (67 to 86 years of age).[46] The results supported Powell's data showing no difference in total body theophylline clearance. Jusko and associates developed nomogram guidelines for theophylline administration in which patients over 50 years of age receive a lower infusion rate.[47] Nielsen-Kudsk et al. studied theophylline pharmacokinetics in 10 elderly patients who had sustained strokes or Parkinson's disease.[48] The elimination half-life ranged from 5.4 to 9.0 hours. The volume of distribution and plasma clearance were both less than established values in younger healthy adult patients. Thus, whether older patients (older than 60 years of age) are characterized by a reduced clearance of the drug remains in dispute. Regardless of age, theophylline disposition in the geriatric population would be expected to be as variable as in a young adult population, therefore necessitating that administration be conservative and be guided by the use of routine serum level determinations.

Various illnesses have been shown to decrease theophylline clearance, necessitating a dosage reduction (Table 4–1). These conditions have great importance and implications when theophylline is used in acutely ill patients. Clearance is decreased (half-life increased) in hepatic dysfunction, severe congestive heart failure, acute pulmonary edema, and critically ill patients with severe obstructive pulmonary disease, renal failure, pneumonia and fever, and chronic obstructive pulmonary disease complicated by cor pulmonale[45,49-55] Powell et al. measured clearance and half-life in 31 volunteers and 26 acutely ill patients with airway obstruction within 24 hours after hospital admission and again when the intravenous administration of aminophylline was discontinued two to 10 days later.[45]

TABLE 4–1. Conditions That Alter Plasma Clearance of Theophylline

Decrease in clearance
    Critically ill patients with severe obstructive airway disease or cor pulmonale
    Acute pulmonary edema
    Severe congestive heart failure
    Hepatic dysfunction
    Pneumonia with fever
    Renal failure
    Alcoholism
Increase in clearance
    Heavy smokers

Clearance values were 40 per cent less in patients with severe bronchial obstruction and congestive heart failure as compared with a previously established value measured in otherwise healthy adult asthmatic patients.[56] Other studies have reported similar results.[52,59]

Vozeh et al. described a two- to threefold decrease in clearance changes as the illness becomes worse and a threefold increase in clearance as the patient's illness responds to treatment.[53] It appears that the alteration in clearance results from a change in the liver's capacity to metabolize the drug.

Theophylline clearance is significantly increased (40 to 50 per cent) in heavy smokers as compared with nonsmokers.[60,61] The clearance in exsmokers (two years' duration) has been measured and tends toward the clearance value in nonsmokers, but it is not significantly different statistically from that in heavy smokers.[60] Thus, the effect of smoking or of having smoked within two years has important implications in the clinical use of the drug.

Nearly all studies in which an apparent volume of distribution has been calculated show no significant difference between patients with decreased clearance and control patients. A study by Resar et al. did show that acidemic patients (pH < 7.3) had an increased volume of distribution, which accounted for low serum levels after a loading dose.[62] Whether the volume of distribution decreased after correction of the acidemia was not stated. The clinical significance of this finding is unclear.

Interaction Potential. The macrolide antibiotics, erythromycin and troleandomycin, and also lincomycin and clindamycin have been documented to decrease theophylline clearance when given in the usual dose.[63,64] In the case of troleandomycin, a 50 per cent decrease in clearance was measured in eight adult patients with severe intractable asthma. Although the mechanism is unknown, this interaction was thought to be responsible for a theophylline induced seizure in one of the eight patients. Aminophylline may increase excretion of lithium carbonate and may antagonize the effects of propranolol. Cimetidine decreases theophylline clearance by approximately 40 per cent.[174,175]

In summary, many pathologic conditions and drugs can alter theophylline clearance in adults. This in addition to the wide variation in clearance in healthy adults must be taken into consideration when a dosage regimen is designed.

Toxicity. The accepted therapeutic range for plasma theophylline is 10 to 20 mcg. per ml.[30,52,57] Theophylline concentrations greater than 10 mcg. per ml. are associated with optimal bronchodilation (Fig. 4–1), and toxic effects are common when 20 mcg. per ml. is exceeded.[20,38,52,56,65] Theophylline toxicity is primarily related to the dose and plasma concentrations. Toxic episodes may be classified into three groups, which are summarized in Table 4–2.[52] Generally the most serious side effects, namely, seizures or supraventricular tachycardia, require levels exceeding 30 mcg. per ml.

Although severe toxic side effects (cerebral seizures, cardiac arrhythmias, or cardiorespiratory arrest) are infrequent, Zwillich and coworkers reported eight patients who developed grand mal seizures during intravenous aminophylline therapy.[20] None of the eight had a history of a neurologic disorder, and all were acutely ill with severe pulmonary or cardiovascular disease. Blood theophylline concentrations obtained within one hour after the seizure ranged from 25 to 70 mcg. per ml., with a mean value of 53 ± 14.8 mcg. per ml.—more than twice the upper limit of the recommended therapeutic concentration (20 mcg. per ml.). Factors predisposing to the high serum concentrations in the patients with seizures were a significantly higher drug dosage compared with other patients without seizures, and hepatic dysfunction.

TABLE 4–2. Therapeutic and Toxic Plasma Theophylline Concentrations

Therapeutic level 10–20 mcg./ml.

Mild toxicity 18–30 mcg./ml.
    Gastrointestinal: Nausea, vomiting, diarrhea, anorexia
    Central nervous system: Nervousness, insomnia, headache
    Cardiac: Tachycardia (≥ 120 beats per minute)

Potentially serious toxicity 25–40 mcg./ml. (all the foregoing, and)
    Cardiac: Occasional premature ventricular contractions

Severe toxicity 40 mcg./ml. or greater (all the foregoing, and)
    Cardiac: Ventricular tachycardia
        Frequent premature ventricular contractions
        Runs of premature ventricular contractions
        Cardiorespiratory arrest
    Central nervous system: Grand mal seizures

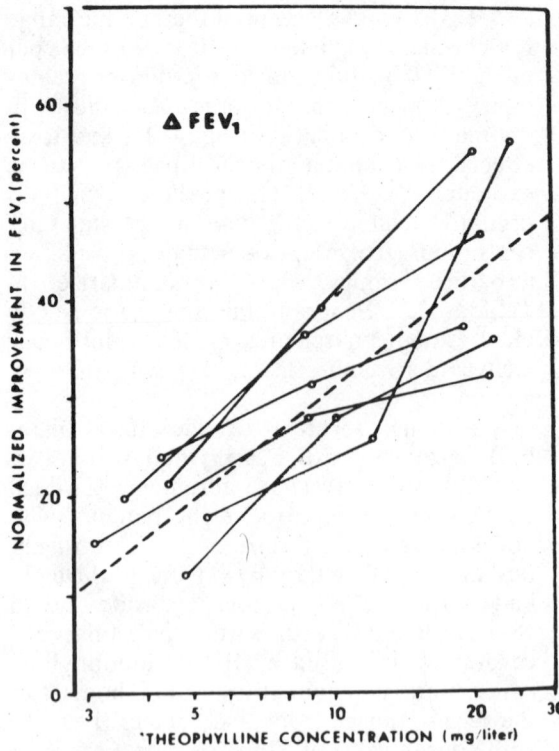

Figure 4–1. Dose-response relation for changes in forced expiratory volume in the first second ($\triangle FEV_1$) against the plasma theophylline concentration plotted semilogarithmically. Plots for each subject are presented individually (—), as well as the unweighted least squares regression line for the whole group (---). For each subject the $\triangle FEV_1$ is normalized by division of the mean difference from the placebo value at each drug concentration plateau by the predicted value minus the placebo value. (From Mitenko, P.A., and Ogilvie, R.L.: Rational intravenous doses of theophylline. N. Engl. J. Med., 289:600–603, 1973.)

In summary, theophylline plasma levels between 10 and 20 mcg. per ml. provide optimal bronchodilation without toxicity in most patients. Mild toxic complaints—headache, nausea, anorexia, and diarrhea—begin at about 15 mcg. per ml. in a few patients and become common over 20 mcg. per ml. Some patients tolerate much higher levels, but deliberate use of higher levels is not advisable. Levels of over 30 mcg. per ml. lead to the possibility of seizures, sometimes not preceded by any complaints, while levels over 40 mcg. per ml. may lead to serious cardiac rhythm disturbances and seizure disorders.

Intravenous Theophylline Administration. For the patient who needs immediate relief and who is not already receiving theophylline therapy, a loading dose is necessary to promptly produce a therapeutic serum level (Table 4–3). Without a loading dose, an interval of 4 to 5 half-lives will elapse before a steady state level is achieved following intermittent therapy or a continuous intravenous infusion. A recommended loading dose for adult patients is 4 to 5 mg. per kg. of theophylline (or 6 mg. per kg. of aminophylline) to achieve a serum level of 10 mcg. per ml.[45,56] If a serum level of 15 to 17 mcg. per ml. is desired, the loading dose of aminophylline should be 7 to 8 mg. per kg. As mentioned previously, a serum level of 10 mcg. per ml. may not be achieved in acidemic patients with a standard loading dose.[62] Nielsen-Kudsk et al. recommend a loading dose of 4.4 mg. per kg. of aminophylline in

TABLE 4–3. Intravenous Aminophylline Dosage Recommendations in Acutely Ill Patients*

Loading infusion 7–8 mg./kg.†	
Maintenance infusion	
Asthma—heavy smoker, otherwise healthy	1 mg./kg./hr.
Asthma—nonsmoker, otherwise healthy	0.5–0.9 mg./kg./hr.
Asthma—over 65, otherwise healthy	0.5 mg./kg./hr.
Chronic obstructive pulmonary disease with:	
Severe obstruction with cor pulmonale	0.25–0.5 mg./kg./hr.
Pneumonia	0.25–0.5 mg./kg./hr.
Cardiac decompensation with acute pulmonary edema	0.25 mg./kg./hr.
Liver dysfunction	0.25 mg./kg./hr.

*Infusion rate to achieve and maintain plasma theophylline level close to 15 mcg./ml.
†Assumes no pre-existing or coexisting disease or circumstance that will complicate therapy.

patients over 65 in order to achieve a serum level of 10 mcg. per ml.[48] Further studies are needed to confirm these recommendations.

If a higher serum level is desired, the loading dose is calculated as follows:

$$LD = Cp(d) \times Vd$$

where LD is the loading dose, Cp(d) is the desired serum level, and Vd is the apparent volume of distribution in L. per kg. The average Vd value for theophylline is 0.45 L. per kg. (0.3 to 0.6 L. per kg.) and usually does not change significantly with age, illness, or disease. The volume of distribution does not necessarily reflect any real volume or anatomic space, but is the factor required that relates the amount of a drug in the body to the concentration. Thus, if a level of 15 mcg. per ml. is desired in a 70 kg. person, the loading dose would be:

$$LD = (15 \text{ mg. per L.})(70 \text{ kg.} \times 0.4 \text{ L. per kg.})$$
$$= 420 \text{ mg. theophylline}$$
$$= 495 \text{ mg. aminophylline}$$

Grossly obese patients should be dosed according to the ideal body weight in order to avoid excess plasma levels.

If the patient has been receiving theophylline-containing drugs during the previous 24 hour period and no evidence of toxicity is present, one-third to one-half the standard loading dose can be given cautiously over 30 to 45 minutes. Rapid intravenous injection through a central venous catheter has resulted in cardiac arrest and sudden death.[66] Giddiness, weakness, and diaphoresis are common when the drug is administered too rapidly.

Patients who have taken a theophylline containing preparation in the previous 24 hours and show signs or symptoms of toxicity should not receive a loading dose. In these individuals a theophylline serum level should be obtained promptly to guide further intravenous aminophylline therapy.

Maintenance intravenous therapy, given as a continuous drip, should be instituted immediately following the loading dose. Continuous rather than intermittent administration is recommended, since the airway response is dependent on the theophylline serum level. Continuous administration can be accomplished by the standard intravenous drip method. However, an infusion pump to provide a constant rate of administration is the best method because of the practical difficulty in maintaining a well regulated intravenous drip.

Table 4–3 provides recommendations for initial intravenous maintenance infusion of aminophylline dosage based on experience in critically ill patients.[52,61] The infusion rate is variable, for the previously recommended fixed value of 0.9 mg. per kg. per hr. to maintain a serum concentration of 10 mcg. per ml. proved inappropriate in many clinical situations. Studies have shown that this fixed infusion rate can result in theophylline serum levels sufficiently high to place certain patients at risk for serious adverse effects, including seizures.[52,57–59]

Theophylline serum levels should be obtained in patients maintained on intravenous therapy with aminophylline for more than 24 hours because of the variable plasma clearances referred to earlier. Often a hospitalized patient may have received a continuous intravenous infusion of aminophylline for 24 hours and may not show much symptomatic improvement. If the patient is at risk for adverse effects (Table 4–1), a serum theophylline level should be determined before increasing the infusion rate. The clinician should always check to make certain that the patient received the medication. Personal experience has shown that when questions are asked, there are a number of reasons why the intravenous infusion was not started on time, interrupted, or discontinued. These circumstances make a difference in the decision to adjust the infusion rate.

If the serum level is below the therapeutic range and the appropriate infusion rate has been continued long enough to produce a steady state plasma concentration (24 to 48 hours in most adults), the infusion rate can be adjusted upward (Table 4–3). The adjustment can be made empirically. For example, if the level was 7 mcg. per ml. and a level of 14 mcg. per ml. is the goal, the infusion rate can be doubled. This is acceptable because theophylline demonstrates linear kinetics within the therapeutic range; i.e., doubling the infusion rate will double the concentration at steady state. There are some suggestions that at higher serum levels (toxic range) theophylline will exhibit dose dependent kinetics.[69,70] One has to remember that it will take four to five half-lives to reach the new steady state; therefore a supplemental bolus dose can be given to raise the level immediately. The equation is:

Dose = (desired Cp − measured Cp) (Vd)

Additional information can be gained by applying pharmacokinetic equations to patient specific data. When a steady state level has been achieved and a measured serum level is above the therapeutic range, the approximate half-life of the drug can be calculated. This will guide the clinician in determining how long the infusion should be continued. For example, if a level returns to 30 mcg. per ml. after 48 hours of a continuous infusion at 60 mg. per hr., the half-life can be calculated as follows (assuming a near steady state condition has been reached):

$$\text{Infusion rate} = (\text{clearance})(\text{Cp steady state})$$
$$= (kd \times Vd)(\text{Cpss})$$
$$= \left(\frac{0.693}{t_{1/2}} \times Vd\right)(\text{Cpss})$$

Therefore,

$$t_{1/2} = \frac{0.693 \times Vd \times \text{Cpss}}{\text{infusion rate }(0.85)}$$

$$t_{1/2} = \frac{0.693 \times 0.5 \text{ L./kg.} \times 70 \text{ kg} \times 30 \text{ mg./L.}}{60 \text{ mg./hr. aminophylline} \times 0.85\%}$$

$$t_{1/2} = 14 \text{ hours}$$

Therefore, the infusion should be discontinued for 14 hours (one half-life), and the serum level will decrease by 50 per cent to 15 mcg. per ml. At that time the infusion can be restarted at 30 mg. per hr. to maintain a level of 15 mcg. per ml.

Oral Theophylline Therapy. Patients stabilized on an intravenous infusion can be switched to an oral preparation when the clinical situation permits. The most convenient method for converting is to multiply the hourly infusion rate by the desired dosing interval (e.g., 50 mg. per hr. × eight hours = 400 mg. every eight hours). If an oral preparation is chosen that contains 100 per cent theophylline, the conversion factor of 0.85 must be used.

The pharmaceutical industry has produced many oral theophylline dosage forms. A major source of confusion among the various theophylline products is that equal weights of different salts provide greatly different

TABLE 4–4. Theophylline Equivalents of Commercially Available Methylxanthines

Methylxanthine	Percentage Theophylline	Equivalent Dose (mg.)
Theophylline anhydrous	100	100
Theophylline monohydrate	91	110
Aminophylline anhydrous	86	116
Aminophylline dihydrate	79	127
Theophylline mono-ethanolamine	75	133
Oxtriphylline	64	156
Theophylline sodium glycinate	49	200
Theophylline calcium salicylate	48	208

amounts of theophylline (Table 4–4). When choosing an oral dosage regimen, these differences must be accounted for.

Many clinicians prefer either USP uncoated tablets of aminophylline (85 per cent theophylline) or an anhydrous theophylline sustained release preparation that is 100 per cent absorbed. The uncoated tablets produce a peak effect in one to two hours.[22] Since optimal bronchodilation is serum level dependent, it is best to give these preparations on an every six hour basis. The sustained release products provide much less fluctuation between peak and trough serum levels. These products will help minimize bronchoconstriction breakthrough at the end of a dosing interval. For patients with impaired theophylline clearance, a sustained release product is not necessary because the plain uncoated tablets are 100 per cent absorbed and elimination is prolonged enough to provide adequate serum levels. The uncoated tablets are also useful for "occasional asthmatic" patients.

The liquid preparations are an adequate alternative to intravenous doses of aminophylline for providing prompt relief secondary to acute attacks of bronchoconstriction. The hydroalcoholic and aqueous solutions produce the most rapid onset of action with clinical response noted in approximately 15 to 30 minutes.[67] They are the dosage form of choice for patients with nasogastric tubes. Under no circumstances should sustained release tablets or capsules be crushed for administration via a nasogastric tube.

Combination products have been quite popular, especially for mild "occasional" asthma. It must be realized, however, that the combination preparations contain only one-fourth to one-half the optimal dose of theophylline for most patients.

In a significant number of patients an oral theophylline preparation can be given initially on an outpatient basis. Wyatt et al. determined that a starting oral dosage of 13 mg. per kg. per day or 900 mg. per day of theophylline, whichever is less, has little potential for exceeding a serum concentration of 10 mcg. per ml.[68] Patients who are at risk for severely depressed clearance should not be started with more than 400 mg. per day of aminophylline administered in divided doses. Adverse effects such as nausea, vomiting, headache, and diarrhea are common at serum concentrations over 20 mcg. per ml. Since seizures, which are rare at serum concentrations less than 30 mcg. per ml., have occurred without prior warning, the dosage should not be increased in anticipation that minor symptoms may serve as an end point of therapy. Beyond a total theophylline dosage of 13 mg. per kg. per day, 10 to 20 per cent of adult patients will be at risk for exceeding 20 mcg. per ml.[68] Thus, adults can be titrated to this dose, if tolerated, and then a serum theophylline measurement can aid in further dosage adjustment.

Sympathomimetic Drugs

The mechanism of action of sympathomimetic bronchodilator drugs has already been discussed. The older drugs, epinephrine and ephedrine, stimulate both alpha and beta receptors, whereas isoproterenol affects only the beta receptors.[71] Subsequent to the subdivision of beta receptors in 1967 by Lands into beta$_1$ and beta$_2$ categories, new drugs with beta$_2$ specificity have become available.[72] The effects of alpha, beta$_1$, and beta$_2$ stimulation are listed in Table 4–5. The molecular structure of the adrenergic agonist dictates physiologic activity and receptor site specificity. Development of a pure beta$_2$ receptor agonist has not been successful as yet because both beta receptors share some characteristics.

In addition to the effects on adrenergic receptor sites, the major differences between epinephrine or isoproterenol and the new beta$_2$ selective drugs, metaproterenol, terbutaline, albuterol, salbutamol, and fenoterol, are that they are active when given orally and have a longer duration of action (Table 4–6).[73–75]

With the exception of isoetharine, which must be given by inhalation, the beta$_2$ specific drugs are not catecholamines and thus are not subject to rapid inactivation in the gut and lung by catechol-ortho-methyl-transferase (COMT).[71,74,76] This accounts for the longer duration of action (four to seven hours) than that of epinephrine and isoproterenol. Isoetharine is subject to inactivation by COMT, thus shortening its duration of action to one to three hours.[77]

Ephedrine is unaffected by COMT but is nonspecific with respect to receptor site activity.[71] Its use as a bronchodilator is of questionable value, and even though the central nervous system effects are not measurably different from those of some beta$_2$ drugs when used in equal doses, its use has been relegated to that of a second line drug by most authorities. The alpha receptor stimulation augmenting urinary retention precludes its use in many elderly males.

With the exception of epinephrine for status asthmaticus, the beta$_2$ specific drugs have virtually replaced the older sympathomimetic drugs. The use of epinephrine and its effects on airway smooth muscle are well known.[71] Isoproterenol is the standard by which the newer drugs are tested. Isoproterenol's absorption by the sublingual route is erratic, and its intravenous use has great potential for causing adverse cardiac effects.[78] Prolonged isoproterenol use as an aerosol is associated with drug tolerance.[79] This is thought to be correlated with the accumulation of a 3-methoxymetabolite, which has a weak beta blocking action.[73]

The route of administration of the beta$_2$ drugs has a greater impact on treatment of obstructive airway disorders than does the choice of the drug itself. The major differences among the beta$_2$ drugs are their durations of action and dosage forms. Unlike theophylline,

TABLE 4–5. Adrenergic Receptors and Selected Responses

Receptor	Clinical Effect
Alpha	Urinary retention
Alpha	Hypertension
Beta$_1$	Lipolysis
Beta$_1$	Tachycardia
Beta$_1$	Cardiac contractility
Beta$_2$	Tremor
Beta$_2$	Bronchodilation
Beta$_2$	Glycogenolysis

TABLE 4–6. Beta$_2$ Sympathomimetics

Drug	Receptor	Onset of Action	Duration of Effect	Usual Dose
Isoetharine (Bronkosol, Bronkometer)	$B_2 > B_1$	5–10 min.	1–3 hours	Bronkosol, diluted: 4 puffs every 3–4 hours Bronkometer: 1–2 puffs every 3–4 hours
Metaproterenol (Alupent, Metaprel)	$B_2 > B_1$	5–10 min. (inhalation) 15–30 min. (oral)	4–5 hours 4–6 hours	Aerosol: 1–3 puffs every 4 hours Oral: 10–20 mg. every 6 hours
Terbutaline (Brethine, Bricanyl)	$B_2 > B_1$	30 min. (oral) 30–45 min. (subcutaneous)	5–7 hours 1.5–4 hours	Oral: 2.5–5.0 mg. every 6 hours Subcutaneous: 0.25 mg. every 4–6 hours
Albuterol (Proventil, Ventolin)*	$B_2 >> B_1$	Within 15 min. (aerosol) Within 30 min. (oral)	3–4 hours 4–6 hours	Aerosol: 1–2 puffs every 4–6 hours; Oral: 2–4 mg. three to four times daily. Start low with the elderly.
Fenoterol†	$B_2 >> B_1$		5–7 hours	Oral: 5–10 mg. every 6 hours

*Same as salbutamol.
†Not available in the United States.

there is no method for measuring the blood levels of active drug to which a therapeutic range can be assigned. The clinician must base dosage changes on objective and subjective changes in pulmonary function and observe for signs of toxicity.

Terbutaline is currently the only beta$_2$ injectable drug available in the United States. Freedman suggests that 0.25 mg. given subcutaneously will be as efficacious as 2.5 to 5.0 mg. orally.[80] The maximal effect is seen in 45 minutes following a 0.25 mg. subcutaneous dose, and the duration of effect is 1.5 to 4.0 hours. The subcutaneous administration of terbutaline in acute asthma is controversial. Both epinephrine, 0.25 and 0.5 mg. and terbutaline, 0.25 mg., show similar significant increases in the FEV$_1$ value and peak expiratory flow rate (PEFR) after 15 minutes. At four hours terbutaline maintains a significantly greater increase in PEFR over epinephrine.[81] At both recommended and higher than recommended subcutaneous doses, terbutaline significantly increases the heart rate to a degree greater than that with subcutaneous doses of epinephrine.[81-83] Because of these studies one must question whether the subcutaneous administration of terbutaline is advantageous over subcutaneous epinephrine for the treatment of acute asthma in patients prone to develop cardiac arrhythmias from hypoxia and acid-base imbalances. The tachycardia is thought to be the result of stimulation of intracardiac beta$_1$ receptors and a reflex mechanism from peripheral vasodilation from beta$_2$ receptor activity.[82]

Fenoterol, a beta$_2$ agonist used extensively in the United Kingdom, is also reported to cause a significantly greater increase in heart rate than epinephrine when administered subcutaneously.[76]

The oral route of administration of beta$_2$ agonists provides a convenient approach to treatment. A significant amount of beta$_2$ specificity is maintained by this route, with minor cardiac stimulation occurring. However, a significant number of patients experience hand tremor, which can be quite bothersome.

Five milligrams of terbutaline given orally has a maximal effect on the FEV_1 at two to three hours and a duration of approximately five to seven hours.[75,77,84–86] The onset of activity has been measured at 45 minutes to one hour.[75,85,86]

A double blind study in 15 patients (ages 24 to 70 years, mean 45 years) with FEV_1 values 70 per cent below normal (mean 48 per cent) compared single oral doses of terbutaline, 5 mg., ephedrine, 25 mg., and placebo to detect changes in forced vital capacity (FVC), FEV_1, forced midexpiratory flow between expulsion of 25 per cent and 75 per cent of vital capacity (FEF 25 to 75 per cent), airway resistance converted to its reciprocal and expressed as conductance/thoracic gas volume or specific conductance to correct the resistance for the volume at which it was measured, (SG_{AW}), arterial blood gas levels, heart rate, and blood pressure.[87] Terbutaline produced significant changes as compared with placebo responses in all ventilatory functions 30 to 240 minutes after administration. Following ephedrine all ventilatory functions improved but these changes were not statistically significant from those with placebo. The changes in ventilatory functions after terbutaline were significantly greater than with ephedrine at all times. The maximal changes at two to three hours are shown in Table 4–7.

Terbutaline produced a significant increase in the heart rate (10 beats per minute) one to three hours after oral administration. No significant changes in the electrocardiogram or systolic blood pressure were observed. Terbutaline use was accompanied by a significant increase in the blood glucose level from a mean control level of 110 ± 3.8 to 132 ± 5.2 mg. per 100 ml.

Metaproterenol is available in an orally administered dosage form as 10 and 20 mg. tablets; its duration of action is slightly shorter than that of terbutaline. Following the oral administration of metaproterenol at the usual dose of 10 to 20 mg. three to four times daily, the onset of activity has been measured at 15 to 30 minutes, with a peak effect on FEV_1 at two hours. Duration has been measured up to four hours.[88,89]

Albuterol is available as 2 and 4 mg. tablets. The usual adult dose is 2 to 4 mg. three or four times daily not to exceed 32 mg. per day. In the elderly and in those sensitive to beta adrenergic agonists, the initial dose should be 2 mg. three to four times daily. Doses may be increased gradually if necessary.

Fenoterol is not available in the United States, but is similar to terbutaline with respect to bronchodilating capacity and duration of action when used in equipotent doses.[74] Fenoterol holds promise as a useful drug because several studies have demonstrated that it elicits side effects about half as frequently as terbutaline when given orally or by inhalation.[75,76,89]

Inhalation of $beta_2$ agonists offers a major advantage, since low doses of the drug are deposited topically at the site of bronchial smooth muscle. This provides an excellent mechanism for treating early stages of mild to moderate acute airway obstruction, with little risk of toxicity. The inhalation drugs available generally have an onset of action of 15 seconds (isoproterenol and fenoterol) to several minutes (albuterol and metaproterenol).[76,78,89–91] The duration of action for metaproterenol and albuterol is approximately four to six hours.[78,91]

Isoetharine combined with phenylephrine (Bronkosol) has a duration of action of one to two hours. The rationale for the addition of phenylephrine is questionable, since it has been shown that it does not potentiate or prolong the duration of isoetharine itself.[92,93] The peak effect has been reported at 15 to 45 minutes after inhalation.[92,93] Isoetharine alone is available and has replaced most isoetharine-phenylephrine combinations.

With the current drugs available for inhalation, it is important to also consider the administration technique and the maximal number of inhalations consistent with good therapy. These considerations apply to steroid inhalers and cromolyn powder as well.

The particle size of most inhalant aerosols is 10 μm. or less. The factors that determine aerosol particle deposition in the lung include size, shape, flow rate, tidal volume, respiratory frequency, and airway caliber.[94,95] In patients with partial or total airway occlusion, particle deposition is severely compromised. Asymp-

TABLE 4–7. Changes in Ventilatory Function with Terbutaline and Ephedrine

	FVC	FEV_1	$FEF_{25-75\%}$	SG_{AW}
Terbutaline	21%	42%	79%	73%
Ephedrine	10%	16%	29%	40%

tomatic smokers with normal FEV_1 and maximal midexpiratory flow rate (MMFR) values show abnormal aerosol deposition, which may be related to narrowing of the small airways.[95] Thus, it is questionable whether aerosols used in acutely obstructed patients reach the site necessary for bronchial smooth muscle relaxation.

Patients using metered dose inhalers should be instructed about the proper use of the device. Before placing the mouthpiece, the patient is instructed to exhale to his relaxed end tidal volume. The mouthpiece is then placed just inside the lips. As the patient inhales slowly to vital capacity, one dose of the inhalant is dispensed. Holding the breath at end of inspiration allows for deposition of particles less than 3 μm. into the small airways.

If the inhalation flow rate is excessive, the larger 5 to 10 μm. particles are deposited in the upper respiratory tract. Deposition results from the relatively high inertia of these particles, which makes it difficult for them to follow the air stream as it changes direction. Smaller aerosol particles remain airborne to penetrate beyond the tenth bronchial division and are deposited mainly by sedimentation.[95]

Despite the widespread use of intermittent positive pressure breathing as a delivery mechanism for beta adrenergic drugs such as Bronkosol, there is no evidence that it is superior to the aerosol metered dose in delivering medication to the bronchial tree.[96] A significant amount of drug is retained in the mouthpiece, nebulizer, and tubing. The study by Weber et al. demonstrated that six to eight times as much terbutaline was required for the same degree of improvement when intermittent positive pressure breathing was used as compared to the metered dose aerosol response.[97] Intermittent positive pressure breathing is useful when the patient is unable to breathe adequately on his own. It cannot be overemphasized that proper patient instruction about the use of aerosols can make the difference between therapeutic success and failure.

Toxicity. As with most drugs, side effects are of special consideration in the elderly population, and the adrenergic drugs are no exception. Patients with cardiovascular disease, hyperthyroidism, and diabetes are more susceptible to side effects of these drugs.[78]

All beta adrenergic drugs, whether specific for $beta_2$ receptors or not, will increase heart rate as a dose dependent response. Older patients, especially those who are hypoxic or who have an irritable myocardium from cardiac disease, are at high risk. There are conflicting reports as to whether oral administration of terbutaline can increase the frequency of premature ventricular beats.[86,98] Banner et al. indicated that terbutaline tended to increase premature ventricular beats in patients with chronic obstructive lung disease more so than either ephedrine or aminophylline.[98] Tachycardia and palpitations seem to occur most often with oral or subcutaneous administration.

As mentioned previously, hand tremor is a common complaint more often with orally administered drugs than with aerosols. This usually appears after the first few doses and is the result of stimulation of $beta_2$ receptors in the skeletal muscle.[99] Fortunately tolerance develops after three to six weeks of continued use. Starting at a low dose may help to lessen this bothersome effect. The dosage should be increased gradually to the full dosage level.

Other side effects that patients may experience include nervousness, insomnia, headache, dizziness, and giddiness. Metabolic effects noted in single dose studies of $beta_2$ drugs include an increased blood glucose level and a fall in the serum potassium level.[76,87] The significance or frequency of this is unknown, but electrolyte and serum glucose levels should be checked in any debilitated patient receiving a beta adrenergic agent for acute airway obstruction.

Development of Tolerance. The development of reduced drug effectiveness, measured by the decline in FEV_1, PEFR, and SG_{AW} values, for isoproterenol is well documented.[73,79,101] This could be related to the accumulation of the 3-o-methylisoproterenol metabolite. Whether tolerance to the $beta_2$ specific drugs develops with continued use is controversial, and conflicting results have been reported.[101,103,104] Studies in which tolerance has developed have also found that recovery of the bronchodilator response appears to occur after one to two weeks off therapy.[100] Sacker et al. studied the development of tolerance after 90 days of oral metaproterenol therapy in asthmatic children;[101] he noted no significant tolerance.

Effects on Mucociliary Clearance. The adrenergic drugs give an added benefit of increasing tracheal mucus velocity when given in therapeutic doses orally, by injection or by inhalation.[102] This effect is usually seen 30 to 60 minutes after administration and lasts for up to two hours. This could be of potential benefit to patients with chronic bronchitis. The mechanism is thought to be an effect of increased ciliary activity rather than a change in mucus production or an increase in pulmonary vascular blood flow.

In summary, the beta$_2$ adrenergic drugs are useful therapeutically when used alone for the treatment of mild to moderate obstructive airway disease or occasional asthma. Severe obstruction necessitates the addition of theophylline, a theophylline derivative, or a corticosteroid.

Anticholinergic Drugs

The effects of atropine or atropine-like compounds in the treatment of asthma and chronic bronchitis have been known for many years.[105] As discussed earlier, the role of the parasympathetic branch of the autonomic nervous system in the generation of airway obstruction is quite significant. Parasympathetic stimulation releases acetylcholine from vagal nerve endings, causing mediator release from sensitized mast cells, enhancement of mucus production, and increases in bronchial smooth muscle tone. Atropine antagonizes these vagally mediated actions in patients with hyperirritable airways.[106] Several studies suggest that these compounds act predominantly in the large airways rather than in peripheral airways, since the FEV_1 value is increased more than the FEF 25 to 75 per cent value.[107,108]

In 1959 Herxheimer gave patients with bronchial asthma and emphysema atropine cigarettes to smoke.[105] The vital capacity increased 5 to 48 per cent. The point was made then, as it is in nearly all the recent studies using anticholinergic drugs in treating asthma, that when they are applied topically by inhalation to the bronchial tree, the elicitation of well known atropine side effects are minimal although they are occasionally present. The drying effect on secretions leading to airway plugging has not been established in study publications.

A double blind crossover study by Klock et al. demonstrated that 1 mg. of inhaled atropine sulfate was as effective as 1 mg. of inhaled isoproterenol hydrochloride in significantly improving the FEV_1 and SG_{AW} values in 15 patients with chronic bronchitis.[109] The mean response to both drugs was the same. It is of particular interest that the mean increase in the SG_{AW} value with atropine was 68 per cent, whereas in previous studies in normal subjects the increases in the SG_{AW} values were 38 per cent and 42 per cent. These results suggest that atropine may be beneficial in chronic bronchitis because of the possible increased cholinergic activity in patients with chronic bronchitis. Five subjects reported increased difficulty in starting urination during atropine treatment. Other complaints were blurred vision and dry mouth.

A study by Brady and Easton confirmed atropine's effect in improving pulmonary flow rates, and also demonstrated that the combination of atropine plus isoproterenol produced significantly greater increases in FEV_1 and FEF 25 to 75 per cent values than either drug alone.[110] No adverse cardiovascular effects were reported.

An atropine-like drug, ipratropium bromide (also known as SCH1000), developed in the 1960's as an aerosol bronchodilating drug, is now undergoing clinical trials. It is a quaternary ammonium radical, thus eliminating central nervous system and anticholinergic effects. Studies to date indicate that it may be useful in chronic bronchitis or intrinsic asthma, with less reported extrapulmonary anticholinergic effects than atropine.[111] The drug has not been shown to alter blood gas levels or heart rate. Like atropine, SCH1000 in combination with a beta$_2$ agonist is more effective than either drug alone.[113,114]

Exactly where anticholinergic compounds fit into the treatment plan of obstructive airway disease is not known. As mentioned, preliminary results indicate that they may be useful in chronic bronchitis. A 1 per cent solution of atropine sulfate may be administered as an aerosol in a dosage range of 0.05 to 0.1 mg. per kg. of body weight up to four times a day.[106] The duration of action is four to six hours. There are no commercial preparations available, thus necessitating the use of aseptic technique in preparation of the solution. It should be noted that this is not an FDA approved use of atropine and may require special consent forms.

To date the majority of instances of use would be confined to refractory hospitalized patients. As usual, caution is emphasized in the geriatric patient with regard to anticholinergic effects. One must keep the patient adequately hydrated without producing fluid overload. The patient's cardiovascular status must be monitored because low doses slow the heart rate slightly owing to central stimulation of the center of the medulla, whereas higher doses increase the heart rate and atrioventricular conduction time owing to its vagal inhibitory effect. Studies to date with aerosolized atropine report an insignificant effect on systolic or diastolic blood pressure, although some patients have complained of flushing. Other side effects that should be monitored include constipation, urinary retention or hesitancy, drowsiness, and restlessness. The drug is contraindicated in narrow angle glaucoma.

Cromolyn Sodium

Cromolyn sodium (Intal) is not a bronchodilator and should not be used as such. It is thought to prevent the release of mediators (histamine, SRS-A, serotonin) from mast cells in the lung by stabilizing cell membranes.[115,116] Cromolyn is ineffective in the treatment of acute asthmatic episodes, thus limiting its role to prophylactic treatment.

Those who benefit most from cromolyn are usually young, have symptoms related to a specific allergen, are affected by occupational dust, fumes, and animal hairs, or have hyperactive airways as a result of exercise. Not all patients with the extrinsic type of asthma respond, and in fact it is impossible to predict who will respond. Many patients with the extrinsic type of disease do show benefit; thus in asthmatic patients who are not controlled on bronchodilators, a trial of cromolyn is useful.[118] Berstein recommends that all patients with chronic perennial asthma be given a therapeutic trial with cromolyn therapy before corticosteroid therapy is instituted.[117] Therapeutic benefit has also been noted in aspirin intolerant patients. A response may not be seen for two to four weeks after initiating therapy, however. Although subjective improvement may be marked, patients may show no improvement in FEV_1 or PEFR values after using cromolyn.[119] Cromolyn's use in patients with pure chronic bronchitis or emphysema has not been studied, but patients with obstructive airway disease who demonstrate an allergic component may benefit. If a response is not seen after four weeks, the drug should be discontinued.

Cromolyn sodium is available as a dry powder in capsular form administered in a spinhaler and as a solution for inhalation. The 20 mg. capsule is placed in the spinhaler, which punctures the capsule. As the patient inhales, the capsule spins, releasing the powder. Less than 10 per cent of a 20 mg. capsule reaches the airways, the rest being deposited in the oropharynx and trachea and eventually swallowed. One capsule (20 mg.) is administered four times a day at regular intervals. Cromolyn is poorly absorbed from the gastrointestinal tract (approximately 1 per cent) but is absorbed from the lungs (approximately 9 per cent) when inhaled as a fine powder or as an aerosol. The majority of the absorbed drug is excreted unchanged in the urine and bile.[120]

The route of administration of the capsule for inhalation is a major drawback to using this drug. Unlike the beta adrenergic aerosols requiring one to two puffs every four to six hours, each capsule may require up to 10 inhalations to empty the entire contents of the capsule. This would preclude its use in debilitated patients or patients with a poor respiratory effort. Like other aerosols, a considerable amount of coaching in regard to correct administration techniques might be required. Compliance problems as well as high cost impose significant limitations on the use of this drug. The solution for use in a nebulizer is a much more convenient and effective dosage form. The solution is available as 20 mg per 2 ml. ampule.

A major advantage of the drug is that patients can reduce concurrent steroid usage.[117,119,121,122] This should be done slowly with frequent monitoring to prevent Addisonian crises. As usual, the patient should be instructed to take oral doses of corticosteroids if an exacerbation in the disease becomes apparent.

The other primary advantage is the high benefit to risk ratio. Side effects are a minor problem. They include throat irritation, nasal congestion, dryness of the mouth, acute cough, and mild bronchospasm occurring immediately after inhalation.[122] The use of a $beta_2$ agonist aerosol before cromolyn inhalation can minimize the bronchospasm and allow deeper penetration into the lungs. Because of its irritating properties, patients should be instructed never to use cromolyn in an acute episode of airway obstruction because it could provoke the problem into a more serious situation. Initiation of therapy should begin one to two weeks after an acute exacerbation has settled.

The place of cromolyn in the treatment of an elderly person with airway obstruction is limited to outpatients with demonstrated ability to master use of the spinhaler or a nebulizer. Patients with an allergic component respond most often, but this should not limit a trial use in patients with hyperactive airways who are poorly controlled with bronchodilator treatment.

Corticosteroids

Corticosteroids almost always provide dramatic relief in severe refractory asthma.[123-125] The use of steroids in chronic bronchitis and emphysema is controversial because of the lack of objective evidence of improvement in many patients. A double blind randomized study comparing 44 patients with the diagnosis of chronic bronchitis with severe airflow obstruction with patients receiving similar bronchodilators with either methylprednisolone, 0.5 mg. per kg. every six hours for 72 hours, or placebo indicated that the methylprednisolone treated patients did better clinically as measured by spirometry than placebo treated controls.[145] However, without objective evidence for improvement, clinicians are reluctant to begin the maintenance use of steroids because of their adverse effects. Whether the geriatric patient with asthma or chronic obstructive pulmonary disease receives more or less benefit from prolonged steroid use is unknown. As with patients of any age, the elderly patient with obstructive airway disease who also has other diseases that can be worsened by steroids must be monitored closely.

There are many steroids available on the market today, and they can be given orally, intravenously, intramuscularly, and by inhalation. Obviously the drug chosen depends on the anti-inflammatory potency, mineralocorticoid activity, and route of administration (Table 4–8).

Injectable hydrocortisone is the steroid most commonly used to break an acute severe asthmatic attack. Because of its potent mineralocorticoid effect, it should not be used in patients with a poor cardiac reserve, however. The dosage is from 300 mg. up to 2 gm. per day. Collins et al. recommend 3 to 4 mg. per kg. given intravenously every six hours to maintain a cortisol level of 100 to 150 mcg. per ml., the necessary level to achieve a therapeutic response in severe asthma.[126] Patients who have been taking maintenance therapy with corticosteroids have increased cortisol metabolism and may require 500 to 1000 mg. of hydrocortisone every six hours to maintain cortisol levels above 100 mcg. per ml.[127]

Prednisone is the most popular orally administered steroid. After absorption it is metabolized in the liver to the active compound, prednisolone. There is evidence to suggest that there is a delay in the biotransformation of prednisone to prednisolone in patients with hepatic dysfunction, but the clinical significance of this is unclear.[128] The usual oral dosage of prednisone is 5 to 80 mg. per day. The advantage over hydrocortisone is less sodium retaining activity.

Methylprednisolone sodium succinate may be given intravenously for acute asthma. The soluble succinate ester is reported to have a rapid onset of action.[129] Methylprednisolone has 50 per cent of the sodium retaining properties of hydrocortisone and is four to five times more potent in anti-inflammatory activity. Doses are variable; usually 40 to 125 mg. is given intravenously every six hours initially and then the dose is tapered over the next three to five days.

Dexamethasone is one of the most potent anti-inflammatory drugs available for injection and oral administration. Although it has no mineralocorticoid activity, its parenteral use in refractory asthma has not been well studied. Dexamethasone, parametasone, betameth-

TABLE 4–8. Clinical Characteristics of Selected Orally Administered Corticosteroids

Drug	Biologic Half-life (Hours)	Approximate Equivalent Dose (Mg.)	Relative Sodium Retaining Property
Cortisone	1.5	25.0	2+
Hydrocortisone	1.5	20.0	2+
Prednisone	18–36	5.0	1+
Prednisolone	18–36	5.0	1+
Triamcinolone	18–36	4.0	0
Methylprednisolone	18–36	4.0	0
Paramethasone	36–54	2.0	0
Fluprednisolone	36–54	1.5	0
Dexamethasone	36–54	0.75	0
Betamethasone	36–54	0.6	0

asone, and fluprednisolone would not be drugs of choice for oral maintenance therapy because of their long biologic half-life, suppressing the hypothalamic-pituitary-adrenal axis, thus preventing the conversion to an alternate day dosing regimen.

Beclomethasone dipropionate (Vanceril, Beclovent) is the most efficacious available steroid for inhalation. Its topical anti-inflammatory effect is many times greater than that of dexamethasone.[129] When it is given by inhalation at the recommended daily dosage of 800 mcg. (50 mcg. per puff), there is evidence of minimal or no adrenal suppression and a lack of systemic side effects.[130,131] At a level of 2000 mcg. per day or more, adrenal suppression is reported.[132,133]

Patients taking oral doses of 10 mg. of prednisone or less per day have the greatest chance for success with complete replacement of oral steroid use with aerosol beclomethasone.[134,135] Pulmonary function test improvement in asthmatic patients may be observed in one to four weeks after the initiation of treatment. Like cromolyn, beclomethasone is not indicated for acute asthmatic attacks and may actually worsen the event.

Deaths have been reported in asthmatic patients during transfer from prolonged systemic steroid use to a beclomethasone inhalant. Patients should be instructed to continue the usual oral steroid dose during the first one to two weeks of treatment with beclomethasone and then to reduce the systemic dose by no more than 2.5 mg. of prednisone or its equivalent per week. It may take as long as 36 weeks to complete recovery of hypothalamic-pituitary-adrenal function.[130] During acute exacerbations or in stress producing situations it is necessary to cover the patient with systemic doses of steroids, which can then be tapered over one to two weeks to the previous dosage regimen.

The reappearance of steroid suppressed allergic problems such as eczema, rhinitis, hay fever, and nasal polyps may worsen during the steroid withdrawal period. If addisonian symptoms appear (nausea, lethargy, weakness and arthralgias) or asthma worsens during or after withdrawal of the systemic doses of steroid, the patient should inform his physician. The rapid ACTH test can be helpful in indicating whether systemic use of steroids should be reinstated.[136]

Asymptomatic oral candidiasis has been found in 45 to 77 per cent of the patients in whom cultures were done while beclomethasone was being administered.[137] No pulmonary infections have been reported to date, but the utmost care should be used in seriously debilitated patients who are using or have received beclomethasone in the recent past. The asymptomatic Candida infection can be treated with oral doses of nystatin or amphotericin. Rinsing the mouth or gargling with water after inhalation may reduce the colonization of Candida.

The only indication for beclomethasone is in patients who require or have a demonstrated need for continuous systemic doses of steroids to control bronchial asthma. Patients who require systemic doses of steroids infrequently or patients whose disorders are controlled by bronchodilators are not candidates.

Considerations in the Elderly When Using Corticosteroids. Steroids should never be withheld in any patient who has refractory bronchospasm, particularly in those who have required steroids in the past. Any delay can be life threatening, since improvement in pulmonary function may not be seen for four to six hours after the dose.[126,138,139] Methylprednisolone is the drug of choice in geriatric patients because of its quick onset of action and minimal mineralocorticoid effect. When sympathomimetic drugs are contraindicated, as in patients with arrhythmias, steroids are the only practical alternative.

Maintenance steroid therapy in the elderly asthmatic patient has the same indications and benefits as for a younger patient. The goal of therapy is to keep the patient as symptom free as possible, out of the hospital, and on the smallest possible dose to minimize side effects. For patients currently taking systemic doses of steroids daily, alternate day therapy is desirable. The change-over should be gradual and should be consistent with the needs of the patient. A number of patients may require a minimal dose on the off day. Whether oral alternate day therapy is superior or inferior to beclomethasone aerosol therapy is controversial, but either is less of a toxicity risk than daily oral steroid doses greater than 10 mg. of prednisone or its equivalent.[140] Improvement in pulmonary function test results and decreased sputum eosinophilia are useful guidelines to follow in patients taking maintenance doses of steroids. Horn et al. suggest that a total eosinophil count less than 80 to 100 per cu. mm. indicates adequate steroid administration.[141] Symptomatic improvement and loss of auscultatory signs of airway obstruction may precede spirometric evidence of improvement.

The indications for steroids in the management of chronic bronchitis and pulmonary emphysema in the elderly are debatable and much more vague than for patients with asthma. This poses a special problem for clinicians dealing with elderly patients with obstructive airway disease, since most present with a mixed obstructive illness.

Many studies in which this problem has been examined have not been well designed, have lacked control groups, have used questionable measurements to substantiate objective improvement, or have involved patients in whom there was an allergic component to the disease. To cloud the issue, the question of a steroid induced euphoric effect leading to subjective improvement without significantly improving pulmonary function has been raised. A 1978 review of 17 studies pointed out that although a number of studies have been poorly designed, the majority concluded that corticosteroids are not objectively helpful in most patients with chronic obstructive pulmonary disease.[142] However, there are numerous such patients who do respond to steroid therapy. Kettel and Morse indicated that a patient who has not responded to a trial of corticosteroids while in a chronic state is not likely to do so when he suddenly becomes worse.[143]

As yet, the spirometric measurement that accurately reflects objective improvement in airway disease following administration of steroids to chronic bronchitis patients has not been conclusively decided. Williams and McGavin's study concluded that the patient's assessment of breathlessness and walking distance correlates best with an increase in the forced vital capacity value.[144] Albert et al. conducted a controlled double blind trial in patients with chronic bronchitis with acute respiratory insufficiency.[145] Their results showed that methylprednisolone in a dose of 0.5 mg. per kg. of body weight added to standard bronchodilator therapy significantly improved the FEV_1 value by 72 hours when compared to placebo. More long term studies with both effort dependent and effort independent spirometric measurements are needed to completely assess the contribution of corticosteroids to the relief of airway obstruction in patients with chronic obstructive pulmonary disease. There are no data to support the use of either prolonged or short term use of steroid therapy in patients with pure emphysema. Certainly patients with chronic obstructive pulmonary disease in whom there is an asthmatic component and whose symptoms are not controlled by bronchodilators deserve a short term trial of corticosteroids if the potential benefit outweighs the risk of adverse effects.

Toxicity. The list of adverse effects from corticosteroids is long and well known (Table 4–9). Elderly patients and patients with low serum albumin concentrations are potentially more susceptible to the adverse effects of corticosteroids.[146,147] Hydrocortisone is bound to cortisol binding globulin and albumin. The free fraction is the active compound accounting for tissue effects. Patients with hypoalbuminemia, as in liver disease, have an increased level of free glucocorticoid. When exogenous corticosteroids are given to such patients, there is an increase in adverse effects.

TABLE 4–9. Corticosteroid Induced Adverse Effects*

Endocrine	Adrenal supression, pituitary unresponsiveness, hyperglycemia, cushingoid state
Gastrointestinal	Abdominal distention, ulcerated esophagitis, nausea, peptic ulcer, increased appetite, weight gain, pancreatitis
Musculoskeletal	Muscle weakness, tendon rupture, osteoporosis, aseptic necrosis of femoral and humeral heads, long bone fracture, vertebral compression fracture, muscle atrophy
Cardiovascular	Sodium retention and edema, thrombophlebitis, hypertension, necrotizing angiitis
Central nervous system	Insomnia, nervousness, euphoria, depression, psychoses, increased intracranial pressure with papilledema, vertigo, headache
Ophthalmic	Glaucoma, posterior subcapsular cataracts
Dermatologic	Impaired wound healing, erythema, increased perspiration, subcutaneous fat atrophy, purpura, striae, hyperpigmentation, hirsutism, acneiform eruptions, urticaria, angioneurotic edema
Metabolic	Negative nitrogen balance due to protein catabolism

*Some steroid products contain tartrazine dye, which can cause allergic type reactions (including bronchial asthma) in sensitive patients. Tartrazine sensitivity is often seen in patients with aspirin hypersensitivity.

Several of the side effects listed in Table 4–9 deserve elaboration with respect to potential problems in geriatric patients. Carbohydrate intolerance is usually mild, although diabetic coma and acidosis have been reported.[148,149] The elderly insulin dependent diabetic patient with chronic obstructive pulmonary disease in whom corticosteroid therapy is begun should be instructed to follow urine or blood glucose test results more closely.

The subject of steroid induced gastric ulcer is controversial and inconclusive. In hospitalized asthmatic patients or those with chronic obstructive pulmonary disease with acute respiratory failure who are receiving high doses of corticosteroids, prophylactic therapy probably should be undertaken against ulceration with antacids, cimetidine, or ranitidine. The same considerations should be given to patients with major postsurgical steroid dependent obstructive airway disease. Other steroid induced adverse effects that would be hazardous to elderly patients include development of cataracts and increased risk of long bone fractures and vertebral compression fractures.[150]

In addition to producing numerous adverse effects, the corticosteroids may interact with a number of other drugs. Phenytoin, phenobarbital, ephedrine, and rifampin may enhance the metabolic clearance of corticosteroids, thus requiring an increased dose of corticosteroid to achieve the desired effect. Corticosteroids may inhibit the normal response to coumarin anticoagulants. Patients receiving corticosteroids with mineralocorticoid activity who concurrently receive potassium depleting diuretics should be observed closely for the development of hypokalemia. Steroid induced hypokalemia may enhance the possibility of digitalis toxicity.

In summary, corticosteroids give marked relief in asthma, but their role in chronic obstructive pulmonary disease is unclear. The decision to use steroids should be made on an individual basis with controlled objective assessments as indicators of effectiveness. If the trial is with low to moderate doses for a short period of time, the benefit to risk ratio should be high. Under no circumstance should a patient be maintained on corticosteroid therapy if objective ventilatory improvement has not been demonstrated. Whenever possible, the patient should be given the beclomethasone aerosol preparation when steroids are indicated.

Special Considerations in Therapy of Obstructive Airway Diseases in the Elderly

Asthma

The overall goal in treating the outpatient asthmatic is to keep the patient symptom free and out of the hospital or emergency room. This preventive management approach consists of the avoidance of irritants and allergens, the maintenance of adequate hydration, and optimal drug therapy without producing adverse effects. No single treatment modality precludes the use of the other. The first two measures are well known and do not require elaboration for specific application to the elderly population.

Optimizing drug therapy is a multistep scheme, which requires subjective and objective measurements at each level. Simple spirometric tests and sputum and blood eosinophil counts should serve as objective guides by which drug therapy decisions are made. After the diagnosis of asthma is made and treatment with drugs is deemed necessary, therapy should start with a theophylline compound or a beta$_2$ agonist sympathomimetic drug.

The initial dose of the theophylline derivative is 100 to 300 mg. four times daily, depending on the patient's estimated ability to clear the drug from the body (Table 4–1). One must remember that minor toxicities (nausea and vomiting) do not always appear before major toxicities (arrhythmias and seizures). Alternatively one can start therapy with a sustained release theophylline preparation, which will minimize peak-trough differences and may improve drug compliance. Serum theophylline levels should be obtained periodically to ascertain compliance and achievement of the therapeutic range. If the patient is asymptomatic on a theophylline dose that produces a serum level slightly below or in the low therapeutic range, there is no need to increase the dose further to achieve a level in the higher end of the therapeutic range. Trough serum levels will indicate whether the dose is sufficient to keep the serum level in a therapeutic range throughout the dosing interval, whereas peak serum levels will indicate presence of toxicity. Obviously a trough level in the high therapeutic range may require a reduction in dose, since the serum level would be above 20 mcg. per ml. for the majority of the dosing interval. In the elderly patient the peak serum level is usually what is obtained, since decreased drug metabolism may quickly lead to toxic serum levels. Sustained release preparations with a peak in the midtherapeutic range almost always have a therapeutic trough level. In addition, sustained release theophylline preparations are helpful for patients experiencing nocturnal asthma. As mentioned previously, in patients with disease states associated with low theophylline clearance, a plain uncoated aminophylline tablet will suffice, since the half-life will be prolonged.

A question that is commonly asked is whether the dosage in an elderly asthmatic patient not controlled by theophylline alone should be pushed to the higher end of the therapeutic range before the addition of a second drug. Certainly a patient with a history of tachyarrhythmias would not be a good candidate for high serum levels (15 to 20 mcg. per ml.), since drug induced tachycardia is very common in this range. If the patient is a healthy asthmatic, does not have heart disease, and does not have a history of acute obstructive airway decompensation that would change theophylline clearance, the drug level could be pushed to achieve a serum level of 15 to 20 mcg. per ml. The elderly patient with asthma and cardiovascular disease is at less of a risk of theophylline induced arrhythmias if a target serum level of 10 to 15 mcg. per ml. is achieved in conjunction with the use of a beta$_2$ agonist. Wolfe et al. have demonstrated that improvement in the FEV$_1$ value can be achieved with low dose theophylline therapy combined with low dose terbutaline therapy similar to that with high dose theophylline alone (Fig. 4–2).[151]

The beta$_2$ agonist can be given orally or by inhalation. If the adverse cardiovascular effects present a problem, the inhalation route should be used. Shim and Williams have recently shown that metaproterenol given by inhalation (five puffs) achieved a significantly greater increase in the FEV$_1$ value than did metaproterenol given orally (20 mg).[152] Unlike many previous studies, the five inhalations were given 20 minutes apart. This presumably allowed deeper penetration of each successive inhalation. The FEV$_1$ value leveled off after the third puff. No side effects were noted in the patients using only aerosol therapy.

Optimizing drug therapy requires rigorous patient education. Patients should be taught the significance of maintaining a theophylline blood level close to the therapeutic range. If an aerosol device is used, proper technique is a necessity. The patient should be asked to demonstrate the use of the inhaler during routine office visits.

The most common method of stepwise addition of antiasthmatic drugs is that the first two drugs be a theophylline compound and a beta$_2$ agonist. Cromolyn sodium or beclomethasone aerosol would be added next. If the patient has an allergic component that causes the airway to be hyperactive, cromolyn is worth a trial. If no improvement is seen in four to six weeks, the drug should be discontinued. Beclomethasone aerosol has provided

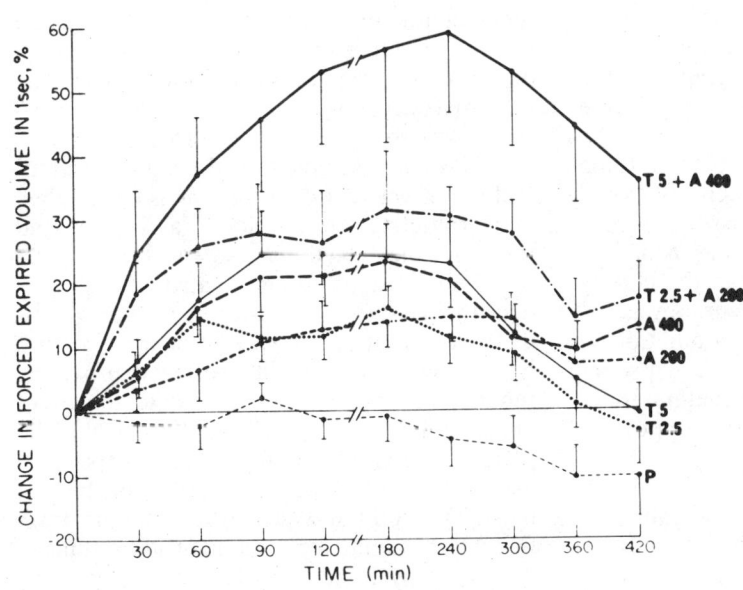

Figure 4–2. Mean percentage changes in forced expired volume in one second with time after oral administration of drug or placebo. A denotes aminophylline, P denotes placebo, T denotes terbutaline, and the numbers after those letters show the dose in milligrams. Note that the combination T 2.5 + A 200 is comparable to A 400 or T 5 alone, and T 5 + A 400 appears to yield best results. (From Wolfe, J.D., et al.: Bronchodilator effects of terbutaline and aminophylline alone and in combination in asthmatic patients. N. Engl. J. Med., 298:363, 1978.)

many perennial asthmatic patients with continued bronchospastic relief that was unobtainable with theophylline and a $beta_2$ drug combined. A $beta_2$ aerosol used prior to the beclomethasone will allow deeper penetration of the steroid than if the steroid is used alone.

There are a number of patients in whom the combination of theophylline and a $beta_2$ agonist (inhaled or oral) produces intolerable cardiac side effects. In these individuals either theophylline or the $beta_2$ drug can be used in conjunction with beclomethasone. If the theophylline agent is chosen, the $beta_2$ aerosol can be reserved for occasions when the patient has bronchospastic flare-ups.

In patients who frequently experience mild flare-ups while taking theophylline and a $beta_2$ drug at therapeutic doses, the beclomethasone aerosol can be started. It should be explained to the patient that relief may not be noted for one to four weeks, and that the steroid inhaler is not for immediate relief of bronchospasm. If the airway obstruction is severe enough to require more prompt attention, oral doses of corticosteroids can be given for one to two weeks, after which a changeover to beclomethasone is appropriate. Prednisone is usually given in doses of 20 to 60 mg. the first two to three days, and then the dose is tapered over the next week as improvement occurs. It must be stressed that the clinician should not let possible steroid induced euphoric effects interfere with subjective and objective measurements of improvement.

Patients currently consuming daily systemic doses of steroids are candidates for alternate day therapy or the beclomethasone aerosol. As mentioned previously, the changeover to either alternate day therapy or the aerosol should be gradual, and any acute exacerbations that occur must be covered by oral doses of steroids during the episode. Long term maintenance therapy with steroids should be tapered to the lowest dose possible. It may take many attempts to achieve this goal.

Treatment of acute asthma in the elderly may require hospitalization to accurately assess the clinical course that follows. In addition to medication, treatment should include proper assessment of monitoring parameters, adequate oxygenation, ventilatory support if needed, and nutritional support.

The choice of drug therapy in the elderly person with acute bronchospasm is similar to that in a younger person. Some practitioners prefer the subcutaneous administration of epinephrine (0.3 ml. of a 1:1000 solution) or terbutaline (0.25 mg.) initially. If the patient does not have a history of an arrhythmia disorder, this method is acceptable in most cases. Other practitioners prefer initial treatment with the intravenous administration of aminophylline. A careful patient history is a necessity. Elderly patients who have taken theophylline in the last 24 hours do not require a full loading dose. If there is any question about the patient's use of theophylline in the previous 24 hours and no signs of toxicity exist, a blood level determination should be done and then one-third to one-half the usual loading dose given. One must remember that in patients who are acutely obstructed or have severe heart failure, theophylline does not clear from the body as readily as when these problems are corrected; thus if the patient has been taking theophylline regularly before and during the early stages of the severe attack, chances are the drug is accumulating. This in addition to a bolus of aminophylline would put the patient at risk for toxicity. When this situation occurs and theophylline levels are readily available, the level should be known before the aminophylline is given.

The maintenance infusion should follow the guidelines listed in Table 4–3. Unstable asthmatic patients who are susceptible to theophylline toxicity could benefit from theophylline serum level determinations as frequently as every 24 to 36 hours while taking intravenous therapy.

Intravenous corticosteroid doses are given for status asthmaticus and to patients with severe obstruction who have responded to them in the past. The drug of choice in an elderly patient is methylprednisolone in doses of 40 to 125 mg. every six hours. With the administration of corticosteroids, responsiveness to beta agonists returns.

Periodic assessment of the patient's status and the effectiveness of therapy is undertaken by spirometry, arterial blood gas studies, and fluid and electrolyte assessment.

Nebulized solutions of atropine may reduce the need for corticosteroids, although this is unproven. It is known that atropine with a $beta_2$ agonist has an additive effect in providing relief of airway obstruction. To date, the use of anticholinergic drugs is investigational. The patient with antigen induced bronchospasm or a component of chronic bronchitis may benefit most. The point at which anticholinergic drugs fit into the multistep system of antiasthmatic drug therapy remains to be established.

Respiratory physical therapy may be helpful to remove secretions. When physical symptoms, chest x-ray examination, and Gram staining of sputum indicate the presence of infection, antibiotics are necessary. Yearly influenza vaccination is recommended for patients over 65, especially those with disabling diseases such as asthma or chronic obstructive pulmonary disease.

Sedatives should be avoided unless mechanical ventilation is under way. The use of intermittent positive pressure breathing to deliver a sympathomimetic drug is controversial and to date has offered no advantage over the hand held nebulizer unless the patient is unable to breathe deeply on his own.

Chronic Bronchitis and Emphysema

Chronic bronchitis and emphysema often coexist in the same patient. Emphysema in its pure form is not responsive to bronchodilators. Chronic bronchitis often has a reversible component, although the gain in FEV_1 post isoproterenol inhalation may only be 10 to 15 per cent. Patients with chronic bronchitis sometimes do not respond to an aerosolized $beta_2$ agonist because of severe mucus plugging, poor inspiration, or acute bronchospasm. This does not mean they are not candidates for bronchodilator therapy because they may respond after several weeks of continued use.

The guidelines determining the bronchodilator drug to choose first are vague and unclear. The important point is that after a long enough trial is given, objective evidence be obtained to document the benefits. As a rule, unnecessary drugs are costly and have greater potential for adverse effects in the elderly than in a younger age group.

Patients with chronic obstructive pulmonary disease with occasional bronchospasm may benefit from an aerosolized $beta_2$ agonist. As always, proper use of the device is essential. Patients with excessive mucus production may benefit from the oral administration of sympathomimetic drugs owing to their stimulating effect on the rate of mucus clearance.[102]

Theophylline compounds have not been well studied in chronic obstructive pulmonary disease, but their clinical benefits have been observed often. The same guidelines that are suggested for use in asthma should be followed.

As mentioned previously, corticosteroid use in patients with chronic obstructive pulmonary disease is controversial and unclear. If the patient's symptoms are not controlled by a standard bronchodilator regimen, a two to four week trial of orally administered prednisone is reasonable if there are no absolute contraindications. It is not unusual for patients with chronic bronchitis who did not respond to isoproterenol to respond to oral doses of prednisone. Spirometry testing is essential to document benefit. If the patient does not improve after four weeks, the prednisone dosage can be tapered rapidly. Beclomethasone aerosol can be initiated in patients who do respond to the prednisone. The oral doses of prednisone should then be tapered over several weeks.

In addition to bronchodilators, antibiotics are extremely important in patients with chronic obstructive pulmonary disease. Increases in wheezing and breathlessness, purulent sputum, and symptoms of lower respiratory tract infection should be signals for aggressive treatment. *Diplococcus pneumoniae* and *Haemophilus influenzae* are the most likely organisms, although positive sputum cultures are hard to document. The administration of properly chosen antibiotics (e.g., tetracycline, erythromycin) for seven to 10 days will clear the infection in most instances.

Reduction and facilitated removal of secretions in chronic bronchitis have been the claim of many pharmacologic preparations. The most effective method to reduce secretions is the discontinuation of smoking and the avoidance of dusty or polluted air.

The use of mucolytics and expectorants is widespread, although the evidence for beneficial results is lacking in the majority of cases. Guaifenesin, an expectorant found in many cough preparations, has never been shown to be effective in the dosage range used (100 to 200 mg. three or four times daily). A saturated solution of potassium iodide is thought to increase the volume and decrease the viscosity of secretions and activate proteolytic enzymes. Although some patients show benefit, guidelines for use are unclear. Potassium iodide is excreted renally and therefore would not be recommended in patients with renal insufficiency. Other problems encountered with long term iodide use include rhinorrhea, sneezing, hypothyroidism, parotid gland enlargement, acneiform eruptions, and an unpleasant metallic taste.[153] In most patients the risks outweigh the possible benefits.

Mucolytic drugs can help in removing secretions that are not easily eliminated by coughing. Acetylcysteine (Mucomyst) has been demonstrated in vivo and in vitro to reduce the viscosity of bronchial secretions.[153] Evidence suggests that disruption of disulfide bonds in glycoproteins is the mechanism of action. The 10 per cent or 20 per cent commercially available solution can be combined with an equal volume of saline and administered via nebulization. Frequently bronchospasm necessitates the combined use with an aerosolized bronchodilator. Clinical benefits from acetylcysteine use in emergency situations have been observed by many. Suctioning may be required to remove large amounts of sputum when the drug is administered. Prolonged use of acetylcysteine in patients with chronic obstructive pulmonary disease has not been reported. Whether altering the sputum viscosity on a long term basis will decrease the number of acute exacerbations is unknown.

In summary, the mucolytic drugs may be useful in certain cases, and a significant improvement in airway caliber may result. They work best in well hydrated patients who are also encouraged to cough and breathe deeply and are given postural drainage therapy. Modification of bronchial secretions in stable chronic obstructive pulmonary disease is questionable.

TREATMENT OF HEART FAILURE IN CHRONIC OBSTRUCTIVE PULMONARY DISEASE

Long standing chronic obstructive pulmonary disease is frequently associated with both right and left sided heart failure. Cor pulmonale is thought to result from pulmonary artery hypertension in chronic bronchitis and pulmonary emphysema. Pulmonary hypertension develops as a result of hypoxia, polycythemia, chest infection, thromboembolism, and a reduction in the pulmonary vascular bed.[154,155] Left sided failure is usually a result of coronary artery disease or cardiovascular hypertension; otherwise the left ventricular ejection fraction is normal in chronic obstructive pulmonary disease.[156]

Aminophylline increases both the right and the left ventricular ejection fraction in chronic obstructive pulmonary disease.[18,19] The serum levels and dosage considerations are the same as for treating asthma. Diuretics can improve alveolar gas exchange, reduce peripheral venous congestion, and decrease pulmonary vascular resistance. The use of digitalis to improve right side performance is controversial, since the benefit is not yet known and COPD patients are susceptible to digitalis toxicity.[157] Digitalis is indicated in supraventricular tachyarrhythmias and left sided failure.*

Low flow oxygen therapy for cor pulmonale is now considered the major emphasis of therapy. Benefits include the correction of hypoxia, a decrease in the hematocrit level, a decrease in pulmonary artery pressure, improvement of right ventricular performance, and improvement in the quality of life.[158,159] Most patients require 12 to 15 hours of continuous therapy to receive significant benefit.[160] A recent study indicates that patients with chronic obstructive pulmonary disease who receive 24 hours of continuous low flow oxygen have a mortality rate half that of patients receiving 12 hours of continuous therapy.[161]

PULMONARY EMBOLISM

Pulmonary embolism, resulting from occlusion of a portion of the pulmonary vascular bed by thrombi (or nonthrombotic material occasionally) is not a primary disease but rather a complication of another disorder. Venous thrombi in the deep veins of the lower extremities account for 80 to 90 per cent of pulmonary emboli. Pulmonary embolism, next to pneumonia, is the most common acute pulmonary lesion seen in hospitalized patients. The elderly are particularly at risk for the development of pulmonary embolism because of the immobilization, inactivity, and cardiovascular disease prevalent in this group.

Pulmonary emboli may be single or multiple and extremely variable in size. Emboli lodging in the arterial tree potentially result in four primary events. There is less blood flow through the pulmonary circuit to the left heart and systemic circulation, a damming back of blood behind the physical obstruction, hemorrhagic necrosis of the ischemic area, and impaired pulmonary function. The clinical consequences of pulmonary emboli depend on a number of factors, such as the number of emboli, the degree of obstruction of the pulmonary arterial bed, the size of the emboli and vessel(s) occluded, and the prior state of the lungs and the circulatory system. The average adult, with some exceptions, can withstand

---

*See Chapter 5 on cardiovascular disease for a discussion of the use of digitalis in the elderly.

considerable obstruction of the pulmonary arterial bed without serious consequences.

Massive pulmonary embolism, which is defined as occlusion of 50 per cent or more of the pulmonary arterial circulation, may produce a symptom complex consisting of sudden dyspnea, tachypnea, cyanosis, substernal pain, evidence of right sided heart failure, syncope, anxiety, tachycardia, and hypotensive episodes. With massive embolism, death may occur suddenly or be delayed for several hours. Shock with cardiovascular collapse is often a component of massive pulmonary embolism. Recovery becomes more likely when the blood pressure spontaneously returns to normal. With occlusion of less than 50 per cent of the pulmonary circulation when medium sized or smaller vessels are involved, symptoms vary from transient episodes of dyspnea to life threatening symptoms. With submassive embolism the prognosis is good if adequate treatment is employed and the patient has no history of prior embolism or severe cardiopulmonary disease.

Treatment

Supportive Management

Although anticoagulant therapy is the mainstay of treatment, numerous supportive measures also may be employed to attenuate the symptoms produced by pulmonary emboli. Bed rest, analgesics for pain, and oxygen should be employed as soon as possible. In severe cases, continuous positive pressure oxygen may prove useful, particularly when pulmonary edema is present. Prophylactic antimicrobial therapy is not indicated. Patients should be advised to avoid all sudden effort, especially straining at defecation. The prophylactic use of fecal softeners (Colace) may prove useful. Digitalis is indicated if cardiac failure appears to worsen. Cardiac arrhythmias and shock should be treated appropriately.* Aminophylline may prove useful if dyspnea is prominent or pulmonary edema is present.

Anticoagulants

Heparin. In the absence of any absolute contraindications (e.g., uncontrolled bleeding, hemorrhagic lesions, allergy to heparin, malignant hypertension), heparin therapy should be instituted immediately in all patients with pulmonary embolism. Heparin acts at multiple sites in the normal coagulation system. It inhibits the formation of fibrin clots but does not markedly alter the concentrations of the normal clotting factors of blood. The clotting time is prolonged by therapeutic doses, but the bleeding time is usually unaffected. Because heparin does not have fibrinolytic activity, it will not lyse existing clots but can prevent their extension.

Heparin is not active orally because it is readily inactivated by gastric acid. It should be administered intravenously or subcutaneously. The intravenous route is preferred during the first several days of therapy owing to better antithrombotic effects as compared to those with the subcutaneous route. Intramuscular injections are strongly discouraged owing to the frequent complications of local pain and hematomas.

The duration of action of heparin is dose dependent. When it is administered subcutaneously, therapeutic effects may be maintained for eight to 12 hours. Once absorbed, heparin is distributed in the plasma where it is about 95 per cent protein bound. The average plasma half-life of heparin is 60 to 90 minutes. The plasma half-life may be increased to approximately 2.5 hours at doses of 400 units per kg. The plasma clearance and volume of distribution in patients with deep vein thrombosis may be about twice that in normal individuals. The normal plasma clearance rate of heparin is about 1.6 ml. per kg. per min., with a mean volume of distribution of 127 ml. per kg. The plasma clearance is increased and the half-life shortened in patients with pulmonary emboli; therefore larger than "normal" doses may be required. The dosage of heparin should be adjusted by monitoring the Lee-White clotting time and activated partial thromboplastin time. The Lee-White clotting time should be maintained at a range 2.0 to 2.5 times normal, and the activated partial thromboplastin time should be maintained at a range 1.5 to 2.5 times normal. Heparin is believed to be partially metabolized by liver heparinase and the reticuloendothelial system. Heparin is excreted in the urine as unchanged drug (20 to 50 per cent) and as uroheparin, which possesses mild anticoagulant activity. Heparin clearance is decreased in elderly patients with renal disease.

Numerous precautions should be observed during heparin therapy. Because heparin is derived from bovine lung and porcine intes-

---

*See Chapter 5.

tinal mucosa, a trial dose of 1000 units may be advisable in patients with a history of allergy if the clinical situation allows. Cumulation may occur in patients with hepatic or renal disease. Patients with hypertension or indwelling catheters should receive heparin with caution. Heparin has been reported to produce thrombocytopenia as a result of platelet aggregation. If abnormal platelet aggregation occurs, heparin should be discontinued immediately. Antiplatelet drugs such as aspirin, dipyridamole, or dextran may be helpful in reversing this phenomenon. Heparin should be used with extreme caution when there is increased danger of hemorrhage—subacute bacterial endocarditis, arterial sclerosis, dissecting aneurysm, spinal anesthesia, surgery, shock, hypertension, thrombocytopenia, inaccessible ulcerative lesions, ulcerative colitis, and biliary disease.

Numerous interactions have been reported between heparin and other drugs. The most significant interaction is with drugs that may prolong the prothrombin time or delay coagulation (e.g., aspirin, dextran, phenylbutazone, ibuprofen, indomethacin, dipyridamole, and hydroxychloroquine). Heparin may slightly antagonize the action of ACTH, insulin, and corticosteroids. Digitalis, tetracycline, and nicotine may partially counteract the anticoagulant action of heparin. Heparin also may prolong the one stage prothrombin time. When it is administered with coumarin anticoagulants (e.g., warfarin sodium or dicumarol), a period of four to five hours after the last intravenous dose or 12 to 24 hours after the last subcutaneous dose should elapse if a valid prothrombin time is to be obtained.

A host of adverse effects have been associated with heparin use. Hemorrhage is the chief complication and may occur in as many as 50 per cent of women over age 60. Minor bleeding or an overly prolonged clotting time usually can be controlled by withdrawing the drug. Significant gastrointestinal or urinary tract bleeding may indicate the presence of an occult lesion. The drug should be discontinued immediately in patients who develop symptoms of adrenal insufficiency secondary to adrenal hemorrhage. A variety of hypersensitivity reactions have been reported; these include chills, fever, urticaria, bronchospasm, rhinitis, lacrimation, and anaphylaxis. Other adverse effects include arthralgia, headache, acute reversible thrombocytopenia, osteoporosis (with long term therapy), delayed transient alopecia, and rebound hyperlipemia.

Administration via continuous intravenous infusion is the preferred mode of anticoagulant therapy in the early stage of pulmonary embolism. Intermittent injections produce periods of overcoagulation or undercoagulation and generally require higher daily dosages to achieve an adequate response. A suggested procedure is to begin by administering a loading dose of 75 units per pound of body weight (165 units per kg.) followed by a continuous infusion of 10 units per pound per hour (22 units per kg.) through an indwelling plastic catheter. Subsequent dosing should be adjusted to maintain the activated partial thromboplastin time at 1.5 to 2.5 times normal and the Lee-White clotting time at 2.0 to 2.5 times normal. Heparin requirements may drop after two to three days of therapy. If the intermittent injection technique is employed, it is suggested that the dosage be 10,000 units every four hours the first day and then regulated on the basis of coagulation determinations. Coagulation tests should be performed one hour prior to each dose during the first 24 to 48 hours of intermittent heparin therapy and daily thereafter. If a continuous infusion is to be used, an intravenous infusion pump is beneficial to insure accuracy of dosage. Heparin therapy is recommended for periods of seven to 10 days before relying solely on orally administered anticoagulants.

If a patient is overheparinized, heparin effects can be negated by protamine sulfate (1.0 per cent solution) by slow infusion. Each milligram of protamine sulfate neutralizes approximately 100 heparin units, although decreasing amounts of protamine are required as the time from last heparin injection increases. For example, 30 minutes after a dose of heparin, approximately 0.5 mg. of protamine sulfate is sufficient to neutralize each 100 units of heparin administered. Protamine sulfate has anticoagulant activity and a longer half-life than heparin; therefore no more than 50 mg. should be administered by slow infusion in any 10 minute period.

Orally Administered Anticoagulants (Coumarin and Indanedione Derivatives). Oral anticoagulation (perferably with warfarin) should be instituted several days before heparin therapy is discontinued and continued for up to six months. If the emboli are associated with immobilization, oral doses of anticoagulants should be continued until physical activity is resumed. If emboli recur upon discontinuation of oral anticoagulant therapy, long term prophylactic therapy may be necessary. These drugs act by depressing hepatic synthesis of vitamin K dependent clotting factors through inhibition of vitamin K_2, 3-epoxide reductases. The resultant in vivo effect is a depression of factors II, VII, IX, and X. The degree of depression of these clotting factors is dose dependent. Orally administered anticoagulants have no direct effect on an established thrombus but may prevent further extension of the formed clot and prevent secondary thrombotic complications.

Anticoagulant serum levels are readily achieved, but therapeutic anticoagulant effects are not observed until there has been a significant depletion of clotting factors from the plasma. A maximal anticoagulant effect is usually seen in two to three days, which is the time required to reach steady state plasma levels. Table 4–10 lists the half-life, time required to achieve peak anticoagulant effect, and duration of effect following discontinuation of the coumarin and indanedione derivatives.

Dicumarol has erratic bioavailability owing to its poor water solubility. The other orally administered anticoagulants are more rapidly and more completely absorbed. Additionally dicumarol has a dose dependent half-life that increases with increasing dose. All the orally administered anticoagulants are highly but weakly bound to plasma proteins, primarily warfarin (97 per cent). The orally administered anticoagulants are metabolized by hepatic microsomal enzymes and are excreted primarily in the urine as inactive metabolites. Elderly patients are more sensitive to the anticoagulant effects of these drugs, although the precise mechanism of this hypersensitivity has not been defined.

There are numerous contraindications to the oral use of anticoagulants. Any hemorrhagic diathesis due to a reduction in plasma coagulation factors, platelet number, or platelet function (e.g., hemophilia, leukemia, thrombocytopenic purpura) is a contraindication. The drugs are contraindicated in recent or contemplated surgery of the eye and central nervous system. Patients bleeding from the gastrointestinal, respiratory, or genitourinary tract or patients with lesions that are likely to bleed should not receive the drug. Other contraindications are abortion (threatened), aneurysm, acute nephritis, suspicion of a hemorrhagic cerebrovascular accident, bleeding granuloma, diverticulitis, blood dyscrasias, uncontrolled hypertension, hepatic insufficiency, pericardial effusion, polycythemia vera, subacute bacterial endocarditis, ulcerative lesions, and visceral carcinoma.

Numerous precautions should be observed when oral doses of anticoagulants are prescribed. The treatment of each patient is highly individualized. The dosage should be regulated to prolong the one stage prothrombin time by 1.5 to 2.0 times the control time by the Quick test. Prothrombin times that are 1.5 times the control value or less may not be effective. Prothrombin times that are 2.5 times or greater than the control value are usually associated with an increased incidence of bleeding. Prothrombin times should be monitored daily during initiation of therapy and whenever a drug is added to or deleted from the regimen. Once the patient is stabilized, prothrombin times should be monitored every two weeks. Patients should be advised to report any signs of easy bruising, bleeding, red or dark urine, and black or red stools. The drug should be discontinued at the earliest sign of a bleeding disorder. Abrupt cessation of routine therapy with no complications is not recommended and doses should be tapered gradually.

The orally administered anticoagulants have the greatest potential of any pharmacologic class of drugs for clinically significant interactions with other drugs. Patients should be advised against taking any drug

TABLE 4–10. Activity Characteristics of Orally Administered Anticoagulants

Drug	Half-life	Peak Activity	Duration
Coumarin derivatives			
Dicumarol	1–2 days	1–4 days	2–10 days
Phenprocoumon	6–7 days	2–3 days	4–7 days
Warfarin	1.5–2.0 days	1.5–3.0 days	4–5 days
Indanedione derivatives			
Phenindione	5 hours	1–2 days	2–4 days

(legend or over the counter) without consulting with their physician or pharmacist. Numerous drugs may enhance the anticoagulant properties of orally administered anticoagulants. They may do this by decreasing endogenous vitamin K (oral doses of antibiotics, cholestyramine), displacing the anticoagulant from plasma proteins (phenylbutazone, salicylates, sulfonamides, sulfonylureas, ethacrynic acid, mefenamic acid, nalidixic acid, oxolinic acid, diazoxide, and other acidic drugs), and inhibiting the metabolism of orally administered anticoagulants (chloramphenicol, allopurinol, nortriptyline, disulfiram, metronidazole, alcohol [acute ingestion], phenylbutazone, and colfibrate). Other drugs may increase bleeding tendencies in patients taking oral doses of anticoagulants by inhibiting platelet aggregation (salicylates, phenylbutazone, oxyphenbutazone, sulfinpyrazone, indomethacin, and dipyridamole), inhibiting procoagulant factors (quinidine, antimetabolites, alkylating agents, salicylates) and inducing ulcer formation (phenylbutazone, oxyphenbutazone, sulfinpyrazone, salicylates, indomethacin, and adrenal corticosteroids). Although most drug-drug interactions result in an increased anticoagulant effect, some interactions result in a decreased hypoprothrombinemic effect by inducing hepatic microsomal enzymes and subsequent metabolism of the anticoagulant (barbiturates, glutethimide, etchlorvynol, griseofulvin, phenytoin, carbamazepine, rifampin, and chlorinated insecticides) and producing increased procoagulant factors (estrogens, orally administered estrogen-containing contraceptives, and vitamin K).

The principal adverse drug reaction associated with oral doses of anticoagulants is hemorrhage. Overdosage or an enhanced effect from drug interactions may produce hematuria, hemorrhage from wounds or ulcerative lesions, bleeding from mucous membranes, widespread petechiae and ecchymotic hemorrhages, and adrenal hemorrhage with associated acute adrenal insufficiency. The coumarin derivatives seldom produce side effects other than hemorrhage, but these may include alopecia, urticaria, nausea, vomiting, abdominal cramping, diarrhea, fever, agranulocytosis, leukopenia, and nephropathy. The indanedione derivatives, particularly phenindione, cause a substantially greater incidence of nonhemorrhagic adverse effects than the coumarin derivatives, particularly hepatic, hematopoietic, and cutaneous reactions. Hematopoietic adverse effects of the indanediones include aplastic anemia, leukopenia, red cell aplasia, anemia, and thrombocytopenia. Dermatologic reactions range from rash to exfoliative dermatitis. Hepatitis and jaundice may also be induced by the indanediones. The indanediones may discolor the urine orange-red; the patient should be advised that this can be differentiated from blood by its disappearance on acidification of the specimen with vinegar or other acid.

The dosage, as mentioned previously, should be individualized and adjusted according to the one stage prothrombin time. A suggested regimen would be to give 10 to 15 mg. of warfarin daily until the desired effect on prothrombin time is achieved and then adjust the dose accordingly to maintain that level. In patients who are being switched from heparin to warfarin, a period of overlap is necessary because of the significant delay in onset of the antithrombotic effect of warfarin. A suggested procedure is to administer warfarin, 10 to 15 mg. daily, for two to three days (until desired prothrombin time is reached) and then, while continuing the maintenance dose of warfarin, progressively reduce heparin over three to four days to a point of discontinuing heparin therapy.

If minor bleeding or excess hypoprothrombinemia should occur, one or more doses should be omitted until the prothrombin time returns to normal therapeutic range and the bleeding stops. Early manifestations of overdosage include microscopic hematuria, excessive menstrual bleeding, melena, petechiae, oozing from shaving nicks, and bleeding from the gums. If minor bleeding persists or progresses, vitamin K (phytonadione) may be given orally in doses of 1 to 10 mg. If overt bleeding occurs, 20 to 40 mg. of parenteral vitamin K may be required. The parenteral administration of vitamin K should not be used unless absolutely necessary because it may produce a hypercoagulable state which complicates subsequent anticoagulant therapy.

Thrombolytic Enzymes. Thrombolytic enzymes are indicated in the lysis of acute massive pulmonary emboli causing obstruction or severe filling defects involving two or more lobar pulmonary arteries or an equivalent amount of emboli in other vessels, and for the lysis of pulmonary emboli characterized by unstable hemodynamics, such as failure to maintain blood pressure without supportive measures. Treatment should be instituted as soon as possible after the onset of symptoms and no later than five days after the onset of symptoms.

These clot dissolving drugs provide the only medical means for directly lysing a formed thrombus. The thrombolytic enzymes act on the endogenous fibrinolytic system by converting plasminogen to the enzyme plasmin (fibrinolysin). Plasmin degrades fibrin clots as well as fibrinogen and other plasma proteins. Because plasminogen is present in the thromboembolus, activation by thrombolytic enzymes occurs both within and on the surface of the thromboembolus. The most useful thrombolytic enzymes are streptokinase and urokinase.

Because the products of plasmin degradation of fibrin have an anticoagulant effect, bleeding complications may be difficult to control. The risk of hemorrhage should be weighed against the potential benefits of therapy. Bleeding complications are more frequent with thrombolytic enzyme therapy than with heparin or orally administered anticoagulants. When bleeding occurs, it is difficult to manage; therefore thrombolytic enzymes should be used only by physicians who are experienced in the management of thrombotic diseases in hospitals where clinical and laboratory monitoring can be performed. Situations that put the patient at risk for hemorrhagic complications secondary to thrombolytic enzyme therapy are surgery within 10 days of therapy, lumbar puncture, thoracentesis or paracentesis, invasive diagnostic tests (e.g., liver or kidney biopsy), recent trauma with possible internal injury, thrombocytopenia, recent cerebral embolism, malignant disease, hepatic or renal insufficiency, ulcerative wounds, chronic lung disease with cavitation, rheumatic valvular disease, and severe hypertension.

Concurrent use of anticoagulants is not recommended and may be hazardous. In patients who have been treated previously with heparin, the effects of heparin should be allowed to diminish. A thrombin time of less than twice the normal control value is adequate for starting infusions safely. Heparin should not be started following therapy until the thrombin time has returned to less than twice the normal control value (usually three to four hours with streptokinase). Intramuscular injections should be avoided because of the high probability of hematoma formation. Some patients may be resistant to the effects of streptokinase. When resistance levels are greater than 1,000,000 I.U., streptokinase should not be administered. The concurrent use of drugs that may alter platelet function (e.g., aspirin, indomethacin, phenylbutazone) should be avoided.

Because urokinase is a protein of human origin, allergic reactions are extremely rare and mild. Streptokinase is highly antigenic, however. Reactions that represent possible anaphylaxis have been observed in approximately 2.5 percent of the patients treated with streptokinase. The spectrum of allergic reactions ranges from mild symptoms occurring in approximately 12 per cent of the patients (urticaria, itching, flushing, nausea, headache, and musculoskeletal pain) to more severe allergic reactions, such as bronchospasm and angioneurotic edema. Mild or moderate reactions should be managed with concomitant antihistamine or corticosteroid therapy. Severe allergic reactions require immediate discontinuation of streptokinase and symptomatic management as required. Febrile episodes occur in 2.0 to 3.0 per cent of the patients treated with urokinase. Symptomatic treatment is usually sufficient, and acetaminophen should be used rather than aspirin. If phlebitis occurs near the site of streptokinase infusion, further dilution of the solution is usually adequate for management. In cases of serious bleeding secondary to streptokinase or urokinase administration, the drug should be discontinued. If blood loss has been substantial, packed red cells are indicated. Plasma volume expanders (other than dextran) are indicated to replace the blood volume deficit. The use of aminocaproic acid as an antidote for thrombolytic enzymes has not been well documented; it may be considered, however, if the hemorrhage is life threatening and unresponsive to blood replacement.

Streptokinase therapy is usually begun with a loading dose of 250,000 I.U. infused into a peripheral vein over a 30 minute period. A maintenance dose infusion at the rate of 100,000 I.U. per hour should be continued for 24 hours for pulmonary embolism (up to 72 hours for deep vein thrombosis). The thrombin time should be monitored regularly. Urokinase should be given by administering a priming dose of 2000 units per lb. (4400 units per kg.) by infusion into a peripheral vein over a 10 minute period. This dose should be followed by a continuous infusion at the rate of 2000 units per lb. per hour (4400 units per kg. per hour) for 12 hours. At the end of urokinase therapy, treatment with a continuous infusion of heparin should begin, but not until the thrombin time has decreased to less than twice the normal control value.

DRUG INDUCED PULMONARY DISEASE

Drugs are readily suspected of being the etiologic agent when patients suffer rash, nausea, vomiting, diarrhea, and assorted minor symptoms. The physician's index of suspicion relative to drug induced pulmonary disease is often not high, however. The situation is further complicated by the fact that adverse drug induced effects on the lungs may closely resemble various respiratory diseases. Finally, the elderly population is at greater risk than the population at large for drug induced pulmonary complications because they are more likely to be suffering from disease requiring treatment with many drugs having pulmonary toxicity, and they are more likely to have compromised respiratory function secondary to aging or progressive respiratory disease.

Table 4–11 presents the drugs known to produce pulmonary toxicity, and Table 4–12 presents selected drug induced pulmonary responses.[162–165] Of all drug induced respiratory complications, asthma (bronchospasm) is the most common and aspirin is most commonly implicated. Many of the anticancer drugs are likely to produce pulmonary responses, the most prevalent being interstitial pneumonitis and interstitial fibrosis. There is no sharp distinction between these two patterns of response, and one may progress to the other. All central nervous system depressants are capable of producing respiratory depression, and the degree of respiratory depression is primarily dose related. The risk of respiratory depression with aminoglycosides and neuromuscular blockers is markedly potentiated when these drugs are administered together, and such combinations should be avoided.

The lupus-like syndrome may be induced by numerous drugs, but procainamide, hydralazine, phenytoin, and isoniazid account for over 90 per cent of the well documented cases. With a drug induced lupus-like syndrome there is pleural or lung involvement in approximately 80 per cent of the cases. Pleural effusion may occur secondary to hypersensitivity pneumonitis, and therefore most drugs that produce interstitial pneumonitis may be implicated in

TABLE 4–11. Drugs Causing Pulmonary Toxicity*

Drug Class	Drugs
Adjuncts to anesthesia	Pancuronium bromide and other nondepolarizing neuromuscular blockers
Analgesics	Antipyrine, aspirin, fenoprofen, ibuprofen, indomethacin, mefenamic acid, naproxen, phenylbutazone, propoxyphene
Antibiotics	Cephalothin, colistin, gentamicin, kanamycin, neomycin, penicillins, polymyxin B, streptomycin, tetracycline, tobramycin, viomycin
Anticoagulants	Warfarin sodium
Anticonvulsants	Ethosuximide, mephenytoin, phenytoin, primidone, trimethadione
Antifungals	Griseofulvin
Antihypertensives	Hydralazine, methyldopa, reserpine
Anti-infectives (nonantibiotic)	Isoniazid, nitrofurantoin, para-aminosalicylic acid, sulfonamides
Antineoplastics	Bleomycin, busulfan, carmustine, chlorambucil, cyclophosphamide, melphalan, mercaptopurine, methotrexate, mitomycin, nitrogen mustard, procarbazine
Cholinergic drugs	Pilocarpine, neostigmine
Endocrine agents	Chlorpropamide, contraceptives (oral, estrogen containing), corticosteroids, estrogens
Sympathomimetics	Ephedrine, epinephrine, isoproterenol, propranolol
Tricyclic antidepressants	Amitriptyline, imipramine
Miscellaneous	Acetylcysteine, amaranth (FD & C red No. 2), azathioprine, calcium excess, colchicine, cromolyn sodium, fluorescein, gold salts, hydrochlorothiazide, illicit drugs (contaminated and administered intravenously), iodinated diagnostic contrast media, mineral oil (aspirated), methysergide, paraquat, penicillamine, phosphorus (excess), potassium iodide, propylthiouracil, tartrazine (FD & C yellow No. 5), vitamin D excess

*Adapted from references 162 to 165.

TABLE 4–12. Selected Adverse Pulmonary Responses Attributable to Various Drugs*

Adverse Pulmonary Response	Drugs Implicated
Bronchospasm	Acetylcysteine, amaranth (FD & C red No. 2), antipyrine, antifungals, antibiotics (hypersensitivity reaction), aspirin, cromolyn sodium, fenoprofen, ibuprofen, indomethacin, iodinated diagnostic contrast media, isoproterenol (overuse), mefenamic acid, naproxen, phenylbutazone, tartrazine (FD & C yellow No. 5)
Interstitial pneumonitis and fibrosis	Alpha adrenergic nasal sprays, carmustine, bleomycin, busulfan, carbamazepine, chlorambucil, cyclophosphamide, drugs that can induce the lupus-like syndrome, gold salts, illicit drugs (intravenous, contaminated), iodinated diagnostic contrast media, melphalan, mercaptopurine, methotrexate, methysergide, mineral oil (aspirated), mitomycin, nitrofurantoin, paraquat, penicillamine, procarbazine
Lupus-like syndrome	Ethosuximide, gold salts, griseofulvin, hydralazine, hydrochlorothiazide, isoniazid, mephenytoin, methyldopa, oral contraceptives, para-aminosalicylic acid, penicillin, phenylbutazone, phenytoin, primidone, procainamide, propylthiouracil, reserpine, streptomycin, sulfonamides, tetracycline, trimethadione
Mediastinal lymphadenopathy	Phenytoin, potassium iodide, methotrexate
Noncardiogenic pulmonary edema	Aspirin, colchicine, fluorescein, hydrochlorothiazide, illicit drugs (intravenous, contaminated), nitrogen mustard, propoxyphene
Parenchymal hemorrhage	Anticoagulants, estrogens, mineral oil, penicillamine
Pleural effusion	Anticoagulants, bleomycin, busulfan, drugs that can induce the lupus-like syndrome, ibuprofen, methotrexate, methysergide, mitomycin, nitrofurantoin, para aminosalicylic acid, penicillin, procarbazine
Pulmonary angiitis	Busulfan, corticosteroids, illicit drugs (intravenous, contaminated), sulfonamides
Pulmonary hypertension	Alpha adrenergic nasal sprays, estrogens, illicit drugs (intravenous, contaminated)
Pulmonary infiltrates as manifestation of hypersensitivity response	Amitriptyline, bleomycin, busulfan, chlorpropamide, imipramine, isoniazid, methotrexate, nitrogen mustard, para-aminosalicylic acid, penicillamine, penicillin, phenytoin, procarbazine, sulfonamides
Pulmonary parenchymal calcification	Calcium containing antacids (excess), phosphorus, vitamin D excess
Respiratory depression	Aminoglycoside antibiotics (gentamicin, kanamycin, neomycin, streptomycin, tobramycin), narcotics, nondepolarizing neuromuscular blockers (pancuronium bromide), polymyxin antibiotics (colistin, polymyxin B), sedative-hypnotics (barbiturates, benzodiazepines), miscellaneous (viomycin)

*Adapted from references 162 to 165.

the genesis of pleural effusion as a secondary complication.

The clinician cannot prevent drug induced pulmonary complications without compromising the value of drug therapy in many instances. What is required, therefore, is a high degree of awareness of what respiratory complications may occur secondary to drug therapy and conscientious monitoring of patients at risk for drug induced pulmonary toxicity. By following these broad procedures the physician will be able to render more informed risk-benefit decisions while reducing drug induced morbidity or mortality without markedly compromising the desired pharmacologic response. The lowest possible dose that will yield the desired therapeutic response should be utilized.

ASPIRATION

Acute or chronic pulmonary aspiration may be a significant cause of morbidity and mortality in the elderly.[166] In many people, as part of the aging process, there are depressed cough and gag reflexes. Patients with arteriosclerotic vascular disease may have cranial nerve dysfunction, thus further diminishing these reflexes. During periods of protracted illness, nasogastric feeding tubes may be placed. There may be delayed gastric emptying and tube feedings quickly fill the stomach. The tube may render the gastroesophageal sphincter incompetent, thus allowing regurgitation and potential aspiration.

Sudden aspiration of a large piece of food can lead to sudden death by asphyxiation. The suddenness of this occurrence has led to the incorrect diagnosis of acute myocardial infarction with sudden death. When one is confronted with a person who is suffering this catastrophic event while eating, aspiration of a large piece of food into the larynx or trachea should be quickly considered. A brisk, sudden hug around the chest with the hands pushing in and upward in the subxyphoid area, the Heimlich maneuver, may dislodge a large particle from the glottic opening.[167] Aspiration of a less massive foreign body usually requires bronchoscopy for removal. Otherwise a smaller bronchus may be obstructed with resultant atelectasis and infection.

A common cause of chemical pneumonitis is the aspiration of gastric acid. Animal models have suggested that the pH of the aspirate must be ≤ 2.5.[168] Initial pathologic changes include atelectasis, hemorrhage within the bronchial wall, and pulmonary edema.[168] Marked hypoxemia is usually seen. Therapeutically one should give supplemental oxygen and, if necessary, intubate and ventilate the patient using positive end expiratory pressure.[169]

Much has been written about the efficacy of corticosteroids. Most studies using animal models have failed to show a marked benefit.[169-170] Wynne and Modell believe after reviewing all the available studies, that there are no conclusive data proving that corticosteroids are of significant value.[169] If steroids are to be used, many advocates suggest that they be used as early as possible.[171,172] Finally, they should be given for only 48 to 72 hours.

If food particles are aspirated, an extensive hemorrhagic pneumonia may be seen in about six hours. This is followed by a widespread granulomatous reaction with macrophages and giant cells. In about five days granulomas are found around food particles. With repeated food aspiration the x-ray findings may be similar to those seen in miliary tuberculosis.

Many aspirations fail to cause significant disorder. Examples are saline, barium, and most nasogastric feeding solutions. Other aspirations cause a significant problem only because of continued aspiration over a long period of time. The oral use of mineral oil to lubricate and soften stools is a common practice in the elderly. If it is taken immediately before bedtime, continued low level aspiration can cause chronic lipoid pneumonia. This is best treated by prevention. Patients of any age should be warned against taking mineral oil habitually, especially near bedtime. This warning is particularly important as patients grow older and acquire other diseases that may inhibit gastric emptying or decrease the gag and cough reflexes.

Treatment

Minimizing the factors predisposing to aspiration is the best treatment. Patients with altered states of consciousness should not be fed orally. They should be placed in bed to facilitate drainage of upper airway secretions and gastric contents. A patient should never be restrained flat on his back. If a patient is fed orally or through a nasogastric tube, he should be observed for delayed gastric emptying. Positioning closer to the sitting position after feeding may prevent regurgitation.

If a patient is observed aspirating, he should be positioned head down to facilitate drainage. Upper airway and endotracheal suctioning should be attempted to clear the upper airway and stimulate coughing. If particulate matter is aspirated, bronchoscopy should be performed as soon as possible with an attempt to remove all particles. This may require bronchial lavage. Both aspiration and bronchial lavage cause hypoxemia. Thus, support should be provided with supplemental oxygen and mechanical ventilation if necessary.

Bartlett and Gorbach have reviewed the role of antibiotics.[172,173] They believe that antibiotics should not be given at the time of aspiration, but should be reserved for cases in which there is evidence of infection.

CONCLUSION

As this chapter indicates, drugs can be extremely valuable in the management of pulmonary diseases. The same drugs serve as two edged swords, however, for they all possess significant toxicity. Particularly at risk for drug induced toxicity are elderly patients with altered physiology or coexisting disease processes that not only skew the dose-response curve away from the norm but, in fact, may predispose the patient to drug induced toxicity if appropriate dosage adjustments are not made. Furthermore, numerous drugs consumed for the treatment of diseases other than pulmonary disease may produce pulmonary morbidity. To optimize therapeutic benefits while minimizing the risk of toxicity, the clinician should develop highly defined therapeutic goals, monitor patients appropriately, and scrupulously adjust dosages. Precision in the drug therapy process can pay tremendous dividends in terms of health benefits.

REFERENCES

1. Lehnert, B.E., and Schachter, E.N.: Characterization of obstructive disorders. In The Pharmacology of Respiratory Care. St. Louis, The C.V. Mosby Co., 1980, pp. 269–289.
2. Lee, H.Y., and Stretton, T.B.: Asthma in the elderly. Br. Med. J., 4:93, 1972.
3. Conrad, W.M., et al.: Chronic cough as the sole presenting manifestation of bronchial asthma. N. Engl. J. Med., 300:633, 1979.
4. Costello, J.F.: Asthma. In Hinshaw, H.C., and Murray, J.F. (Editors): Diseases of the Chest. Ed. 4. Philadelphia, W.B. Saunders Company, 1980, pp. 524–559.
5. Hinshaw, H.C., and Murray, J.F.: Diseases of the Chest. Ed. 4. Philadelphia, W.B. Saunders Company, 1980, pp. 560–590.
6. Advances in the understanding of asthma. (Medical Staff Conference, University of California, San Francisco.) West. J. Med., 130:43, 1979.
7. Dunnill, M.S.: The contribution of morphology to the study of chronic obstructive lung disease. Am. J. Med., 57:506, 1974.
8. Austen, K.F.: A review of immunological, biochemical, and pharmacological factors in the release of chemical mediators from human lung. In Austen and Lichtenstein (Editors): Asthma. New York, Academic Press, Inc., 1973, Ch. 8.
9. Gold, W.: Cholinergic pharmacology in asthma. In Austen and Lichtenstein (Editors): Asthma. New York, Academic Press, Inc., 1973, Ch. 11.
10. Mellon, M., et al.: An approach to the treatment of asthma—University of California, School of Medicine, and the University of California Medical Center, San Diego (specialty conference). West. J. Med., 128:408, 1978.
11. Boushey, H.A., et al.: State of the art: bronchial hyperactivity. Am. Rev. Resp. Dis., 121:389, 1980.
12. Paterson, J.W., et al.: State of the art: bronchodilator drugs. Am. Rev. Resp. Dis., 120:1149, 1979.
13. Tager, L., and Speizer, F.E.: Role of infection in chronic bronchitis. N. Engl. J. Med., 292:563, 1975.
14. Diener, C.F., and Burrows, B.: Further observations on the course and prognosis of chronic obstructive lung disease. Am. Rev. Resp. Dis., 111:719, 1975.
15. Matsuba, K., and Thurlbeck, W.M.: Disease of the small airways in chronic bronchitis. Am. Rev. Resp. Dis., 107:552, 1973.
16. Hanna, C.J., and Eyre, P.: On the action of combination bronchodilators. Agents Actions, 9:301, 1979.
17. Yarnell, P.R., and Chu, N.: Focal seizures and aminophylline. Neurology, 25:819, 1975.
18. Matthay, R.A., et al.: Effects of aminophylline upon right and left ventricular performance in chronic obstructive pulmonary disease. Am. J. Med., 65:903, 1978.
19. Matthay, R.A., et al.: Oral theophylline improves biventricular performance in chronic obstructive pulmonary disease. Am. Heart J. 104:1022, 1982.
20. Zwillich, C.W., Matthay, R.A., and Weinberger, M.M.: Theophylline induced seizures in adults: correlation with serum concentrations. Ann. Intern. Med., 82:781, 1975.
21. Hendeles, L., et al.: Absolute bioavailability of oral theophylline. Am. J. Hosp. Pharm., 34:525, 1977.
22. Weinberger, M., et al.: The relation of product formulation to absorption of oral theophylline. N. Engl. J. Med., 299:852, 1978.
23. Trembath, P.W. and Boobis, S.W.: Plasma theophylline levels after sustained-release aminophylline. Clin. Pharmacol. Ther., 26:654, 1979.
24. Dasta, J., Martallo, J.M., and Altman, W.: Comparison of standard and sustained-release theophylline tablets in patients with chronic obstructive pulmonary disease. Am. J. Hosp. Pharm., 36:6B, 1979.
25. Tinkelman, D., et al.: Use of a twelve hour theophylline preparation in chronic adult asthmatics. Ann. Allergy, 43:155, 1979.
26. Welling, P.G., et al.: Influence of diet and fluid on bioavailability of theophylline. Clin. Pharmacol. Ther., 17:475, 1975.
27. O'Malley, K., et al.: Geriatric clinical pharmacology and therapeutics. In Avery, G.S. (Editor): Drug Treatment: Principles and Practice of Clinical Pharmacology and Therapeutics. Sydney, Australia, Adis Press, 1980, pp. 158–181.
28. Lillehei, J.P.: Aminophylline; oral vs. rectal administration. J.A.M.A., 205:305, 1968.
29. Kern, J.W., and Lipman, A.O.: Rational theophylline therapy. A review of the literature with a guide to pharmacokinetic and dosage calculations. Drug Intell. Clin. Pharm., 11:144, 1977.
30. Jenne, J.W.: Rationale for methylxanthines in asthma. In Stein, M.S. (Editor): New Directions in Asthma. Park Ridge, Illinois, American College of Chest Physicians, 1975, pp. 391–414.
31. Weinberger, M., and Hendeles, L.: Formulations and dosage requirements for theophylline in the treatment of asthma. Curr. Med. Res. Opinion, 6 (Suppl. 6):116, 1979.
32. Thompson, R.D., et al.: Determination of theophylline and its metabolites in human urine and serum by high pressure liquid chromatography. J. Lab. Clin. Med., 84:584, 1974.
33. Miech, R.P., and Lohman, S.M.: Metabolism and pharmacokinetics of theophylline. In Stein, M. (Editor): New Directions in Asthma. Park Ridge, Illinois, American College of Chest Physicians, 1979, pp. 391–414.

34. Jenne, J.W., et al.: Relationship of urinary metabolites of theophylline to serum levels. Clin. Pharmacol. Ther., *19:*375, 1976.
35. Lohman, S.M., and Miech, R.P.: Theophylline metabolism by the rat liver microsomal system. J. Pharmacol. Exp. Ther., *196:*213, 1976.
36. Jacobs, M.H.: Theophylline toxicity due to impaired theophylline degradation. Am. Rev. Resp. Dis., *110:*342, 1974.
37. Vozeh, S., et al.: Influence of allopurinol on theophylline disposition in adults. Clin. Pharmacol. Ther., *27:*194, 1980.
38. Jenne, J.W., et al.: Pharmacokinetics of theophylline: application to adjustment of the clinical dose of aminophylline. Clin. Pharmacol. Ther., *13:*349, 1972.
39. Mitenko, P.A., and Ogilvie, R.I.: Pharmacokinetics of intravenous theophylline. Clin. Pharmacol. Ther., *14:*509, 1973.
40. Piafsky, K.M., et al.: Theophylline kinetics in acute pulmonary edema. Clin. Pharmacol. Ther., *21:*310, 1977.
41. Walson, P.D., et al.: Interpatient variability in theophylline kinetics. J. Pediatr., *91:*321, 1977.
42. Ellis, E.F., et al.: Pharmacokinetics of theophylline in children with asthma. Pediatrics, *58:*452, 1976.
43. Levy, G., and Koyssoko, R.: Pharmacokinetic analysis of the effect of theophylline on pharmacy function in asthmatic children. J. Pediatr., *80:*789, 1975.
44. Zaske, D.E., et al.: Oral aminophylline therapy: increased dosage requirements in children. J.A.M.A., *237:*1453, 1977.
45. Powell, J.R., et al.: Theophylline disposition in acutely ill hospitalized patients. The effect of smoking, heart failure, severe airway obstruction and pneumonia. Am. Rev. Resp. Dis., *118:*229, 1978.
46. Cusack, B., et al.: The effect of age and smoking on theophylline kinetics. Br. J. Clin. Pharm., *4:*384, 1980.
47. Jusko, W.J., et al.: Intravenous theophylline therapy: nomogram guidelines. Ann. Intern. Med., *86:*400, 1977.
48. Nielsen-Kudsk, F., et al.: Pharmacokinetics of theophylline in ten elderly patients. Acta Pharmacol. Toxicol., *42:*226, 1978.
49. Piafsky, K.M., et al.: Theophylline disposition in patients with hepatic cirrhosis. N. Engl. J. Med., *296:*1495, 1977.
50. Mangione, A., et al.: Pharmacokinetics of theophylline in hepatic disease. Chest, *73:*616, 1978.
51. Jenne, J.W., et al.: Apparent theophylline half-life fluctuations during treatment of acute left ventricular failure. Am. J. Hosp. Pharm., *34:*408, 1977.
52. Hendeles, L., et al.: Frequent toxicity from IV aminophylline infusions in critically ill patients. Drug Intell. Clin. Pharm., *11:*12, 1977.
53. Vozeh, S., et al.: Changes in theophylline clearance during acute illness. J.A.M.A., *240:*1882, 1978.
54. Piafsky, K.M., et al.: Theophylline kinetics in acute pulmonary edema. Clin. Pharmacol. Ther., *21:*310, 1977.
55. Vicuna, N., et al.: Impaired theophylline clearance in patients with cor pulmonale. Br. J. Clin. Pharmacol., *7:*33, 1979.
56. Mitenko, P.A., and Ogilvie, R.L.: Rational intravenous doses of theophylline. N. Engl. J. Med., *289:*600–603, 1973.
57. Weinberger, M.W., et al.: Intravenous aminophylline dosage: use of serum theophylline measurement for guidance. J.A.M.A., *235:*2110, 1976.
58. Hendeles, L., Weinberger, M., and Bighley, L.: Disposition of theophylline after a single intravenous infusion of aminophylline. Am. Rev. Resp. Dis., *118:*97, 1978.
59. Kordash, T.R., et al.: Theophylline concentrations in asthmatic patients: after administration of aminophylline. J.A.M.A., *238:*139, 1977.
60. Hunt, S.N., et al.: Effect of smoking on theophylline disposition. Clin. Pharmacol. Ther., *19:*546, 1976.
61. Powell, J.R., et al.: The influence of cigarette smoking and sex on theophylline disposition. Am. Rev. Resp. Dis., *116:*17, 1977.
62. Resar, R.K., et al.: Kinetics of theophylline: variability and effect of arterial pH in chronic obstructive lung disease. Chest, *76:*11, 1979.
63. Kozak, P.P.: Administration of erythromycin to patients on theophylline. J. Allergy Clin. Immunol., *60:*149, 1977.
64. Weinberger, M., et al.: Inhibition of theophylline clearance by troleandomycin. J. Allergy Clin. Immunol., *59:*228, 1977.
65. Jacobs, M.H., Senior, R.M., and Kessler, G.: Clinical experience with theophylline: relationships between dosage, serum concentration and toxicity. J.A.M.A., *235:*1983–1986, 1976.
66. Camarata, S.J., et al.: Cardiac arrest in the critically ill. 1. A study of predisposing causes in 132 patients. Circulation, *44:*688, 1971.
67. Sherter, C., Walter, M., Brousseau, D., and Ponder, J.: Pharmacokinetics and pulmonary function studies after oral and intravenous aminophylline administration in asthmatics. Am. Rev. Resp. Dis., *117:*177, 1978.
68. Wyatt, R., Weinberger, M., and Hendeles, L.: Oral theophylline dosage for the management of chronic asthma. Am. J. Dis. Child., *132:*876, 1978.
69. Weinberger, M., and Ginchansky, E.: Dose dependent kinetics of theophylline disposition in asthmatic children. J. Pediatr., *91:*820, 1977.
70. Jacobs, M.H., and Senior, R.M.: Theophylline toxicity due to impaired theophylline degradation. Am. Rev. Resp. Dis., *110:*342, 1974.
71. Innes, I.R., and Nickerson, M.L.: Norepinephrine, epinephrine and the sympathomimetic amines. *In* Goodman, L.S., and Gilman, A.G. (Editors): The Pharmacological Basis of Therapeutics. Ed. 5. New York, Macmillan Publishing Co., Inc., 1975, pp. 477–494.
72. Lands, A.M., et al.: Differentiation of receptor systems activated by sympathomimetic amines. Nature, *214:*597, 1967.
73. Lehnert, B.E., and Schachter, E.N.: Adrenergic receptors and amines. *In* The Pharmacology of Respiratory Care. St. Louis, The C.V. Mosby Co., 1980, pp. 117–143.
74. Alexander, M.R., et al.: The beta-2 agonist bronchodilators. Drug Intell. Clin. Pharm., *11:*526, 1977.
75. Miller, W.C., and Rice, D.L.: A comparison of oral terbutaline and fenoterol in asthma. Ann. Allergy, *44:*15, 1980.
76. Heel, R.C., et al.: Fenoterol: a review of its pharmacological properties and therapeutic efficacy in asthma. Drugs, *15:*3, 1978.
77. Freedman, B.S., and Hill, G.B.: Comparative study of duration of action and cardiovascular effects of bronchodilator aerosols. Thorax, *26:*46, 1971.

78. Webb-Johnson, D.C., et al.: Drug therapy: bronchodilator therapy. N. Engl. J. Med., *297*:476, 1977.
79. Miller, J., et al.: Double-blind one-year clinical study of fenoterol metered dose inhaler: preliminary results of a cooperative study. Ann. Allergy, *39*:418, 1977.
80. Freedman, B.J.: Trial of a new bronchodilator, terbutaline, in asthma. Br. Med. J., *1*:633, 1971.
81. Sly, M.R., et al.: Comparison of subcutaneous terbutaline with epinephrine in the treatment of asthma in children. J. Allergy Clin. Immunol., *59*:128, 1977.
82. Smith, P.R., et al.: A comparative study of subcutaneously administered terbutaline and epinephrine in the treatment of acute bronchial asthma. Chest, *71*:129, 1977.
83. Amory, D.W., et al.: Comparison of the cardiopulmonary effects of subcutaneously administered epinephrine and terbutaline in patients with reversible airway obstruction. Chest, *67*:279, 1975.
84. Kanarek, D.J., et al.: The effect of oral terbutaline in asthma. Acta Allerg., *27*:302, 1972.
85. Tashkin, D.P., et al.: Double-blind comparison of acute bronchial and cardiovascular effects or oral terbutaline and ephedrine. Chest, *68*:155, 1975.
86. Pierson, D.J., et al.: Cardiopulmonary effects of terbutaline and a bronchodilator combination in chronic obstructive pulmonary disease. Chest, *77*:176, 1980.
87. Geumel, A., et al.: Evaluation of a new oral B2-adrenoceptor stimulant bronchodilator, terbutaline. Pharmacology, *13*:201, 1975.
88. Kerr, A., and Givvie, T.: Comparison of orciprenaline, ephedrine and methoxyphenamine as oral bronchodilators. N.Z. Med. J., *77*:320, 1973.
89. Emirgil, C., et al.: Fenoterol: clinical trial of a new lung acting bronchodilator. Ann. Allergy, *39*:415, 1977.
90. Ruffin, R.E.: Response of asthmatic patients to fenoterol inhalation: a method of qualifying the airway bronchodilator dose. Clin. Pharmacol. Ther., *23*:338, 1978.
91. Beck, G.J.: Controlled clinical trial of a new dosage form of metaproterenol. Ann. Allergy, *44*:19, 1980.
92. Spector, S.L., et al.: Effect of Bronkosol and its components on cardiopulmonary parameters in asthmatic patients. J. Allergy Clin. Immunol., *59*:371, 1977.
93. Kaimal, S., et al.: Aerosol bronchodilator therapy: a comparison of the effects of bronkometer with isoetharine, isoproterenol and phenylephrine. Ann. Allergy, *43*:151, 1979.
94. Lehnert, B.E., and Schachter, E.N.: Basic drug science. *In* The Pharmacology of Respiratory Care. St. Louis, The C.V. Mosby Co., 1980, pp. 97–116.
95. Newhouse, M.T., and Ruffin, R.E.: Deposition and fate of aerosolized drugs. Chest, *73* (Suppl.):936, 1978.
96. Murray, J.F.: Review of the state of the art in IPPB. *In* Proceedings of the Conference on the Scientific Basis of Respiratory Therapy. Am. Rev. Resp. Dis., *110*:132, 1974.
97. Weber, R.W., et al.: Aerosolized terbutaline in asthmatics: comparison of dosage strength, schedule, and method of administration. J. Allergy Clin. Immunol., *63*:116, 1979.
98. Banner, A.S., et al.: Arrhythmogenic effects of orally administered bronchodilators. Arch. Intern. Med., *139*:434, 1979.
99. Larsson, S., and Svedmyr, N.: Tremor caused by sympathomimetics is mediated by beta$_2$-adrenoreceptors. Scand. J. Resp. Dis., *58*:5, 1977.
100. Plummer, A.L.: The development of drug tolerance to beta$_2$ adrenergic agents. Chest, *73* (Suppl.):949, 1978.
101. Sackner, M., Silva, G., Zucker, C., and Marks, M.: Long-term effects of metaproterenol in asthmatic children. Am. Rev. Resp. Dis., *115*:945, 1977.
102. Sackner, M.A.: Effect of respiratory drugs on mucociliary clearance. Chest, *73* (Suppl.):958, 1978.
103. Svedmyr, N.L., et al.: Development of resistance in beta-adrenergic receptors. Chest, *69*:479, 1976.
104. Miller, W.C.: Long-term beta$_2$ bronchodilator therapy and the question of tolerance. Chest, *73* (Suppl.):1000, 1978.
105. Herxheimer, A.: Atropine cigarettes in asthma and emphysema. Br. Med. J., *16*:167, 1959.
106. Lehnert, B.E., and Schachter, E.N.: Pulmonary muscarinic antagonist. *In* The Pharmacology of Respiratory Care. St. Louis, The C.V. Mosby Co., 1980, pp. 144–157.
107. Chick, T.W., And Jenne, J.W.: Comparative bronchodilator responses to atropine and terbutaline in asthma and chronic bronchitis. Chest, *72*:719, 1977.
108. Ashutosh, K., et al.: Density dependence of expiratory flow and bronchodilator response in asthma. Chest, *77*:68, 1980.
109. Klock, L.E., et al.: A comparative study of atropine sulfate and isoproterenol hydrochloride in chronic bronchitis. Am. Rev. Resp. Dis., *112*:371, 1975.
110. Brady, R.E., and Easton, S.G.: The value of atropine in the documentation of reversible airways obstruction. Ann. Allergy, *42*:211, 1979.
111. Ruffin, R.E., et al.: Aerosol therapy with Sch 1000: short-term mucociliary clearance in normal and bronchitic subjects and toxicology in normal subjects. Chest, *73*:501, 1978.
112. Storms, W.W., et al.: Aerosol Sch 1000: an anticholinergic bronchodilator. Am. Rev. Resp. Dis., *111*:419, 1975.
113. Casali, L., et al.: Clinical pharmacology of a combination of bronchodilators. Int. J. Clin. Pharm. Biopharm., *7*:277, 1979.
114. Marlin, G.E., et al.: Combined cholinergic antagonist and B$_2$ adrenoceptor agonist bronchodilator therapy by inhalation. Aust. N.Z. J. Med., *9*:511, 1979.
115. Dykes, M.H.M.: Evaluation of an antiasthmatic agent, cromolyn sodium (Aarane, Intal). J.A.M.A., *227*:1061, 1974.
116. Cox, J.S.G.: Disodium cromoglycate(FPL 67C): a specific inhibitor of reagenic antibody-antigen mechanisms. Nature, *216*:1378, 1967.
117. Berstein, I.L., et al.: Therapy with cromolyn sodium. Ann. Intern. Med., *89*:228, 1978.
118. Turner-Warwick, M.: Long term study of disodium cromoglycate in treatment of severe extrinsic or intrinsic bronchial asthma. Br. Med. J., *4*:383, 1972.
119. Irani, F.A., et al.: Evaluation of disodium cromoglycate in intrinsic and extrinsic asthma. Am. Rev. Resp. Dis., *106*:179, 1972.
120. Powell, J.R.: Asthma, chronic bronchitis, and emphysema. *In* Applied Therapeutics for Clinical Pharmacists. Ed. 2. San Francisco, Applied Therapeutics, Inc., 1978, pp. 266–300.
121. Crisp, J., et al.: Cromolyn sodium therapy for chronic perennial asthma. J.A.M.A., *229*:787, 1974.

122. Webb-Johnson, D.C., et al.: Bronchodilator therapy. Drug therapy. N. Engl. J. Med., *297:*758, 1977.
123. Baxter, J.D., and Forsham, P.H.: Tissue effects of glucocorticoids. Am. J. Med., *53:*573, 1972.
124. Fauci, A.S., Dale, D.C., and Balow, J.E.: Glucocorticosteroid therapy: mechanism of action and clinical considerations. N. Engl. J. Med., *84:*304, 1976.
125. Azarnoff, D.L. (Editor): Steroid Therapy. Philadelphia, W.B. Saunders Company, 1975.
126. Collins, J.V., et al.: The use of corticosteroids in the treatment of acute asthma. Quart. J. Med., *44:*259, 1975.
127. Dwyer, J., Lazarus, L., and Hickie, J.: A study of cortisol metabolism in patients with chronic asthma. Aust. Ann. Med., *16:*297, 1967.
128. Powell, L.W., et al.: Corticosteroids in liver disease: studies on the biological conversion of prednisone to prednisolone and plasma protein binding. Gut, *13:*690, 1972.
129. Lehnert, B.E., and Schachter, E.N.: Corticosteroids. *In* The Pharmacology of Respiratory Care. St. Louis, The C.V. Mosby Co., 1980, pp. 191–213.
130. Davies, G., et al.: Steroid-dependent asthma treated with inhaled beclomethasone dipropionate: a long term study. Ann. Intern. Med., *86:*549, 1977.
131. Ballin, J.C.: Evaluation of a new aerosolized steroid for asthma therapy, beclomethasone dipropionate. J.A.M.A., *236:*2891, 1976.
132. Costello, J.F., et al.: Response of patients receiving high dose beclomethasone dipropionate. Thorax, *29:*571, 1974.
133. Gaddie, J., et al.: Aerosol beclomethasone dipropionate: a dose response study in chronic bronchial asthma. Lancet, *2:*280, 1973.
134. Hodson, M.E., et al.: Beclomethasone dipropionate aerosol in asthma. Transfer of steroid-dependent asthmatic patients from oral prednisone to beclomethasone dipropionate aerosol. Am. Rev. Resp. Dis., *110:*403, 1974.
135. Holst, P.E., et al.: A controlled trial of beclomethasone dipropionate in asthma. N.Z. Med. J., *79:*769, 1974.
136. Dixon, R.B., and Christy, N.P.: On the various forms of corticosteroid withdrawal syndrome. Am. J. Med., *68:*224, 1980.
137. Milne, L.J.R., et al.: Beclomethasone dipropionate and oropharyngeal candidiasis. Br. Med. J., *3:*397, 1974.
138. Klasutermeyer, W.B., and Hale, F.C.: The physiologic effect of an intravenous glucocorticoid in bronchial asthma. Ann. Allergy, *37:*80, 1976.
139. Ellul-Micallef, R., et al.: Time-course of response to prednisolone in chronic bronchial asthma. Clin. Sci., *47:*105, 1974.
140. Wyatt, R., et al.: Effects of inhaled beclomethasone dipropionate and alternate day prednisone on pituitary-adrenal function in children with chronic asthma. N. Engl. J. Med., *299:*1387, 1978.
141. Horn, B.R., et al.: Total eosinophil count in obstructive pulmonary disease. N. Engl. J. Med., *292:*1152, 1975.
142. Sahn, S.A.: Corticosteroids in chronic bronchitis and pulmonary emphysema. Chest, *73:*389, 1978.
143. Kettel, L.J., and Morse, J.O.: Corticosteroids in the treatment of pulmonary disease. *In* Azarnoff, D.L. (Editor): Steroid Therapy. Philadelphia, W.B. Saunders Company, 1975, pp. 287–312.
144. Williams, I.P., McGavin, C.R.: Corticosteroids in chronic airways obstruction: can the patient's assessment be ignored? Br. J. Dis. Chest, *74:*142, 1980.
145. Albert, R.K., et al.: Controlled clinical trial of methylprednisolone in patients with chronic bronchitis and acute respiratory insufficiency. Ann. Intern. Med., *92:*753, 1980.
146. Lieberman, P., et al.: complications of long-term steroid therapy for asthma. J. Allergy Clin. Immunol., *49:*329, 1972.
147. Lewis, G.P., et al.: Prednisone side effects and serum protein levels. Lancet, *2:*781, 1971.
148. Pierce, L.E., and O'Brien, J.J.: Hyperglycemic coma associated with corticosteroid therapy. N.Y. J. Med., *69:*1785, 1969.
149. Alavi, I.A., et al.: Steroid-induced diabetic ketoacidosis. Am. J. Med. Sci., *262:*15, 1971.
150. Bond, W.S.: Toxic reactions and side effects of glucocorticoids in man. Am. J. Hosp. Pharm., *34:*479, 1977.
151. Wolfe, J.D., et al.: Bronchodilator effects of terbutaline and aminophylline alone and in combination in asthmatic patients. N. Engl. J. Med., *298:*363, 1978.
152. Shim, C., and Williams, M.H.: Bronchial response to oral versus aerosol metaproterenol in asthma. Ann. Intern. Med., *93:*428, 1980.
153. Irwin, R.S., et al.: Cough. A comprehensive review. Arch. Intern. Med., *137:*1186, 1977.
154. Bishop, J.M.: Cardiovascular complication of chronic bronchitis and emphysema. Med. Clin. N. Am., *57:*771, 1970.
155. Robin, E.D., and Gaudio, R.: Cor pulmonale. Disease A Month, May 1970.
156. Steele, P.P., et al.: Left ventricular ejection fraction in chronic obstructive pulmonary disease. Am. J. Med., *59:*21, 1975.
157. Green, L.H., and Smith, T.W.: The use of digitalis in patients with pulmonary disease. Ann. Intern. Med., *87:*459, 1977.
158. Flick, M.R., and Block, A.J.: Chronic oxygen therapy. Med. Clin. N. Am., *61:*1397, 1977.
159. Steward, B.N., et al.: Long-term results of continuous oxygen therapy at sea level. Chest, *68:*486, 1975.
160. Stark, R.D., et al.: Daily requirement of oxygen to reverse pulmonary hypertension in patients with chronic bronchitis. Br. Med. J., *3:*724, 1972.
161. Nocturnal Oxygen Therapy Trial Group: Continuous or nocturnal oxygen therapy in hypoxemic chronic obstructive lung disease. Ann. Intern. Med., *93:*391, 1980.
162. Ribon, A., and Parikh, S.: Drug induced asthma: a review. Ann. Allergy, *44:*220–233, 1980.
163. Demeter, S.L., et al.: Drug induced pulmonary disease. Part I. Patterns of response. Cleveland Clin. Quart., *46:*89–99, 1979.
164. Demeter, S.L., et al.: Drug induced pulmonary disease. Part II. Categories of drugs, Cleveland Clin. Quart., *46:*101–112, 1979.
165. Rosenow, E.C.: Drug-induced pulmonary disease. Clin. Notes Resp. Dis., *16:*3–11, 1977.
166. Cameron, J., and Zuidema, G.: Aspiration pneumonia. J.A.M.A., *219:*1194, 1972.
167. Heimlich, H., Hoffmann, K., and Canestri, F.: Food choking and drowning deaths prevented by external subdiaphragmatic compression. Physiological basis. Ann. Thorac. Surg., *20:*188, 1975.
168. Greenfield, L., et al.: Pulmonary effects of experi-

mental graded aspiration of hydrochloric acid. Ann. Surg., *170:*74, 1969.
169. Wynne, J., and Modell, J.: Respiratory aspiration of stomach contents. Ann. Intern. Med., *87:*466, 1977.
170. Chapman, R., et al.: The ineffectiveness of steroid therapy in treating aspiration of hydrochloric acid. Arch. Surg., *108:*858, 1974.
171. Downs, J., Chapman, R., Modell, J., and Ian Hood, C.: An evaluation of steroid therapy in aspiration pneumonitis. Anesthesiology, *40:*129, 1974.
172. Bartlett, J.: Aspiration pneumonia. Clin. Notes Resp. Dis., *18:*3, 1980.
173. Bartlett, J., and Gorbach, S.: The triple threat of aspiration pneumonia. Chest, *68:*560, 1975.
174. Roberts, R.K., et al.: Cimetidine impairs the elimination of theophylline and antipyrine. Gastroenterology, *81:*19, 1981.
175. Lalonde, R.L., et al.: The effects of cimetidine on theophylline pharmacokinetics at steady state. Chest, *83:*221, 1983.

CHAPTER 5

CARDIOVASCULAR DISORDERS
Robert H. Hoy and Charles D. Ponte

HYPERTENSION

Aging and High Blood Pressure

Hypertension in the elderly, as defined by a systolic pressure greater than 160 mm. Hg and a diastolic pressure greater than 95 mm. Hg, is very common, affecting perhaps 45 per cent of persons over the age of 60.[1-4] Hypertension in the elderly affects a significantly higher percentage of blacks (55 per cent) than of whites (40 per cent). Moreover, hypertension is approximately 20 per cent more prevalent in elderly women than in men.

Although systolic as well as diastolic blood pressure increases with advancing age, systolic blood pressure tends to increase more sharply than diastolic pressure. Two forms of hypertension are most likely to be encountered in the elderly—isolated systolic hypertension and systolic-diastolic hypertension. Isolated systolic hypertension is characterized by a systolic blood pressure greater than 160 mm. Hg and a diastolic pressure less than 95 mm. Hg. Systolic-diastolic hypertension is the classic hypertension in which the systolic pressure exceeds 160 mm. Hg and the diastolic pressure exceeds 95 mm. Hg. Elevated diastolic or systolic blood pressure correlates with the presence of cardiovascular disease (e.g., cerebral infarction, myocardial infarction, renal insufficiency, congestive heart failure, retinopathy, ischemic heart disease). Cardiovascular disease is three to four times more common in the elderly hypertensive than in the elderly normotensive.

Many internal and external factors play a role in the genesis of hypertension in the elderly.[1-13] Decreased elasticity of the arteries due to the arteriosclerotic process (possibly secondary to decreased levels of high density lipoproteins and increased levels of low density lipoproteins) or calcification and fibrous tissue replacement of the elastic tissue lead to increased peripheral vascular resistance. Arteriosclerosis appears to be the major factor related to isolated systolic pressure elevation. One principal consequence of an elevated systolic pressure is an increase in the cardiac work load, thus increasing wall stress and wall thickness, which leads to left ventricular hypertrophy. An age related decrease in the renal mass, glomerular filtration rate, renal blood flow, and overall kidney function may contribute to hypertension in the elderly because the kidneys' regulatory impact on homeostasis is reduced.

An age related decrease in the lean muscle mass with a proportionate increase in adipose tissue results in a net decrease in the total body water as a percentage of the total body weight. The plasma volume shrinks also, and there is a subsequent lowering of plasma renin activity. Most elderly hypertensive patients have a low renin form of hypertension.

Numerous extrinsic factors such as situational stress, smoking, lack of exercise, obesity, and excessive salt intake play a definite role in the etiology of hypertension. These factors should be controlled whenever possible.

Treatment Objectives

Before treatment is begun, hypertension should be properly diagnosed, with an accurate assessment of the true blood pressure. This should involve six readings on three consecutive days if possible. Two readings should be taken with the patient standing and sitting. A reading with the patient in the standing position is very important because the age associated decline in baroreceptor sensitivity may impair the body's ability to respond to shifts of position. Blood pressure may decline 20 mm. Hg or more on standing in approximately 20 per cent of elderly patients. The true blood pressure would be between the sitting and standing values. If the patient is diagnosed as hypertensive, the diagnosis should be confirmed by follow-up one month later. Follow-up every six to nine months is appropriate. Most cases of hypertension in the elderly are not related to renovascular disease or hypertension secondary to hyperaldosteronism or pheochromocytoma. If the patient's hypertension worsens or is refractory to standard treatment modalities, further diagnostic steps would become necessary.

The physician should examine the patient for target organ damage secondary to the excessive resistive pressure associated with hypertension. A history of angina pectoris, myocardial infarction, peripheral vascular disease, cerebrovascular impairment, congestive heart failure, cardiac arrhythmias, renal impairment, or retinopathies suggests target organ damage from hypertension. The degree of damage to specific organs can provide considerable insight into the duration and severity of the hypertension and the proper treatment of the blood pressure elevation.

Traditionally, isolated systolic hypertension in the elderly was considered a normal part of the aging process and generally was not treated. To a lesser degree this has been true with elevated systolic and diastolic blood pressures in the geriatric patient. Several recent, large scale surveys of elderly hypertensive Americans have demonstrated significant risk associated with an elevation in the systolic and diastolic blood pressure.[3,4,10] Longitudinal analysis of patient data indicates clearly that the higher the blood pressure and the greater the age, the greater the danger of cardiovascular morbidity and mortality.[3,4,10] Cardiovascular disease is overwhelmingly the major cause of illness and death in the elderly. The question related to the treatment of hypertension in the elderly is therefore not whether to treat but rather when and how to treat.[11]

O'Malley and O'Brien consider treating elderly patients with more than one reading of 160/100 mm. Hg.[3] Some clinicians believe that elderly patients with only an elevated systolic pressure, with no symptoms of cardiovascular disease, should not be treated.[4] The National Institutes of Health Report of the Joint National Committee on Detection, Evaluation, and Treatment of High Blood Pressure makes no distinction between elderly and younger adult patients. Lamy states that the risks from hypertension in the elderly are as great or greater than in young adults, and a more conscientious approach to diagnosis and management is warranted.[1]

The consensus evolving with regard to the treatment of hypertension in the elderly is toward treatment in an individualized manner, taking into account pre-existing disease and risk factors. The trend is toward treatment when the diastolic pressure is higher than 95 mm. Hg. Most clinicians would seriously consider treating patients with systolic levels above 160 to 180 mm. Hg. Blood pressure reduction must be effected gradually and carefully, however, to avoid impairment of cerebral and myocardial perfusion, which is more likely in the elderly.

The general goals of treatment are to keep blood pressure within established limits, to prevent target organ damage, to minimize progression of previously existing target organ damage, to eliminate or minimize extrinsic risk factors contributing to hypertension, and to use the step therapy approach with medication, keeping drug induced adverse effects to a minimum.

Treatment

The first approach to the treatment of hypertension is to attempt to avoid or minimize the influence of extrinsic risk factors. These include such factors as smoking, situational stress with associated anxiety, lack of exercise, obesity, and excessive salt intake. Most of the extrinsic risk factors are established components of a life style. The elderly patient is less inclined to change his life style than a young adult. A substantial effort to educate the patient about the risk associated with a certain situation or behavior and the benefits of changing that situation or behavior in terms of quality of life and longevity is fundamental to success. Clinicians should not despair if success is not immediate or frequent. The dividends for the clinician in terms of professional satisfaction when successes are recorded can be very rewarding, however.

Secondly, if drug therapy is to be employed in an attempt to control blood pressure, the physician should be aware of several pathologic, physiologic, and pharmacokinetic factors that may influence the response to drug therapy. Antihypertensive medications as a class have many adverse effects associated with their use. Pre-existing diseases or disorders (e.g., depression, hypokalemia, dehydration, gout, diabetes) may be aggravated by these drugs. A thorough knowledge of the potential of each antihypertensive medication to produce adverse effects is paramount to optimal management of high blood pressure.

The pharmacokinetics of antihypertensive drugs may be changed by the altered physiology in the elderly patient. Absorption of drugs may be impaired as a result of age related decreases in the vascularity, surface area, and motility of the small intestine. Decreases in plasma volume, extracellular fluid volume, and serum protein levels may change drug distribution. Metabolism may be impaired by decreased liver function. The glomerular filtration and creatinine clearance rates are decreased substantially in the elderly, therefore impairing the elimination of drugs and drug metabolites. Also, the elderly patient frequently consumes several prescription and over the counter drugs to treat medical disorders other than hypertension. One should be mindful of the potential of antihypertensive drugs for interacting with other drugs and the possible consequences of such interactions.

Specific antihypertensive therapy in the elderly should begin only after a reliable baseline evaluation of the blood pressure is obtained, routine laboratory tests are performed, the extent of target organ damage has been determined, and all risk factors associated with the drug therapy have been considered. In general, one should initiate therapy with lower doses and make gradual increases (start low—go slow). The treatment regimen should be as simple as possible to maximize compliance.

If the desired blood pressure is not achieved through other means, drugs should be added to the regimen sequentially, one drug at a time, in a stepwise fashion. Step therapy is traditionally begun with a thiazide diuretic.

Step 1. Diuretic Therapy

A diuretic alone often provides adequate blood pressure control. A short to intermediate acting thiazide may be preferred at the onset of therapy. Table 5–1 presents some of the pharmacologic properties of the thiazide and thiazide-like diuretics. The exact mechanism by which the thiazide diuretics lower the blood pressure is not known. The immediate antihypertensive action is associated with diuresis and contraction of the extracellular and intravascular fluid volume, which decreases cardiac output and peripheral vascular resistance. Thiazides may produce their long

TABLE 5–1. Selected Pharmacologic Properties and Equivalent Doses of the Thiazide Diuretics*†

	Onset	Peak	Duration	Equivalent Dose
Chlorothiazide	2 hr.	4 hr.	6 to 12 hr.	500 mg.
Flumethiazide	2 hr.	4 to 6 hr.	12 to 18 hr.	500 mg.
Hydrochlorothiazide	2 hr.	4 hr.	6 to 12 hr.	50 mg.
Benzthiazide	2 hr.	4 to 6 hr.	12 to 18 hr.	50 mg.
Hydroflumethiazide	1 to 2 hr.	2 to 4 hr.	6 to 12 hr.	50 mg.
Bendroflumethiazide	1 to 2 hr.	6 to 12 hr.	18 to 24 hr.	5 mg.
Cyclothiazide	Within 6 hr.	7 to 12 hr.	18 to 24 hr.	2 mg.
Methyclothiazide	2 hr.	6 hr.	24 hr.	5 mg.
Trichlormethiazide	2 hr.	6 hr.	24 hr.	2 mg.
Polythiazide	2 hr.	6 hr.	36 hr.	2 mg.
Quinethazone	2 hr.	6 hr.	18 to 24 hr.	50 mg.
Metolazone	1 hr.	2 hr.	12 to 24 hr.	5 mg.
Chlorthalidone	2 hr.	Within 2 hr.	48 to 72 hr.	50 mg.

*Reprinted with permission from Facts and Comparisons, 1982, p. 137a.
†Metolazone and quinethazone (quinazolone derivatives) and chlorthalidone (a phthalimidine derivative) are included because of their structural and pharmacologic similarity to the thiazides.

term blood pressure lowering effect via a vasodilator action on the vascular wall.

Elderly patients are sensitive to small doses of thiazides. An initial dose of 25 mg. of hydrochlorothiazide once daily in the morning is recommended. Elderly patients are particularly at risk if excessive diuresis is undertaken because of the diminished capacity to correct volume depletion. Occasionally elderly patients have a diminished thirst reflex, which may be worsened by such drugs as the phenothiazines. Overdiuresis in an elderly patient could shrink the plasma volume too quickly and predispose to orthostatic episodes, dizziness, syncope, falls, or fractures; fractures secondary to falls are even more likely if the patient also has senile osteoporosis.

The thiazides may lower the serum potassium level, elevate the serum glucose level, and elevate the serum uric acid level. For these reasons the thiazides should be used with caution in hypokalemic patients, borderline or known diabetics, and persons susceptible to gout. Attention should be directed to periodic urine glucose tests, serum electrolyte evaluation (sodium, chloride, and bicarbonate as well as potassium), and serum uric acid and fasting blood glucose determinations. Urate levels greater than 12 mg. per 100 ml. may warrant allopurinol therapy.

The potential for the loss of sodium, potassium, chloride and bicarbonate is dose related. The monitoring of potassium levels is especially important, because marked hypokalemia (2.5 mEq. per L. or less) may predispose the patient to cardiac arrhythmias, especially if the patient is concurrently taking a digitalis glycoside. If the potassium level drops to an unacceptable level and is uncorrectable by dietary means, 50 mg. of spironolactone or triamterene or 5 mg. of amiloride as potassium sparing diuretics may be added to the regimen. A more acceptable therapeutic approach, however, would be potassium replacement.

When potassium replacement is required, caution must be observed because the elderly patient has a lower lean body mass and total body potassium level and therefore lower potassium replacement requirements. Additionally, with the physiologic loss of renal function with advancing years, the potassium supplements provided may be conserved. No more than 10 to 20 mEq. of potassium per day would generally be required if a patient were receiving 25 to 50 mg. of hydrochlorothiazide daily. The most physiologic potassium supplement is potassium chloride. The principal considerations in selecting a potassium supplement should be palatability and cost.

Loop Diuretics. Use of the more powerful "loop diuretics," bumetanide, ethacrynic acid and furosemide, is seldom necessary. These drugs may be utilized if there is a marked degree of renal failure or congestive heart failure. The thiazides are generally considered to be superior to the loop diuretics as antihypertensives, substantially less risk being associated with their use.

Potassium Sparing Diuretics. Use of the potassium sparing diuretics (amiloride, spironolactone, and triamterene) is generally not warranted in the management of hypertension unless there is intolerance or a contraindication to the use of thiazides. The potassium sparing diuretics are weak antihypertensives, work poorly in renal insufficiency, produce many side effects, and have the potential for interacting with many other drugs. Potassium supplementation and the heavy use of salt substitutes in patients receiving potassium sparing diuretics may produce severe hyperkalemia. Osmotic diuretics, mercurial diuretics, and carbonic anhydrase inhibitor diuretics have no place in antihypertensive drug therapy.

Aggressive treatment with diuretics to lower the blood pressure to "normal" is not recommended. Twenty-five to 50 mg. of hydrochlorothiazide or an equivalent dose of another thiazide or thiazide-like diuretic should produce the optimal response consistent with the lowest incidence of adverse effects. The thiazides should be administered in a single dose as early in the day as possible to minimize nocturia. If pressure elevations or fluid retention is noted in the evening, a longer acting thiazide may be employed.

A reasonable treatment goal with diuretic therapy is a blood pressure of 150 to 160/90 to 100 mm. Hg. If this is not attained, the clinician may choose to go to the second step of antihypertensive therapy.

Step 2. Diuretic Therapy as Well as Adrenergic Inhibiting Drugs (Clonidine, Methyldopa, Guanabenz, Prazosin, Beta Blockers, Reserpine)

If diuretics alone do not control the elevated blood pressure and further lowering is desired, adrenergic inhibiting drugs may be added to the regimen.[17] Selected pharmacologic characteristics of these drugs are presented in Table 5–2. Combination therapy

TABLE 5–2. Selected Pharmacologic Effects of Step 2 Antihypertensive Drugs*

Drug	Peak Effect (Hours)[1]	Duration of Action (Hours)[2]	Plasma Volume	Plasma Renin Activity	RBF/GFR[3]	Peripheral Resistance	Cardiac Output	Heart Rate	Usual Maintenance Dosage Range	Dosage Interval	Comments
Antiadrenergic drugs—centrally acting											
Methyldopa	4–6	12–24	↑	→	0	→	↓sl/0	↓sl/0	250–500 mg.	Two to four times daily	Maximal recommended dose: 500 mg. every 6 hours; single daily dose possible
Clonidine	2	12–24	↑sl	→	0	→	↓/0	→	0.1–0.4 mg.	Twice daily	2.4 mg. daily is maximal effective dose; do not discontinue abruptly; single daily dose possible
Guanabenz	2–4	6–12	0	0	0	→	0	→	4–8 mg.	Twice daily	Maximal studied dose: 32 mg. twice daily
Antiadrenergic drugs—peripherally acting											
Reserpine	6–12	6–24	↑	↓	0	→	0/↓	→	0.1–0.25 mg.	Once daily	
Prazosin	3	6–12	↑sl	→	→	→	0	0	2.0–5.0 mg.	Two to three times daily	20 mg. daily is maximal effective dose; initial dose should be 1.0 mg. two to three times daily
Antiadrenergic drugs—beta blockers											
Metoprolol	2–4	13–19	↓sl/0	→	↓sl/0	0/↓	→	→	50–200 mg.	Twice daily	Initial dose: 50 mg. twice daily
Nadolol	2–4	17–24	↓sl/0	→	0	0	→	→	80–320 mg.	Once daily	Initial dose: 40 mg. once daily
Propranolol	2–4	8–12	↓sl/0	→	→	0	→	→	40–120 mg.	Two to four times daily	Initial dose 40 mg. twice daily; up to 640 mg. daily may be required; long acting capsule may be given once daily
Atenolol	2–4	24+	↓sl/0	→	↓/0	0	→	→	50–100 mg.	Once daily	Initial dose: 50 mg. once daily
Timolol	1–3	12	↓sl/0	→	?	0	→	→	10–20 mg.	Twice daily	Initial dose: 10 mg. twice daily; up to 60 mg. daily may be required
Pindolol	1–2	24+	—	0	0	→	→	→	10–20 mg.	Twice daily	Maximal recommended dose: 60 mg./day; intrinsic sympathomimetic activity

*Adapted with permission from Facts and Comparisons, 1982, p. 160.
[1] Peak clinical effect following a single oral dose.
[2] Duration of action is frequently dose dependent.
[3] Renal blood flow/glomerular filtration rate.

with a diuretic and an antiadrenergic drug may contribute significantly to minimizing side effects common if higher doses of a single drug are used. The antiadrenergic drugs also may lead to secondary fluid accumulation, which is retarded by concurrent diuretic therapy.

Methyldopa. Methyldopa probably exerts its antihypertensive effect through its metabolism to alpha-methylnorepinephrine, which then lowers the arterial pressure by stimulation of central inhibitory alpha-adrenergic receptors, false neurotransmission, or reduction of plasma renin activity. Methyldopa has no significant direct effect on cardiac function and usually does not reduce the glomerular filtration rate, renal blood flow, or the filtration fraction value. These characteristics are positive factors in the elderly patient with pre-existing cardiovascular or renal disease. Approximately two days are required to achieve a maximal antihypertensive response at a given dose.

A positive Coombs test result is seen in 10 to 20 per cent of the patients with prolonged therapy. This is seldom associated with hemolytic anemia. Baseline blood work (hematocrit, hemoglobin, and red cell count) prior to the initiation of therapy is encouraged. A follow-up blood count and Coombs test every six to 12 months after the initiation of therapy may be useful. Liver disorders occur rarely. If previous methyldopa therapy has been associated with liver disorders, the drug is contraindicated in any form of active hepatic disease (e.g., hepatitis or cirrhosis). Sedation is the most common side effect encountered and is usually transient. Other early transient adverse effects are headache, orthostatic episodes, and weakness. Overall, methyldopa is well tolerated. In fact, if insomnia is a problem, 50 to 60 per cent of a daily dosage may be given one to three hours before bedtime.

Clonidine. Clonidine appears to be a central alpha adrenergic stimulant. It produces inhibition of bulbar sympathetic cardioaccelerator and sympathetic vasoconstrictor centers, thereby causing a decrease in the sympathetic outflow from the brain. The most common adverse effects associated with clonidine therapy are dry mouth (40 per cent), drowsiness (35 per cent), and sedation (8 per cent). Constipation, dizziness, headache, and fatigue have been reported. Generally these effects tend to diminish after four to six weeks of therapy. Orthostatic episodes are mild and infrequent. Cardiac output may be reduced moderately (15 to 20 per cent) in the supine position but tends to return to pretreatment levels with continued therapy. The renal blood flow and glomerular filtration rate remain essentially unchanged with clonidine therapy.

The phenomenon of rebound hypertension has been associated with abrupt cessation of clonidine therapy. Therapy should be discontinued by reducing the dose gradually over two to four days to avoid a rapid and possibly severe rise in blood pressure and an increase in associated symptoms.

Reserpine. Reserpine probably exerts its antihypertensive effect by depleting norepinephrine through inhibition of catecholamine storage in postganglionic adrenergic nerve fibers. The onset of action is slow, for it takes days for norepinephrine stores to be depleted. The antihypertensive effect of reserpine may be associated with bradycardia. Generally there is no significant alteration in cardiac output or renal blood flow. The carotid sinus reflex is inhibited, but episodes of postural hypotension are rarely seen.

Reserpine has been largely replaced in antihypertensive therapy by more potent and more specific drugs with a lower incidence of side effects. Side effects associated with reserpine therapy include anorexia, diarrhea, gastric hypersecretion, gastrointestinal bleeding, arrhythmias, bradycardia, drowsiness, depression, nightmares, dermal reactions, nasal congestion, dry mouth, decreased libido, impotence, weight gain, gynecomastia, and breast engorgement.

Reserpine is contraindicated in patients with mental depression, active peptic ulcer, and ulcerative colitis and in patients receiving electroconvulsive therapy. Cardiac arrhythmias are more likely to occur if, in addition to reserpine, the patient is taking digitalis or quinidine. The long term use of reserpine as an antihypertensive may be associated with an increase in the incidence of carcinoma of the breast.

Prazosin. Prazosin is especially useful in geriatric patients because of its specificity and relatively low incidence of side effects. Prazosin reduces peripheral vascular resistance and blood pressure by selective blockade of postsynaptic alpha-adrenergic receptors. It dilates both resistance (arterioles) and capacitance (veins) vessels. The blood pressure is lowered in both the supine and standing positions; this effect is most pronounced on the diastolic blood pressure. Therapeutic lowering of blood pressure occurs without clinically significant changes in cardiac output, heart rate, renal blood flow, and glomerular filtration rate.

The "first dose phenomenon" or first dose effect may result in syncope with sudden loss of consciousness. In most cases this is due to an excessive postural hypotensive effect. Syncopal episodes usually occur within 30 to 90 minutes after the initial dose. The incidence of syncopal episodes is approximately 1 per cent in patients given an initial dose of 2.0 mg. or more. Syncopal episodes may be minimized by limiting the initial dose to 1.0 mg. and increasing the dosage slowly. The initial dose and the first dose at an increased level may best be administered at bedtime to minimize possible adverse sequelae of a hypotensive episode. The patient should be advised to not drive or operate machinery for four hours after the first dose. The first dose effect is self-limiting and does not usually recur.

Other side effects associated with prazosin therapy include dizziness (10.3 per cent), headache (7.8 per cent), drowsiness (7.6 per cent), lack of energy (6.9 per cent), palpitations (5.3 per cent), and nausea (4.9 per cent). In most instances the side effects disappear with continued therapy. Prazosin has the tendency to produce sodium and water retention, and therefore it should routinely be administered with a diuretic. The drug is 97 per cent bound to plasma proteins and may theoretically interact with other highly bound drugs.

Guanabenz. Guanabenz is an orally active antihypertensive drug that is thought to act via stimulation of central $alpha_2$ receptors. This results in a decrease in sympathetic outflow from bulbar vasoconstrictor centers, similar to the mechanism of action proposed for clonidine and methyldopa. Guanabenz is extensively metabolized; less than 1 per cent of a dose is recovered unchanged in the urine. The effects of the age related decline in renal and hepatic function on the disposition of guanabenz in the elderly have not been adequately studied. However, a knowledge of the pharmacokinetics of the drug suggests that the dosage of guanabenz should be reduced in patients with a significant decrease in hepatic function.

Clinically guanabenz has proven to be as effective as methyldopa and clonidine in the treatment of hypertension. A potential advantage of guanabenz over clonidine and methyldopa in elderly patients is that it reportedly causes a smaller degree of orthostatic hypotension. Unlike methyldopa and clonidine, guanabenz does not cause significant sodium and fluid retention, even when used as sole therapy for several months. This could be a potential benefit in elderly patients with congestive heart failure.

The two most common adverse effects associated with the administration of guanabenz include dry mouth and sedation (20 to 30 per cent). The incidence and severity of these side effects seem to be dose related, and they may be particularly troublesome in elderly patients. Other reported side effects include weakness, dizziness, nausea, nasal congestion, depression, and gynecomastia. However, there have been no reports of significant hepatic, renal, cardiac, or biochemical abnormalities associated with the use of guanabenz.

A "withdrawal syndrome" similar to that seen with clonidine has been reported in patients receiving large doses of guanabenz (24 mg. twice daily) following abrupt discontinuation of the drug. Symptoms included marked anxiety, nervousness, insomnia, diaphoresis, palpitations, and a rapid rise in blood pressure. Reinstitution of the drug promptly resulted in the resolution of symptoms.

The recommended starting dosage of guanabenz is 4 mg. twice daily. The dosage may be increased by 4 to 8 mg. per day every one to two weeks, depending on the patient's response and tolerance of adverse effects.

Beta-adrenergic Receptor Blocking Drugs. The beta-adrenergic receptor blocking drugs (metoprolol, nadolol, propranolol, atenolol, pindolol, and timolol) compete with beta-adrenergic agonists for available beta receptor sites.[16] Propranolol, nadolol, and timolol inhibit both beta-1 and beta-2 receptors. Metoprolol and atenolol are cardioselective and preferentially inhibit beta-1 receptors. Pindolol is a nonselective beta-adrenergic antagonist, which possesses intrinsic sympathomimetic activity. The clinical response to beta blockade includes slowing of the heart rate, depression of atrioventricular conduction, decreased cardiac output at rest and following exercise, reduction of systolic blood pressure following exercise, general reduction of supine and standing blood pressure, and reduction of reflex orthostatic tachycardia. All the beta-blockers are virtually equivalent in antihypertensive efficacy. They are particularly useful in treating selected elderly patients with pre-existing cardiovascular complications, since they are also useful in the treatment of angina pectoris and may prevent myocardial infarction. Pindolol has very little effect on resting cardiac output and may cause a smaller decrease in pulse rate than other beta-blockers.

Propranolol and metoprolol are extensively metabolized by the liver; nadolol and atenolol are excreted unchanged by the kidneys; and timolol and pindolol are partially metabolized by the liver and excreted by the kidneys.[15] Nadolol and atenolol have longer half-lives than metoprolol, pindolol, propranolol, and timolol and may be administered in single daily doses.

Most adverse effects with the beta blockers are mild and transient and rarely require withdrawal of therapy.[14,15] Beta blockade may mask premonitory signs of acute hypoglycemia. Nonselective beta blockers may potentiate insulin induced hypoglycemia. Because hypoglycemic attacks may be accompanied by a precipitous elevation of blood pressure, these drugs should be used with caution, particularly in labile diabetics. Propranolol, nadolol, and timolol are contraindicated in patients with any type of bronchospastic disease because of their beta-2 activity. Because of their relative beta-1 selectivity, atenolol and metoprolol should be used with caution in patients with bronchospastic disease who do not respond to or cannot tolerate other antihypertensive treatment. Pindolol may be useful in patients with resting bradycardia who require beta blockade, as it does not usually lower heart rate because of its intrinsic sympathomimetic activity.

All these drugs should be used with caution in cases of impaired hepatic or renal function. The half-life of propranolol, metoprolol, and timolol may be markedly prolonged in hepatic disease. The half-life of nadolol and atenolol would be markedly increased in renal failure. If the creatinine clearance rate is 15 to 35 ml. per min. per 1.73 sq. m., the maximal daily dosage of atenolol is 50 mg.; if the creatinine clearance rate decreases below 15 ml. per min. per 1.73 sq. m., the dosage should be 50 mg. every other day. With nadolol the dosage interval is every 24 hours if the creatinine clearance rate is greater than 50 ml. per min., every 24 to 36 hours at a rate of 31 to 50 ml. per min., every 24 to 48 hours at a rate of 10 to 30 ml. per min., and every 40 to 60 hours at a rate of less than 10 ml. per min.

Nadolol and atenolol do not readily pass the blood-brain barrier and therefore are associated with a lower incidence of central nervous system side effects than metoprolol, pindolol, propranolol, and timolol.

The antiadrenergic beta blockers have the potential for interacting with many drugs.[14-16] These include the catecholamine depleting drugs, monamine oxidase inhibitors, aminophylline, clonidine, prazosin, intravenous doses of phenytoin, digoxin, calcium channel blockers, and sympathomimetic drugs.

The effects of beta-adrenergic blocking drugs can be reversed by the administration of isoproterenol, norepinephrine, dopamine, or dobutamine. If the bradycardia from the beta blockers is excessive, atropine may be administered intravenously. Drug induced bronchospasm warrants administration of a beta-2 stimulant or theophylline derivative.

Step 3. Diuretic Therapy as Well as a Adrenergic Inhibiting Drug and Hydralazine (Vasodilator)

When maximal therapy with a combination of a thiazide diuretic and an antiadrenergic drug fails to control hypertension adequately or leads to undesirable side effects, hydralazine (a vasodilator) may be utilized. Hydralazine is most effective when used with beta-adrenergic blockers because hydralazine produces reflex tachycardia caused by decreased peripheral vascular resistance.

Hydralazine lowers the blood pressure by effecting direct relaxation of vascular smooth muscle (primarily arteriolar), with little effect on venous capacitance vessels. This results in a decrease in arterial blood pressure (diastolic more than systolic), decreased peripheral vascular resistance, reflex tachycardia, increased stroke volume, and increased cardiac output. Hydralazine also maintains or increases renal and cerebral blood flow. Hydralazine has a peak effect one hour after oral administration and a duration of action of six to 12 hours.

Hydralazine is contraindicated in coronary artery disease and mitral valvular rheumatic heart disease. In a few patients hydralazine may produce a clinical picture simulating acute systemic lupus erythematosus. This syndrome is most likely dose related, is associated with long term therapy, and occurs more frequently in slow acetylators. Symptoms usually regress when the drug is discontinued.

The adverse effects most commonly associated with hydralazine therapy include headache, palpitations, anorexia, nausea, vomiting, diarrhea, tachycardia, and angina. A host of other adverse effects that occur rarely have been reported.

Therapy should be initiated in gradually increasing dosages. The initial dosage should be 10 mg. four times daily. Further dosages should be based on the clinical response. After two to four days the dosage may be increased to 25 mg. four times daily. The dosage may be increased to 50 mg. four times daily in the second week. Up to 400 mg. daily may be required in some patients. The dosage should be adjusted to the lowest effective level.

Step 4. Diuretic Therapy as Well as Adrenergic Inhibiting Drug and Guanethidine, Minoxidil, or Captopril

In refractory hypertension that is unresponsive to step 3 drug therapy, a diverse group of drugs known for their potency and toxicity may be employed if the potential benefits outweigh the risks. These drugs are guanethidine, minoxidil, and captopril.

Guanethidine. Guanethidine is the most often used of the step 4 drugs. In fact, some physicians use guanethidine as a step 2 drug in low doses. Guanethidine exerts its potent antihypertensive action by inhibiting norepinephrine release and depleting norepinephrine stores in adrenergic nerve endings. Guanethidine's long half-life (approximately five days) requires a two week interval to adequately evaluate the response.

Guanethidine may produce severe episodes of orthostatic hypotension, which is particularly dangerous in the elderly. Postural hypotension is most marked in the morning and is worsened by alcohol, hot weather, and exercise. Dizziness and weakness may be particularly bothersome. Reduced dosages are required in renal failure. Guanethidine must be administered with a diuretic lest the sodium retention and compensatory fluid retention lead to serious symptomatology. Other frequently occurring and particularly troublesome adverse effects include bradycardia, profuse diarrhea, inhibition of ejaculation, lethargy, urinary incontinence, and despondency.

Guanethidine interacts in a potentially adverse way with numerous drugs. These include reserpine, digitalis, sympathomimetics, tricyclic antidepressants, phenothiazines, orally administered contraceptives, and monoamine oxidase inhibitors.

Treatment should begin with a daily dosage of 10 mg. Dosage adjustments should not be made more often than every seven days in the elderly. The dosage should be increased only if there is no decrease in standing blood pressure. The average dosage is 25 to 50 mg. given once daily.

Minoxidil. Minoxidil is an orally effective, direct acting peripheral vasodilator that reduces both systolic and diastolic blood pressure. Minoxidil has positive virtues in that it does not interfere with vasomotor reflexes and therefore does not produce significant orthostatic hypotension, does not adversely affect central nervous system function, and preserves the renal blood flow and glomerular filtration rate. A number of predictable adverse effects are elicited as a result of the drug's vasodilator properties. These include increased cardiac rate and cardiac output, and salt and water retention.

Minoxidil may produce serious adverse effects, including pericardial effusion progressing to tamponade in approximately 3 per cent of the patients. If the blood pressure is controlled too rapidly with minoxidil, myocardial infarction or cerebrovascular accidents may occur. Approximately 7 per cent of the patients taking minoxidil therapy develop temporary edema. Approximately 80 per cent of the patients will develop elongation, thickening, and enhanced pigmentation of fine body hair within three to six weeks after the initiation of therapy. Upon discontinuation of the drug, one to six months may be required for the pretreatment appearance to return. Breast tenderness (less than 1 per cent), rash (less than 1 per cent), nausea, fatigue, and headache have also been reported. The hematocrit and hemoglobin levels and the erythrocyte count usually fall about 7 per cent initially and then recover to pretreatment levels.

Minoxidil should be reserved for severely hypertensive patients who do not respond adequately to maximal therapeutic doses of a diuretic and two other antihypertensive drugs. The physician should be notified if the pulse rate increases 20 beats or more per minute over normal; if a rapid weight gain of 5 pounds or more is noted; if there is unusual swelling of the extremities, face, or abdomen; if difficulty in breathing is reported; or if there are new or aggravated symptoms of angina, dizziness, or syncope.

The recommended initial dosage is 5 mg. per day given as a single dose. The daily dosage then may be increased to 10, 20, and then 40 mg. in single or divided doses if required. The maximal recommended dosage is 100 mg. per day. When used properly, minoxidil produces a mean diastolic blood pressure reduction of 20 mm. Hg; there is a reduction to 90 mm. Hg in approximately 75 per cent of the patients. The initial dose should be titrated according to individual response. The interval between dosage adjustments should be at least three days.

Captopril. Captopril appears to lower the blood pressure through suppression of the renin-angiotensin-aldosterone system, yet it is antihypertensive even in low renin hypertension. Renin is synthesized by the kidneys and released into the circulation to produce angiotensin I. Angiotensin I is then converted to a potent endogenous vasoconstrictor, known as angiotensin II, by angiotensin converting enzyme. Captopril appears to inhibit angiotensin converting enzyme, thus preventing conversion of angiotensin I to angiotensin II.

The serious side effects associated with captopril therapy restrict its use to step 4 therapy. A total urinary protein level greater than 1.0 gm. per day was seen in 1.2 per cent of the patients receiving captopril. The nephrotic syndrome occurred in about one-fourth of these cases. Prior renal disease predisposes to this adverse effect. Neutropenia (less than 300 per cu. mm.) associated with myeloid hypoplasia has been observed in approximately 0.3 per cent of the patients treated with captopril. Baseline and routine differential counts should be performed during captopril therapy. Neutropenia usually appears after three to 12 weeks of therapy. Patients should report mouth sores, sore throat, fever, edema, palpitations, or chest pain to the physician immediately. A rash with pruritus and occasional fever and eosinophilia occurs in about 10 per cent of the patients during the first four weeks of therapy. The rash is usually mild and frequently disappears with dosage reduction or treatment with antihistamines.

Other troublesome adverse effects include hypotension (2 per cent), reversible loss of taste perception (7 per cent), gastric irritation, abdominal pain, nausea, vomiting, diarrhea, anorexia, peptic ulcer, dizziness, headache, fatigue, insomnia, dry mouth, and paresthesias.

Captopril may interact with concomitant diuretic therapy to produce a precipitous drop in blood pressure within three hours after the first dose. This response is somewhat transient and is not a contraindication to further therapy. Other antihypertensive drugs that cause renin release augment the effects of captopril. All drugs that decrease sympathetic activity may lead to enhanced antihypertensive effects if given with captopril. Potassium sparing diuretics or potassium supplements should be administered with caution because captopril decreases aldosterone production, which may lead to an elevation of the serum potassium level.

Captopril should be administered one hour before meals. The initial dosage is 25 mg. three times daily. If this dosage does not lead to satisfactory control after one to two weeks, the dosage may be increased to 50 mg. three times daily. If further reduction in blood pressure is desired, the dosage may be increased at one to two week intervals to 100 mg. three times daily and ultimately to 150 mg. three times daily. The maximal dosage of 450 mg. per day should not be exceeded.

ANGINA PECTORIS

Coronary artery disease can give rise to a number of painful conditions, including angina pectoris and its variant forms, and acute myocardial infarction and its occasional companion, pericarditis. The etiology of angina rests in those conditions that lead to myocardial ischemia. It is not a condition that is caused by, or results in, myocardial necrosis, as with an acute myocardial infarction. Angina is the pain associated with oxygen deprivation. The severe pain classically presents as a pressure-like sensation, a crushing, or, as angina means, a suffocating sensation. It is not typical for angina to be described as a stabbing or knifelike pain. Angina has the peculiar quality of radiating from the heart or sternum toward the shoulder and then down the left arm. It may radiate to the neck, right arm, abdomen, or elsewhere, but these courses are less typical in their presentation. The pain may be accompanied by great anxiety, diaphoresis, dyspnea, a tense quick pulse, or an elevation in blood pressure during the attack. Exertion, either physical or emotional, can bring on the attack. Rest, relaxation, or sedation may stop the attack. Peripheral vasodilators that reduce the preload, such as sublingually administered nitrates, can stop the attack by decreasing myocardial oxygen demand. The duration of the acute attack is usually a few seconds to a few minutes, depending in part upon steps taken by the patient to decrease exertion or tension, or by using nitrates sublingually.

Drugs of three pharmacologic classes are used prophylactically for angina—nitrates, beta blockers, and calcium channel blockers.

The nitrates, in all forms, indirectly decrease myocardial oxygen demand through venous dilation or preload reduction. The beta blockers prevent exercise induced increases in heart rate and stroke volume. In doing so, they avoid an increased myocardial oxygen demand when the patient with angina attempts to exercise. This effect of keeping the "brakes" on cardiac output with beta blockers necessarily limits the patient's exercise tolerance.

A variant form of angina called Prinzmetal's angina responds to the calcium channel blockers nifedipine, verapamil, and diltiazem, as does the more common angina pectoris. Prinzmetal's angina is provoked by coronary artery vasospasm and is associated with chest pain at rest and a reversible ST segment elevation with or without organic obstructive lesions. Nifedipine, verapamil, and diltiazem block or reduce vasospasm by relaxing arteriolar smooth muscle tone. A strong argument can be made that typical angina as well as Prinzmetal's angina might be relieved best by using calcium channel antagonists rather than beta adrenergic blockers.[18] The role of these new drugs in typical angina is evolving.

Treatment of Stable Angina in the Elderly

The conditions that cause angina are those that lead to myocardial tissue ischemia. These include inadequate circulation, increased oxygen demand, decreased perfusion pressure, hypermetabolic conditions, coronary spasm, and other causes.

The prevention of angina is the most effective approach to its treatment in the elderly. The measures that reduce myocardial oxygen consumption include weight reduction, cessation of cigarette smoking, avoidance of emotional stress, and avoidance of sudden physical effort, strenuous arm activity, or sudden changes in the environmental temperature. Correction of underlying conditions contributing to angina should be attempted. These conditions include cardiac arrhythmias, anemia, diabetes, gout, hypertension, and hyperthyroidism.[19] Instructions to the patient, especially if the angina is of recent onset, should encourage a more relaxed style of life. If the angina remains stable, a gradual increase in physical activity should then begin.[19]

Nitrates

Relaxation of vascular smooth muscle is the principal pharmacologic action of nitrates. Although venous effects predominate, nitroglycerin in a dose related manner produces dilation of arterial and venous beds. Dilation of the postcapillary vessels, including large veins, promotes peripheral pooling of blood and decreases the venous return to the heart, reducing left ventricular end diastolic pressure (preload). Arteriolar relaxation reduces systemic vascular resistance and arterial pressure (afterload). Myocardial oxygen consumption or demand is decreased by both the arterial and venous effects of nitroglycerin. In the coronary circulation the nitrates redistribute the circulating blood flow along collateral channels so that the inner layers of the myocardium are better perfused.

Nitroglycerin and isosorbide dinitrate are well absorbed sublingually. Nitroglycerin is also absorbed through the skin; nitroglycerin ointments and transdermal systems provide a gradual release of the drug, which reaches target organs before hepatic inactivation. Transmucosal nitroglycerin passes directly into the blood through the oral mucosa. Orally administered nitrates undergo significant first pass biotransformation in the liver by nitrate reductase to inactive metabolites. Approximately one-third of an inhaled dose of amyl nitrite is excreted in the urine. The dosage forms available, onset, and duration of action of the various nitrates are included in Table 5–3.

Amyl nitrite, sublingual doses of nitroglycerin, and sublingual or chewable isosorbide dinitrate are indicated for the relief of acute anginal episodes. They may also be used to prevent or minimize anginal attacks when taken immediately prior to events likely to provoke an attack. Long acting nitrates and topically, transdermally, transmucosally, and orally administered sustained release nitroglycerin are used in the prophylaxis and long term management of patients with recurrent angina. Intravenous doses of nitroglycerin may be employed in individuals who have not responded to recommended doses of organic nitrates or a beta blocker.

These drugs may increase intracranial pressure; therefore they should be used with great caution, if at all, in patients who have sustained head trauma or cerebral hemorrhage. Intravenously administered nitroglycerin is contraindicated in hypotension or uncorrected hypovolemia. Tolerance and cross tolerance with other nitrates may develop with repeated use over prolonged periods of time. Tolerance may be minimized by using the

TABLE 5–3. Dosage Forms and Selected Pharmacologic Effects of the Nitrates*

Drug	Dosage Form	Onset	Duration
Amyl nitrite	Inhalant	30 seconds	3 to 5 minutes
Nitroglycerin	Intravenous	Immediate	Transient
	Sublingual	3 minutes	10 to 30 minutes
	Transmucosal	3 minutes	6 hours
	Oral, sustained release	Slow	8 to 12 hours
	Topical ointment	30 to 60 minutes	4 to 6 hours
	Transdermal	30 to 60 minutes	24 hours
Isosorbide dinitrate	Sublingual and chewable	2 to 5 minutes	1 to 2 hours
	Oral	15 to 30 minutes	4 to 6 hours
	Oral, sustained release	Slow	12 hours
Erythrityl tetranitrate	Sublingual and chewable	5 minutes	2 hours
	Oral	30 minutes	Variable
Pentaerythritol tetranitrate	Oral	30 minutes	4 to 5 hours
	Oral, sustained release	Slow	12 hours

*Reprinted with permission from Facts and Comparisons, 1982, p. 143.

smallest effective dose and alternating with other nitrates. Patients with gastric hypermotility should take sublingual or oral doses rather than sustained release forms. Excessive dosing may produce a violent headache; lowering the dose and using analgesics help control the headache. The nitrates should be discontinued if blurring of vision or dry mouth occurs.

When discontinuing prolonged therapy, withdrawal should be gradual owing to the possibility of precipitating angina following abrupt cessation. The elderly are more susceptible to episodes of postural hypotension, and appropriate precautions should be observed.

Among the more common adverse effects is cutaneous vasodilation with flushing. Headache is also common and may be severe and persistent during initial therapy. Transient episodes of dizziness, palpitation, vertigo, and weakness, as well as other signs of cerebral ischemia associated with postural hypotension, may develop occasionally. These effects may be minimized if the patient takes the medication while in a sitting or recumbent position. Rarely an individual exhibits marked sensitivity to the hypotensive effects of nitrates, and significant responses, including nausea, vomiting, abdominal pain, hypotension, pallor, and perspiration, may occur. Alcohol may enhance this effect. Drug rash or exfoliative dermatitis has been reported rarely.

The sublingual use of nitroglycerin tablets requires careful attention to detail. The tablets are best absorbed from the buccal mucosa. Swallowing the tablets or the saliva containing the dissolved tablet defeats the purpose of using the sublingual preparation. If the patient is capable of secreting sufficient saliva, he should be instructed to put the tablet under the tongue or chew the tablet, but not to swallow the saliva for several minutes. A stinging or burning sensation under the tongue results from dissolution of fresh tablets. The development of a headache after the sublingual tablet dissolves and is absorbed is another indicator of tablet potency.

The pharmacist should dispense nitroglycerin tablets for sublingual administration in the manufacturer's original dark brown glass bottle. The cotton should be discarded upon opening the bottle for the first time. Nitroglycerin potency may be lost by sublimation from the tablets to the cotton. Because sublingual nitroglycerin tablet degradation is accelerated by light, heat, and moisture, the patient should be instructed to keep the bottle tightly capped. He should not transfer the tablets to a plastic bottle, a pillbox, or any other container. Six months after opening the bottle, any unused nitroglycerin tablets should be considered subpotent and discarded. The physician should instruct the patient to keep the bottle of potent nitroglycerin tablets with him at all times.

In the hospital the order for "Nitroglycerin sublingual tablets at the patient's bedside" should instead be written, "Nitroglycerin sublingual tablets *with the patient*" in order to avoid the situation in which the patient is in the x-ray department while the tablets are at his bedside. If the patient finds the headaches to be predictable and disconcerting, he may be tempted to discontinue taking the sublingual doses of nitroglycerin. The use of acetaminophen or aspirin one-half hour before taking the sublingual dose of nitroglycerin may prevent the headache.

Titration of the sublingual dose needed for relief of anginal symptoms is done by the patient. A 0.3 mg. dose initially would be a proper starting point. Doses may be repeated every five minutes until relief is obtained. If the patient has to use a third dose within 15 minutes with no significant relief, the patient should go to an emergency room or consult his physician as soon as possible.

Nitroglycerin applied topically as a 2 per cent ointment prevents angina for four to six hours after application. Its slow onset of action, about 30 minutes, precludes its use in the treatment of acute attacks of angina. The 2 per cent ointment provides approximately 15 mg. of nitroglycerin per inch of application. Application should be done so as to maximize absorption while delivering a constant amount each time it is applied. The site of application should be washed clean at the end of the dosing interval. A new site should be chosen utilizing skin surfaces that are not covered by hair, scars, or burns and that are not abraded, broken, or inflamed. The ointment does not have to be applied directly over the heart.

A major factor affecting topical absorption is the surface area over which the ointment is spread. Only the molecules touching the skin can be absorbed; no migration of nitroglycerin occurs through a thick layer of ointment. The ointment may be spread according to the guideline outlined in Table 5–4.

Larger ointment pads are available on request from the pharmaceutical manufacturer. The use of an occlusive dressing increases absorption but also increases the incidence of dermatologic reactions. The person applying the ointment needs to take precautionary steps to prevent absorption by wearing gloves or using a tongue depressor to spread the ointment. The beneficial effects of topically applied nitroglycerin are the result of reduced ischemia and reduced myocardial oxygen demand. Because these effects last considerably longer than when the sublingual form is used, nitroglycerin paste is useful in the prophylaxis of recurrent angina, especially nocturnal angina. The usual therapeutic dose is 1 to 2 inches every eight hours. Some patients may require as much as 4 to 5 inches or application every four hours.

A third formulation of nitroglycerin used to treat or prevent angina is the orally administered sustained release capsule. Because the liver extracts a high percentage of oral doses of nitroglycerin during the first pass, much larger doses must be given by mouth than when given by the sublingual route. The oral form has a delayed onset of action, and effects last for up to eight to 12 hours.

The transmucosal dosage form contains nitroglycerin in an inert polymer base, which releases the drug for absorption by the oral mucosa over a period of time. When administered under the upper lip or bucally, the tablets adhere to the mucosa. The tablet should be allowed to dissolve; they should not be chewed or swallowed. It normally takes three to four hours for the tablet to dissolve. If continuous nitration is desired, the next tablet should be taken within one hour after the previous one dissolves.

The usual dose is one tablet three times daily (upon arising, after lunch, and after the evening meal). Treatment should be started with the 1.0 mg tablets. The dosage may be titrated upward if necessary. If angina occurs while the tablet is in place, the dose may be increased. If angina occurs between tablet administration when no tablet is in place, the frequency of dosing may be increased to four times daily.

The transdermal nitroglycerin system is applied to the skin, and nitroglycerin is predictably and continuously absorbed into the systemic circulation for a minimum of 24 hours. Therapeutic plasma levels are generally attained within one hour and remain in the therapeutic range for 24 hours.

The patches should be applied once daily to a skin site free of hair and not subjected to excessive movement. The application site should be changed each time to avoid undue skin irritation. A new patch should be applied if the product loosens. Table 5–5 lists the commercially available transdermal media and

TABLE 5–4. Topical Application of Nitroglycerin Ointment

Nitroglycerin	Surface Area
1.0 inch	4 inch diameter area
1.5 inches	5 inch diameter area
2.0 inches	6 inch diameter area

TABLE 5-5. Transdermal Nitroglycerin Systems and Release Rates*†

Product	Release Rate
Transderm-Nitro (Ciba)	5 mg./24 hours (8 sq. cm.—16 mg. total content) 10 mg./24 hours (16 sq. cm.—32 mg. total content)
Nitro-Dur (Key Pharmaceutical)	2.5 mg./24 hours (5 sq. cm.—26 mg. total content) 5.0 mg./24 hours (10 sq. cm.—51 mg. total content) 7.5 mg./24 hours (15 sq. cm.—77 mg. total content) 10 mg./24 hours (20 sq. cm.—104 mg. total content) 15 mg./24 hours (30 sq. cm.—154 mg. total content)
Nitrodisc (Searle)	5.0 mg./24 hours (10 sq. cm.—25 mg. total content) 10.0 mg./24 hours (20 sq. cm.—50 mg. total content)

*Adapted with permission from Facts and Comparisons, 1982, p. 143g.
†Direct data comparing serum levels and clinical response to various products not currently available.

their release rates. The optimal dosage regimen should be based upon the clinical response, side effects, and the heart rate. The dosage may be increased by applying a larger surface area or a system with a higher release rate.

The intravenous administration of nitroglycerin is seldom indicated in angina. If administered for refractory angina, it should be diluted in 5 per cent dextrose injection U.S.P., or 0.9% sodium chloride injection U.S.P., prior to infusion. Nitroglycerin infusions may be used in dilutions ranging from 25 to 400 mcg. per ml.; concentration of the infusion should be based on individual patient fluid requirements.

The initial dosage should be 5 mcg. per min. delivered through an infusion pump capable of exact and constant delivery. The subsequent infusion rate should be based on clinical response in 5 mcg. per min. increments.

Oral and sublingual doses of isosorbide dinitrate act similarly to nitroglycerin. The usual dose of the sublingual form is 2.5 to 10.0 mg., although doses up to 30 mg. have been administered. Doses may be taken as needed for the prompt relief of anginal pain or every four to six hours prophylactically. The oral tablet is for prophylactic management of angina. The average dose with the oral tablet is 10 to 20 mg. four times daily. The usual dose of the sustained release dosage form is 40 mg. every six to 12 hours.

Beta Blockers

The beta-adrenergic receptor blocking drugs (as presented under the section on hypertension) compete with beta-adrenergic agonists for available beta receptor sites and vary in their selectivity for beta-1 and beta-2 receptors. Although not the most cardioselective of this group of drugs, propranolol and nadolol are the only beta-adrenergic blockers approved for use in the management of angina at this time.[20]

Propranolol and nadolol appear to exert their antianginal effect by reducing the oxygen requirement of the heart at any given level of effort by blocking catecholamine induced increases in heart rate, systolic blood pressure, and the velocity and extent of myocardial contraction. Conversely, these drugs may increase oxygen requirements by increasing left ventricular fiber length, end diastolic pressure, and systolic ejection period, particularly in patients with heart failure. If the net physiologic effect of beta-adrenergic blockade in angina is advantageous, it would be expected to manifest itself during exercise as a delayed onset of pain.

Propranolol and nadolol, because of their capacity to inhibit beta-2 receptors, are contraindicated in elderly patients with asthma or severe chronic obstructive lung disease. These drugs should be used with extreme caution in the elderly who suffer cardiac failure, because the beta blockade could depress myocardial contractility and worsen the failure.

The beta blockers should not be withdrawn abruptly. There have been numerous reports of a period of catecholamine hypersensitivity following abrupt withdrawal, including exacerbation of angina, myocardial infarction, ventricular arrhythmias, and transient symptoms including tremulousness, perspiration, palpitation, headache, and malaise. Because coronary artery disease may be unrecognized in the elderly, it is advisable to taper therapy with beta blockers even if the drugs are being used to treat hypertension.

The dosage of beta blockers should be reduced gradually over a one to two week period. If angina worsens markedly during the withdrawal, therapy should be reinstituted temporarily and other drugs employed to manage the unstable angina.

The physician should be notified if an unusually slow pulse rate, dizziness, lightheadedness, mental confusion, or depression occurs during therapy. Propranolol should be taken with food to enhance absorption; nadolol may be taken without regard to meals.

The usual initial dosage of nadolol in the treatment of angina is 40 mg. given once daily. The dosage may be increased gradually in 40 to 80 mg. increments at three to seven day intervals until the desired response is achieved. The usefulness and safety of doses exceeding 240 mg. per day have not been established. The usual maintenance dosage range is 80 to 240 mg. administered once daily. Most patients respond to a daily dosage of 160 mg. or less. The section on hypertension provides guidelines for giving nadolol in patients with marked renal impairment.

The usual initial dosage of propranolol in the treatment of angina is 10 to 20 mg. three or four times daily. The dosage may be increased at three to seven day intervals until the desired response is achieved. The value and safety of dosages beyond 320 mg. daily have not been established. Dosing should be individualized; the average optimal daily dosage is 160 mg. Twice daily doses of propranolol are also effective in the management of angina pectoris.

Calcium Channel Blockers

The calcium channel blocking drugs (also known as calcium antagonists and slow channel inhibitors) are an entirely new class of drugs receiving widespread acceptance in this country in the management of various cardiovascular disorders, including angina pectoris.

The predominant action of the calcium channel blockers (nifedipine, verapamil, and diltiazem) is to oppose calcium fluxes at specific cellular membranes. Calcium plays a critical role in cardiac function, and the effect of impeding calcium flux has numerous effects. Calcium plays a key role in linking the electrical depolarization of a cell to contraction. The excitation-contraction coupling is initially triggered by a small amount of calcium, which enters the cell during the plateau phase of the action potential. Calcium also plays a key role in cardiac electrical activity, particularly at the sinoatrial and atrioventricular nodal cells where sodium channels exert a lesser influence. The smooth muscle tone in the coronary arteries is critically influenced by alterations in the influx of calcium. The intracellular actions of catecholamines operate by influencing calcium. The uncontrolled influx of calcium may be one of the early cellular events that cause ischemic cells to die.

The calcium channel blockers of greatest interest in the United States are verapamil (Calan, Isoptin), nifedipine (Procardia), and diltiazem (Cardizem). Table 5–6 summarizes and compares selected pharmacologic and pharmacokinetic characteristics of these drugs. These calcium channel blockers are heterogeneous in chemical structure and action. Nifedipine, verapamil, and diltiazem are currently the only calcium channel blockers approved for use in the United States in the treatment of angina.

Nifedipine, verapamil, and diltiazem are indicated for the treatment of both vasospastic (Prinzmetal's or variant) angina and chronic stable (classic effort induced) angina. The precise mechanism by which calcium channel

TABLE 5–6. Selected Pharmacologic and Pharmacokinetic Characteristics of Calcium Channel Blockers*

	Verapamil	Nifedipine	Diltiazem
Pharmacokinetics			
Oral bioavailability (%)	30–35	65–70	40–60
Onset of action oral (min.)	30[1]	20[2]	30
Protein binding (%)	90	>90	70–85
Therapeutic serum levels (mcg./ml.)	0.12–0.4	—	0.05–0.2
Excreted unchanged in urine (%)	<5	<5	<4
Half-life (hours)	2–5	2–4	4–9
Pharmacology			
SA node automaticity[3]	↓↓	0	↓
AV node conduction[3]	↓↓↓	0/↓	↓↓
Myocardial contractility[3]	↓↓	↓	↓
Peripheral vascular resistance	↓↓	↓↓↓	↓
Heart rate	↑↓	↑	0/↓
Cardiac output	↓↑	↑	0/↑

*Reprinted with permission from Facts and Comparisons, 1983, p. 148g.
[1]Onset is rapid with IV use.
[2]Onset is 3 minutes sublingually.
[3]Direct effects may be counteracted by reflex sympathomimetic activity.

blockers relieve the symptoms of angina has not been fully defined, but two primary events occur.[21] These are relaxation of coronary arteries and prevention of vasospasm, and reduction of oxygen utilization. The drugs dilate coronary arteries in both ischemic and non-ischemic areas and are very effective inhibitors of coronary artery vasospasm. Thus, these drugs increase myocardial oxygen delivery in both vasospastic and stable types of angina. They also reduce arterial pressure at rest and with exercise by dilating peripheral arterioles and reducing the total peripheral resistance (afterload) against which the heart works, thus decreasing myocardial energy consumption and the oxygen requirement. This probably accounts for the effectiveness of the drugs in chronic stable angina.

Contraindications to the use of the calcium channel blockers is known hypersensitivity to the drug, hypotension, and second or third degree atrioventricular block. Adverse effects occur frequently but are seldom serious enough to warrant discontinuation of therapy or dosage adjustment. Most of the adverse effects are associated with the vasodilator effects of the drugs and include dizziness, lightheadedness, giddiness, flushing, headache, weakness, lassitude, dyspepsia, muscle cramps, peripheral edema, nasal congestion, and sore throat. Nausea, arrhythmias, headache, rash, and transient hypotension have also been reported. Transient hypotension appears to be most probable in patients who are concurrently consuming beta-adrenergic blocker drugs. Syncope occurs in about 0.5 per cent of nifedipine treated patients. Hypotensive and syncopal episodes have important safety implications in the elderly. To minimize the possibility of falls and fractures during initial therapy or periods of upward dosage adjustment, elderly patients should be monitored very closely and the smallest possible dose consistent with acceptable management of angina utilized.

Peripheral edema, as well as transient hypotension, appears to be a dose related adverse effect. Edema occurs most commonly in the lower extremities and responds well to diuretics. Fewer than 2 per cent of the patients reported the following adverse effects: shortness of breath, diarrhea, constipation, joint stiffness, muscle cramps, sleep disturbances, urticaria, fever, or sexual difficulties.

Occasionally a patient reports increased frequency, duration, or severity of angina on initiation of therapy or at the time of dosage increases. The mechanism of this response is poorly defined, but it could result from decreased coronary perfusion associated with decreased diastolic pressure and increased heart rate or from increased demand resulting from increased heart rate alone.

Patients recently withdrawn from beta blockers may develop a withdrawal reaction, with increased angina. The initiation of treatment with calcium channel blockers does not prevent this occurrence and may exacerbate it by provoking reflex catecholamine release. There is no acceptable alternative to tapering the dosage of beta blockers prior to withdrawal.

Calcium channel blockers may be safely coadministered with long acting nitrates. The antianginal effectiveness and benefits of the combination have not been fully evaluated, however.

The typical starting dosage of nifedipine is 10 mg. three times daily. Patients with vasospastic angina respond best to larger or more frequent doses. In such patients dosages of 20 to 30 mg. three to four times daily may be required. Dosages above 120 mg. daily are rarely necessary; dosages above 180 mg. per day are not recommended.

Diltiazem is available as 30 and 60 mg. tablets. The dosage should be adjusted to each patients' needs. The usual starting dosage is 30 mg. four times daily before meals and at bedtime. The dosage may be increased gradually to 240 mg. given in divided doses three or four times daily. The dosage should be increased in small increments at one to two day intervals.

Verapamil is available as 80 and 120 mg. tablets and an injectable form containing 5 mg. per 2 ml. The dosage should be individualized and may be increased at daily or weekly intervals until an optimal clinical response is achieved. The maximal effect of any given dose would normally be apparent during the first 24 to 48 hours of therapy. The usual initial dosage is 80 mg. three to four times daily. The value and safety of dosages exceeding 480 mg. per day in angina have not been determined.

Generally a seven to 14 day titration period is necessary to assess the response at the various dosage levels while monitoring the blood pressure. Hospitalized patients may be started on an accelerated titration schedule. Sublingual doses of nitroglycerin may be taken as required to control the acute manifestations of angina during titration. No rebound effect to abrupt withdrawal has been noted, but gradual tapering of the dosage is recommended.

CONGESTIVE HEART FAILURE

Congestive heart failure represents a continuum of disease from asymptomatic pump failure to the brink of cardiogenic shock. When the heart is unable to adequately pump blood to vital organs, a number of compensatory mechanisms bring about the physical changes leading to congestion of the circulatory system with excess fluid accumulation. An understanding of this process is fundamental to proper therapy. Even with a number of therapeutic measures available, the five year mortality rate is over 50 per cent. When we consider this prognosis, the need is apparent for a thorough understanding of the elderly patient's altered sensitivity to the disease and the drug therapy.

Pathophysiology

In their review, Elenbaas and Covinsky emphasize the importance of understanding the pathophysiology of heart failure in order to apply complex therapy.[22] The etiology of congestive heart failure is most commonly essential hypertension, ischemic heart disease, or rheumatic heart disease. Less commonly pulmonary embolism, thyrotoxicosis, chronic anemia, renal disease, bacterial endocarditis, rheumatic fever, persistent cardiac arrhythmias, or myocardiopathy may play a part in its development. The reason the myocardial cells lose their contractile strength in heart failure is not well understood.

When the heart begins to fail, a number of compensatory processes begin. The decreased systolic pressure causes the carotid baroreceptors to increase the sympathetic impulses to the heart, increasing the heart rate and the strength of contraction. Decreased renal artery perfusion pressure causes a reflex increase in renin release from the juxtaglomerular apparatus of the kidney. This eventually leads to an increase in angiotensin II and aldosterone levels. Angiotensin II increases peripheral vascular resistance, and aldosterone causes sodium and fluid retention in the distal nephron. The heart enlarges as the intravascular fluid volume expands. Failure of the left ventricle causes the excess intravascular volume to accumulate behind it in the lungs; right ventricular failure causes congestion of fluid in the systemic venous circulation.

A shift occurs in the osmotic balance between the capillary lumen and interstitial space. The systemic venous congestion increases the hydrostatic pressure and dilutes the colloid osmotic pressure. Both these changes favor the movement of fluid from the capillary lumen to the interstitial space. The result of this process is the formation of peripheral edema in right sided failure and pulmonary fluid retention in left sided failure. The clinical manifestations of this process are diagramed in Figure 5-1.

Other changes may occur, including peripheral cyanosis, fatigue, and weakness. The edema is gravity dependent, forming in the ankle and pretibial areas in ambulatory patients and in the sacral area in bedridden patients.

Drugs can exacerbate congestive heart failure by several mechanisms. As with foods that are high in sodium content, some medicinals (e.g., androgens, corticosteroids, estrogens, lithium carbonate, phenylbutazone) contain or cause retention of sodium. Like sodium, other substances (e.g., albumin, glucose, mannitol, saline, urea) are osmotically active and can increase the intravascular volume, worsening failure. Drugs that act as sympatholytics can diminish the heart rate or stroke volume that is reflexly increased by sympathetic tone.

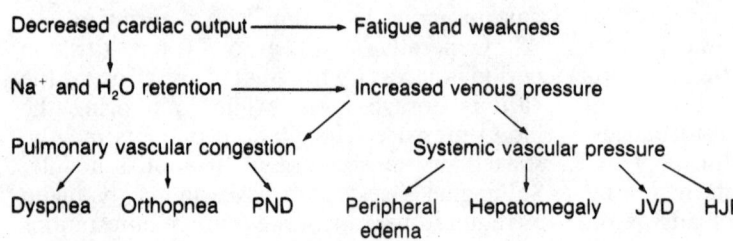

Figure 5-1. Clinical manifestations of heart failure. PND, paroxysmal nocturnal dyspnea. JVD, jugular venous distention. HJR, hepatojugular reflex. (From Elenbaas, R.M., and Covinsky, J.O.: Approaches to the management of acute, chronic and refractory congestive heart failure. J.C.E. Hosp. Clin. Pharm., 11, Jan./Mar. 1979.)

Treatment

The principal considerations in the management of congestive heart failure include elimination of etiologic factors precipitating the failure, reducing the workload on the heart, increasing myocardial contractility and performance, and decreasing sodium and water retention.[22] Thus, the medical management of congestive heart failure includes correction of underlying disease states (e.g., hypertension), bed rest, a sodium restricted diet, and the administration of digitalis glycosides, diuretics, and possibly vasodilators. We will follow this scheme in this chapter, discussing nondrug therapy, digoxin, diuretics, and the potential role of vasodilators and sympathomimetics in the treatment of refractory congestive heart failure.

Nondrug Treatment

Limited activity and bed rest are very effective in reducing the cardiac workload. Significant weight loss in obese patients assists in achieving compensation. Control of elevated blood pressure leads to afterload reduction and is always effective in improving performance of the left ventricle. Reduction of salt and water intake is part of the treatment of numerous cardiovascular diseases. Restricting cooking salt and elimination of table salt can bring the daily sodium chloride intake down to about 4 grams (approximately 2 grams of sodium). In the normal American diet containing 10 grams of salt, any reduction in salt intake will be beneficial. Total salt restriction is very difficult to achieve and unacceptably unpalatable to most patients.

Treatment with Digitalis Glycosides

The subject of digoxin therapy is a fascinating one, spanning a 200 year history, filled with controversy and unsettled even today. Several reviews will be of interest to anyone interested in further information.[22-28] This section focuses on which patients with congestive heart failure should be given digoxin as the first drug and who should receive diuretics instead, how the dosing of digoxin changes in the elderly patient, and guidelines for the safe use of digoxin (dosing, toxicity, and drug-drug interactions). Digitoxin and the other digitalis glycosides (deslanoside and lanatoside C) are not presented because they are seldom used.

If the patient with congestive heart failure has a normal sinus rhythm, a controversy currently exists regarding whether the patient should be initially treated with digoxin or with diuretics.[22,24,29] This argument is of particular interest when one is considering the treatment of elderly patients because of their susceptibility to digoxin toxicity.[26] More important, several reports in the literature point to evidence that in many patients taking long term digoxin therapy, withdrawal can be accomplished safely and without the need for resuming digoxin. The percentage of patients in whom this may be done ranges from 14 to 94 per cent.[24,28] The use of diuretics as first line drugs in the treatment of congestive heart failure is gaining popularity as its efficacy is demonstrated.[29] Digoxin remains an important drug for initial therapy if dietary restriction of salt intake controls fluid accumulation.

The use of digoxin in elderly patients with congestive heart failure is commonplace, but deserves a review because of the potential for lack of efficacy or toxicity in this patient population if the drug is improperly used. The cardiac glycosides are more effective in some types of failure and less effective in others. For example, digoxin is very effective in biventricular or left ventricular failure associated with excessive hemodynamic burdens produced by hypertension, valvular disease, or ischemic heart disease. Digoxin is less effective in treating heart failure secondary to rheumatic fever, anemia, beriberi, complete atrioventricular block, cor pulmonale, infection, mitral stenosis, and thyrotoxicosis.

Digitalis is contraindicated in patients with ventricular fibrillation, ventricular tachycardia, or second degree or unstable atrioventricular block.[22] The use of digoxin following a myocardial infarction presents two problems. In the first place, it may increase or decrease the myocardial oxygen supply-demand, increasing or decreasing anginal complaints. Because of the transient sensitivity of the peri-infarction zone to inotropic drugs, the use of digoxin should be avoided early in the postinfarction period. Secondly, because ventricular performance often improves after stabilization of the infarction and necrotic process, patients may not need digoxin on a long term basis.

Another difficult aspect of digoxin therapy is in recognizing a useful therapeutic endpoint. Use of the Swan-Ganz catheter and hemodynamic subset theory would be extremely useful but not advisable in most patients with congestive heart failure. Because digoxin improves the cardiac index, signs of pulmonary and systemic interstitial fluid congestion begin to reflect improvement. Edema in the ankle and pretibial areas may be slow to resolve and is not as accurate for monitoring acute changes as pulmonary symptoms (resolution of rales, dyspnea, orthopnea) and cardiac changes (slowed heart rate).

The value of digoxin serum concentrations remains controversial. Some authors carry out routine serum determinations as part of an individualized approach to dosage adjustment, whereas others downplay the usefulness of digoxin concentrations. Aronson notes that "... the plasma digoxin concentration has not been shown conclusively to be correlated either with the quantity of digoxin present in cardiac tissue [or] with various measures of the clinical effects of the drug either in atrial fibrillation or in cardiac failure in sinus rhythm."[23] A middle of the road viewpoint would be to recommend that a trough serum concentration be determined if toxicity is suspected; if malabsorption, noncompliance, or other reasons exist to suspect a "subclinical" concentration; or if confirmatory evidence is desired for a clinical impression following a therapeutic dose.[22] If a peak serum concentration of digoxin is desired, six to eight hours should elapse after the oral dose before a serum level is obtained. Sufficient time must be allowed for distribution of the drug to occur so as to avoid spuriously high serum digoxin levels. Careful adjustment of the digoxin concentration within the therapeutic range may not optimize the clinical effect or avoid toxicity. The diagnosis and management of digoxin's effect or toxicity are best effected clinically. The normal "therapeutic" serum concentration of digoxin is 0.8 to 2.0 ng. per ml.; the toxic range is generally considered to be 2.0 ng. per ml. or greater. Digitoxin is considered therapeutic at a concentration of 14 to 26 ng. per ml. and toxic at serum concentrations of 34 ng. per ml. or higher.

Digoxin is administered differently in the elderly and in the younger patient. In about 12 per cent of digoxin treated elderly patients, 20 to 55 percent of the drug is metabolized.[23] Changes in hepatic function might be expected to change the elimination rate of digoxin in these patients. However, data from one study showed that digoxin elimination was not impaired by the presence of cirrhosis or diabetes insipidus.[27] The volume of distribution of digoxin is apparently reduced in the elderly patient; a lower loading dose (digitalization dose) is recommended in the elderly patient.[23,26] One explanation for this occurrence might be the loss of skeletal muscle mass in elderly patients. Digoxin binds avidly to skeletal muscle, possibly to the extent of 65 per cent. Another major factor influencing the pharmacokinetics of digoxin in the elderly is the decrease in the glomerular filtration rate with advancing age. The figures presented in Table 5-7 indicate the marked normal decline in creatinine clearance with advancing age.

The elderly patient inevitably develops a form of progressive renal dysfunction, which alters the capacity to excrete digoxin. The half-life of digoxin has been shown to increase as much as 40 per cent in the elderly with reduced creatinine clearance rates. Since most patients excrete over 85 per cent of the digoxin unchanged in the urine, alterations in renal function should account for almost all changes in the elimination half-life.[23] In the elderly patient, then, accounting for changes in creatinine clearance is desirable in order to adjust the digoxin dosage. No adjustment of digoxin dosing for changes in hepatic function seems justifiable at this time. The nomogram in Figure 5-2 can be of value in estimating creatinine clearance.

The approximate creatinine clearance rate in ml. per min. also can be derived by using the following formula:*

$$\text{Creatinine clearance rate† (ml./min.)} = \frac{(140 - \text{age}) \text{ (kg. mass)}}{72 \text{ (serum creatinine in mg. per 100 ml)}}$$

The creatinine clearance rate obtained may be utilized to calculate a reduced digoxin maintenance dosage. For example, if the creatinine clearance rate is 50 to 79 ml. per min. a daily maintenance dosage of 0.25 mg. of digoxin is usually appropriate. If the creatinine clearance rate is 26 to 49 ml. per min., a daily digoxin dosage of 0.1875 mg. is more appropriate. If the creatinine clearance is 8 to 25 ml. per min., one would seldom administer more than 0.125 mg. of digoxin daily.

---

*Adapted from Cockcraft, D.W., and Gault, M.H.: Prediction of creatinine clearance from serum creatinine. Nephron, *16*:31-41, 1976.

†Multiply the determined Ccr value by 0.85 to determine the value for females.

TABLE 5-7. Normal Decline of Creatinine Clearance with Advancing Age*

Patient's Age	Creatinine Clearance (ml./min.)	
	Male	*Female*
20–29	117 ± 23	91 ± 19
30–39	98 ± 39	96 ± 25
40–49	98 ± 22	76 ± 26
50–59	81 ± 21	74 ± 24
60–69	76 ± 22	60 ± 15
70–79	64 ± 15	49 ± 12
80–89	45 ± 15	41 ± 14
90–99	35 ± 9	34 ± 8

*Adapted from Kampmann, J., et al.: Rapid evaluation of creatinine clearance. Acta Med. Scand., *196*:518, 1974.

These dosing guidelines represent a starting point for therapy. Clinical evaluation of the patient for safe and effective dosing is the main guide for the clinician. The appropriate use of digoxin may be viewed in three steps. These include careful digitalization, recognition of digoxin toxicity, and recognition of the patient who might be safely withdrawn from the drug.

When initiating digoxin therapy, the safest method takes into account the lower volume of distribution of digoxin in the elderly and the slow distributive phase of the drug. The lowered digoxin volume of distribution may result from renal impairment, as occurs with increasing age. Decreasing the loading dose by one-third to one-half may produce adequate and nontoxic digoxin effects. An oral digitalization dose of 0.25 to 0.75 mg. of digoxin is adequate in most elderly patients.[30] If the loading dose is to be given, dividing it into 0.25 mg. increments and spacing these at least six hours apart reduces the chance of toxicity during the long distributive phase after the drug has been absorbed. If the clinician can justify a more gradual program for initiating digoxin therapy, the safer way to begin digoxin is by starting with the maintenance dose. Therapeutic effects take days to begin, but the risk of toxicity during the loading dose period is greatly reduced.

Monitoring for digoxin toxicity should be a substantial part of a clinician's responsibility in routine use of digoxin. Toxicity is quite common; it may be present in 2 to 20 per cent of the patients taking digoxin regularly.[26] As many as 18 per cent of digitalis toxic patients may die from digitalis induced arrhythmias.[22] The arrhythmias accompanying digitalis toxicity are more common (80 to 90 per cent of all digitalis-toxic patients) than extracardiac manifestations (only half of all digitalis toxic patients).[22,26]

Some common clinical signs and symptoms of digitalis toxicity include anorexia, nausea, vomiting, diarrhea, headache, mental depression, abdominal pain, weight loss, scotoma, blue-yellow vision, and cardiac arrhythmias. Many of the arrhythmias that digitalis glycosides are effective in treating resemble those associated with digitalis toxicity. Digitalis glycosides are indicated for the treatment of atrial fibrillation, atrial flutter, and paroxysmal atrial tachycardia. Cardiac arrhythmias most commonly induced by digitalis glycosides include ventricular arrhythmias, atrioventricular block, atrial arrhythmias, junctional arrhythmias, sinoatrial arrhythmias, and atrioventricular dissociation. If the possibility of digitalis induced arrhythmia cannot be excluded readily, cardiac glycosides should be withdrawn

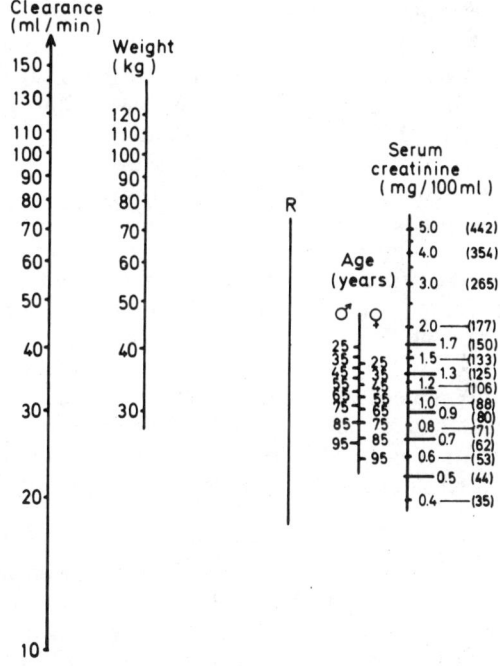

Figure 5–2. Nomogram for evaluation of the endogenous creatinine clearance. *Use of the nomogram:* Connect with a ruler the patient's weight on the second line from the left with the patient's age on the fourth line. Note the point of intersection on *R* and keep the ruler there. Turn the right part of the ruler to the appropriate serum creatinine value and the left side will indicate the clearance in ml/min. Serum creatinine values in μmol/l are given within parentheses. (From Kampmann J., et al.: Rapid evaluation of creatinine clearance. Acta Med. Scand., *196*:519, 1974.)

temporarily, if the clinical situation permits, to determine the extent to which the arrhythmias are drug induced.

Several factors can predispose to digitalis toxicity. Renal insufficiency is of special concern in the patient receiving digoxin therapy. Hypokalemia sensitizes the myocardium to digitalis glycosides. Excess serum calcium increases the effect of cardiac glycosides and may lead to cardiac excitability and arrhythmias. Hypothyroidism (untreated) may predispose the patient to digitalis toxicity.

As mentioned previously, several researchers have concluded that many patients taking digoxin on a long term basis may be safely withdrawn from therapy with no apparent ill effects. The safe use of digoxin might logically include a retrospective analysis of whether the patient needs digoxin on a long term or permanent basis. Patients may be safely withdrawn with no apparent ill effects because the original diagnosis was incorrect, noncompliance in 50 to 60 per cent of the patients amounts to self-withdrawal, inadequate doses were originally prescribed, or initial indications have subsided.[24] It is safe to assume that no ill effects will accompany digoxin withdrawal if the serum digoxin level has been maintained at a level below 0.8 ng. per ml. Two-thirds of the patients taking digoxin and having a "therapeutic" digoxin level can be successfully withdrawn after an appropriate period of time.

It is suggested that the following questions be asked to determine the patient's need for continued digoxin after three months of treatment:

1. Is the patient in normal sinus rhythm? Patients needing digoxin to control the ventricular rate between 70 and 90 beats per minute may need it for life, but patients with normal sinus rhythm may not need digoxin for life.

2. Is there a lack of evidence of cardiac failure? Among this group there is no absolute way to predict whether the patient will require maintenance digoxin therapy. A digoxin free period in asymptomatic patients could be tried. Perhaps a diuretic alone will be sufficient.

3. Is the digoxin level below the "therapeutic range"?

If the answer to all three questions is affirmative, withdrawal may be safe and indicated.[24] Should the patient's cardiac status deteriorate, early resumption of digitalis glycoside therapy is recommended.

Two final points should be made with regard to digoxin therapy. The bioavailability of digoxin varies greatly among different oral preparations. The average bioavailability of digoxin tablets is 50 to 70 per cent.[23,27] Changes from one brand to another should be avoided, and a preparation of proven bioavailability, such as Lanoxin, should be used.[30] Also, drug interactions between digoxin and other drugs can increase or decrease the effect of digoxin. The transit time of the dissolving digoxin tablet as it passes through the gastrointestinal tract is an important factor in determining the percentage absorbed. Propantheline and diphenoxylate with atropine (e.g., Lomotil) decrease gastrointestinal tract motility time, possibly increasing digoxin absorption. Metoclopramide increases gastrointestinal tract motility, leading to a decrease in digoxin absorption. Antacids may cause diarrhea or constipation; this effect does not seem to be a key factor in determining why digoxin absorption is impaired by the concomitant use of antacids. The only antacid that significantly impairs digoxin absorption is magnesium trisilicate. The authors in one study suggested that the digoxin tablets were being coated by the antacid, thus decreasing absorption.[27] This mechanism may explain why there is decreased absorption of digoxin when it is given within a few hours after the administration of kaolin-pectin antidiarrheal preparations or cholestyramine. Merely avoiding the concomitant use of digoxin and antacids, antidiarrheals, or cholestyramine by two to three hours avoids the likelihood of an interaction. Certain antimicrobial drugs such as sulfasalazine, para-aminosalicylic acid, and neomycin may decrease digoxin absorption.

Renal tubular secretion of digoxin can be impaired significantly by concurrent administration of the diuretic spironolactone. A 25 per cent increase in the serum digoxin concentration has been observed with this interaction.[27] A more dramatic example of altered tubular secretion or reabsorption of digoxin occurs in the presence of quinidine. Adding quinidine to the regimen of a patient taking digoxin rapidly (within 24 hours) causes an increase (as much as double) in the serum digoxin level and electrocardiographic evidence of an enhanced digoxin concentration. Although not shown conclusively, a decrease in the volume of distribution, possibly as a result of the displacement of digoxin from tissue protein binding sites, may play a role in this observed interaction. The decreased tubular elimination of digoxin by quinidine is a more plausible explanation of the interaction. A decrease in the maintenance dosage of digoxin by 50 per cent and monitoring for signs and symptoms of digoxin toxicity are recommended in patients taking digoxin in whom quinidine therapy is about to be initiated.[27] Digoxin serum levels may fall below the therapeutic range with the discontinuation of concomitant quinidine therapy.

In summary, because of widely varying absorption rates in different manufacturers' digoxin tablets, a preparation with proven bioavailability should be used when generic substitution is allowed. Drug interactions with digoxin and other drugs include absorption, distribution, and elimination changes. Of great clinical significance is the quinidine-digoxin interaction, wherein the digoxin effect is markedly enhanced when quinidine is added to the regimen.

Treatment with Diuretics

Diuretics are used both as first line drugs and as adjuncts to cardiac glycosides in the treatment of congestive heart failure. By reducing the fluid excess in the central vascular compartment, diuretics decrease the volume of fluid that must be pumped by the failing heart. Any resulting increase in cardiac output will lead to diuresis of interstitial or "third space" fluid, collecting as pulmonary interstitial fluid or peripheral edema. Because of their effect on blood pressure, diuretics are also used to treat hypertension, but the effect sought in the treatment of mild congestive heart failure is the diuretic effect. The use of thiazides, furosemide, ethacrynic acid, triamterene, and spironolactone in the elderly patient is of interest.

As mentioned previously, the prolonged use of digoxin to treat congestive heart failure has been questioned recently. Several studies revealed that about 75 per cent of all patients taking digoxin suffer no ill effects when the drug is discontinued. Digoxin therapy may be ineffective on a long term basis, and it is certainly responsible for a high percentage of toxic complications. For these several reasons, a safer and yet effective alternative for digoxin has been sought.[19]

Diuretics are more difficult to use in the elderly patient than in the younger patient, from the standpoints of both safety and efficacy. Toxicity resulting from digoxin could favor diuretics as first line drug therapy, except that the toxic effects of diuretics also increase with advancing age.

Older persons tend to develop hypovolemia because of decreased dietary intake of liquids and decreased concentrating capacity in the tubules as the renal mass diminishes. Hypovolemia can occur if diuresis is too rapid, even in a patient with peripheral edema and pulmonary congestion.[22] The development of hypovolemia can exacerbate other diuretic complications in the elderly.

Overly rapid diuresis can decrease plasma volume, leading to secondary hyperaldosteronism.[19,22] This can increase sodium reabsorption proximally and exacerbate potassium losses.[19,22] Hyponatremia commonly occurs in patients with decreased glomerular filtration rates, as is frequently seen in the elderly patient.[22] Hyponatremia can occur as a result of a dilutional effect secondary to diuretic induced sodium loss and normal fluid intake. Diuretics that waste sodium or potassium, such as the loop diuretics or the thiazides, also waste chloride ion; replacing potassium losses with potassium chloride is critical to the correction of the hypochloremia and the potential acid-base disturbance (metabolic alkalosis).[22]

Smaller than usual doses of diuretic are usually required in the treatment of congestive heart failure in the elderly. The usual dosing range of hydrochlorothiazide is 12.5 to 100 mg. per day. Its bioavailability is approximately 65 per cent, but this varies widely from patient to patient, increasing with food intake and decreasing in renal failure. The normal elimination half-life of 10 hours can nearly double in patients with cardiac failure.[31]

A drug similar in chemical structure and pharmacologic function to hydrochlorothiazide is chlorthalidone. It binds avidly to erythrocytes, has a resulting volume of distribution that is very large (300 liters), and is eliminated unchanged in the urine. Its very long half-life of 40 to 65 hours allows it to be given once a day or even less often.

The most frequently prescribed loop diuretic is furosemide. Its dosage range is 20 to 3000 mg. per day. Its bioavailability is about 65 per cent, which decreases in uremia or nephrosis by about one-third. The normal half-life is about one hour, but this can increase in patients with renal failure up to three hours. The change in half-life is widely variable from patient to patient exhibiting the same degree of renal failure. Use of the drug in renal failure depends in part upon its capacity to redistribute renal blood flow and decrease renal vascular resistance, improving the diuretic effect in failing kidneys.[22] Congestive heart failure does not change the pharmacokinetics of furosemide.

The potassium sparing diuretic, spironolactone, should be used cautiously in patients with renal failure, congestive heart failure, and liver disease. These disease states prolong the half-life of the drug. Spironolactone is normally a weak diuretic, and in patients with renal failure it can cause hyperkalemia. This holds true for triamterene and amiloride also. Spironolactone is extensively metabolized to active metabolites, undergoes enterohepatic recycling, and acts as an inducer of hepatic metabolism of other drugs. Its active metabolites allow its action to be prolonged such that dosing intervals of 12 to 24 hours are rational.

To make definite conclusions as to the place of diuretic therapy in the initial treatment of congestive heart failure is difficult. Mild congestive heart failure is treatable by using digoxin to improve myocardial pump performance. The substitution of a diuretic as the drug of first choice might be justifiable in a patient with mild right sided failure or in a patient with sinus rhythm.[19,22] Less aggressive diuretic therapy decreases the chance of hypovolemia or hyponatremia. As with digoxin, diuretic therapy in the elderly must be approached cautiously, keeping in mind the fact that the elderly are more apt to experience side effects from the drugs and are less able to compensate for physiologic disruptions.

Treatment with Vasodilators and New Inotropic Drugs

The use of vasodilators and new orally administered inotropic drugs is being evaluated in the management of congestive heart failure. These drugs may be appropriate for use if traditional therapy fails. Vasodilators used in heart failure can be subdivided into arteriolar dilators (e.g., hydralazine, minoxidil) and venodilators (e.g., nitrates). Prazosin dilates both arteriolar and venous vessels. Patients with heart failure have an excessive increase in systemic vascular resistance that further reduces cardiac output. Arteriolar dilation and afterload reduction from a drug such as hydralazine may produce a very substantial increase in cardiac output, even if the patient is already receiving digitalis and diuretics. Venoconstriction is also common in patients with severe heart failure, and venodilation with nitroglycerin, for example, may decrease the preload by redistributing blood from the congested vasculature of the central chest to the periphery. This lowers the right and left atrial pressures and reduces symptoms of pulmonary and systemic congestion.

New inotropic drugs, such as amrinone, are being developed and evaluated. Initial studies indicate important and beneficial hemodynamic effects. Amrinone, for example, increases myocardial contractility and also produces vasodilation.

The role of the vasodilators and new inotropic drugs in the management of heart failure is not clearly defined at this time. There are still questions about when these drugs should be used, how early in the course of the disease they should be used, which drug should be employed, and whether they should be used as adjuncts in combination with traditional therapy. Digitalis and diuretics do not appear to represent the last of the drugs to be developed for the management of heart failure. New drug developments indicate that we can do more. The exact nature of better management through therapeutic intervention with less risk of drug induced side effects remains to be defined.

CARDIAC ARRHYTHMIAS

A cardiac arrhythmia may arise as a result of a disturbance of either impulse formation or impulse conduction. The treatment of cardiac arrhythmias in the elderly is similar in most ways to that in younger patients, the differences being largely in the doses of antiarrhythmic drugs employed. The individual arrhythmias are to be discussed in terms of overall management considerations; then the individual antiarrhythmic drugs are reviewed to emphasize special considerations in their use in the elderly. Emphasis is placed upon the following drugs with antiarrhythmic properties: digoxin, quinidine, procainamide, disopyramide, lidocaine, phenytoin, propranolol, bretylium, and verapamil.

Before an arrhythmia is treated, several goals should be established. These include the following:[32]

1. Making an accurate electrocardiographic diagnosis and repeating electrocardiography

often enough to follow the progress of the disease and therapy.

2. Determining the etiology of the arrhythmia and trying to establish underlying or treatable secondary causes (e.g., electrolyte imbalance, hypoxemia, thyroid disease, and drug toxicity).

3. Establishing therapeutic goals for each patient.

4. In many instances, using drug serum concentrations to determine compliance with selected therapy, confirm whether a subtherapeutic concentration is responsbile for therapeutic failure or whether the drug is not effective in the therapeutic range, confirm the existence of toxicity when clinical evidence implicates it, alter the dose in a patient with liver disease or renal failure, change the dose when a drug-drug interaction has occurred, or confirm the suspicion that the drug is not indicated.

Effects of Aging on Antiarrhythmic Therapy

Stress, drug-drug interactions, changing tissue sensitivity, declining organ function, and other age related changes should be considered when giving antiarrhythmic drugs in the elderly. Aging is most likely to alter a drug's effect via changes in the serum protein concentration, metabolic and excretory pathways, or other effects that alter the serum concentration of the drug in the elderly.

Renal function and liver function decline with age.[33,34] Antiarrhythmic drugs are inactivated and eliminated from the body by both organs, and the progressive organ dysfunction with age leads to elevation of serum concentrations as accumulation occurs in the elderly patient. Liver blood flow and microsomal enzyme activity decline with age.[33] Drugs affected by age related changes in liver function include antiarrhythmic drugs whose major route of elimination is by hepatic metabolism. These include lidocaine, quinidine, phenytoin, and propranolol, as well as other such frequently prescribed drugs as chlordiazepoxide, desipramine, diazepam, lorazepam, and acetaminophen.

Antiarrhythmic drugs affected by age related changes in renal function include those eliminated by renal filtration or secretion. These include digoxin, procainamide (and N-acetylprocainamide), disopyramide, and possibly bretylium.

The effect of other disease states on antiarrhythmic drugs is also important. Congestive heart failure leads to an alteration of blood flow patterns that shunts blood into the central vascular system. This alteration diminishes liver blood flow, lowers the apparent volume of distribution of drugs, and leads to a decrease in the drug required for loading and maintenance doses. Cirrhosis, hepatitis, and other liver diseases, as well as the normal aging process, decrease the body's production of albumin and other plasma proteins. Drugs that have a high affinity for plasma proteins can cause the percentage of unbound, pharmacologically active drug to increase significantly because of an age related decrease in albumin and protein synthesis.

Many misconceptions remain when one is considering antiarrhythmic treatment of the elderly. Among these are that quinidine is safer than propranolol, propranolol is dangerous in the elderly, side effects from antiarrhythmic drugs are more common in the elderly, and indications for and therapeutic effectiveness of antiarrhythmic drugs are different in elderly patients.[35] The following section attempts to clarify these misconceptions and presents treatment alternatives for various arrhythmias.

Treatment of Arrhythmias

The treatment of any arrhythmia initially should include a review of possible factors that may enhance or induce arrhythmias. Pathologic states that may induce or complicate an existing arrhythmia include any organic heart disease (e.g., valvular disease, ischemic disease, myocarditis, pericarditis), hypertension, increased intracranial pressure, seizures, pulmonary embolism, pneumonia, shock, anemia, hypothyroidism, hyperthyroidism, and acid-base disturbances. Drugs known to have the capacity to induce or enhance cardiac arrhythmias include digitalis glycosides, sympathomimetic amines, antidepressants, tranquilizers, tobacco, antihypertensives, halothane, isoproterenol, and theophylline derivatives.

Sinus Bradycardia. Sinus bradycardia (less than 60 beats per minute) is not uncommon in the elderly. It may be due to sinus node ischemia or inflammation; it may be a part of a cardiomyopathy or may result from surgical intervention. Correctable causes should be looked for, including drugs (e.g., digitalis glycosides, propranolol, morphine, antihypertensive drugs, and antiarrhythmic drugs). It may result from vomiting, hypothermia, myxedema, obstructive jaundice, or increased intracranial pressure. If the bradycardia becomes symptomatic, short term relief can be achieved by using atropine or isoproterenol, but the preferred long term treatment is an artificial pacemaker.

Atrial Premature Beats. Atrial premature beats are common in the elderly, appearing on 10 per cent of baseline standard electrocardiograms. Although they are not usually dangerous, treatment may be indicated if they trigger atrial flutter or fibrillation.[19] They serve as a warning in patients with postmyocardial infarction. They may signal pericarditis, atrial enlargement from congestive heart failure, or thyrotoxicosis. Treatment with digoxin, propranolol, or quinidine may be useful.[19]

Sinus Tachycardia. Sinus tachycardia (heart rate greater than 100 beats per minute) is not harmful, and treatment is seldom indicated. It is usually an arrhythmia warning of severe infection or impending heart failure.

Paroxysmal Supraventricular Tachyarrhythmias. Paroxysmal supraventricular tachyarrhythmias represent a family of arrhythmias including atrial tachycardia, the Wolff-Parkinson-White syndrome, atrial flutter, and atrial fibrillation. Atrial tachycardia (heart rate from 150 to 250 beats per minute) may have secondary causes, including drug therapy (atropine, epinephrine, ephedrine, isoproterenol, or thyroid replacement), hyperthyroidism, anemia, pulmonary embolism, infection, hypoxia, and heart failure.

Patients without organic heart disease usually tolerate the rapid ventricular rate. In patients who have sustained a myocardial infarction, atrial tachycardia may precede left ventricular failure. Treatment with verapamil has been successful in 80 per cent of the cases in which it was used.[19] Beta blockers, such as propranolol, or other antiarrhythmic drugs such as procainamide, have been effective; if they are not, timed direct current shock usually leads to reversion. Once the cardiac rhythm returns to normal, digoxin or other antiarrhythmic drugs may be employed.

Tachycardia originating in the sinoatrial node or atria comprises only 10 per cent of all paroxysmal supraventricular tachyarrhythmias. The majority originate from a variety of sources including atrioventricular node re-entry (60 per cent), AV bypass re-entry (15 per cent), sinoatrial or atrial re-entry (10 per cent), and ectopic tachycardia (4 per cent).

The treatment of this mix of paroxysmal supraventricular tachyarrhythmias depends upon a careful electrocardiographic diagnosis, observing the QRS width and whether the P wave falls before, during, or after the QRS complex during tachyarrhythmias. The clinical setting is of equal importance, for it is the patient who is to be treated, not the electrocardiographic record. Some authors emphasize the importance of the electrocardiographic analysis in deciding whether to use one antiarrhythmic drug rather than another, whereas others would say that the choice is still largely empirical, but emphasize the importance of an adequate therapeutic trial before substituting another drug. Both points are well taken, and it is important to re-emphasize the utility of antiarrhythmic drug serum concentrations to adjust doses and rule out toxicity.

Atrial Flutter. Atrial flutter (heart rate from 250 to 350 beats per minute, paroxysmal or sustained, with 2:1, 3:1, or 4:1 AV block) occurs in approximately 2 per cent of the routine instances of electrocardiographic monitoring. Digoxin, propranolol, and verapamil have been used to treat atrial flutter. Higher doses of digoxin or propranolol than required for the treatment of other arrhythmias may be necessary. Verapamil or propranolol may be substituted for digoxin if the latter is being used but hemodynamic deterioration occurs. If verapamil or propranolol is not used, immediate direct current countershock should be used, followed by digoxin and another antiarrhythmic, if necessary.[19]

Atrial Fibrillation. Atrial fibrillation (heart rate greater than 350 beats per minute, irregular with some degree of atrioventricular block) may be seen on 5 to 18 per cent of routine electrocardiograms in elderly patients. It is common after a myocardial infarction in the elderly. Various treatment goals exist. Control of the ventricular rate, thereby improving circulation and cardiac output, is one goal.[19] Re-establishing atrial rhythm restores the atrial contribution to ventricular filling, increasing cardiac output by as much as 10 to 20 per cent. Conversion or control of a rapid ventricular response improves the coronary blood flow by increasing the diastolic interval. Finally, the high risk of pulmonary and systemic emboli is greatly diminished when conversion to a normal sinus rhythm occurs.[19]

Correction of the underlying cause(s) is

important in treating atrial fibrillation. Such conditions include hyperthyroidism, thyrotoxicosis, heart failure, hypertension, pulmonary disease, and myocardial ischemia.

Drug management of atrial fibrillation now includes the decision whether to use digoxin, propranolol, or verapamil. If the heart rate is above 90 beats per minute, some would treat with digoxin, using enough to lower the ventricular rate to between 70 and 90 beats per minute.[24] Adding propranolol may help to achieve this goal.[24,36] In patients with thyrotoxicosis or hypertrophic cardiomyopathy, propranolol may be the drug of choice over digoxin.[19] Most would choose digoxin as the first drug to employ in other situations.[19,24,36] It protects the ventricle by slowing atrioventricular conduction through the bundle of His directly and by indirectly increasing vagal tone.[24] In one-third of the patients the ventricular rate is adequate and treatment is not required. Reversion to a normal sinus rhythm is the exception, not the rule, when using digoxin alone.[24] Even with direct current cardioversion, 70 per cent of the patients converted relapse to atrial fibrillation within one year and approximately 33 per cent relapse within the first month.[36]

Thus, we encounter the second use of digoxin in the treatment of atrial fibrillation, namely, to prevent relapse. It is useful in patients who have undergone successful direct current cardioversion. Some authors recommend the indefinite continuation of digoxin in these patients.[24] The use of direct shock to achieve sinus rhythm will buy time for the slow digoxin loading process as well.[19] If this is not satisfactory in controlling the ventricular rate, propranolol may be added to digoxin.[19,24] Alternatively, disopyramide or verapamil may be used to convert and maintain the patient in sinus rhythm. The approximately 30 per cent risk of showering pulmonary or systemic emboli from a heart in paroxysmal atrial fibrillation leads to recommendations for anticoagulation after cardioversion.[36]

Atrioventricular Block. First degree atrioventricular block (prolonged PR interval) usually requires no therapy; it is common in the elderly. Likewise, Mobitz type I or Wenckebach block usually requires no therapy. Symptomatic Mobitz type II block and complete heart block necessitate the use of an artificial pacemaker.[36] Pacing may reduce the incidence of sudden death in patients with bundle branch block or high degree atrioventricular block following a myocardial infarction.[36]

Ventricular Premature Beats. Ventricular premature beats occur in approximately 18 per cent of elderly patients when examined with routine electrocardiography.[36] They are seen in over 80 per cent of elderly patients with recent acute myocardial infarctions.[19] In patients without underlying heart disease, the ventricular premature beats usually do not require treatment.[19,36] Digoxin intoxication may precipitate ventricular premature beats and should be ruled out with a serum digoxin concentration determination. Hypokalemia should be corrected if present, digoxin stopped, and antiarrhythmic drugs, such as phenytoin or propranolol, used if necessary.[19] In the patient with a myocardial infarction, the ectopic location should be identified by electrocardiography and the frequency of ventricular premature beats monitored. One must determine whether multiple foci are responsible for the ventricular premature beats, whether they occur in couplets or runs, and finally whether they occur in the vulnerable repolarization period (R on T ectopic beat).[19,36] These criteria aid in indicating ventricular premature beats that are more likely to lead to a decreased left ventricular ejection fraction or to sudden, fatal ventricular arrhythmias. Lidocaine is often used in the hospital setting to suppress ventricular premature beats. Procainamide, quinidine, disopyramide, and propranolol have been used in the hospital as well as outside the hospital to suppress ventricular premature beats and lower the incidence of sudden death during the first six months after myocardial infarction.[36] If a patient has not been receiving digoxin and presents with cardiac failure, there is no reason to withhold digoxin because of the presence of ventricular premature beats.[19]

Ventricular Tachycardia. Ventricular tachycardia (ventricular rate from 150 to 250 beats per minute, paroxysmal or sustained) is life threatening and should be treated at once. Lidocaine, direct current countershock, procainamide, and bretylium are used in the acute phase, and suppression after conversion is accomplished with procainamide, phenytoin, propranolol, bretylium, and pacemaker ventricular overdrive.[19]

Ventricular Fibrillation. Ventricular fibrillation is a medical emergency, treated with direct current countershock. If it is unsuccessful, the patient's state of oxygenation is checked, sodium bicarbonate administered to neutralize metabolic acidosis, and countershock attempted again. A bolus of lidocaine, procainamide, or bretylium may facilitate cardioversion. Control following successful cardioversion is possible with the foregoing antiarrhythmic drugs or phenytoin or propranolol.[19]

A review of selected antiarrhythmic drugs and their general effectiveness in particular types of arrhythmic disorders may be found in Table 5–8.

Antiarrhythmic Drugs

It is appropriate to preface the discussion of specific antiarrhythmic drugs with a quotation from a clinical study that illustrates the need to understand the use of pharmacokinetic data in optimizing antiarrhythmic therapy:

One of the chief advantages in the use of quinidine is the accessibility of blood level determinations. Unfortunately, this advantage was often

TABLE 5–8. General Efficacy of Specific Antiarrhythmic Drugs with Various Arrhythmias*[a]

	Quinidine	Procainamide	Disopyramide[i]	Lidocaine	Phenytoin	Propranolol[e]	Bretylium[g,i]	Digitalis[h]
Supraventricular arrhythmias								
Atrial premature beats	1	1	1	4	3	3	N	4[h]
Paroxysmal supraventricular tachycardia								
AV nodal re-entry	1–2[b]	1–2[b,c]	1–2[b]	4	4	2	N	2
AV bypass re-entry	2[b]	2[b]	2[b]	4	3–4	3	N	1–4[j]
SA node and atrium re-entry	2	2	2	4	4	2	N	2–3
Automatic	3	3	3	4	4	3–4	N	N
Atrial flutter: conversion	1–2[b]	1–2[b]	1–2[b]	4[b]	4[b]	3	N	3–4
Control of ventricular response	N	N	N	N	N	1[f]	N	1[f]
Atrial fibrillation: conversion	1[b]	1[b]	1–2[b]	4[b]	4[b]	3	N	3
Maintenance of sinus rhythm	1–2	1–2	—	N	N	3	N	3
Control of ventricular response	N	N	N	N	N	1[f]	N	1[f]
Sinus bradycardia	N	N	N	N	N	N	N	N
Digitalis induced nonparoxysmal supraventricular tachyarrhythmias	3[d]	3[d]	3[d]	2	2	4[d]	N	N
Junctional premature beats	2	2	—	4	4	3	N	4[h]
Ventricular arrhythmias								
Ventricular premature beats	1	1	1	1	3	2	2–3	3[h]
Ventricular tachycardia	2	1–2	1–2	1–2	3	2–3	1–2	N
Ventricular fibrillation	3	2–3	2–3	1	3	2–3	1	N
Escape rhythm with complete heart block	N	N	N	N	N	N	N	N
Digitalis induced ventricular arrhythmias	3[d]	3[d]	3[d]	1	1	3[d]	N	N

*From Mehlman, D.J., and Arusdorf, M.F.: Antiarrhythmic therapy for the elderly: a two-edged sword. Geriatrics, 44–45, May 1979. Reprinted with permission of Geriatrics.

[a]These are general observations. Responsiveness to therapy depends on patient selection and clinical context. Comparative ranking of drugs is tentative and in many instances reflects authors' preferences. Response: 1-excellent, 2-good, 3-fair, 4-poor, N-not recommended.

[b]AV conduction may be enhanced. In the absence of AV nodal disease, propranolol or digitalis is usually needed.

[c]Rarely may enhance antegrade AV node conduction and potentiate induction of re-entrant tachycardia.

[d]Although effective in treating digitalis-excess arrhythmias, these drugs may produce problems with conduction and impulse production, leading to AV dissociation and asystole. If they are used, artificial pacemaking should be considered.

[e]In states of catecholamine excess, propranolol may be more effective than indicated.

[f]Use with caution in the presence of AV nodal disease.

[g]Initial catecholamine release may worsen dysrhythmias or potentiate dysrhythmias related to digitalis toxicity.

[h]By improving cardiac hemodynamics, digitalis may improve rhythm disturbances for which it is not recommended as an antiarrhythmic.

[i]Not approved in the United States for use in supraventricular arrhythmias.

[j]The effects of digitalis on suppressing supraventricular tachycardias using AV bypass re-entry pathways depends on the relative refractory periods of the AV node and accessory pathways.

negated by a lack of understanding of the concept of "steady-state" blood levels as related to half-life. Thus, in one patient ... 8 serum quinidine determinations were performed in 11 days. During this period, (the patient) received at least 6 different daily doses of quinidine and was never maintained with any one dosage for longer than 48 hours. A satisfactory dosage ultimately was found, but the blood level determinations were of no value in establishing it.[35]

The dosing of antiarrhythmic drugs in elderly patients requires careful attention to changes in absorption, distribution, first pass metabolism, protein binding, hepatic metabolism, and renal elimination. Most changes that need to be made in the doses of drugs in the elderly can be described in pharmacokinetic terms. Table 5–9 summarizes some pharmacokinetic and dosing data for several of the antiarrhythmic drugs.[19,23,32,33,37–39] Table 5–10 indicates dosage adjustments to be considered with selected antiarrhythmic drugs that are administered orally when renal dysfunction exists.[40]

TABLE 5–9. Selected Summary of Pharmacokinetic Data and Dosing Guidelines of Antiarrhythmics

Drug	Half-life (Hours)	Half-life in Elderly (Hours)	Therapeutic Serum Concentration	Protein Binding (Percentage)	Route of Elimination	Usual Dose (Adult)
Digoxin	30+	>40	1–2 ng./ml.	25–35	Renal (hepatic)[4]	Oral maintenance dose is: 0.125 mg./d. at Ccr of 10–25 ml./min. 0.1875 mg./d. at Ccr of 26–49 ml./min.
Quinidine	4–8	5–12	3–6 mcg./ml.	60–95	Hepatic (renal)	Maintenance dose should be adjusted to maintain the plasma concentration between 3–6 mcg./ml.; this usually requires 10–20 mg./kg./day in 4–6 divided oral doses.
Procainamide	2–4	4–8[5]	4–8 mcg./ml.[1]	15–20	Renal (hepatic)	IV: 25–50 mg./min. until 0.5–1.0 gm. given, or 500–600 mg. at a constant rate over 25–30 min. then 1–6 mg./min. IV infusion. Oral: ventricular tachycardia—1.0 gm. followed by maintenance dose of 50 mg./kg./day in divided doses every 3 hours; VPB—50 mg./kg./day in divided doses every 3 hours; atrial fibrillation and paroxysmal atrial tachycardia—1.25 gm. followed by 0.75 gm. in one hour if no ECG change occurs. Suggested maintenance dose is 0.5–1.5 gm. every 4–6 hr.
N-acetylprocainamide[8]	4–15	8–9	10–30 mcg./ml.	—	Renal	
Disopyramide	5–8	8–43	2–6 mcg./ml.	40–50	Renal (hepatic)[4]	Oral: 300 mg., then 100–150 mg. every 6 hours; for patients weighing less than 50 kg. the dose should be 100 mg. every 6 hr.

TABLE 5–9. Selected Summary of Pharmacokinetic Data and Dosing Guidelines of Antiarrhythmics (*Continued*)

Drug	Half-life (Hours)	Half-life in Elderly (Hours)	Therapeutic Serum Concentration	Protein Binding (Percentage)	Route of Elimination	Usual Dose (Adult)
Lidocaine	1–2	1.5–2.5	1.5–5 mcg./ml.	40–80	Hepatic	IV: 50–200 mg. bolus at a rate of 20–50 mg./min. Second bolus of 1/3 to 1/2 the initial dose may be used in 20–40 min.; then IV infusion at a rate of 1.0–4.0 mg./min. to maintain therapeutic plasma levels.[6]
Phenytoin	8–60[2]	—	10–20 mcg./ml.	~90	Hepatic	IV: 25–50 mg./min. to 100 mg.; repeat every 5 min. until response, toxicity, or 100 mg. given. Oral: 1000 mg. over first 24 hours; then 200–400 mg./day in two divided doses.
Propranolol	3–6	Approximately 30% longer	50–100 ng./ml.	90–95	Hepatic	IV: 1–3 mg. A second dose may be given if necessary after 2 min. Do not administer more propranolol IV for 4 hours. Convert to oral therapy as soon as possible. Oral: 10–40 mg. 3 to 4 times daily; increase as necessary. Dosage requirements highly variable.
Bretylium	6–12	16[3]	0.6–20 mcg./ml.	—	Renal	For life threatening arrhythmia: IV, slow push, 5–10 mg./kg.; IV infusion, 1–2 mg./min. May repeat initial dosing up to 30 mg./kg. max. Maintenance dose 5–10 mg./kg. over 10–30 min. every 6 hr.
Verapamil	3–8	—	50–200 ng./ml.	90	Hepatic[7]	IV: 5–10 mg. as bolus over 1–3 min. May repeat dose in 30 minutes if initial response is not adequate. Elderly patients should receive the IV bolus over 3 minutes to minimize untoward effects.

[1]Up to 12 mcg./ml. in 10% of patients.
[2]Dose dependent.
[3]At Ccr of 21 ml./min.
[4]Primarily eliminated by renal excretion.
[5]As high as 20 hours with severe renal impairment.
[6]Infusion should be terminated as soon as cardiac rhythm stabilizes or at the earliest sign of toxicity. Change patient to oral antiarrhythmic as soon as possible. IV infusions are seldom necessary for more than 24 hours. Maintenance infusions should be reduced in patients with heart failure or liver disease and in those over the age of 60.
[7]In patients with marked hepatic insufficiency, elimination half-life may be prolonged up to 14–16 hours.
[8]N-acetylprocainamide (NAPA) is a cardioactive metabolite of procainamide. Approximately one-fourth of administered procainamide is converted to n-acetylprocainamide in the liver.

TABLE 5–10. Dosing Guidelines for Oral Administration of Selected Antiarrhythmics in Patients with Renal Failure[1]

Drug	Normal Dose Interval	Adjustment for Renal Failure Creatinine Clearance Rate		
		> 50 ml./min.	10–50 ml./min.	< 10 ml./min.
Digoxin[2]	Every 24 hours	No change	Decrease dose by 25–75%	Decrease dose by 75–90%
Procainamide	Every 4–6 hours	No change	Change dosing interval to every 6–12 hr.	Change dosing interval to every 8–24 hr.
Disopyramide	Every 6 hours	No change	Change dosing interval to every 12–24 hr.	Change dosing interval to every 24–40 hr.
Bretylium	Every 6–8 hours	No change	Decrease dose by 50–75%	Not recommended

[1]The kinetics of quinidine, lidocaine, phenytoin, propranolol, and verapamil are not markedly influenced by renal disease.
[2]See Table 5–9.

Digoxin. Digoxin is used primarily to treat supraventricular arrhythmias, mainly atrial flutter and atrial fibrillation, and to control the ventricular response. Patients who have cardiomegaly or left ventricular failure stand to benefit most from digoxin because it protects the ventricle against ectopic impulses. Recent studies demonstrate that in as many as 75 per cent of elderly patients taking digoxin on a long term basis the drug can be safely withdrawn. Caution should be used when withdrawing digoxin, and some recommend that patients with atrial fibrillation in addition to left ventricular failure be maintained with digoxin for life.[37]

When atrial fibrillation with a rapid ventricular response is not treated adequately with digoxin alone, propranolol or possibly metoprolol should be cautiously added.[24,32] The oral administration of 10 to 40 mg. of propranolol every six hours or 50 mg. of metoprolol every 12 to 24 hours is generally most effective. The higher the heart rate, the more benefit is derived from the beta blockers. Dosing should be individualized and cautious, for in some patients exercise tolerance may be reduced when a beta blocker is added to the regimen.

The treatment of atrial flutter with digoxin and then with a beta blocker is recommended. Treatment with digoxin may convert atrial flutter to atrial fibrillation or, in over half the patients, to a sinus rhythm.[24]

The use of digoxin in one particular type of the Wolff-Parkinson-White syndrome is contraindicated. If impulses are traveling anterograde down the accessory bundle, digoxin may worsen the condition by accelerating anterograde conduction. Considerable caution should be exercised in using digoxin in the Wolff-Parkinson-White syndrome generally.

The heart is more susceptible to the cardiac effects of digoxin following direct current cardioversion. When possible, one should discontinue digoxin three days prior to elective cardioversion. When this is not possible, one should start with lower voltage shocks in the digitalized patient.[24]

The serum potassium concentration must be monitored and corrected in patients receiving digoxin. Hypokalemic patients may exhibit digoxin toxicity at serum concentrations as low as 1.0 ng. per ml.[37] The treatment of suspected digoxin toxicity should include adjustment of the serum potassium concentration. Drugs that lower the serum potassium concentration may produce clinically significant interactions with digoxin.

Another important drug-drug interaction

occurs when quinidine is added to a digitalized patient's regimen. By impairing renal digoxin clearance, quinidine has the effect of lowering digoxin maintenance dosage requirements by approximately 50 per cent. Serum digoxin concentrations may double following the addition of quinidine to the regimen. Potassium sparing diuretics such as spironolactone, amiloride, and triamterene may reduce the cardiac effects of digitalis, particularly in a patient who previously had been hypokalemic. Digoxin should be administered with caution in patients receiving thyroid preparations, for this may lead to increased susceptibility to the toxic effects of digitalis glycosides. Digoxin may be additive to cardiac effects induced by concurrently administered quinidine, procainamide, and propranolol.

Aging brings with it a loss of skeletal muscle and renal function. The loading dose and the maintenance dose should be lowered in the elderly according to the guidelines presented herein. The dosing of digoxin in the elderly for the treatment of atrial fibrillation is made more difficult by the need for higher serum concentrations of digoxin to control supraventricular arrhythmias. Digoxin doses high enough to produce steady state serum concentrations of 2 to 4 ng. per ml. may be needed.[37]

Quinidine. Quinidine is used primarily to prevent paroxysmal supraventricular tachyarrhythmias, to maintain sinus rhythm after direct current cardioversion, and to prevent life threatening ventricular tachyarrhythmias and premature ventricular beats in the postmyocardial infarction period.[41] Approximately 30 per cent of the patients receiving quinidine experience significant side effects. This population tends to comply poorly because of the side effects. Gastrointestinal side effects are most common. These include diarrhea, nausea, and vomiting. The effect is not dose related, but can be decreased by the use of the gluconate or polygalacturonate salt, which decreases gastrointestinal symptoms by prolonging the absorption phase. Use of these salts results in lower peak concentrations, however. One must be aware that the absolute bioavailability of these two salts (60 per cent) is lower than with the sulfate salt (70 per cent).[38] Also the amount of quinidine gluconate or polygalacturonate must be adjusted to deliver the same amount of quinidine as the sulfate salt. Dosage forms containing quinidine as the sulfate contain 83 per cent anhydrous quinidine. Preparations containing quinidine gluconate contain 62 per cent anhydrous quinidine, and quinidine polygalacturonate dosage forms contain 60 per cent anhydrous quinidine.

The administration of quinidine with food or antacids does not decrease the bioavailability of the drug, but does prolong the absorption phase, decreasing gastrointestinal symptoms, nasal congestion, and palpitations.[38,42] The effect of quinidine in a patient with compromised cardiac output is to further depress cardiac output and lower arterial pressure. Also patients with heart failure appear to require a smaller dose of quinidine because the apparent volume of distribution of quinidine decreases.[38] Whether this concern is clinically significant is open to question. Most authors state that in patients with heart failure the maintenance quinidine dosage should be reduced, possibly by as much as 30 per cent.[32,38]

The anticholinergic effect of quinidine enhances conduction through the atrioventricular node. The use of quinidine alone in the treatment of atrial fibrillation or atrial flutter might worsen the situation by enhancing the number of depolarizations able to pass through the node.[37,41] It is recommended that the atrioventricular node be adequately blocked (with digoxin, for example) before starting quinidine in these patients.[41] Anticholinergic drugs administered concurrently with quinidine produce additive vagolytic effects.

Four or more active metabolites of quinidine are found in the serum during prolonged quinidine therapy; their serum levels may increase, especially in patients with renal failure.[38] The metabolites are active and should be considered when one is assessing the efficacy and toxicity of quinidine therapy. The serum assay of quinidine commonly used (double extraction–fluorometric) measures quinidine and one active metabolite, dihydroquinidine.[38] Other new assays being used measure only quinidine (thin layer chromatography, high pressure liquid chromatography, and EMIT). The results with the latter assay method cannot be compared to those with the double extraction–fluorometric assay, which gives falsely high values as evidence of quinidine concentration.[38] Clinicians are advised to know the method and therapeutic range for the quinidine assay currently used in their institution. Patients with renal failure are more apt to accumulate active metabolites, which may or may not be reflected by the quinidine assay but contribute to the drug's effect and toxicity.

Quinidine binding to albumin and other serum proteins is extensive (up to 95 per cent).

The percentage bound decreases in patients with hepatic insufficiency or cirrhosis or with the concomitant use of aspirin, phenytoin, or tolbutamide. Unbound quinidine is pharmacologically active; the response to quinidine is enhanced by conditions increasing this unbound fraction.[32,38]

Renal clearance of quinidine is only 15 to 40 per cent. There is disagreement whether anything except severe renal dysfunction has an important effect on quinidine clearance.[38] The same disagreement occurs in considering the effect of heart failure on quinidine clearance.[32,38] Liver disease seems to lower quinidine clearance.[32,41] Overall, the aging process lowers the total body clearance of quinidine.[38,43] It is suggested that in all persons receiving long term quinidine therapy, serum quinidine concentrations be determined to correlate with clinical impressions.[38] After an oral dose, the peak serum concentration occurs 1 to 1.5 hours later.

In addition to serum concentrations, an electrocardiogram may be useful in detecting quinidine toxicity. A QRS interval wider than 25 per cent of the baseline (before quinidine therapy) indicates quinidine toxicity.[32] Arrhythmias induced by excessive quinidine also include ventricular premature beats, ventricular tachycardia, QT prolongation, PR prolongation, and atrioventricular block. Only 0.5 per cent of the instances of quinidine toxicity are fatal. Nonserum concentration related toxicities includes rash, fever, thrombocytopenia, hepatic dysfunction, hemolytic anemia, agranulocytosis, thrombocytopenic purpura, and drug induced systemic lupus erythematosus.

The intravenous use of quinidine can be carried out safely by an experienced clinician.[38] Intramuscular injections are painful, damaging to muscle, and erratically absorbed. Oral loading doses of twice the oral maintenance dose achieve a steady state serum concentration quickly; it may take 24 to 48 hours if only the oral maintenance dose is given.[38] The dosing interval for sustained release preparations is every eight to 12 hours, instead of every six to eight hours as with the sulfate salt.

Additional drug-drug interactions include decreased serum quinidine concentrations when phenobarbital, rifampin, or phenytoin induces its liver metabolism; an additive vasodilatory effect with peripheral vasodilators; an added antiarrhythmic effect with propranolol; displacement of warfarin from plasma protein by quinidine; and enhanced renal tubular reabsorption of quinidine if the urine is alkalinized by acetazolamide or sodium bicarbonate.[32,38]

Procainamide. Procainamide is widely used to treat paroxysmal supraventricular tachyarrhythmias, atrial premature beats, atrial flutter, atrial fibrillation, and ventricular arrhythmias. Long term use is associated with undesirable side effects, especially a systemic lupus-like syndrome. Two diseases that must be considered when giving procainamide in the elderly are cardiac failure and renal failure.

Cardiac failure lowers the apparent volume of distribution of procainamide.[19] In initiating therapy, infusions or initial oral dosing should be done cautiously; the maintenance dose may also need to be reduced when the apparent volume of distribution is lowered. A 25 per cent reduction in the procainamide dose in patients with mild heart failure has been recommended. Absorption of procainamide from the gut and from intramuscular injection sites may be slow and incomplete in patients with heart failure. Acetylation of procainamide and renal clearance are diminished in patients with cardiac failure.[22]

Because procainamide is eliminated mainly by the kidney (50 per cent excreted unchanged), alterations in renal function significantly reduce its elimination.[19,34] The elderly patient exhibits an age related decrease in renal function and procainamide clearance as well. Thus the dosage of procainamide must be individualized in the elderly to correct for deteriorating renal function. No standard dosage nomograms exist, but a starting dose 30 to 50 per cent less than the usual adult dose may be necessary. The dose can then be titrated on the basis of electrocardiographic findings, the serum concentration of the drug, and overall clinical response.

The active metabolite of procainamide is n-acetylprocainamide. Fifteen to 25 per cent of orally administered procainamide is converted to n-acetylprocainamide.[44] Approximately 84 per cent of the latter is excreted unchanged in the urine.[19,44] The half-life of n-acetylprocainamide is two to five times that of procainamide; it increases in patients with renal failure and coronary artery disease and in the elderly.[41,44] Dosing procainamide in patients who are elderly or have renal or cardiac disease should be done utilizing both procainamide and n-acetylprocainamide serum concentrations.

Procainamide serum concentrations associated with an antiarrhythmic effect range from 4 to 10 mcg. per ml.[19] Toxicity begins at concentrations above 8 mcg. per ml. and is much more likely above 12 mcg. per ml. N-acetylprocainamide levels are still being investigated but are generally in the range of 10 to 30 mcg. per ml.

Cardiovascular side effects from procainamide include hypotension, conduction block, and arrhythmias when an intravenous dose is given too rapidly. Its effect in enhancing atrioventricular nodal conduction is similar to that of quinidine. Of particular interest is the systemic lupus-like syndrome that may be seen with procainamide administration. Fast acetylators, who produce more n-acetylprocainamide, are less apt to develop the lupus-like syndrome. The syndrome is associated with pleural and pleuropulmonary involvement more frequently than in typical systemic lupus erythematosus. Arthralgias, fever, and pleuritis develop, but renal and cerebral involvement is not seen with the procainamide induced lupus-like syndrome.[19] Restricting the length of therapy to under six months has been advocated to avoid this syndrome. Other adverse effects associated with procainamide therapy include anorexia, nausea, diarrhea, urticaria, pruritus, thrombocytopenia, and agranulocytosis.

Disopyramide. Disopyramide is effective for preventing and treating numerous rhythm disturbances (see Table 5–8). It is, however, less effective than quinidine or procainamide in atrial arrhythmias, with the exception of the Wolff-Parkinson-White syndrome. By prolonging the refractory period of impulses traveling anterograde down accessory pathways, it can abolish a Wolff-Parkinson-White arrhythmia that responds poorly to verapamil, quinidine, procainamide, or lidocaine. Because it is eliminated partially by hepatic metabolism and excreted unchanged (40 to 60 per cent) in the urine, changes in both liver or renal function may prolong the half-life of disopyramide.[19,41] Low cardiac output states or heart failure leads to a decreased apparent volume of distribution. Some clinicians recommend the reduction of the loading dose and maintenance dose in such patients.

Disopyramide has mild negative chronotropic activity. The effect is enhanced in patients with pre-existing cardiac failure. Patients taking beta blockers and disopyramide should be observed for hypotension.[32]

Hypokalemia decreases the antiarrhythmic effect of disopyramide, and hyperkalemia increases the drug's potential for causing myocardial depression.[32] The negative inotropic effect is more pronounced after an intravenous dose. This may be diminished by giving the injection over a 10 minute period.[19]

The most common side effect of disopyramide is its anticholinergic effect; it occurs in 10 to 40 per cent of all patients receiving the drug. Although this usually causes tolerable symptoms (blurred vision, dry mouth), the elderly patient is particularly susceptible to urinary retention caused by disopyramide. The anticholinergic effects on the myocardium can be serious. Ventricular tachycardia, fibrillation, or flutter has been unmasked by disopyramide alone or in combination with quinidine, procainamide, or lidocaine therapy. Syncope, atrioventricular block, QRS widening, and QT interval prolongation have occurred after the administration of disopyramide. The most serious adverse reactions to disopyramide therapy are hypotension and congestive heart failure. Other adverse reactions include constipation, nausea, headache, dizziness, fatigue, weakness, syncope, chest pain, anorexia, rash, and insomnia.

Lidocaine. Lidocaine is effective in treating ventricular arrhythmias, in preventing the recurrence of arrhythmias after direct current cardioversion, in treating digitalis induced ventricular arrhythmias, and in the postmyocardial infarction period for suppressing premature ventricular beats. Dosing and development of central nervous system toxicity depend in part upon changes in the liver blood flow rate, renal function, and the existence of heart failure.

The elimination of lidocaine is decreased in elderly patients; the lidocaine half-life in young patients is approximately 1.3 hours but increases to approximately 2.3 hours in older patients.[36] The incidence of lidocaine toxicity rises from 4 per cent in patients less than 50 years old to 8 per cent in patients over 70 years old.[36]

Patients with liver disease, congestive heart failure, or a recent myocardial infarction exhibit a decrease in lidocaine elimination. Heart failure decreases the apparent volume of distribution of lidocaine. The metabolism of lidocaine is highly dependent upon liver blood flow. As one or more insults to the liver and its circulation occur, the half-life of lidocaine increases. The half-life after an uncomplicated myocardial infarction has been reported in the range of 3.2 to 4.3 hours. If congestive heart failure accompanies the myocardial infarction, the half-life can be 10 hours.[32] Recommendations have been made to decrease the dose by 50 per cent in cases of poor liver blood flow. Although the effect of aging on liver blood flow can be demonstrated, pathologic variables changing liver blood flow make a more significant contribution to the changes in the lidocaine serum half-life than age related changes.

Another consideration in dosing lidocaine as a continuous infusion results from the accumulation of active metabolites in patients with renal failure. The metabolite of lidocaine (MEGX) has antiarrhythmic properties and accumulates in cases of postmyocardial infarction with congestive heart failure, even when the serum lidocaine concentration is within the therapeutic range. The metabolite GX is not a potent antiarrhythmic, is eliminated in part by renal excretion, and accumulates in renal failure.[19] In patients with congestive heart failure experiencing renal dysfunction and receiving a continuous infusion of lidocaine, a decrease in the infusion rate of 30 to 50 per cent should be considered in patients after 12 to 24 hours.[19] Serum levels above 7.0 mcg. per ml. usually produce toxicity.

Lidocaine coadministered with propranolol can lead to reduced renal clearance of lidocaine. An intravenous dose of phenytoin administered concurrently with a lidocaine infusion may produce excessive cardiac depression. Additive neurologic effects may occur if lidocaine and procainamide are administered concomitantly.

Manifestations of lidocaine toxicity in the central nervous system include lightheadedness, dizziness, tinnitus, blurred or double vision, vomiting, sensations of heat or cold, numbness, tremors, convulsions, respiratory arrest, and cardiovascular collapse. Allergic reactions are rare.

Phenytoin. Phenytoin is the antiarrhythmic drug of choice in the treatment of digitalis induced ventricular arrhythmias.[19] Nondigitalis induced atrial arrhythmias do not usually respond, nor do arrhythmias secondary to myocardial ischemia. Phenytoin may be tried as an alternate antiarrhythmic for nondigitalis induced arrhythmias, but the response is variable.[32] It should be avoided in atrial flutter because it often enhances atrioventricular and occasionally intraventricular conduction.[19,37] Phenytoin has numerous pharmacokinetic properties that make it difficult to use properly.

Phenytoin is highly bound (90 per cent) to plasma albumin; binding decreases in patients with hypoalbuminemia, uremia, and cirrhosis and with increasing age. Phenytoin assays for unbound and total drug are useful in an attempt to adjust for protein binding alteration. The serum half-life increases as the total daily dosage or serum concentration increases. Saturation of elimination can occur within the usual therapeutic concentrations, but is more likely with toxic plasma concentrations. As the clinician increases the dose of phenytoin, extra caution should be taken to observe the patient and the serum concentrations for signs of toxicity. Bioavailability from some oral products and absorption from intramuscular injections are erratic. A high bioavailability product (Dilantin, for example) should always be used. Because of its long half-life (20 to 30 hours), a loading dose is often used. Because of plasma protein binding and other variables, there is wide interindividual variation in response to the loading dose. Furthermore, elderly and hemodynamically unstable patients are more susceptible to toxicity and generally require a smaller dose. Most ventricular arrhythmias respond to phenytoin in serum concentrations of 10 to 20 mcg. per ml.; toxic effects are more likely to be seen at concentrations greater than 25 mcg. per ml. Large intravenous boluses (more than 50 mg. per minute) may be cardiotoxic. Manifestations of cardiac toxicity include atrioventricular block, bradycardia, hypotension, and cardiac arrest. Central nervous system toxicity is the most common and may include nystagmus, ataxia, drowsiness, dysarthria, slurred speech, motor twitching, mental confusion, insomnia, depression, tremor, and headache. Other adverse effects include nausea, vomiting, diarrhea, constipation, drug fever, rash, and on rare occasions thrombocytopenia, agranulocytosis, and toxic hepatitis. Additionally, phenytoin interacts adversely with many drugs.

With all the foregoing pharmacologic difficulties and the narrow spectrum of antiarrhythmic activity, it is not difficult to see why phenytoin has a limited role in antiarrhythmic therapy. On a risk-benefit basis, it is seldom considered as a first line drug in arrhythmia management.

Propranolol. Propranolol has a growing number of indications in managing arrhythmias. Because of its beta blocking activity, it is effective for arrhythmias caused by or associated with excessive catecholamine or sympathomimetic activity. It is used for ventricular and supraventricular arrhythmias. It has been used to treat stress or emotion provoked sinus tachycardia and paroxysmal atrial tachycardia. It is contraindicated in the "sick sinus" syndrome. A beta blocker such as propranolol is useful in treating atrial fibrillation or atrial flutter when digoxin alone cannot bring the heart rate below 90 beats per minute, while it protects the ventricle by slowing atrioventricular conduction.[24,32] Propranolol slows atrioventricular and re-entry conduction and is effective for suppressing ventricular arrhythmias, especially when due to catecholamines or digitalis toxicity. Because some patients require a high sympathetic tone to compensate for heart failure, beta blockers used to treat arrhythmias should be given cautiously to avoid precipitation of heart failure. Beta blockers may precipitate congestive heart failure by decreasing myocardial contractility. Although not the drugs of choice for ventricular tachycardia and ventricular fibrillation, beta blockers may work in exercise induced arrhythmias when quinidine or digoxin fail. In suppressing adrenergic stimulation of ectopic pacemakers, beta blockers may be most effective when the arrhythmia is induced by excess catecholamines, digitalis toxicity, or myocardial infarction.[21]

Adequate beta blockade can be judged clinically. If the heart rate cannot be increased above 100 to 125 beats per minute with exercise or, less reliably, the resting heart rate is less than 60 beats per minute, the patient has been given a beta blocking dose.[32]

Changes occur in the autonomic nervous system with age. The heart rate becomes resistant to effects of circulating and exogenous catecholamines. The elderly exhibit a decreased sensitivity to the effect of propranolol on the heart rate and cardiac output. In response to stress, older patients secrete more epinephrine than younger patients and have a greater blood pressure response than young patients.[45] The incidence of propranolol related toxicity (bradycardia, pulmonary edema, hypotension) is greater in patients older than 60 years. This is complicated by atherosclerotic cerebrovascular disease, decreased renal function with azotemia and the use of multiple cardiovascular drugs. Thus, there exists the dilemma of the elderly patient with higher circulating catecholamine levels, less physiologic response to those catecholamines, and more susceptibility to the adverse effects of beta blockers, which need to be given in amounts adequate to overcome the increased concentrations of catecholamines. Elderly patients must be given beta blockers in a most careful manner.

Propranolol is well absorbed but undergoes significant hepatic metabolism (the "first pass effect").[32] Propranolol is a drug with intermediate hepatic extraction when it is given for a long period; its clearance is dependent upon both liver blood flow and intrinsic enzyme activity.[33] Hepatic extraction of propranolol is reduced in the elderly, and liver blood flow decreases with age.[33] The elderly patient has a diminished "first pass effect" and the drug has a prolonged half-life (approximately 30 per cent longer).[33] Cirrhosis increases the free fraction of propranolol by as much as 38 per cent, increasing the effect of the drug. The dosage should therefore be lowered in patients with liver disease or diseases that lower serum protein levels.

In the elderly, one should begin oral therapy with a low dosage (10 mg. every six hours) and increase the dosage as needed. Most patients receive 20 to 100 mg. orally every six hours.[32] Intravenous therapy avoids the "first pass effect." If intravenous therapy is required, 0.5 to 0.75 mg. is given every two minutes until the patient responds favorably or a dose of 0.1 to 0.15 mg. per kg. has been given.[32] The blood pressure, heart rate, and electrocardiographic response should be monitored regularly. If an overdose is given, bradycardia, atrioventricular block, or asystole can be reversed with atropine, isoproterenol, or a cardiac pacemaker.

The side effects of propranolol include bronchospasm, bradycardia, heart failure, intermittent claudication, Raynaud's phenomenon (peripheral vascular vasospasm), nightmares, vivid dreams, exacerbation of hypoglycemia in diabetics, and allergic symptoms. Metoprolol, atenolol, and other cardioselective beta blockers may improve Raynaud's phenomenon and decrease the incidence of bronchospasm. Abrupt cessation of beta blockers in patients with angina may exacerbate angina or cause ventricular fibrillation or a myocardial infarction. If therapy is discontinued, the dose should be tapered over a two week period.

The role of beta blockers as antiarrhythmic drugs is evolving. Their use in elderly patients requires particular attention to avoid toxicity and its potentially serious consequences.

Bretylium. Bretylium is indicated for life threatening arrhythmias such as refractory ventricular tachycardia and ventricular fibrillation, especially postmyocardial infarction.[32] It is not useful in atrial arrhythmias. Bretylium has defibrillatory properties and, by acting to a greater degree in noninfarcted tissue, tends to restore rhythm control to normal tissue.[41] It is often effective in preventing ventricular tachyarrhythmias when lidocaine, procainamide, phenytoin, and propranolol may have failed. It may be given by slow intravenous push, intravenous infusion, or intramuscular injection (see Table 5–9).

Immediate side effects include nausea and vomiting in most patients and in some patients an increase in blood pressure.[32,41] As norepinephrine release is inhibited, the supine and standing blood pressures drop. This effect may be overcome by increasing the dose or by careful use of fluids or norepinephrine.[41] Norepinephrine or any catecholamine used to counteract hypotension must be administered with the awareness that bretylium may sensitize the heart to the effects of catecholamines.[32] Other side effects include parotid gland tenderness and the possibility that bretylium may worsen arrhythmias caused by digoxin toxicity.[32]

Verapamil. Verapamil (Galan, Isoptin) is the first of the new class of drugs categorized as calcium antagonists approved for use in the treatment of cardiac arrhythmias. It has been suggested that excitation of cardiovascular tissue occurs as a result of the movement of positive ions in two channels of the cell membrane. Sodium ions generate a rapid surge of current in the fast channel, and calcium ions generate a slow current in the slow channel. Although both currents are involved in the initiation of contraction of the myocardial and vascular musculature, the pacemaker cells in the sinoatrial node and the proximal part of the atrioventricular node are activated primarily by the slow calcium current. By slowing conduction velocity through the atrioventricular node, verapamil has been demonstrated to be effective in the treatment of supraventricular tachyarrhythmias.

Administered intravenously, verapamil is effective in rapidly converting paroxysmal supraventricular tachycardia (including the Wolff-Parkinson-White and Lown-Ganong-Levine syndromes) to normal sinus rhythm. These tachycardias have been terminated in 60 to 80 per cent of the patients, conversion usually occurring within two to five minutes. Verapamil is also indicated for the temporary control of a rapid ventricular rate in atrial flutter or atrial fibrillation, although conversion to normal sinus rhythm occurs in only about 10 per cent of the patients. Verapamil appears to be less effective than other currently available antiarrhythmic drugs in the treatment of ventricular arrhythmias.

In addition to slowing conduction through the atrioventricular node, verapamil produces systemic arterial dilation and diminishes myocardial contractility by inhibiting calcium influx into contractile and conductile myocardial cells and vascular smooth muscle. Verapamil is of potential value, therefore, in the management of angina and hypertension.

Verapamil is contraindicated in patients with severe hypotension, cardiogenic shock, second or third degree atrioventricular block, and severe congestive heart failure. Unlike the beta-adrenergic blocking drugs, verapamil is not likely to cause bronchoconstriction, and may be used safely in patients with such conditions as asthma and other chronic obstructive pulmonary diseases.

Verapamil has the potential for interacting adversely with other antiarrhythmic drugs, although no serious effects of such interactions have been noted. It has been suggested that verapamil may elevate digoxin levels by as much as 50 to 70 per cent if given concomitantly over a week or more.

Verapamil has been administered intravenously to patients receiving oral doses of beta-adrenergic blocking drugs without the occurrence of serious adverse effects. Both drugs, however, depress myocardial contractility or atrioventricular conduction, and serious reactions have been reported when both drugs were administered intravenously. It is recommended that verapamil and beta blockers not be administered intravenously within a few hours of one another. It is also advised that disopyramide not be administered within 48 hours before or 24 hours after verapamil administration, because information regarding the safety of this combination is not currently available.

Beta-adrenergic agonists such as isoproterenol can be expected to oppose the action of verapamil, and there is preliminary evidence that methylxanthines such as caffeine and theophylline may produce a similar response. Verapamil is highly bound to plasma proteins and must be used with caution in patients receiving other highly protein bound drugs (e.g., warfarin, acetylsalicylic acid, amitriptyline, and phenytoin). Verapamil can be given with nitroglycerin.

The usual initial parenteral adult dose of

verapamil in the elderly is 5 to 10 mg. administered as an intravenous bolus over a period of at least three minutes. A repeat dose (10 mg.) may be administered 30 minutes later if the initial response is not adequate. The oral dosage form is generally used in the management of angina.

The dosage of verapamil should be adjusted downward in elderly patients with hepatic dysfunction because the drug is highly metabolized by the liver. The normal half-life of verapamil is three to five hours, but it may be extended to 14 to 16 hours in severe hepatic dysfunction. As little as one-third of the normal dose may be all that is required if hepatic failure is marked.

In conclusion, the use of antiarrhythmic drugs in the elderly patient requires careful diagnostic interpretation, appreciation of the disease states that alter the serum concentrations of these drugs, and an awareness of side effects from antiarrhythmic drugs that are more commonly seen in the elderly patient. Careful use of antiarrhythmic drugs can be as helpful in the control of arrhythmias in the elderly as during any other time of life.

REFERENCES

1. Lamy, P.P.: Prescribing for the Elderly. Littleton, Massachusetts, PSG Publishing Company, 1980.
2. Simpson, F.O: Hypertensive disease. In Avery, G.S. (Editor): Drug Treatment—Principles and Practice of Clinical Pharmacology and Therapeutics. New York, ADIS Press, 1980, pp. 638–682.
3. O'Malley, K., and O'Brien, E.: Management of hypertension in the elderly. N. Engl. J. Med., 302:1397–1401, 1980.
4. Amery, A., et al.: Aging and the cardiovascular system. Acta Cardiol., 33:443–467, 1978.
5. Simpson, F.O.: Combination therapy in hypertension. Drugs, 20:69–73, 1980.
6. Kannal, W.B., et al.: Components of blood pressure and risk of atherothrombotic brain infarction: the Framingham study. Stroke, 7:327–331, 1976.
7. Spence, J.D., et al.: Pseudohypertension in the elderly. Clin. Sci., 55:399–402, 1978.
8. Hammond, J.J., and Kirkendall, W.M.: Antihypertensive drugs for the aging. Geriatrics, 34:27–36, 1979.
9. Waern, U., and Aberg, H.: Blood pressure in 60-year-old men. Findings in a health survey and some comparisons with 50-year-old men in the same community. Acta Med. Scand., 78:99–105, 1979.
10. Ostfeld, A.M.: The elderly hypertensive patient. Epidemiologic review. N.Y. J. Med., 78:1125–1129, 1978.
11. Amery, A., et al.: Antihypertensive therapy in patients above age 60. (Fourth interim report of the European working party on high blood pressure in the elderly: EWPHE). Clin. Sci., 55:263s–270s, 1978.
12. Finnerty, F.A.: Hypertension in the elderly. Special considerations in treatment. Postgrad. Med., 65:119–125, 1979.
13. Drayer, J.M., and Weber, M.: Hypertension in the elderly: a new understanding. Drug Ther. Bull., 39–44, 1981.
14. MacLoed, S.M., et al.: Antihypertensive efficacy of propranolol given twice daily. Can. Med. Assoc. J., 121:737–740, 1979.
15. Heel, R.C., et al.: Nadolol: a review of its pharmacological properties and therapeutic efficacy in hypertension and angina pectoris. Drugs, 20:1–23, 1980.
16. Waal-Manning, H.J.: Beta blockers in hypertension: how to get the best results. Drugs, 17:129–133, 1979.
17. Drugs for hypertension. Med. Lett. Drugs Ther., 23:45–48, 1981.
18. Stone, P.H., et al.: Calcium channel blocking agents in the treatment of cardiovascular disorder. Part II. Hemodynamic effects and clinical applications. Ann. Intern. Med., 93:886–904, 1980.
19. O'Malley, K., Judge, T.G., and Crooks, J.: Geriatric clinical pharmacology and therapeutics (158–181), and Sloman, J.G., and Manolas, E.: Cardiovascular disease (569–637). In Avery, G.S., (Editor): Drug Treatment—Principles and Practice of Clinical Pharmacology and Therapeutics. New York, ADIS Press, 1980, pp. 663–682.
20. Segal, B.: The management of unstable angina pectoris. Geriatrics, 34:43–45, 1979.
21. Karlsberg, R.P.: Calcium channel blockers for cardiovascular disorders. Arch. Intern. Med., 142:452–455, 1982.
22. Elenbaas, R.M., and Covinsky, J.O.: Approaches to the management of acute, chronic and refractory congestive heart failure. J.C.E. Hosp. Clin. Pharm., 9–34, 1979.
23. Aronson, J.K.: Clinical pharmacokinetics of digoxin. Clin. Pharmacokinet., 5:137–149, 1980.
24. Taggart, A.J.: Digitalis: its place in modern therapy. Drugs, 20:398–404, 1980.
25. Ewy, G., et al.: Digoxin metabolism in the elderly. Circulation, 39:449–453, 1969.
26. Anderson, G.J.: Clinical clues to digitalis toxicity. Geriatrics, 35:57–65, 1980.
27. Brown, D.D.: Drug interactions with digoxin. Drugs, 20:198–206, 1980.
28. Whiting, B.: Computer-assisted review of digoxin therapy in the elderly. Br. Heart J., 40:8–13, 1978.
29. Hutcheon, D., et al.: The role of furosemide alone and in combination with digoxin in the relief of symptoms of congestive heart failure. J. Clin. Pharmacol., 20:59–70, 1980.
30. Johnston, G.D.: Digoxin dose precision: prescribing aids or intuition? Drugs, 20:494–499, 1980.
31. Beerman, B., et al.: Clinical pharmacokinetics of diuretics. Clin. Pharmacokinet., 5:221–245, 1980.
32. Moses, H.W., and Yu, P.N.: Antiarrhythmic drugs. J. Clin. Pharmacol., 20:598–618, 1980.
33. Vestal, R.E., et al.: Influence of age and smoking on drug kinetics in man. Clin. Pharmacokinet., 5:137–149, 1980.
34. Reidenberg, M.M.: Aging and renal clearance of procainamide and acetylprocainamide. Clin. Pharmacol. Ther., 28:732–735, 1980.
35. Berman, N.D.: The elderly patient in the coronary care unit. I. Acute myocardial infarction. II. Incidence

and treatment of arrhythmias. J. Am. Geriatr. Soc., 27:145–151, 203–207, 1979.
36. Mehlman, D.J., and Armsdorf, M.F.: Antiarrhythmic therapy for the elderly: a two edged sword. Geriatrics, 29–62, 1979.
37. Opie, L.: V. Digitalis and sympathomimetic stimulants. Lancet, 1:912–918, 1980.
38. Ochs, H.R., et al.: Clinical pharmacokinetics of quinidine. Clin. Pharmacokinet., 5:150–168, 1980.
39. Schwartz, J.B., Keefe, D., and Harrison, D.C.: Adverse effects of antiarrhythmic drugs. Drugs, 21:23–45, 1981.
40. Bennett, W.M., et al.: Drug therapy in renal failure: dosing guidelines for adults. Part II. Ann. Intern. Med., 93:286–325, 1980.
41. Kessler, K.M.: Pharmacologic basis of cardiovascular drug action. Hosp. Formul., 15:457–463, 1980.
42. Woo, E., et al.: Effect of food on enteral absorption of quinidine. Clin. Pharmacol. Ther., 27:188–193, 1980.
43. Drayer, D.E., et al.: Prevalence of high (3S)-3-hydroxyquinidine/quinidine ratios in serum, and clearance of quinidine in cardiac patients with age. Clin. Pharmacol. Ther., 27:72–75, 1980.
44. Kates, R.E., et al.: Intravenous N-acetylprocainamide disposition kinetics in coronary artery disease. Clin. Pharmacol. Ther., 28:52–57, 1980.
45. Palmer, G.J., et al.: Response of norepinephrine and blood pressure to stress increases with age. J. Gerontol., 33:482–487, 1978.

CHAPTER 6

GASTROINTESTINAL DISORDERS
Arthur I. Jacknowitz

The management of all gastrointestinal disorders in the elderly demands careful evaluation including a history, a physical examination, and a myriad of appropriate diagnostic maneuvers. The management becomes even more complex when one considers the host of management possibilities that do not involve the use of drug therapy or a surgical procedure. Although the emphasis in this chapter is on drug therapy in the management of selected gastrointestinal disorders, emphasis is placed on selection of the appropriate drug to treat a specific disorder with consideration given to dosing, adverse drug reaction potential, drug-drug interaction potential, precautions and warnings to be observed, and contraindications to use of the drug.

CONSTIPATION

Constipation is prevalent among the elderly for numerous reasons. Many of these individuals have deep rooted traditions and beliefs that a daily bowel movement is not only the desired state of "normalcy" but also that it is necessary to maintain proper health. The erroneous concept of "autointoxication," the absorption of toxic substances into the body as a result of lack of production of a daily stool, is very prevalent. In addition to the production of a daily bowel movement, cathartics have been used in the treatment of various diseases, including the common cold, depression, and weakness. Laxatives have also been used in the management of abdominal cramps, a particularly dangerous practice.

A major factor leading to constipation in the elderly is lack of mobility due to stroke, depression, senility, and other chronic debilitating diseases. Poor nutrition and a decreased fluid intake may also produce constipation. Lack of appetite, poor dentition, inability to pay for meals, and a psychologic unwillingness to prepare and eat a meal alone are underlying reasons for constipation in the aged. Numerous medications taken for chronic illnesses may also be constipating. Anticholinergics, phenothiazines, tricyclic antidepressants, sedatives, opiates (especially codeine), iron salts, and calcium containing antacids are but a few of the most frequently implicated drugs.

Since laxatives are nonprescription products, they are commonly viewed as being relatively harmless. Continuous use and abuse of irritant laxatives is another cause of constipation. Ingestion of large amounts of purgative laxatives for a prolonged period of time can result in the "cathartic colon." This condition resembles chronic ulcerative colitis both radiologically and pathologically.[1]

Definition

Constipation is defined as a decrease in the frequency of bowel movements accompanied by a prolonged and difficult passage of stool. This is usually followed by a sensation of incomplete evacuation.[2]

In one study over 98 per cent of 1445

patients, which included elderly patients, had bowel movements in the range of three per day to three per week.[3] A bowel movement that occurs at least once a week is still considered to be within the normal range.

Colon Physiology

The normal activity of the colon involves mixing movements, which are nonpropulsive, and mass movements, which are propulsive. The mixing movements cause segmentation of the lumen of the large intestine, which allows for increased absorption of water. These effects are essentially obstructive and prevent the forward movement of fecal material. These movements are also increased by constipating drugs such as morphine.

Mass movements, a form of propulsion, are stimulated by meals and physical activity. This is also known as the duodenocolic or gastrocolic reflex. The mass propulsive movements drive the feces into the rectum, and rectal distention produces the urge to defecate. This reflex may be voluntarily inhibited.

The bedfast, immobile, elderly patient is particularly at risk of developing constipation, since he must depend on another individual to allow a response to rectal distention. If this opportunity is not afforded at the appropriate time, the urge to defecate may pass. Later it may not be possible for the individual to defecate at will.[4] Lack of physical activity enhances this problem. Even if the patient is mobile and active, increased age by itself may also delay transit time.

Approach to Management

Anyone who presents with true constipation should undergo a complete workup in a search for reversible organic causes, such as hypothyroidism, hypercalcemia, or intestinal obstruction. One must also check the medication history for drugs that commonly cause this side effect. Specific questions should be asked concerning the possibility of laxative abuse.

Concerning the choice of a laxative, it is first important to determine whether a laxative is necessary at all. There is a tendency to indiscriminately prescribe laxatives for every patient in long term care facilities. An increase in the amount of bran in the daily diet can be effective in the treatment and prevention of constipation in up to 60 per cent of elderly individuals. (A study by Hull et al. documented this finding.[5] Following implementation of this dietary program, the institution's pharmacy reported a saving of $44,000 in expenditures for laxative drugs.) Subjects with atonic constipation (full rectum) are not always responsive to treatment with bran, since such therapy may actually add to the problem by increasing the bulk of an already distended colon. These individuals often have neuromuscular damage because of age, chronic disability, or chronic laxative abuse. This condition is usually treated by mechanical disimpaction and enemas. It is usually necessary to give an enema, such as a hypertonic phosphate enema, daily for a period of approximately seven to 10 days. Care must be taken during the administration of the enema to prevent damage to the mucosa of the anus or rectum. Another method that has been proposed is the administration of a saline solution via a nasogastric tube.[6] However, there is great concern that such a solution may precipitate or aggravate congestive heart failure even though a diuretic is administered concurrently.

Once this form of constipation has been alleviated, the weekly use of an enema or a bisacodyl or glycerin suppository may be necessary.

In the postoperative period and following a myocardial infarction, it is desirable to prevent straining at the stool. Bran or bulk laxatives are probably the agents of choice, although surfactant laxatives have been commonly employed for this purpose. Various laxative combinations affecting both the small intestine and the colon have been employed prior to barium enema radiologic examinations.

Bulk Forming Laxatives

By increasing the amount of fiber residue in the form of bran in the diet, constipation frequently can be alleviated or prevented.

Bulk laxatives include methylcellulose, sodium carboxymethylcellulose, polycarbophil, and psyllium. The laxative effect results from absorption and retention of large amounts of water. Owing to this particular property, these drugs are also paradoxically effective in the management of diarrhea. The mechanical distention caused by these laxatives promotes peristalsis and facilitates passage of the stool. Effects are normally seen within 12 to 24 hours, but it may take up to three days for a full laxative effect.

Some individuals cannot tolerate bran and should avoid these products. Patients with pseudo- or partial intestinal obstruction and disabling adhesions can develop complete bowel obstruction, especially if there is a diminished intake of fluid.

Patients should be instructed to mix bulk laxatives with water and to drink at least 8 ounces of fluid. Tablets should not be chewed or swallowed without water. Special care should also be taken with diabetic patients and those receiving sodium restricted diets. Most psyllium containing bulk laxatives contain up to 50 per cent dextrose. Konsyl is an exception. Diabetics often have decreased gastric emptying and other motor disturbances of the bowel, which may complicate the use of bulk laxatives. Individuals receiving sodium restricted diets should avoid using Metamucil instant mix, which contains 250 mg. of sodium per pack.

Polycarbophil is a recent addition to the bulk laxative category. It is a synthetic hydrophilic polyacrylic resin, which can absorb up to 60 times its weight in water. Although polycarbophil is probably just as effective as other bulk forming compounds in the management of constipation, comparative clinical trials are required to document this premise.

Side effects are infrequent with bulk laxatives. Adverse effects include flatulence, borborygmi, and the formation of soft bulky stools.

Stimulants

The stimulant laxatives can induce a relatively mild laxative action or in high dosages can produce severe cramping and fluid and electrolyte imbalance. Stimulant cathartics as a group are the most abused by the public, and excessive use can result in "cathartic colon." With chronic abuse, enteric loss of protein and malabsorption can occur.

Although these laxatives are termed stimulants, they have other actions as well, such as the production of water and electrolyte loss. When used judiciously, they are useful for acute constipation secondary to other medications, constipation due to prolonged bed rest or hospitalization, and as preparation for x-ray examination of the abdomen.

This large group of laxatives can be further subdivided into the following categories: castor oil, anthraquinones, and diphenylmethanes.

Castor oil is hydrolyzed by lipase enzymes to produce the active ingredient, ricinoleic acid. Although some of this active compound is absorbed, it is metabolized like other fatty acids. Chronic use of castor oil can cause erosion of the intestinal villi, leading to malabsorption of nutrients.

Cascara sagrada, danthron, senna, and aloe belong to the group of anthraquinone laxatives. Colonic bacteria hydrolyze these laxatives into their active forms. A portion of the dose is absorbed and subsequently acts on the colon. Melanosis coli, a darkened pigmentation of the colon mucosa, has been observed in chronic users of these laxatives. Aloe has the reputation of being the most irritating of the laxative compounds.

The diphenylmethane group of stimulant laxatives includes bisacodyl and phenolphthalein. These laxatives supposedly act directly on the mucosal nerve plexus of the colon, inducing fluid and electrolyte loss.

Bisacodyl is unique in that it can be administered orally and rectally. The suppository takes 15 minutes to one hour to produce its effects. Antacids or cimetidine should not be administered with oral doses of bisacodyl, since an increase in gastric pH will dissolve the enteric coating of the tablet, leading to abdominal cramping and possibly vomiting. Chewing of these enteric coated tablets is also to be avoided.

Up to 15 per cent of a dose of phenolphthalein is absorbed systemically and undergoes enterohepatic circulation. For this reason the cathartic effect may last for up to three or four days. In the presence of an alkaline urine, phenolphthalein will produce a pink to red color. Excessive and prolonged use of this particular laxative can induce osteomalacia secondary to impaired absorption of vitamin D and calcium. Any patient who develops a bullous skin reaction or a fixed eruption should be questioned concerning the use of phenolphthalein, since this drug has been one of the products most frequently implicated in this type of reaction.

Other members of this group of laxatives are mentioned only to be avoided, since they are very irritating. Compounds in this category include calomel (mercurous chloride) and podophyllum.

Saline Laxatives

The sulfate salts are considered to be the most potent of this group of laxatives, followed by magnesium salts; phosphate and tartrate salts are the weakest. Osmotic forces were once thought to be the only way in which catharsis was induced with these products. More recent findings suggest that saline cathartics stimulate the release of cholecystokinin, which inhibits the absorption of fluid and electrolytes from the jejunum and ileum. Because of the osmotic activity of these compounds, the patient should be advised to take them with at least a full glass of water so that dehydration does not occur. All formulations produce their laxative effect within three to six hours in most patients. Rectal administration produces a more rapid action.

Magnesium hydroxide is a mild saline cathartic. Approximately 20 per cent of the magnesium contained in this product is absorbed. In an elderly patient, especially one with renal impairment, toxic serum levels of magnesium may result. Hypermagnesemia is characterized by central nervous system depression, hypotension, muscle weakness, and electrocardiographic changes. For these reasons magnesium laxatives are contraindicated in cases of renal failure.

Phosphate salts are available both in oral and rectal forms. The normal laxative dose contains 96.5 mEq. of sodium. Depending upon bowel function, up to 10 per cent or more of this sodium content may be absorbed. This product should be administered cautiously to elderly patients who have congestive heart failure or renal impairment.

Hyperosmotic Laxatives

The two major products within this category are glycerin and lactulose. Glycerin in the form of a suppository usually produces a bowel movement within one-half hour. Oral doses of glycerin are ineffective, since it is rapidly absorbed and broken down systematically.

Lactulose is a nonabsorbable synthetic disaccharide, which was used previously only in the treatment of hepatic encephalopathy. Since its major side effect is diarrhea and it produces relatively few other side effects, lactulose may prove to be an especially useful drug in the elderly. One double blind study appears to confirm this hypothesis.[7]

Surfactant Laxatives

By a detergent activity, dioctyl sulfosuccinates lower the surface tension at the oil-water interface of the stool. This allows the fecal material to be penetrated by water and fat. In addition to this effect, these anionic surface active laxatives cause fluid and electrolyte accumulation in the colon.

These laxatives are useful for conditions in which straining at defecation should be avoided, such as after myocardial infarction and abdominal surgery. When used on a chronic routine basis, they appear to be of little value in the prevention of constipation. The dioctyl sulfosuccinates are available as sodium or calcium salts. Not enough sodium or calcium is contained in these products to be of clinical concern.

In controlled laboratory studies, these anionic surfactants have been found to facilitate the absorption of other poorly absorbable substances, such as mineral oil, and they may increase the toxicity of such substances. Greater mucosal damage is seen when aspirin and these surfactants are administered concurrently than when either drug is given alone. Further clinical study is necessary to determine the true impact of possible drug interactions associated with the use of surfactant laxatives. Until this information becomes available, it is recommended that drugs with a low therapeutic index and relatively poor absorption characteristics, such as digoxin, not be administered at the same time as these surfactants.

Emollient Laxatives

Owing to the availability of equally effective laxatives and its potentially serious side effects, mineral oil should be avoided in elderly patients. Most of the problems associated with mineral oil result from chronic ingestion. Since it is a lipid solvent, it decreases the absorption of fat soluble vitamins A, D, E, and K. Lipid pneumonitis due to the aspiration of mineral oil is more prevalent in the elderly population. Aspiration can produce acute or chronic pneumonitis, localized granuloma, and pulmonary fibrosis. Patients taking anticoagulants orally should not receive mineral oil.

Conclusion

Obviously laxatives are not innocuous chemical entities. Neither are they therapeutically equivalent. The choice of a laxative depends to a significant degree upon the etiology of the constipation. Table 6–1 presents an array of the pharmacologic properties of laxa-

TABLE 6–1. Pharmacologic Properties of Laxatives

Category	Site of Action	Onset of Action	Specific Drugs	Usual Adult Dose
Bulk formers	Small and large intestine	12–24 hours (may take up to three days)	Methylcellulose	4–6 gm.
			Psyllium	7 gm.
			Polycarbophil	1 gm.
Stimulants				
Castor oil	Small intestine	3 hours	Castor oil	15–30 ml.
Anthraquinones	Small intestine	6–12 hours	Senna	2 ml.
			Cascara sagrada	1 ml.
			Danthron	75 mg.
Diphenylmethanes	Small intestine	6–12 hours	Bisacodyl	10 mg.
			Phenolphthalein	10 mg.
Saline	Small and large intestine	½–3 hours	Magnesium and sodium sulfates	15 mg.
			Magnesium citrate	200 ml.
			Sodium and potassium tartrates and phosphates	10 gm.
Hyperosmotic	Colon	30 minutes	Glycerin	3 gm.
			Lactulose	15–30 ml.
Surfactants	Colon	24–48 hours	Dioctyl sodium and calcium sulfosuccinates	50–500 mg.
Emollients	Colon	6–8 hours	Mineral oil	15–30 ml.

tives, and Table 6–2 is provided as a companion document to Table 6–1 so that appropriate precautions will be exercised with the use of laxatives.

PEPTIC ULCER DISEASE*

Peptic ulcer disease has not been widely recognized as being a significant clinical concern in geriatric patients, since it has been generally accepted that the disease develops most frequently in individuals between the third and fifth decades of life. However, many patients 60 years of age and older seek medical attention because of the distress and complications of gastric and duodenal ulcer, and many clinicians still do not appreciate the extent and severity of this problem.

A number of factors contribute to this lack of awareness of geriatric ulcer disease. In an age group in which other clinical entities such as cardiovascular disease and degenerative disease predominate, little attention may be paid to a disease considered minor by comparison. In addition, the clinical patterns of peptic ulcer disease are altered with age, making recognition more difficult. When the medical histories, symptoms and physical findings in older patients are analyzed, the majority are found to have suffered from ulcer symptoms for many years. However, fewer than half the patients recall previous symptoms. When present, the symptoms tend to be vague and often atypical. A pattern of pain alleviated by the ingestion of food is frequently absent. Rather, pain may be difficult to define and localize and in many instances occurs with misleading patterns of radiation. Nausea, vomiting, anorexia, and weight loss are consistently reported in these patients, and such a history often leads to the mistaken diagnosis of neoplastic disease. In addition, the elderly patient is notorious for the difficulty he has in describing symptoms accurately. The vagueness of the symptoms may discourage adequate investigation or result in the ordering of the wrong diagnostic tests, thus delaying accurate diagnosis.

Unlike the younger patient, the elderly patient is likely to present with a major complication as the first indication of the presence of

---

*The section on peptic ulcer disease and its treatment was contributed by Dr. Jacknowitz, who is solely responsible for its content.

TABLE 6–2. Precautions in the Use of Laxatives

Bulk formers	Contraindicated in patients with esophageal, gastric, small intestinal, and colonic obstruction. Do not swallow or chew tablets without water. Mix powder with water and drink at least 8 ounces of fluid. Diabetics should avoid dextrose based products. Patients given sodium restricted diets should avoid sodium containing instant mix formulations.
Stimulants	Drugs most commonly associated with laxative abuse and "cathartic colon." Abuse of these products may lead to hypokalemia, protein losing enteropathy, and malabsorption. Do not administer antacids or histamine—2 antagonists with enteric coated bisacodyl, since abdominal cramping and vomiting may result. Phenolphthalein is associated with skin hypersensitivity in the form of a fixed drug eruption. If the urine is alkaline, a pink to red color will develop during phenolphthalein ingestion.
Saline	To avoid fluid loss, the patient should ingest at least 8 ounces of fluid. Avoid magnesium containing products in patients with renal impairment. Phosphate laxatives contain 96.5 mEq. of sodium and should be administered cautiously to patients given sodium restricted diets.
Hyperosmotics	Glycerin suppositories are ineffective if fecal impaction with hard dry stool is present.
Surfactants	Appear to be of little value in preventing constipation. May exacerbate gastric mucosal damage induced by aspirin.
Emollients	Avoid in elderly. Can cause lipid pneumonitis secondary to aspiration. Chronic use can decrease absorption of food and fat soluble vitamins. May indirectly induce lung cancer by production of pulmonary fibrosis.

the disease. This frequently results in hospitalization for the treatment of hemorrhage, perforation, persistent and severe nausea and vomiting from pyloric obstruction, and, less commonly, persisting pain with occasional vomiting, constipation, loss of weight, weakness, or anorexia not controlled by diet or drug therapy.

Bleeding is the most common complication of peptic ulcer in the elderly and accounts for one-half to two-thirds of all fatal cases.[8] The increasing tendency for gastrointestinal hemorrhage to develop with age is illustrated by the fact that approximately half of all cases of bleeding ulcer occur after the age of 50. In addition, according to one author, a patient over the age of 50 with peptic ulcer disease is twice as likely to suffer a bleeding episode than a patient less than 50 years of age.[9]

Perforation is the second most frequently reported complication and accounts for approximately one-quarter of all peptic ulcer related deaths.[8] Not only does this complication occur two to three times more commonly in the elderly, but the risk of perforation doubles over the age of 50 and the incidence of death increases dramatically with advancing age.[9]

Pyloric obstruction occurs in about 10 per cent of the patients over 60 years of age. Persistent and severe vomiting is a cardinal symptom of this complication. Furthermore, the elderly are particularly at risk of developing the metabolic consequences of prolonged vomiting. Alkalosis, hypocalcemia, and dehydration often lead to such severe weakness and debilitation that their underlying cause is often overlooked.

Finally, there is a small percentage of elderly patients with symptoms of many years' duration whose tolerance has been exhausted and who are hospitalized in order to obtain relief from the intractability of the peptic ulcer.

Pathophysiology

The pathophysiology of peptic ulcer disease remains incompletely understood. It seems clear, however, that many factors contribute to the pathogenesis of an ulcer in an individual patient.

The major sites of peptic ulceration are the stomach and the duodenal bulb. Although there can be overlap between the two, as many as 40 per cent of the patients with ulcers in the stomach also have evidence of past or present ulcers in the duodenum.[10] Gastric and duodenal ulcers have different etiologies and symptoms and are generally regarded as separate entities.

Gastric Ulcer

Gastric ulcer is considered a disease of later life, reaching its peak incidence a decade later than duodenal ulcer. Although in most instances duodenal ulcers occur more frequently in the elderly, two of every three ulcer deaths in these patients are related to gastric ulcers.[8] The patient with a "textbook" gastric ulcer can be characterized as having epigastric pain occurring within 30 to 60 minutes after eating and lasting 60 to 90 minutes. The pain may increase with eating, and it may even be associated with nausea and vomiting. In many instances weight loss is a direct result of the patient's refusal to eat for fear that the pain will return. In general the symptom pattern is less predictable than in the patient with a duodenal ulcer. This is especially true in the elderly in whom the clinical symptomatology of gastric ulcer is often subdued. Pain may be nonexistent or, conversely, very intense, often with unexplained radiating features. For example, pain may radiate to the left upper or lower quadrant. Somatic pain radiating into the back indicates penetration, perforation, or obstruction. A relationship to meals is not consistent, most elderly patients complaining of pain on ingestion of food. On occasion, profound weight loss may be the primary reason that the patient seeks medical care. Since weight loss is encountered with both benign and malignant gastric ulcers, and the clinical presentation of the two overlaps in other aspects in the elderly, these patients are often initially diagnosed as suffering from neoplastic disease. It is not rare in this age group for the radiating pain to be mistaken for variant angina or even a myocardial infarction. Furthermore, the elderly patient suffering from angina who subsequently develops a gastric ulcer may not be able to differentiate the ulcer pain from that caused by the angina, making a correct diagnosis even more difficult. Since chronic blood loss is not uncommon in gastric ulcer disease, the resultant anemia may lead to cardiac or cerebral symptoms and once again cloud the diagnosis.

Finally, the association or lack of association between the development of gastric ulcer and the chronic ingestion of various drugs has received widespread attention.[11] Until recently aspirin was the only commonly used drug that was associated with a higher incidence of gastric ulcer. Evidence implicating other drugs (e.g., corticosteroids, indomethacin, phenylbutazone, and the newer nonsteroidal anti-inflammatory analgesics) is conflicting, but most well controlled studies have failed to show that their use is consistently associated with an increased incidence of peptic ulcer.[12] In evaluating drug induced ulceration, it should be noted that peptic ulcer disease may be more prevalent in patients with other diseases, such as rheumatoid arthritis, even without drug therapy.

It should be pointed out that with regard to the elderly it is important to determine whether a history of analgesic use (or abuse) exists prior to evaluating symptoms of peptic ulcer disease, since these patients are notorious users of analgesics for minor complaints. The danger becomes more significant when these drugs are used to relieve ulcer pain.

Several theories have been proposed to explain the etiology of gastric ulcer disease. One theory involves a dysfunction in the motility of the pyloric sphincter that causes a reflux of duodenal fluid with bile salts into the stomach. Normally the pyloric sphincter prevents reflux of duodenal contents into the stomach. However, patients with gastric ulcer have a lower basal sphincter pressure than that in normal individuals or patients with duodenal ulcer, thereby permitting duodenogastric reflux. Once refluxed into the stomach, bile salts damage the gastric mucosa by altering gastric permeability to acid, salt, and water. The damaged mucosa next to the acid secreting mucosa is more susceptible to ulceration. That pyloric sphincter dysfunction may be important in the pathophysiology of gastric ulcer is further demonstrated by its response to gastrointestinal hormones. The normally functioning pyloric sphincter tightens after endogenous release or exogenous administration of secretin or cholecystokinin. In patients with gastric ulcers, the pylorus fails to respond normally to either of these hormones, and this effect persists even after ulcer healing. Lastly, cigarette smoking, which has been shown to increase bile acid reflux, decreases basal pyloric sphincter pressure. As attractive as this hypothesis is, bile acid reflux has not been shown to precede either gastritis or gastric ulceration.[13]

A second theory involves an acquired abnormality in the gastric mucosa. It is now well documented that the gastric surface epithelium is relatively impermeable to certain ions. The remarkable resistance of the normal gastric mucosa to damage by hydrogen ions appears to be related to a protective factor, the gastric mucosal barrier. This barrier, which normally maintains a concentration gradient of hydrogen ion with respect to plasma of 1,000,000 to 1, can be impaired, resulting in an increased back diffusion of hydrogen ion into the gastric mucosa. Aspirin, ethanol, and bile salts can disrupt the gastric mucosal epithelial barrier, resulting in mucosal damage, bleeding, and eventually gastric ulceration. This theory has gained wide acceptance as the mechanism by which many drugs, bile salts, and severe stress predispose to gastric ulcer disease. Indeed, atrophic gastritis, common in the elderly, makes the stomach more susceptible to the irritating effects of exogenous and endogenous compounds. An abnormal gastric mucosal barrier, however, appears most likely to be a secondary phenomenon, which results from the effect of noxious substances that often saturate the stomach in patients suffering from gastric ulcer disease.

Finally, it has been hypothesized that gastric ulcers develop because of delayed gastric emptying due to pyloric stenosis. A slow gastric emptying time due to this abnormality leads to distention of the antrum and gastric stasis. This serves as a stimulus for gastrin release and increased gastric acid secretion. However, this theory is highly unlikely, since in most patients with gastric ulcers there is normal emptying and decreased acid secretion, and those with low acid secretion have high serum gastrin levels because there is less acid to inhibit antral gastric release.

All these pieces of evidence strongly support the concept of a causal relationship between an abnormal pyloric sphincter mechanism resulting in increased bile acid reflux, chronic inflammation, an increased permeability of the gastric mucosa to hydrogen ion, and the subsequent development of gastric ulcer disease.

Duodenal Ulcer

Duodenal ulcers, constituting about 80 per cent of all peptic ulcers in the Western world, are deep mucosal lesions, which occur most often in the anterior wall of the proximal end of the duodenum.[10] As in gastric ulcer disease, the salient features of duodenal ulcer are pain and gastrointestinal bleeding; however, significant differences occur in the manner in which symptoms are described. The patient with a duodenal ulcer presents with a discrete pattern of complaints. The pain, which is usually located in the midepigastrum, is rhythmical, periodic, and chronic and is described as burning or hunger-like. Typically the pain is absent or diminished in the morning, is present two to three hours after meals, and is often most severe at night. It is also typical for episodes to be clustered in periods lasting for days or weeks interspersed with pain-free intervals of weeks or months. It is of interest that exacerbations have been found to occur most often in the spring and fall. Duodenal ulcer patients often report pain relief in response to meals. This frequently results in weight gain due to increased food intake.

The most common complications of duodenal ulcer are bleeding, perforation, and obstruction. Iron deficiency anemia and occult blood in the stools occur in chronic disease. Perforation and obstruction are indications for immediate surgical intervention and are characterized by sudden changes in symptomatology.

Perhaps 90 per cent of all perforations involve duodenal ulcers, and the site is frequently the anterior duodenal wall.[10] Perforation with peritoneal involvement is almost always manifested by sudden, nonspecific, and nonremitting abdominal pain. The majority of patients who present with perforated duodenal ulcers have a long history of ulcer disease, but a significant number complain of only a few months of ulcer pain, or in some instances, no ulcer pain at all. Infrequently acute ulcers may perforate in patients who have experienced severe stress. On physical examination the abdomen of the elderly patient with peritonitis may be unimpressive in relation to the patient's distress. Although nonspecific direct and rebound tenderness is usually present, other signs of peritonitis, including muscle guarding and boardlike rigidity, are often absent. Diminished bowel sounds or their absence along with a radiographic demonstration of free air in the duodenal cavity are hallmarks of the diagnosis. The effects on other organ systems, particularly the cardiovascular system, may mask the diagnosis. However, a high index of suspicion, along with a readiness to perform surgery in a critically ill patient, remains the primary means for reducing mortality in this age group.

Penetration of the ulcer crater beyond the duodenal wall into contiguous organs such as the pancreas and liver, but without extension into the peritoneum, occurs fairly often in duodenal ulcer disease. The absence of manifestations of peritonitis in the presence of constant pain in the back, the chest, or the side of the abdomen suggests penetration through the posterior wall of the duodenum, and this is one of the most important causes of the failure of medical treatment. In the elderly it is important to exclude other sources of acute abdominal disease, including myocardial infarction or right lower lobe pneumonia, in reaching an appropriate diagnosis.

Like perforation, obstruction most often occurs as a complication of long standing symptomatic duodenal ulcer disease, and the history and initial physical examination usually indicate the diagnosis. Typically the patient has experienced postprandial fullness and discomfort, alteration of the pain pattern, and nausea and vomiting. Prolonged vomiting of undigested food usually brings the elderly patient to see a physician. On physical examination there is usually evidence of recent weight loss and dehydration, as well as profound anorexia. These disturbing features may lead the clinician to suspect the presence of malignant disease. When the diagnosis is confirmed by gastric aspiration, surgical relief of the obstruction is the sole approach to therapy in this age group.

Whereas gastric ulcer disease is commonly thought of as representing a breakdown in the gastric mucosal barrier, duodenal ulcer is related to the hypersecretion of acid and pepsin from the stomach to the duodenum. Although individual patients with duodenal ulcer may have normal acid secretion, most patients with this disease, especially those whose duodenal ulcer is a severe clinical problem, have increased gastric acid secretion, both at rest and in response to gastric stimulation. However, there appears to be little correlation between the severity of the duodenal ulcer and the amount of acid secreted. Although some variation exists, overall data suggest that active duodenal ulcer disease requires a peak secretory capacity greater than 15 mEq. of acid per hour.[14] This relative hypersecretion in patients with duodenal ulcers is a reflection of an increase in the parietal cell mass, since the maximal secretion correlates directly with the number of parietal cells in the stomach. In addition, it has been suggested that since the stomach secretes maximally for only a few minutes after each meal, increased levels of acid are secreted at rest in duodenal ulcer disease. This increased gastric acid and pepsin secretion, both at rest and in response to gastric stimulation, could reflect an increased vagal "drive" to secrete acid, an abnormality in the rate of gastric emptying, an increased sensitivity to gastric acid stimulants, or a decreased inhibition of acid secretion.

Surgical removal of the vagus nerve decreases the gastric secretory responses to all stimuli of gastric acid secretion. It has long been postulated that increased vagal drive, originating in the higher centers of the central nervous system, leads to an increase in acid secretion, resulting in duodenal ulcer disease. However, such a cause and effect relationship has been questioned in recent years. Indeed it has been shown that the percentage reduction in acid secretion after vagotomy in patients with duodenal ulcer is only slightly less in individuals with a high acid secretion as compared to patients with a low acid secretion.[15] Nonetheless, selective vagotomy with pyloroplasty has been an effective remedy.

Although it has been reported that patients with duodenal ulcer disease have markedly increased gastric emptying, so that there is a rapid loss of the buffering capacity of a meal, the results are contradictory. It has not been definitively established whether patients with duodenal ulcer have normal or increased rates of gastric emptying. The rapid emptying of buffer, acid hypersecretion, and increased parietal cell responsiveness could all be manifestations of a defect in the inhibition of gastric motility and secretion by gastrointestinal hormones.

Information concerning hormonal interrelationships in patients with duodenal ulcer and the mechanism of acid neutralization by the duodenum appear to play an important role in the development of a duodenal ulcer. Gastrin, a potent simulant of gastric acid secretion, is a peptide hormone released primarily from the gastric antrum in response to vagal stimulation, digested protein in the stomach, and distention of the antrum. Patients with duodenal ulcers may have increased serum levels of gastrin, in both the fasting state and after a meal. Release of gastrin is inhibited by the presence of acid in the stomach, so that at a pH of 2.5, release of gastrin is almost completely shut down in normal individuals but is only moderately decreased in duodenal ulcer patients. Hormonal regulation may be the primary means by which gastrin is inhibited. It has been suggested that there is an "autonomy" of gastrin release after gastric stimulation in patients with duodenal ulcer, resulting from a defect in the feedback inhibition of the release of gastrin. The hormones secretin, glucagon, gastrointestinal polypeptide (GIP), and vasoactive intestinal polypeptide (VIP) all inhibit the release of gastrin and the secretion of gastric acid following a meal.[16,17] It is possible that a defect in the release of some or all of these peptides may be responsible for impaired inhibition of gastrin release in duodenal ulcer.

Secretin and cholecystokinin are released by the duodenal mucosa when gastric acid enters the duodenum. These hormones stimulate the release of pancreatic and biliary secretions to dilute and neutralize the acid. Since it has been observed that an increased acid load is delivered to the duodenum in duodenal ulcer disease, a defect in intrinsic cellular defenses may cause digestion of the duodenal mucosa.

Although each of the previous factors may be involved in the etiology of duodenal ulcer disease, prevailing concepts suggest that regardless of the actual cause, a basically similar pathogenesis exists for all peptic ulcers, namely, too much acid-pepsin (the aggressive factor) for the degree of local tissue resistance (the protective factor).[18]

Treatment

The elderly patient presents a challenge to the clinician in terms of both recognition of peptic ulcer disease and long term management. After the diagnosis has been made, a great deal of controversy remains regarding the therapeutic modalities that affect healing, pain, recurrence, and complications in elderly patients with peptic ulcers.

Antacids

Antacids remain the cornerstone of medical therapy of peptic ulcer disease. Their usefulness is based on the capacity of antacids to reduce gastric acidity by neutralizing secreted gastric acid. When the total acid load is reduced, less hydrogen ion is available for back diffusion through the gastric mucosa, and less acid is delivered to the duodenum for neutralization. When the intragastric pH is increased from 1.0 to 3.3, 99 per cent of the gastric acid secreted is neutralized. In addition, since the optimal range of pepsin activity occurs at a pH of 1.5 to 2.5, raising the pH reduces the activity of pepsin, resulting in a progressive neutralization of proteolytic action.

The rationale for antacid therapy is to alleviate pain and promote healing. Antacids may relieve peptic ulcer pain by either providing immediate relief of a specific episode of pain, or providing long term relief in which a patient is free of pain episodes for a longer period of time.

Five controlled studies that evaluated either the long term relief or the immediate alleviation of gastric or duodenal ulcer pain have been reported.[19-23] Although long term pain relief in ambulatory patients with gastric ulcer has been demonstrated, no such relief was found in a similar group of patients with duodenal ulcer disease.[22,23] In the latter study a liquid antacid regimen was administererd one and three hours after each meal and at bedtime. At the end of four weeks 69 per cent of the patients taking the antacid formulation and 62 per cent of those taking a placebo were free of pain. In related studies in which hospitalized patients participated, neither gastric ulcer nor duodenal ulcer pain was influenced by the use of antacids.[19-21] In a study in which immediate pain relief in male patients with duodenal ulcer was evaluated, there were no significant differences between antacid and placebo in the time of onset, degree, or duration of pain relief.[21] This finding led the authors to suggest that factors other than the reduction of gastric acidity may be important in the immediate relief of duodenal ulcer pain. However, other investigators found, in contrast, that antacid was significantly better than placebo in relieving the pain of duodenal ulcer when it was instilled directly into the stomach.[24] Finally, a recent report concluded that a liquid antacid offered only a modest therapeutic advantage when compared to placebo in the immediate relief of epigastric pain in patients with duodenal ulcers.[25]

Although their efficacy in relieving the pain of peptic ulcer disease has been a topic of controversy and further studies are needed, there is agreement at the present time that intensive high dose antacid therapy facilitates healing of duodenal ulcers, although promotion of gastric ulcer healing has been questioned.

Several clinical studies have been reported in which endoscopic verification of healing was used to establish the usefulness of antacids in the treatment of duodenal ulcer disease. One study found that after four weeks of treatment with large doses—i.e., 30 ml. of antacid one and three hours after meals and at bedtime— there was a statistically significant difference in complete ulcer healing when the antacid treated group was compared to placebo.[23] Thus, although symptomatic improvement in ulcer pain occurred equally in both groups, it was not a useful indicator of ulcer healing. After four weeks, 78 per cent of the antacid treated ulcers had healed whereas only 45 per cent of the placebo treated ulcers had healed. Another study compared cimetidine with the same antacid regimen.[26] After four weeks of treatment, antacid appeared as effective as cimetidine in healing duodenal ulcer, but with a higher incidence of side effects, usually in the form of disordered gastrointestinal function. Both studies helped to confirm the efficacy of the age-old use of antacids in duodenal ulcer disease. However, they left unanswered the question whether this large dose regimen is necessary for ulcer healing. In this regard a double blind controlled study of duodenal ulcer healing revealed antacid tablets to be significantly more effective than placebo.[27] The antacid, given in a dosage of two tablets one and three hours after meals and at bedtime (just as with the liquid antacid studies cited previously, but with only one-sixth of the neutralizing capacity of the latter), achieved healing in 77 per cent of the patients within four weeks as compared to a 33 per cent rate of healing in placebo treated patients.

Obviously more studies are needed to determine the optimal dose and perhaps the dosage form of antacid necessary to facilitate healing in duodenal ulcer disease. These findings will be of considerable practical importance to the elderly, because the high cost and the high incidence of untoward gastrointestinal problems with large doses are likely to result in therapeutic noncompliance in this population of patients.

Unlike duodenal ulcer, there is no threshold level of acid secretion required for the development of gastric ulcers. Indeed the disease may occur in patients who have minimally detectable acid secretion. Therefore, gastric acid output may have to be reduced to an almost negligible level in order to bring about gastric ulcer healing.

A recent multicenter trial comparing cimetidine with low dose antacid (15 ml. of Maalox one hour after meals and at bedtime) and placebo found cimetidine to be of greater benefit in producing more rapid healing of gastric ulcer than antacid when measured endoscopically. In addition, the side effects of cimetidine were minimal (5 per cent) compared to 6 per cent with placebo and 22 per cent with low dose antacid therapy.[28]

The authors suggest that the choice of treatment should be dictated by treatment goals. If rapid healing is desired, cimetidine appears best to minimize cost and toxicity. If the goal is to relieve symptoms, low doses of antacids appear adequate. Regardless, the authors suggest that eight weeks is a prudent time for first follow-up endoscopy, since almost all gastric ulcers that eventually heal do so by then.

Despite the advent of newer gastric antisecretory drugs, antacids remain the standard of practice, and in 1980 Americans spent more than one-half billion dollars on antacid products.[29] To meet this demand, a variety of antacids are available commercially (Tables 6–3, 6–4). All contain at least one of the four primary neutralizing ingredients—sodium bicarbonate, calcium carbonate, aluminum salts, and magnesium salts.

Ideally a clinician should choose an antacid preparation based upon the following considerations:

1. Efficiency, so that small amounts of the drug will neutralize relatively large amounts of gastric acid.

2. Absence of interference with electrolyte balance when administered in therapeutic concentrations. In addition, the sodium and sugar content of antacids must be taken into account when elderly patients are treated.

3. Exertion of a prolonged therapeutic effect without producing a secondary rise in gastric acid secretion (acid rebound).

4. Palatability, based upon aroma, taste, and texture.

5. Convenience of administration.

6. Inexpensiveness. Since administration may be prolonged, the antacid should neutralize the greatest amount of gastric acid per unit cost.

7. Neither constipation nor diarrhea as a result of therapy.

8. Absence of release of carbon dioxide after reaction with gastric acid; this may increase distention and discomfort and lead to perforation.

No single antacid preparation fulfills all these "ideal" considerations. Therefore, each product must be evaluated individually to determine its capacity to meet each of the aforementioned criteria.

Neutralizing capacity is perhaps the most clinically useful guideline to the selection of an appropriate antacid. However, because degrees of reactivity of commercially available antacids may vary depending upon the specific method of manufacture, it may not be possible

TABLE 6–3. Neutralizing Capacity, Sodium Content, and Cost Effectiveness of Liquid Antacids*

Antacid	Acid Neutralizing Capacity (mEq./ml.)	Volume (ml.) Containing 140 mEq. of Acid Neutralizing Capacity	Sodium Content (mg./5 ml.)	Monthly Cost of Therapy ($)	Composition	Manufacturer
Maalox TC	4.2	33	1.2	44	Aluminum hydroxide, magnesium hydroxide	W.H. Rorer, Inc., Fort Washington, Pennsylvania
Titralac	4.2	33	11.0	35	Calcium carbonate, glycine	Riker Laboratories, Inc., Northridge, California
Delcid	4.1	34	1.5	57	Aluminum hydroxide, magnesium hydroxide	Merrell-National Labs, Cincinnati, Ohio
Mylanta II	3.6	39	1.1	63	Aluminum hydroxide, magnesium hydroxide, simethicone	Stuart Pharmaceuticals, Wilmington, Delaware
Camalox	3.2	44	2.5	55	Aluminum hydroxide, magnesium hydroxide, calcium carbonate	W.H. Rorer, Inc., Fort Washington, Pennsylvania
Gelusil II	3.0	47	1.3	74	Aluminum hydroxide, magnesium hydroxide, simethicone	Parke-Davis, Morris Plains, New Jersey
Basaljel ES	2.9	48	23.0	101	Aluminum carbonate	Wyeth Laboratories, Philadelphia, Pennsylvania
Maalox Plus	2.3	61	2.5	67	Aluminum hydroxide, magnesium hydroxide, simethicone	W.H. Rorer, Inc., Fort Washington, Pennsylvania
Gelusil	2.2	64	0.7	80	Aluminum hydroxide, magnesium hydroxide	Parke-Davis, Morris Plains, New Jersey
Riopan Plus	1.8	78	0.7	78	Aluminum hydroxide, magnesium hydroxide, simethicone	Ayerst Laboratories, New York, New York
Amphojel	1.4	100	7.0	114	Aluminum hydroxide	Wyeth Laboratories, Philadelphia, Pennsylvania
Phosphajel	0.3	466	12.5	498	Aluminum phosphate	Wyeth Laboratories, Philadelphia, Pennsylvania

*From Drake, D., and Hollander, D.: Neutralizing capacity and cost effectiveness of antacids. Ann. Intern. Med., 94:215–217, 1981.

to determine their effective potency accurately from the listed ingredients. Furthermore, neutralizing capacity in vitro does not necessarily reflect the clinical usefulness of antacids. Nevertheless it has been demonstrated that the amount of 0.1N hydrochloric acid that can be added over a two hour period to 1 ml. of liquid antacid suspension without decreasing the pH below 3.0 closely correlates with the relative antacid potency in vivo in patients with peptic ulcer disease. This correlation has made possible the comparison of various high potency antacids with highly concentrated neutralizing capacities (Table 6–3).[30] In this report there was a 14-fold difference in gastric acid neutralizing capacity between the least and the most effective liquid antacids. When acid neutralizing capacity is expressed in terms of the amount of antacid required to neutralize 140 mEq. of acid (in vivo studies suggest that this concentration is needed to control gastric acid secretion in duodenal ulcer disease), the discrepancies in volume contradict previously held views that there is little difference in the effectiveness of various liquid antacids. These differences are further delineated in the wholesale cost of one month of therapy with various antacids.

Chewable antacid tablets are a more convenient dosage form, but must be chewed thoroughly before swallowing and then followed with a glass of water for the patient to receive full therapeutic benefit. Although equal gastric acid neutralization can be ob-

TABLE 6-4. Neutralizing Capacity, Sodium Content, and Cost Effectiveness of Tablet Antacids*

Antacid	Acid Neutralizing Capacity (mEq./Tablet)	Dose Containing 140 mEq. of Acid Neutralizing Capacity (Tablets)	Sodium Content (mg./Tablet)	Monthly Cost of Therapy ($)	Composition	Manufacturer
Camalox	16.7	8	1.5	54	Aluminum hydroxide, magnesium hydroxide	W.H. Rorer, Inc., Fort Washington, Pennsylvania
Basaljel	15.4	9	2.0	68	Aluminum carbonate	Wyeth Laboratories, Philadelphia, Pennsylvania
Mylanta II	11.0	13	1.3	85	Aluminum hydroxide, magnesium hydroxide, simethicone	Stuart Pharmaceuticals, Wilmington, Delaware
Tums	10.5	13	2.7	56	Calcium carbonate	Norcliff Thayer, Inc., Tuckahoe, New York
Alka II	10.5	13	2.0	58	Calcium carbonate	Miles Laboratories, Inc., Elkhart, Indiana
Riopan Plus	10.0	14	0.3	76	Aluminum hydroxide, magnesium hydroxide, simethicone	Ayerst Laboratories, New York, New York
Titralac	9.5	15	0.3	57	Calcium carbonate, glycine	Riker Laboratories, Inc., Northridge, California
Gelusil II	8.2	17	2.1	107	Aluminum hydroxide, magnesium hydroxide, simethicone	Parke-Davis, Morris Plains, New Jersey
Rolaids	6.9	20	53.0	86	Aluminum carbonate	Warner Lambert Company, Morris Plains, New Jersey
Maalox Plus	5.7	25	1.4	106	Aluminum hydroxide, magnesium hydroxide, simethicone	W.H. Rorer, Inc., Fort Washington, Pennsylvania
Digel	4.7	30	10.6	101	Aluminum hydroxide, magnesium hydroxide, simethicone, magnesium carbonate	Plough, Inc., Memphis, Tennessee
Amphojel	2.0	70	7.0	360	Aluminum hydroxide	Wyeth Laboratories, Philadelphia, Pennsylvania

*From Drake, D., and Hollander, D.: Neutralizing capacity and cost effectiveness of antacids. Ann. Intern. Med., 94:215–217, 1981.

tained with tablets and liquids, the major difference is the very large number of tablets required to achieve the desired neutralizing capacity (Table 6–4). Since most tablets are mint flavored, the need to chew them continuously may become so unpleasant because of the mint taste or the sensation of grittiness that patients may stop taking them. Therefore, when frequent use is needed, liquids may be more acceptable.

Since liquid antacids must be taken repeatedly and in relatively large quantities, their palatability seems likely to be a critical factor in patient compliance. In two separate studies, Mylanta II and Titralac were the most acceptable, and Ducon, Gelusil, and Amphojel were the least preferred on the basis of aroma, texture, and taste.[31,32] Refrigerating the antacid may help improve the flavor; however, care should be taken to avoid freezing the suspension.

As can be seen from Table 6–3, high sodium content is no longer a significant problem because of the advent of high potency liquid antacids. Indeed "the lowest in sodium of all leading antacid suspensions" at present, based upon acid neutralizing capacity, is Maalox Therapeutic Concentrate. Table 6–4 indicates the sodium content of antacid tablets. In an elderly patient given a sodium restricted diet who finds antacid tablets the preferred dosage form, Riopan Plus tablets provide the lowest concentration of sodium.

Although some antacid preparations contain considerable quantities of sugar or saccharin per therapeutic dose, these ingredients are not required to be listed on the product label. In the elderly diabetic patient who is being treated concomitantly for peptic ulcer disease, the sugar present in various antacids could interfere with diabetic control. Table 6–5 indicates the sugar and saccharin content as reported by the manufacturers for various antacids.[33]

Since there is a wide choice of antacid preparations and conflicting claims regarding the merits of one preparation over another, a brief discussion of the four primary neutralizing ingredients is warranted.

Sodium Bicarbonate. Sodium bicarbonate, the active ingredient in baking soda and certain effervescent analgesic tablets, is a potent, rapidly acting, effective antacid with a short duration of action. However, because it is readily absorbable, its usefulness is limited, since large doses or prolonged therapy may lead to sodium overload or systemic alkalosis. Each gram of sodium bicarbonate contains 12 mEq. of sodium. This concentration of sodium can present a problem for patients with decreased renal function, hypertension, or congestive heart failure. For this reason and because it is often used in large doses by the elderly, the suggested daily dosage is limited to 100 mEq. of sodium for patients 60 years of age and older. Since gastric distention leading to perforation can result from the ingestion of effervescent sodium bicarbonate, it is not recommended for long term use and indeed can present special problems when used for a prolonged period by the elderly.

Calcium Carbonate. Calcium carbonate is a rapid and potent neutralizer of gastric acid. However, the absorption of calcium, although limited, is significant and can affect both serum calcium levels and acid-base balance. About 90 per cent of the reacted portion of an administered dose of calcium carbonate is reconverted in the small intestine to insoluble calcium salts. About 10 per cent escapes chemical conversion by duodenal bicarbonate, is available for absorption, and may lead to elevated serum calcium levels. In fact, enough calcium can be absorbed after several days of therapy to cause hypercalcemia. This increase in calcium may induce neurologic symptoms, the formation of renal calculi, and decreased renal function. In elderly patients with renal disease or in those with high rates of acid secretion who are ingesting large doses of calcium carbonate, enough soluble calcium may be formed and absorbed to produce the milk-alkali syndrome in the absence of either milk or bicarbonate ingestion.

TABLE 6–5. Sugar and Saccharin Content of Various Antacids*†

Antacid	Sugar	Saccharin
Alternagel liquid	2000	—
Aludrox liquid	150	5.25
Aludrox tablets	368	1.9
Amphojel liquid	60	—
Amphojel tablets, 0.3 gm.	24	0.155
Amphojel tablets, 0.6 gm.	48	0.31
Basaljel liquid	—	1.5
Basaljel capsules or tablets	41	—
Basaljel extra strength liquid	375	7.5
Camalox liquid	—	2.25
Camalox tablets	—	1.5
Gaviscon liquid	1500	2.4
Gaviscon tablets	1200	—
Gaviscon-2 tablets	2400	—
Gelusil liquid	—	2.25
Gelusil tablets	280	—
Gelusil M tablets	265	—
Gelusil II tablets	116	1.0
Maalox liquid	—	4.2
Maalox No. 1 tablets	—	1.0
Maalox No. 2 tablets	145	3.0
Maalox Plus liquid	—	3.3
Maalox Plus tablets	575	1.5
Maalox Therapeutic Concentrate liquid	—	—
Mylanta liquid	2000	—
Mylanta tablets	275	—
Mylanta-II liquid	2000	—
Mylanta-II tablets	805	—
Oxaine liquid	150	1.5
Phillips' Milk of Magnesia, flavored	—	5.78
Phillips' Milk of Magnesia, tablets	195	—
Phosphajel liquid	—	—
Riopan liquid	—	4.05
Riopan chew tablets	70	—
Riopan swallow tablets	—	0.1
Riopan Plus liquid	—	4.05
Riopan Plus chew tablets	610	—
Silain-Gel liquid	—	0.75
Simeco liquid	129	—
Trisogel tablets	—	—

*Adapted from Stolinsky, D.C.: Sugar and saccharin content of various antacids. N. Eng. J. Med., *305*:166–167, 1981. Reprinted by permission of the New England Journal of Medicine.

†Expressed in milligrams per 15 ml. of liquid or per tablet. Hexitols are included if they are listed by the manufacturer.

Calcium carbonate is the only antacid known to produce the reflex hypersecretory state known as "acid rebound." This is probably a direct effect of calcium on the gut mucosa and not due to calcium absorption, since the infusion of calcium has been reported to increase the serum gastrin level and hypergastrinemia in turn may be responsible for gastric hypersecretion.

Although it is frequently thought of as causing constipation, recent findings suggest that calcium carbonate not only may not be constipating, but it may even at times act as a laxative. There is some evidence that the constipation seen in patients taking calcium carbonate for peptic ulcer disease may be caused by the ulcer rather than the calcium.

Calcium carbonate may be used in small doses (e.g., 500 mg.) for immediate symptomatic relief of peptic ulcer disease. However, despite its potency, this antacid causes too many severe side effects to be recommended for long term use in the elderly.

Aluminum Salts. Aluminum salts, such as aluminum hydroxide, aluminum phosphate, and aluminum carbonate, are considered weak neutralizers of gastric acid when compared to the other primary neutralizing ingredients present in commercially available antacids. Aluminum hydroxide is the most potent of the three salts, and when present in excess, it raises the gastric pH to 4 to 4.5, neutralizing approximately 28 to 30 mEq. of hydrogen ion per gram. Aluminum hydroxide can be prepared in either a reactive or a nonreactive form. Therefore, depending upon the manufacturer's process, there are large differences in the solubility of different preparations in solutions of gastric acid and consequently, wide variations in the rate of acid neutralization.

When administered alone, aluminum hydroxide delays gastric emptying, presumably by inhibiting gastric smooth muscle contractions. Free aluminum concentrations decrease significantly as the pH is increased, declining by a factor of 1000 as the pH changes from 4.2 to 8.1. Therefore, the delay in gastric emptying, which is dependent upon the presence of aluminum ion, does not occur when aluminum hydroxide is combined with other neutralizing ingredients that increase the gastric pH and reduce the concentration of free aluminum. This delay in gastric emptying as well as the capacity of aluminum hydroxide to bind bile acids is presumably responsible for the constipating property of aluminum salts, an effect that may limit its use by the elderly. Intestinal obstruction has been reported in patients with decreased bowel motility or relative dehydration and in those in whom fluids are restricted. These characteristics are not unusual in a geriatric population.

Although aluminum previously was thought to be poorly absorbed from the gastrointestinal tract, a three-fold increase in the plasma aluminum concentration and a 10- to 20-fold increase in the urinary aluminum excretion have been reported in normal individuals who were given the equivalent of 2.2 grams of aluminum as aluminum hydroxide gel. Specific tissue concentrations of aluminum may be increased in a number of conditions, including Alzheimer's disease, a syndrome of diffuse cerebral atrophy most frequently observed in the elderly. Aluminum may be neurotoxic in patients with chronic renal failure who are receiving aluminum hydroxide for prolonged periods of time to bind phosphate in the gut, thus preventing hyperphosphatemia. This disorder, occurring primarily in uremic patients maintained on long term dialysis and referred to as "dialysis dementia," is characterized by speech abnormalities, dyspraxia of movement, asterixis, myoclonus, personality changes, dementia, and psychosis. Aluminum absorption may be parathyroid hormone dependent, since a positive correlation between serum parathyroid hormone levels and plasma aluminum levels has been demonstrated in patients with chronic renal disease. This observation may account for the increased aluminum retention in patients undergoing dialysis who are receiving aluminum hydroxide therapy, since they frequently develop secondary hyperparathyroidism. It should be noted that neurologic sequelae of aluminum toxicity have not been demonstrated in patients with unimpaired renal function.

Aluminum forms insoluble complexes with dietary phosphate, which becomes unavailable for absorption. Although they may be useful in treating hyperphosphatemia accompanying chronic renal failure, ingestion of large amounts of antacids may be associated with a phosphorus depletion syndrome and osteomalacia. This syndrome includes not only hypophosphatemia, hypophosphaturia, hypercalciuria, and bone pain, but also debility, anorexia, muscle weakness, and malaise. This syndrome may occur within two weeks after beginning therapy with aluminum containing antacids and is aggravated by the intake of a low protein diet having a low phosphorus content. This applies particularly to elderly patients who are in a poor nutritional state.

Phosphorus depletion can be prevented by increasing the intake of phosphorus. It is believed that phosphorus depletion may not occur if the urinary excretion of phosphorus is maintained at 300 mg. per day or higher. However, the amount of dietary or added phosphorus required to achieve this goal has not yet been documented. In addition, serum phosphate determinations may be necessary bimonthly during prolonged therapy with aluminum containing antacids. The use of aluminum phosphate suspension may minimize the phosphorus depletion syndrome. However, aluminum phosphate as well as aluminum carbonate contains significant amounts of sodium and may cause fluid retention in patients with cardiovascular or renal disease (Table 6–3).

Magnesium Salts. Magnesium salts, such as the hydroxide, carbonate, and trisilicate, are effective antacids with acid neutralizing potencies greater than that of aluminum hydroxide but less than that of sodium bicarbonate and calcium carbonate. Magnesium containing compounds are presumably converted in the small intestine to soluble but poorly absorbed salts, which produce osmotic diarrhea and can lead to fluid and electrolyte depletion. Antacid mixtures containing magnesium hydroxide and a constipating antacid such as aluminum hydroxide have been introduced to minimize the cathartic effects of magnesium, but still retain acid neutralizing capacity. Although constipation and diarrhea may be counterbalanced, other side effects or complications are not.

Although it is excreted mainly in the feces, 10 to 20 per cent of the magnesium is absorbed, filtered in the glomeruli, and excreted in the urine. With normal renal function, magnesium retention does not occur. However, hypermagnesemia manifested by hypotension, central nervous system depression, respiratory depression, and coma can occur in patients with renal failure. Indeed significant increases in the serum magnesium concentration can occur within three to five days after the initiation of therapy. Since magnesium retention is potentially hazardous in such patients, no more than 50 mEq. should be administered daily to a patient with renal disease, and magnesium containing antacids should not be used at all in patients with severe renal failure.

Magnesium trisilicate, like magnesium hydroxide, is excreted primarily in the feces, but it is also absorbed, filtered in the glomeruli, and excreted in the urine. With magnesium trisilicate about 7 per cent of the silica present is absorbed, which may lead to the formation of silica containing kidney stones after chronic antacid use.

Antacid therapy should be individualized. Patient compliance is enhanced if the preparation is palatable, is prescribed in therapeutic doses on an acceptable schedule, and is relatively free of troublesome side effects. The presence of renal disease, cardiovascular disease, or poor nutritional status or the simultaneous administration of other medications must be taken into account prior to selecting a specific antacid or designing a therapeutic regimen. Indeed the rate and completeness of absorption of a number of drugs can be altered when they are administered together with aluminum and magnesium containing antacids (Table 6–6). Finally, the cost to the patient, especially in the elderly patient on a fixed income, is another important factor in antacid use.

Magnesium hydroxide is the safest and most potent substitute for calcium carbonate and sodium bicarbonate. In the absence of renal failure it should be selected for most elderly patients with peptic ulcer disease. Because of its alteration of bowel habits, it is best prescribed in combination with a constipating drug, such as aluminum hydroxide gel, either in the form of combination antacid or in an alternating dosage regimen. In contrast to aluminum hydroxide, which cannot raise gastric pH above 5, or magnesium hydroxide, which may increase the gastric pH to greater than 9, physical combinations of these components maintain the pH at a maximum of 6.5 to 7.5.

Sucralfate

Antacids, although effective ulcer therapy, are often poorly accepted by the patient, and noncompliance is a common problem. Cimetidine has replaced antacid therapy in the management of duodenal peptic ulcer disease to a significant extent, but adverse effects and expense do not indicate its use in every situation. Sucralfate (Carafate), a unique complex of sulfated sucrose and aluminum hydroxide, is a useful alternative to cimetidine or antacids in treating peptic ulcers and has initially been

TABLE 6–6. Effect of Antacids on Absorption of Some Other Drugs*

Drug	Antacid Type	Effect	Clinically Important?
Aminophylline	Mg-Al	Decrease in rate (not extent)	No
Atropine and hyoscine	Mg	Decrease in extent	Possibly
Chlordiazepoxide	Mg	Decrease in rate (not extent)	No
Clorazepate	Mg	Decrease in extent†	Yes
Cimetidine	Mg	Decrease in extent‡	Possibly
Diazepam	Mg-Al	Decrease in rate (not extent)	No
Digoxin	Mg-Al	Decrease in extent	Uncertain
Indomethacin	Mg-Al	Decrease in extent	?
Levodopa	Mg-Al	Decrease in extent	?
Isoniazid	Al	Decrease in peak level	?
Nitrofurantoin	Mg	Decrease in peak level	?
Phenothiazines	Mg-Al	Absorbed in vitro	?
Tetracyclines	Al	Absorbed in vitro	Yes
Warfarin	Mg	Absorbed in vitro	Yes

*From Henry, D.A., and Langman, M.J.S.: Adverse effects of antiulcer drugs. Drugs, 21:444–459, 1981.

†Activity of drug depends on liberation of desmethyldiazepam in the acidic conditions of the gastric contents.

‡Variable effects from person to person.

approved by the FDA for the short term (up to eight weeks) treatment of duodenal ulcers.

Sucralfate exerts its antiulcer effect by binding with proteinaceous material, neutralizing local acidity without affecting the gastric pH, and forming a protective barrier at the ulcer site. It may also inhibit the diffusion of hydrogen ions, inhibit the action of pepsin, and adsorb bile acids. Sucralfate appears to form an ulcer adherent complex with a proteinaceous exudate at the ulcer site that protects the lesion from further attack by acid, pepsin, and bile salts. It does not work by neutralizing gastric acid.

Objective clinical trials indicate that sucralfate is as effective as cimetidine for the short term healing of duodenal ulcer. Sucralfate is not approved for long term maintenance therapy, however. Preliminary results indicate that after nine months of therapy with sucralfate, only 37 per cent of the patients relapsed compared to 78 per cent receiving placebo. Likewise, although favorable responses to sucralfate in the treatment of gastric ulcer have been suggested by several reports in the foreign literature, no data from the United States have appeared to date to support such use.[160]

Sucralfate possesses the virtue of producing few adverse effects because it is not absorbed. The most frequently reported side effect is constipation, with an incidence of 3 to 4 per cent. Less than one person in 350 reported any other adverse effect (e.g., nausea, diarrhea, gastric discomfort, indigestion, dry mouth, rash, pruritus, back pain, dizziness, sleepiness, and vertigo). No drug-drug interactions have been reported. The risk of overdosage is negligible. Lethal doses in animals exceed 12 gm. per kg.

The recommended adult dosage for duodenal ulcer is 1.0 gm. four times daily on an empty stomach one hour before each meal (or two hours after meals) and at bedtime. Sucralfate may be combined with antacids if pain relief is indicated, but antacids should not be administered within 30 minutes of a sucralfate dose because the antacid may interfere with the binding of sucralfate at the site of action. Studies are currently in progress to determine the effect of administering both cimetidine and sucralfate to patients with duodenal ulcers. Treatment with sucralfate should be continued for four to eight weeks unless earlier healing is demonstrated by x-ray or endoscopic examination.

Anticholinergic Drug Therapy

Although antacids are the mainstay of symptomatic therapy in peptic ulcer disease, an alternative approach to neutralizing the acid already present is to reduce secretion, and this is the pharmacologic basis for anticholinergic drug therapy. By blocking vagally mediated smooth muscle contraction, these drugs delay gastric emptying, slow intestinal motility, and inhibit the cholinergic component of gastric acid secretion. Despite their widespread use, there is no clear evidence that anticholinergic drugs relieve symptoms or facilitate healing in peptic ulcer disease. It is of interest, therefore, that a 1982 study reported no significant differences in ulcer healing, relief of ulcer symptoms, antacid consumption, or patient compliance between mixed groups of ulcer patients (duodenal ulcer, pyloric ulcer, and prepyloric ulcer) treated with 15 mg. of propantheline three times daily and 30 mg. at bedtime as compared to 200 mg. of cimetidine three times daily and at bedtime. The final anticholinergic dosage was adjusted to suppress salivary secretion by at least two-thirds.[161] In a commentary preceding this report, the results of the study were analyzed utilizing the following criteria—evaluation of the trial, deciding whether inductive inference of the conclusions from the trial was appropriate, and deciding among competing statements. In each area there were believed to be significant problems that would minimize the use of anticholinergics in treating duodenal ulcers.

Additionally the anticholinergic drugs are associated with a high incidence of side effects in the elderly, including urinary retention in patients with prostatic hypertrophy, blurring of vision, the precipitation of glaucoma, gastroesophageal reflux due to reduction of lower esophageal sphincter pressure, gastric retention in patients in whom there is a pre-existing delay in gastric emptying, and constipation.

Since anticholinergic drugs delay gastric emptying and slow intestinal motility, they inhibit the absorption of rapidly absorbed drugs, such as acetaminophen, and enhance the net absorption of slowly absorbed drugs, including digoxin. Moreover, anticholinergic drugs prolong the duration of action of antacids. However, they should not be combined because antacids reduce absorption of anticholinergic drugs. Furthermore, anticholinergic drugs cannot decrease acidity to a greater extent than the buffering or acid neutralizing capacity of the antacid.

Gastric acid production is under control of the hormone gastrin, which is released from the gastric mucosa on mechanical distention of the stomach, such as occurs after a meal. The effects are not blocked by anticholinergic drugs because gastrin acts independently of vagal innervation. Nevertheless both physiologic mechanisms may have a final common pathway, and this pathway may involve histamine as a mediator. One postulate is that gastrin and acetylcholine act by increasing histamine production or release in the gastric mucosa, which in turn stimulates acid secretion. A second explanation holds that gastrin, acetylcholine, and histamine, by an as yet unidentified mechanism, are mutual potentiators of acid secretion. Blocking any one of the three mediators of gastric secretion should greatly diminish the effect of the remaining two.

In health, histamine is synthesized, stored, and released (it quickly breaks down following release) in special cells located near a variety of effector cells. For instance, histamine is found in gastric and intestinal glands where it regulates various secretory processes and in the myocardium where it affects the frequency and amplitude of heart contraction. Generally there are three types of histamine producing cells, basophils, mast cells, and an unidentified type in the gastric mucosa, the latter near parietal cells.

The acid producing cells in the gastric mucosa release acid upon stimulation via impulses from vagal nerve fibers by gastrin, food, and other mechanisms not thoroughly understood. Histamine is also released and may be the common mediator in the stimulation of acid secretion by the factors already mentioned. Stimulated by histamine, the receptor sites on the parietal cells trigger the release of gastric acid by those cells.

There are two types of receptor site—the H_1 sites associated with histamine and its effector cells in the upper respiratory tract and the H_2 sites associated not only with gastric acid secretion but also with cardiac contractility. The classic antihistamines used to treat allergic reactions are H_1 receptor antagonists; cimetidine and ranitidine block H_2 receptor sites.

Cimetidine

Few drugs have had as great an impact on the medical community as has cimetidine. Within a year after its release nearly 1 per cent of the American population had received this drug, and in 1980 worldwide sales amounted to approximately 700 million dollars.[34]

Cimetidine inhibits, and in high dosage abolishes, gastric acid secretion in response to every known gastric acid stimulant. There is a clear relationship between levels after single doses and the degree of inhibition of gastric acid secretion. A 50 per cent inhibition of acid output during nocturnal fasting is obtained by a cimetidine blood level of about 0.5 mcg. per ml., whereas after meals about 0.6 mcg. per ml. is needed to achieve the same effect.[35] However, neutralization and dilution of gastric acid by a meal contribute to the overall therapeutic effect of cimetidine in reducing gastric acid secretion.[36] Cimetidine therefore appears to be best administered with meals because during the time between ingestion of the drug and the onset of its therapeutic effect, gastric acidity is lowered by the meal itself and because cimetidine blood levels are sustained longer with more prolonged inhibition of gastric acid secretion.

Cimetidine is readily absorbed after oral administration, peak blood concentrations in fasted subjects occurring about 60 to 90 minutes after ingestion. Blood concentrations are dose related in single doses up to 400 mg., but blood levels are disproportionately increased after an 800 mg. dose.[37]

Peak blood concentrations are lower and occur later when cimetidine is given with food than when given after fasting, but the total bioavailability does not appear to be significantly lowered over a six hour period. Intensive antacid therapy can decrease the absorption of cimetidine when the two are administered concomitantly, but total bioavailability remains approximately the same. It is best to give antacids one hour before or after cimetidine administration.

There have been few reports relating to the distribution pattern of cimetidine, but the large apparent volume of distribution (approximately 50 liters) suggests that this drug is widely distributed in human tissue.[37] Since cimetidine is plasma protein bound to the extent of only 15 to 20 per cent, tissue distribution may play a significant role in the therapeutic efficacy of this drug.

The elimination half-life of cimetidine is 1.9 hours, renal excretion of unchanged drug being the major elimination pathway. About 5 per cent of a dose of cimetidine is excreted in the urine as the hydroxymethyl metabolite and about 10 per cent as the sulfoxide. As the dose is increased above 400 mg., a higher fraction of the drug is metabolized to polar metabolites before elimination by the kidneys. This may account for the disproportionately high blood levels of cimetidine after an 800 mg. dose.

Since cimetidine is cleared primarily by the kidneys, approximately 70 per cent of an unchanged dose appears in the urine within six hours after ingestion. Elimination characteristics change with alterations in renal function. In patients with end stage renal disease who are undergoing hemodialysis, a 200 mg. dose twice daily results in blood levels similar to those obtained after a 1 gram daily dose is administered to individuals with normal renal function.[38] An increase in the elimination half-life to about five hours occurs in functionally anephric patients. In accord with these and other findings, the dosage schedule presented in Table 6–7 was prepared for patients with varying degrees of renal failure.[39] Hemodialysis and peritoneal dialysis are effective in removing circulating cimetidine, but the total quantity of unchanged drug in the dialysate is only about 10 per cent. Until more definitive evidence is presented, however, even on the day of dialysis, cimetidine blood levels should be closely monitored.

The worldwide experience with cimetidine has clearly shown the efficacy of this drug in promoting acute gastric and duodenal ulcer healing, and this constitutes its primary use at present. The results of numerous clinical trials indicate that the drug heals duodenal ulcers in approximately 70 to 80 per cent of the patients as compared with a 30 to 40 per cent healing rate in placebo treated control subjects.[40] In most cases the advantage of cimetidine over placebo has been found to be greatest after four to six weeks of continuous therapy. Although foreign investigators have favored slightly lower dosages and less frequent administration of cimetidine, a dosage of 300 mg. four times daily has been used in most clinical trials in the United States and appears to be appropriate for most ulcers in patients with normal renal function.

It is of interest that the severity or duration of symptoms, the presence of single or multiple ulcerations, and the ability of the patient to withstand surgery are factors that do

TABLE 6–7. Dosage Schedule for Patients in Renal Failure

	Creatinine Clearance	Cimetidine Dosage
Mild renal failure	50–87 ml./min.	300 mg. every 6 hours
Moderate renal failure	20–35 ml./min.	300 mg. every 8 hours
Severe renal failure	0–9 ml./min.	300 mg. every 12 hours

not appear to influence the probability of response to cimetidine therapy. A recent study indicates that favorable circumstances for healing by cimetidine include an age over 50 years (with a particular probability of success in retired individuals), a sedentary occupation, no relevant family history of peptic ulcer disease, no smoking, no abuse of analgesic drugs and alcohol, and an acid secretory rate within normal limits.[41] In addition, the authors speculate that reports of resistance to cimetidine treatment may reflect a number of factors, including differences in pathophysiology, interference with the natural healing capability of the gastrointestinal mucosa, differences in absorption of the drug, or differences in parietal cell responsiveness.

The Food and Drug Administration has added cimetidine (a 400 mg. dose at bedtime) for the prevention of recurrent duodenal ulcer to its official list of approved indications. The concept of maintenance therapy for all patients with duodenal ulcers is controversial, since the long term prognosis for their disease is usually benign, with symptomatic improvement or lasting remission occurring in many. There is also some controversy concerning whether repeat courses in patients with recurrent ulcers are as effective as the initial cimetidine therapy. In addition, we do not know how long to continue maintenance therapy with cimetidine in the patient known to be susceptible to recurrent duodenal ulcer disease. Although the risks of long term toxicity are a very real concern in the elderly, a recent report indicates that the safety profile of cimetidine maintenance is favorable.[173] Indications are that if cimetidine is discontinued once the ulcer is healed and maintenance therapy is not utilized, the ulcer may recur. This recurrent ulcer may require higher dosages of cimetidine for longer periods of time (e.g., 1600 mg. daily for eight weeks).[42]

Finally, with regard to duodenal ulcer disease, it remains uncertain whether acute disease heals faster with cimetidine than with antacid therapy, but current evidence suggests that it does not.[43] If cimetidine and intensive antacid therapy are equally effective and produce analogous healing rates in acute duodenal ulcer disease, the choice of treatment then becomes a matter of patient acceptability and therefore compliance, safety, and cost.

Major problems with antacid use are patient compliance and cost. Patients take only an average of 30 to 40 per cent of the quantity of antacid prescribed when they are not subjected to rigorously controlled clinical trials.[44] Moreover, compliance tends to decline with time, so that a regimen of long term antacid therapy is often followed only when symptoms recur. This obviously prolongs the time required for the ulcer to heal.

The problem of patient acceptability results from a number of factors. As indicated previously, antacids are not very palatable. Indeed the administration of therapeutic doses of antacids seven times a day (one and three hours after each meal and at bedtime) is inconvenient and tends to impair the taste and enjoyment of food and beverages. The patient, moreover, must have available large quantities of antacid, identifying him as an "ulcer patient" to his friends and associates. This may be especially troublesome to an elderly patient who is also concerned about other health related problems.

It should be noted that on an empty stomach, that is, at bedtime, antacid administration would be beneficial for only a limited period of time (i.e., 30 to 45 minutes) as compared with cimetidine, which is very effective when no food is present in the stomach. This difference can be of significance in the elderly, since pain might be controlled more effectively, allowing the patient to experience an uninterrupted night's sleep. This is especially important if the patient is known to be a nocturnal hypersecretor of gastric acid.

With regard to the wholesale cost of each of these modalities, one month's therapy with cimetidine costs approximately $37.50 wholesale, as compared to an average of $50.00 for the five most potent antacids if they are administered in dosages adequate to neutralize 140 mEq. of gastric acid. Therefore, although prices vary from pharmacy to pharmacy, cimetidine is no more expensive than antacid therapy and in many cases may be considerably less costly. The obvious economic benefits of such a decreased drug cost in this age group cannot be overemphasized.

It is unlikely that any drug used in the treatment of gastrointestinal diseases has been studied as extensively as has cimetidine. Indeed patient experience with cimetidine has been monitored in the United States by an outpatient surveillance program and throughout the world by a spontaneous adverse reaction reporting system.[45] The overall incidence of adverse effects reported in approximately 10,000 patients treated with cimetidine was 4.4

per cent. The frequencies of adverse reactions reported for more than six million patients treated with cimetidine are shown in Table 6–8.

In addition, in controlled short term studies, side effects requiring the discontinuation of therapy have been noted in approximately 1.5 per cent of the patients receiving cimetidine as contrasted to 1.2 per cent receiving placebo.[46] The most common side effects associated with cimetidine in these studies were, in order of occurrence, diarrhea, tiredness, dizziness, drowsiness, and rash, whereas headache and constipation were more frequently encountered in patients receiving placebos.

Dizziness and mental confusion may develop after inadvertent ingestion of more than the recommended dose of cimetidine, or of normal doses in older patients, since the bioavailability of cimetidine increases with increasing age. Cimetidine associated mental confusion usually begins within 24 to 48 hours after the first dose with signs and symptoms of flushing or sweating, restlessness, confusion, disorientation, and agitation. Hallucinations, focal twitching, seizures, and unresponsiveness may develop. Patients may become belligerent or develop slurring of speech.

Reports of mental confusion, especially in the elderly, have aroused some concern. The susceptibility of individuals in this age group may be partly the result of impaired renal function during senescence, since cimetidine is excreted largely unchanged through the kidneys. It has been shown that by the age of 90, glomerular filtration, renal blood flow, urea clearance, and the capacity to concentrate urine decrease to about half the values found at the age of 30. In addition, histologic studies show that there is a gradual loss of nephrons with advancing age. It would appear prudent to monitor elderly patients closely and adjust the dosage appropriately.

In a pharmacokinetic evaluation of patients with this disorder it was found that six of eight individuals with trough concentrations (i.e., serum cimetidine levels obtained five minutes before each intravenous cimetidine dose) above 1.25 mcg. per ml. experienced mental confusion.[47] The severity of symptoms was directly proportional to the serum cimetidine trough concentrations, the most severe mental symptoms being associated with trough concentrations greater than 2.0 mcg. per ml. It should be noted that all patients exhibiting mental confusion in this study had impaired renal function and liver disease and as a consequence were receiving lower daily dosages of the drug. The relationship between the serum concentration of cimetidine and the onset of mental confusion remains controversial. It has been suggested that symptoms might actually be due to metabolic encephalopathy resulting from underlying renal or hepatic disease.

The occurrence of cimetidine induced changes in mental status seems to be rare, having been reported to occur in 1.1 per 100,000 patients treated. Most involved either elderly patients in intensive care situations or patients with multiorgan disease receiving multidrug therapy, or both.[45] Therefore, elderly patients with severe renal or hepatic dysfunction should be carefully monitored when receiving cimetidine, and the drug should be discontinued if symptoms of mental confusion occur.

Unpleasant immediate side effects are more likely with antacids and may result in discontinuation of therapy by the patient. On the other hand, the possibility of long term side effects may be greater with cimetidine. One such concern, because of the development of the disease in the elderly, is the association of gastric carcinoma with prolonged cimetidine therapy. It is well recognized that the use of cimetidine may mask gastric carcinoma by relieving ulcer symptoms.[48] British investigators reported the discovery of gastric carcinoma in three patients who had been receiving cimetidine for periods up to 11 months and speculated that cimetidine may have been nitrosated to its N-nitroso derivative, thus

TABLE 6–8. Frequencies of Adverse Reactions to Cimetidine

1. Mild central nervous system symptoms
   7.3 per 100,000 patients
2. Gastrointestinal/liver/biliary system
   4.8 per 100,000 patients
3. Skin and musculoskeletal system
   3.1 per 100,000 patients
4. Hematologic system
   2.3 per 100,000 patients
5. Cardiovascular/respiratory system
   1.8 per 100,000 patients
6. Metabolic/endocrine system
   1.4 per 100,000 patients
7. Genitourinary system
   1.0 per 100,000 patients

playing a carcinogenic role in these patients.[49] The authors suggested that the chemical structure of cimetidine makes it a likely molecule for nitrosation.

A flurry of subsequent letters to the editor of *Lancet* both contradicted and concurred with the initial report. All available data relating to N-nitroso compounds and cancer suggest a latency period of 15 to 20 years, rather than the time frame of less than one year originally reported. A 1982 study of almost 10,000 patients who were receiving cimetidine indicated that the risks of developing gastric cancer were no greater in the cimetidine treated population than in the control group not taking the drug.[162] A 1983 study supports this observation.[173]

It is important to re-emphasize that a correct diagnosis be obtained prior to initiation of cimetidine therapy in order not to mask malignant gastric carcinoma. The question of carcinogenicity following H_2 receptor antagonist therapy requires further continued monitoring.

Cimetidine related adverse drug interactions have been noted.[163] Cimetidine has been shown to interact with the cytochrome P-450 dependent drug metabolizing enzyme system, thereby reducing clearance of such drugs as warfarin, diazepam, chlordiazepoxide, phenytoin, and theophylline.[164] The benzodiazepines lorazepam and oxazepam are not significantly affected because their limited hepatic glucuronide conjugation is not influenced by cimetidine.[165,166]

Propranolol clearance is also reduced by cimetidine, apparently by a combination of two processes, inhibition of hepatic microsomal drug metabolizing enzymes and reduced hepatic blood flow.[167] Because cimetidine treatment rapidly reduced hepatic blood flow by approximately 25 per cent, these investigators predicted that drugs such as morphine, lidocaine, and certain beta-adrenergic blockers whose systemic clearance is largely dependent upon hepatic blood flow could also undergo interactions with cimetidine.

When we consider the number of patients who have received cimetidine since its release in August 1977, serious drug reactions and interactions appear to be relatively uncommon. However, the monitoring of the drug's adverse reactions profile continues.

Finally, there is no evidence that combining antacid therapy with cimetidine will produce an additive or synergistic effect on ulcer healing rate. In a multicenter study, patients receiving therapeutic doses of cimetidine combined with sufficient antacid to neutralize 140 mEq. of gastric acid (the latter administered one and three hours after each meal, at bedtime, and as needed for pain) showed no statistical differences in healing when compared with patients treated with cimetidine alone or antacid alone.[50]

Ranitidine

Ranitidine is a new H_2 receptor antagonist, which is related pharmacologically but not structurally to cimetidine. Ranitidine is a nitrofuran and produces effective inhibition of gastric acid secretion. On a mg. for mg. basis ranitidine is significantly more potent than cimetidine; this enhanced potency allows ranitidine to be given twice daily, and the recommended oral dosage in the treatment of peptic ulcer disease is 150 mg. twice daily. Less frequent doses may enhance therapeutic compliance.

Ranitidine may be administered orally or intravenously and is currently available as a 150 mg. tablet. It is bioavailable to the extent of 50 to 75 per cent when consumed orally, and food does not influence overall bioavailability. The elimination half-life of ranitidine in patients with normal renal function is 2.5 to 3.0 hours, and 50 to 70 per cent of the drug is excreted in the urine unchanged. Peak serum concentrations are achieved 60 to 120 minutes after an oral dose.

Clinical experience in the United States regarding adverse effects from ranitidine have been limited largely to phase III trials. Evidence from European studies indicates that ranitidine is associated with a low incidence of toxicity. Adverse effects reported include transient increases in the serum creatinine level, skin rash, headache, diarrhea, dyspepsia, impotence, loss of libido, dizziness, and mental confusion.[187] The incidence of such adverse effects appears to be low.

Clinically significant ranitidine induced mental confusion, gynecomastia, impotence, nephrotoxicity, and cytopenias appear to be extremely rare with the oral dosage form prescribed at approved dosage levels. Hepatotoxicity from the parenteral but not the oral dosage form has been reported. In one report, antiandrogenic side effects disappeared when therapy was changed from cimetidine to ranitidine.[168] In another study leucopenia associated with cimetidine use did not recur with ranitidine.[169] Additionally, ranitidine was better tolerated in a 68 year old male with renal failure who developed agitation, confusion, and delirium after receiving 2400 mg. of cimetidine intravenously over a 48 hour period. Agitation, confusion, and delirium recurred when a lower dosage of cimetidine (300 mg. over 12 hours) was administered. Ranitidine was administered at a dose of 50 mg. intravenously for eight days, followed by 150 mg. twice daily by mouth, and the patient remained alert and free of any mental disorder.[170] Further investigation is needed, however, before ranitidine can be routinely advocated for use in geriatric patients.

Ranitidine, like cinetidine, has been reported to decrease the hepatic blood flow.[171] Interestingly, however, a 1982 report indicates that ranitidine does not significantly alter propranolol elimination, thus suggesting that the effect of ranitidine on hepatic blood flow may not be clinically significant.[172] Liver enzymes may be elevated when the intravenous dosage form of ranitidine is administered. This dose related effect of the intravenous formulation suggests that ranitidine is potentially hepatotoxic. Placebo controlled studies of the oral formulation involving 2437 patients indicate no difference in the incidence of SGOT-SGPT level elevations between the two groups.

Ranitidine does not appear to significantly inhibit the cytochrome P-450 mixed function oxidase enzyme system, and therefore the drug appears unlikely to interact significantly with drugs such as propranolol, warfarin, neophylline, and phenytoin. Additional studies are needed, however, to determine the effects of ranitidine on the cytochrome P-450 enzyme system and hepatic blood flow before conclusions are reached relative to the interaction potential of ranitidine.

As with cimetidine, ranitidine has been initially approved by the FDA for the short term treatment of duodenal ulcer and the Zollinger-Ellison syndrome. The recommended dosage for the treatment of peptic ulcer disease is 150 mg. orally twice daily. The cost of an equivalent daily dosage of ranitidine is approximately 20 per cent higher than that of cimetidine. Because of its long duration of action and twice daily dosage regimen, relatively low interaction potential, and apparently low level of adverse effects, ranitidine will find its place among the modern therapeutic choices for treatment of peptic ulcer disease.

Conclusion

The elderly patient presents a challenge to the clinician both in recognition of peptic ulcer disease and in short term and long term management. Only with close observation and an awareness of the disease and its complications in the elderly can a successful therapeutic approach be developed. The knowledge of the various modalities available, their actions, and reactions will ensure that this disease is adequately treated in this patient population once it is identified.

COLONIC DIVERTICULAR DISEASE

Diverticular disease of the colon, a disease that occurs with increasing frequency in old age, has gained wide recognition in economically developed countries during the past century. Its emergence has been correlated with the removal of cereal fiber from our modern diet.[51] That diverticular disease results from changes in dietary habits has been confirmed by reports describing the disease's widely differing prevalence rates in various geographic areas and among various ethnic groups. Truly "a deficiency disease of Western civilization," diverticular disease is rarely found in nonindustrialized countries, but is prevalent in those societies in which a basic diet consisting of low residue, high fat, and highly refined carbohydrates is found. In this regard it is noteworthy that between 1909 and 1975 the total crude fiber content of the American diet has been reported to have declined by almost 30 per cent, primarily the result of a decreased intake of grains, vegetables, and fruits.[52] Today in the United States, of the estimated 25 million people 70 years or older, 60 per cent have colonic diverticula, and of these, 25 per cent develop complications.[53] These complications account for the morbidity and mortality associated with this condition. Furthermore, in patients with diverticular disease there is a statistically significant increase in the frequency of hemorrhoids, gallbladder disease, varicose veins, hiatal hernia, and coronary artery disease. Studies do not support an association with carcinoma of the colon, and the commonly held notion that diverticular disease is associated with obesity has not been confirmed.

Although there is a marked increase in the incidence of diverticular disease with advancing age, and indeed the probable risk of developing diverticula approaches 50 per cent in the population over the age of 50, the disease is not uncommon in persons under the age of 40. A higher incidence of diverticular disease among females has been suggested.

Pathophysiology

Diverticular disease of the colon can be divided into three phases: the prediverticular state, diverticulosis, and diverticulitis. The prediverticular state is characterized by muscular thickening and luminal narrowing of the colon. Pressure responses in the prediverticular colon are similar to those in colons with established diverticula, emphasizing the fact that the diverticula are not the primary abnormality and that pressure and muscle changes precede their development. These changes persist in 95 per cent of the patients with diverticular disease.

A colonic diverticulum is a herniation of colonic mucosa through an otherwise normal colonic wall, with weakness, abnormalities of intracolonic pressure, or both. The most striking pathologic finding in colon segments involved in diverticular disease is a pronounced thickening of both longitudinal and circular muscle layers. The exaggerated concentrations of the circular muscle layer result in a marked distortion of the colonic lumen, with the appearance of corrugations like those of an accordion and the diverticula occurring between the corrugations (Fig. 6–1).

Most patients who have colonic diverticula remain asymptomatic and are unaware of their presence. A small number of patients come under medical supervision because of the incidental finding of diverticula after barium enema. Others are discovered because of relevant symptoms. The occurrence of diverticula in the colon without complications has been described as diverticulosis. Diverticulitis, on the other hand, implies inflammation in the area of a diverticulum. In the latter phase, associated pericolitis often occurs, for the inflammatory process seldom remains confined to the mucosa. Because of the degree of overlap and the difficulty in differentiating between the two forms, the term diverticular disease of the colon has been adopted to include all aspects of the disease.

Most patients with diverticular disease have few symptoms or signs of colonic disease until they are elderly; then the incidence of

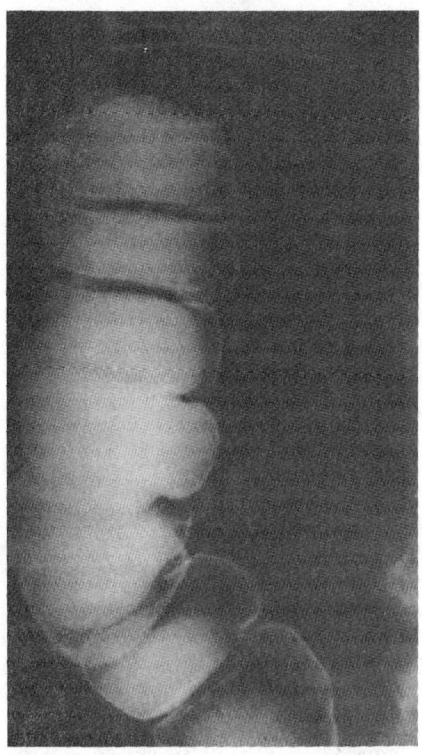

Figure 6–1. Radiographic demonstration of herniation of colonic mucosa and distortion of colonic lumen in diverticular disease.

symptomatology and complications increases. The greater the number of diverticula, the greater the risk of recurrent attacks and complications.

The symptoms of diverticular disease are usually related to the left lower quadrant of the abdomen. In patients with uncomplicated colonic diverticula there may be mild abdominal distention and a minimally tender left lower abdominal quadrant. Barium enema examination is undertaken to evaluate such vague abdominal discomfort, but although it is the primary diagnostic method for identifying diverticula, it is not always definitive. For example, in some patients with diverticulitis the result of the barium enema examination may be completely normal when a single diverticulum is present. In addition, colonic narrowing seen on barium enema examination may resemble fibrotic obstruction or cancer, although the concomitant administration of glucagon during the examination has lessened diagnostic error. Finally, the severe symptoms of acute diverticulitis, including nausea, vomiting, pronounced abdominal distention and fever with leukocytosis, remain a relative contraindication to barium enema examination, and patients often undergo surgery on the basis of clinical findings alone.

Because the symptoms of diverticular disease are often nonspecific, a variety of other conditions must be excluded before the diagnosis of diverticular disease can be made. These include carcinoma of the colon, ulcerative colitis, Crohn's disease of the colon, ischemic bowel disease, infectious bowel disease (amoebiasis, shigellosis, and salmonellosis), irritable bowel syndrome, pseudomembranous colitis, appendicitis, and gynecologic diseases (salpingitis and ovarian tumors).

It is of interest that in 20 per cent of the patients undergoing barium examinations at the Lahey Clinic Foundation, differentiation between cancer of the colon and diverticular disease could not be made definitively.[54] In these individuals a sigmoidoscopic examination was essential to exclude colonic cancer. Crohn's disease and less often ulcerative colitis may coexist with diverticular disease. Crohn's disease may be responsible for precipitating an acute attack of diverticulitis when diverticula are found in the involved portion of the colon.[55] However, in most cases the diagnosis can be made on the basis of the radiologic findings.

Treatment

Once the diagnosis has been made, the association between a lack of dietary fiber and the development of the disease provides a rationale for the treatment of asymptomatic diverticulosis. Indeed the efficacy of high fiber diets in the relief of pain and bowel discomfort and in the prevention of complications of diverticular disease has been shown by numerous clinical studies.[56-58]

Unfortunately there is a great deal of ignorance and confusion about the composition of natural fiber, its dietary occurrence, and the physiologic effects of various fibers. Dietary fiber has been defined as that portion of the diet containing indigestible structural plant material and usually consists of celluloses, hemicelluloses, lignins, and pectins derived from plant cell walls. The relative amounts of these vary accordingly to the age and function of the specific plant from which the fiber is derived. In fact, within an individual species, large differences in the amount of fiber may occur. Regardless of the amount, most dietary fiber is contained in grains, vegetables, fruits, seeds, and nuts. In addition, some processed foods contain synthetic or naturally occurring additives, such as methylcellulose, which along with bulk producing hydrophilic colloids such as psyllium seed also contributes to dietary fiber content.[58]

Physiologically there appears to be little doubt that the addition of fiber to the diet increases the bulk of the stool. This increase is much greater than the dry weight of the added fiber itself and depends primarily on the capacity of the fiber to entrap water. The amount of water that different fibers absorb varies. Cereal bran absorbs three to four times its own weight of water. However, this difference becomes less significant when the actual fiber content is calculated from the total weight. For example, fiber from 10 grams of cereal bran will bind more than 40 grams of water, whereas fiber in 10 grams of raw carrot will absorb approximately 25 grams of water.

It is of interest that the capacity of dietary fiber to increase the bulk of the stool in vitro may not correlate with its capacity to increase the bulk of the stool in vivo. In a recent study, when several different sources of vegetable fiber were compared in human volunteers, the increases in fecal weights were inversely proportional to their capacity to absorb water in vitro, and bran, although least effective in holding water, was the most effective in increasing fecal weight.[59]

Other reported physiologic effects of dietary fiber include softer stools, greater frequency of bowel movements, and decreased intestinal transit time. In rural African natives who eat unrefined whole grain as a staple of the diet, bowel transit time averages 35 hours. This contrasts sharply with a time of more than 75 hours in the average Englishman. With the shorter transit time the stools are moist and bulky and are evacuated without effort about twice daily. The slower passing stools of urban dwellers tend to be small, dry, hard, and constipating, and greater intracolonic pressure is needed to propel them along the bowel. Therefore, the swiftly passed stool resulting from a high fiber diet subjects the sigmoid colon to less strain and does not favor the development of diverticula.

The least expensive, least perishable, and most widely used source of dietary fiber is unprocessed bran, even though in its pure state it looks and tastes like brown sawdust. The efficacy of various bran preparations may be related to the physical state and particle size of the bran used. Indeed the coarser the bran preparation, the more significant the effect on bowel motility. Milling may increase the susceptibility of the plant cell wall material by exposing more surfaces to bacterial action, and this in itself may reduce the capacity of the bran to bind water in the large intestine. Other reported properties of bran include its action as a smooth muscle relaxant in the gut and its capacity to alter bile salt and lipid metabolism and to increase fecal loss of zinc, phosphorus, magnesium, and calcium. High fiber diets are high in phytates. Phytate binding or complexing of minerals in the gut may decrease absorption and increase fecal loss. These mineral losses have not been evaluated to determine their significance in healthy persons given balanced diets. Therefore, no recommendation concerning supplementation with exogenous minerals can be made.

The first study that reported the successful use of a high residue diet that included unprocessed bran in the treatment of symptomatic diverticular disease was published a decade ago.[60] Beginning with 2 teaspoonfuls of unprocessed bran three times daily (6 grams a day) in conjunction with bran cereals, vegetables, fruit, and bread, the amount was increased gradually over two weeks to the level at which soft stools were passed easily once or twice daily. The amount of bran required to accomplish this varied from 10 to 25 grams per day. At first the patients reported flatulence and a feeling of distention, but these symptoms disappeared within four to six weeks. Of 62 patients who continued the diet for an average of 22 months, 88 per cent expressed significant relief of their pretreatment symptoms of abdominal pain and discomfort. On follow-up four years later, all were improved. A sample menu of a high fiber diet is reproduced in Table 6–9. In addition, hydrophilic colloids such as methylcellulose, in tablet form, were reported to decrease high intracolonic pressure, resulting in clinical improvement in patients suffering from diverticular disease. When such substances are used, they should be administered with sufficient fluids to prevent the occurrence of esophageal or bowel obstruction due to the formation of a bolus.

Although natural fiber is useful in the treatment of uncomplicated diverticular disease and the prevention of many of its symptoms, it should be emphasized that no course of therapy for diverticulosis has been proved to reduce the incidence of complications or alter the natural course of the disease.

TABLE 6–9. Sample Menu of High Fiber Diet*

		Fiber (gm.)	Calories
Breakfast	120 gm. fruit or 120 ml. fruit juice	2.5	50
	30 gm. high fiber breakfast cereal or porridge	2.0	100
	30 gm. wholemeal toast	2.9	70
	15 gm. digestive biscuit	0.8	70
Lunch	Meat/cheese/egg	—	200
	60 gm. wholemeal bread	5.8	140
	Salad	3.0	50
	120 gm. apple	2.5	50
	15 gm. digestive biscuit	0.8	70
Evening meal	Meat/fish/cheese/egg	—	200
	120 gm. vegetable	4.0	20
	100 gm. potato	1.0	100
	High fiber pudding	3.0	250
	15 gm. wholemeal biscuit	0.8	70
	Milk—½ pt.; butter—¾ oz.		340
	Bran—20 gm. (2 tablespoons)	8.8	
Total		37.9	1780

*Adapted from Hyland, J.M.P., and Taylor, I.: Does a high fiber diet prevent the complications of diverticular disease? Br. J. Surg., 67:77–79, 1980.

In addition to the use of dietary fiber, other considerations in treating uncomplicated diverticular disease include the following:

1. Explaining to the patient the nature of the disease and reassuring him that this is the only disease causing his discomfort.

2. Informing the patient of the importance of reporting the appearance of blood in the stool, an increase in abdominal pain, alteration of bowel habits if different from what was previously reported, genitourinary tract symptomatology, anorexia, or unexplained weight loss.

3. Directing the patient to avoid foods known to precipitate abdominal pain and distention as well as diarrhea or constipation. In addition, undigestible foods such as corn, popcorn, berries and nuts should be avoided.

4. Reminding the patient that constipation can be controlled by insuring adequate daily exercise, hydration, elimination of drugs that

induce constipation, and the addition of stool softeners.

5. Requesting that the patient avoid large fatty meals because of their role in inducing the secretion of hormones that may alter the muscle tone of the colonic wall.

Other therapeutic measures undertaken in uncomplicated diverticular disease include the use of anticholinergic drugs, antispasmodics, and analgesics. Although the documented hyperactivity of the colon in many symptomatic patients provides a rationale for the use of anticholinergic drugs to decrease motility and hence reduce intracolonic pressure, their usefulness has never been clearly demonstrated. In addition, great care is required when anticholinergic drugs are used in the elderly. Antispasmodics relax smooth muscle and may be useful as adjunctive drugs in controlling symptoms. Of interest is the report of the therapeutic efficacy of glucagon in patients with pain due to colonic muscle spasm.[61] When other measures are not helpful, the use of analgesic drugs is often necessary. Although many patients eventually require more potent therapy, pain may be managed initially by mild analgesics such as acetaminophen. If stronger drugs are required, analgesics, which have been shown to reduce colonic motility while relieving the pain of diverticular disease, are indicated. Meperidine and pentazocine are considered to be the drugs of choice, for both have been shown to decrease the frequency and amplitude of contraction within the colon. However, because of its lesser potential for producing disorientation and confusion in the elderly, meperidine may be preferred.

Complications of diverticular disease occur in approximately 40 per cent of the patients and depend to a large extent on the duration of the disease. About 10 per cent of individuals having the disease for less than 10 years develop complications. About one in four develops diverticulitis. Abscess, perforation, fistula, stenosis and obstruction, and hemorrhage are other complications encountered. These complications are the subject of Figure 6–2.

The development of left lower abdominal quadrant tenderness, cramping pain, a fixed abdominal mass, fever, and leukocytosis in an elderly patient with pre-existing diverticular disease indicates the onset of diverticulitis. It should be noted that the elderly and chronically ill may not show an inflammatory response. Therefore, the diagnosis should be

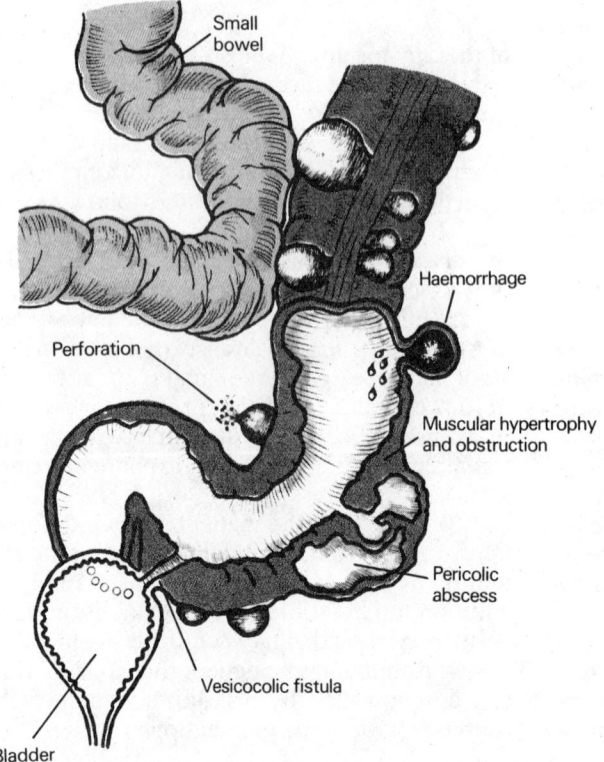

Figure 6–2. Complications of diverticular disease (From Barbezat, G.O.: Rational treatment of diverticular disease. Drugs, 19:63–69, 1980.)

entertained in any elderly patient presenting with abdominal signs and symptoms. In addition, it is important to remember that although the sigmoid colon is almost invariably the site of diverticulitis, the disease is often associated with a variable clinical picture and may coexist with other disease states.

Symptoms suggesting diverticulitis usually indicate that the patient should be admitted to a hospital. The clinical course of the patient dictates the course of treatment to follow. Most often the episode is mild, and as a general rule a conservative course is recommended. Generally, during the acute stage, oral intake is eliminated and hydration is maintained intravenously. Electrolyte and acid-base balance should be closely monitored, particular attention being paid to maintaining adequate urinary output. Antimicrobial drugs are widely used in the management of diverticulitis; some clinicians believe that these drugs are the mainstay of medical treatment. However, although they are used empirically, their benefit has not been adequately assessed. In the absence of bacteremia, specific antibiotics effective against colonic organisms should be administered, the main therapeutic targets being anaerobic and gram negative bacteria. In seriously ill hospitalized patients, ampicillin has been widely used, but an aminoglycoside administered concomitantly with clindamycin provides much more effective coverage of the most likely causative organisms. With the introduction of the parenteral form of metronidazole, which is highly effective against anaerobic organisms, an alternative therapeutic drug became available for the treatment of anaerobic bacteremia; indeed a response can be observed within 24 to 48 hours following the administration of metronidazole.[62] Regardless of the antibiotic used, the risks of drug induced toxicity and colonization of the colon with resistant organisms must be weighed against the expected benefit.

Although in many patients symptoms subside in several days, as many as 30 per cent of hospitalized patients require surgical intervention when complications develop. In addition, although controversial, there has emerged a more aggressive view of the indications for operation in diverticular disease, prophylactic surgical therapy being advised to prevent recurrent complications. With this in mind, the following guidelines can be utilized for selection of patients to undergo elective surgery:

1. Two or more episodes of documented diverticulitis.

2. One attack of diverticulitis, with radiologic evidence of perforation.

3. Diverticulitis accompanied by colonic obstruction or the occurrence of a large intestinal narrowing on barium enema.

4. Clinical evidence of impending or actual colonic fistula.

5. Possibly indicated with previous episode of massive hemorrhage.

6. Inability to exclude associated carcinoma.

7. A patient less than 50 years of age with documented diverticulitis.

Medical management, primarily involving the judicious use of antimicrobial drugs, has its proponents. In addition, it has been suggested that the addition of dietary fiber would prevent recurrence of inflammatory complications. However, in spite of increasingly widespread use of this form of therapy, it has not been critically evaluated.

Conclusion

Truly a disease of the twentieth century, diverticular disease of the colon affects 30 million Americans, causing 200,000 to be hospitalized annually, and incurring annual health care costs exceeding a third of a billion dollars. Only recently has the probable pathophysiology of this disease been clarified along with reports of new ideas regarding its management. There remain many important and unresolved questions to be answered.

CHOLELITHIASIS AND CHOLECYSTITIS

Diseases of the biliary tree are a common medical problem of the elderly and will eventually affect 15 to 20 per cent of all adults. The incidence of biliary tract disease increases with age, and it is the fifth leading cause of hospitalization in this country. Over one-half million cholecystectomies are performed each year.

With the rapid advancements in noninvasive examination of the biliary system by ultrasound and computed tomographic (CT) scanning, an increasing number of unsuspected gallstones are being discovered. Up to 50 per cent of all such stones may be asymptomatic upon initial discovery.[63] If these patients are followed for 10 years, it has been shown that symptomatic cholecystitis will develop in more than half.[64] There is considerable controversy whether "silent" stones should be removed via elective surgery. The mortality risk for "elective" cholecystectomy in patients under 50 years of age is approximately 0.1 per cent. For patients over 65 the risk is somewhat increased. If acute cholecystitis develops, the mortality rate for surgery in patients older than 65 rises dramatically to 10 per cent.[65] Investigational studies are currently under way to determine the feasibility of medical therapy to dissolve gallstones in patients who are poor candidates for surgery because of age or organic disease.

Pathophysiology

Cholesterol is secreted by the liver into the bile, an aqueous medium. For cholesterol to remain soluble, the relative concentrations of each of the three bile components—cholesterol, bile salts, and lecithin—must remain within narrow ranges. The bile salts prevent the precipitation of cholesterol by forming structures called micelles. These circular configurations of bile salt molecules are arranged so that the water soluble region of the molecule faces outward and the lipid soluble area faces the center. Bile salt micelles and lecithin encircle cholesterol and maintain its solubility at a critical micelle concentration. Any disturbance in this critical micelle concentration results in the precipitation of cholesterol gallstones. Gallstones may develop as the result of a decreased rate of bile acid synthesis or an increased rate of production and secretion of cholesterol into the bile. The reason certain individuals develop gallstones is not known, but the tendency may be genetic in origin since certain ethnic groups, such as American Indians, have a very high incidence of gallbladder disease. Certain medications, including clofibrate (Atromid), estrogen, and thiazides, increase the risk of gallstone development.[66]

Approximately 80 per cent of all gallstones contain at least 75 per cent cholesterol and are amenable to medical therapy. Both chenodeoxycholic acid (cheno) and ursodeoxycholic acid (urso) are effective in dissolving these radiolucent stones.

Medical Dissolution of Gallstones

Chenodeoxycholic acid (cheno) and cholic acid are the two primary bile acids found in man. In a classic study concerning the effectiveness of cheno, Danzinger et al. succeeded in dissolving cholesterol gallstones in 60 per cent of their patient population.[67] Since other trials with cholic acid, which differs from cheno only by an additional hydroxyl group, failed to produce similar desaturation or gallstone dissolution, it is theorized that expansion of the bile acid pool is probably not the major mechanism of action of cheno. Chenodeoxycholic acid probably works by interfering with intestinal absorption of dietary cholesterol or by inhibiting cholesterol synthesis. Cheno decreases the amount of hydroxymethylglutaryl–coenzyme A reductase, which is a rate limiting enzyme in the production of cholesterol. Another possible mechanism of action is increased bile flow, which would desaturate bile and prevent stasis.

Although the initial reports with cheno have been promising, the questions of long term efficacy and safety remain to be answered. A National Cooperative Gallstone Study was initiated in 10 medical centers throughout the United States involving 916 patients. The preliminary findings of this trial have been reported.[68] Of the 916 patients in the trial, 305 received 750 mg. per day of cheno, 306 took 375 mg. per day, and 305 were given a placebo. Complete dissolution occurred in 14 per cent of the patients on the high dose, in 5 per cent on the low dose, and in less than 10 per cent of those given placebo. Partial dissolution, defined as at least a 50 per cent decrease in gallstone diameter, occurred in 27 per cent of the patients on high dose cheno, in 19 per cent on low doses, and in less than 10 per cent of the control subjects. The most effective dosage of cheno appears to be 15 mg. per kg. per day. Cheno is well absorbed orally and may be taken with meals.

Side effects of cheno include diarrhea, hepatotoxicity, hypercholesterolemia, and the passage of stones into the cystic or common bile duct. Cheno produces diarrhea by secretion of water and electrolytes in the colon through stimulation of intestinal mucosal cyclic AMP. The diarrhea is dose dependent and usually responds to a reduction of the dose. Elderly patients should be warned to increase the fluid intake to prevent dehydration secondary to diarrhea.

Hepatotoxicity is the major potential problem with cheno. Experiments in laboratory animals have demonstrated the hepatotoxicity of cheno to be due either to a direct effect on hepatic microsomes or to lithocholic acid, a metabolite of cheno produced by intestinal bacteria. Although elevations in serum transaminase levels have been noted in approximately 20 per cent of the patients, this effect is reversible. No clinically significant cases of hepatotoxicity have been reported with the use of cheno. In patients receiving cheno therapy, there is a mean increase in serum cholesterol level of 20 mg. per dl. Migration of stones that decrease in size has occurred in only a few patients taking cheno.

Combination therapy consisting of cheno and phospholipid feedings, lecithin, cholic acid, bran, and phenobarbital has not been shown to be superior to therapy with cheno alone.

Even though cheno is still an investigational product, another compound, ursodeoxycholic acid (urso), may prove to be superior. This 7-beta epimer of cheno is as effective as cheno in one-half to one-third the total daily dosage.[69] It is effective in at least 60 per cent of the patients when given in doses of 250 to 1000 mg. per day. At 1000 mg. per day, urso's success rate is greater than 80 per cent. Urso dissolves gallstones faster than cheno and does not produce diarrhea or serum liver enzyme elevations.[70] The only disadvantage of urso is that it currently costs more to produce than cheno.

When either cheno or urso therapy is chosen for a patient, it may take six months to two years for the gallstones to be dissolved. Once dissolution has occurred, long term or indefinite prophylactic therapy may be necessary to prevent new stone formation.

Acute Cholecystitis

Acute cholecystitis is characterized by anorexia, nausea, vomiting, fever, and severe abdominal pains. The intensity of clinical manifestations loosely parallels the degree of cystic duct obstruction and mucosal inflammation. Most patients show a positive Murphy sign, with pain elicited upon inspiration during gentle palpation in the right subcostal region. In the elderly, perforation may occur without clinical signs of cholecystitis. Early surgical intervention within 72 hours is generally regarded as the therapy of choice, but there is a risk of serious sepsis associated with this disease.

Bile is usually sterile. With the presence of asymptomatic gallstones, the incidence of infected bile is 17 per cent. In patients older than 70 years of age, or if obstructive jaundice or acute cholecystitis is present, the bile is contaminated with bacteria in two-thirds of these cases.[71] The organisms most frequently isolated include *E. coli,* Klebsiella, and enterococci. *Bacteroides fragilis* is isolated in up to one-third of the culture positive specimens. Clostridia is another anaerobe that is sometimes found, especially in cases of emphysematous cholecystitis.

The use of antibiotics is recommended in all individuals requiring operative intervention for acute cholecystitis. In the absence of obstruction, ampicillin, carbenicillin, cefazolin, clindamycin, and nafcillin attain levels equal to or significantly greater than serum levels. Only clindamycin and nafcillin are found in significant concentrations in the bile when obstruction is present. Because obstruction is usually present, effective "in vitro" antibiotics (ampicillin, carbenicillin, and cefazolin) do not attain significant levels in the bile. Conversely, antibiotics that achieve significant bile levels (clindamycin and nafcillin) are effective against only a small percentage of invading organisms.[72]

Numerous antibiotic regimens have been utilized in the treatment and surgical prophylaxis of biliary tract infection. Therapy is aimed at the prevention of secondary spread of the infection. The antibiotic must be effective against *E. coli* and Klebsiella, since the clinical significance of the presence of enterococci remains to be established.[73] Ampicillin or cefazolin alone, or in combination with an aminoglycoside, has been employed frequently. A single 1 gm. intramuscular dose of cefazolin given one hour prior to surgery is superior to placebo or cefazolin given preoperatively and continued for five postoperative days.[74] Wound sepsis in the placebo group was 16.9 per cent, 5.5 per cent in the five day antibiotic regimen, and only 3.2 per cent on the single dose cefazolin protocol. In elderly patients with obstructive jaundice, the addition of clindamycin may be warranted to "cover" *B. fragilis*. Gram staining and a culture of bile at the time of surgery are useful in identifying the infecting organism and in selecting an appropriate antibiotic regimen.

Acute Cholangitis

Presenting clinical features of jaundice, abdominal pain, and chills and fever represent the triad of Charcot, which can aid in the diagnosis of acute cholangitis. Gram negative enteric organisms and anaerobes are frequently isolated. Antibiotic regimens that have been recommended include clindamycin and an aminoglycoside, penicillin and an aminoglycoside, and carbenicillin alone.

Common Bile Duct Stones

Retained bile duct stones are discovered in at least 2 to 6 per cent of the patients who have undergone cholecystectomy and choledochotomy. If a T tube is in place, mechanical removal of the stone with a Dormia basket catheter is the treatment of choice. Endoscopic sphincterotomy can also be employed for the mechanical removal of retained stones. In elderly patients who are high surgical risks, chemical dissolution through the T tube can be attempted.[74] Heparin, sodium cholate, and mono-octonoin have been evaluated for this condition. Heparinized saline has been reported to be successful in 72 per cent of the patients. However, in vitro studies have shown that such solutions do not dissolve gallstones and that the success of the infusion was probably due to a mechanical flushing of the duct. Sodium cholate is an effective gallstone solvent in approximately 65 per cent of the patients but is associated with numerous adverse effects, including fever, elevated liver enzyme levels, cholangitis, pancreatitis, and death.[74]

Mono-octonoin, a commercial emulsifying agent, dissolves gallstones twice as fast as sodium cholate solutions. Each milliliter of mono-octonoin can solubilize 174 mg. of cholesterol. In one study some or all of the common bile duct stones disappeared in 10 of 12 patients when this solvent was administered via a T tube for four to 21 days.[75] In the two patients who failed to respond, the stones were later found (postoperatively) to be insoluble in mono-octanoin. Diarrhea is the only major side effect that is encountered. Mild anorexia, nausea, vomiting, and upper abdominal and back discomfort have also been noted. At the current time the use of mono-octonoin appears to be the most effective and safest way in which to dissolve common duct stones.[76]

Conclusion

Major advances are occurring in the detection and management of gallbladder disease. An awareness of various contemporary treatment modalities will ensure more effective management of gallbladder disease in the elderly.

DIARRHEA

Diarrhea is a common disease in the elderly. These individuals are often intolerant of this condition and can rapidly become dehydrated. Over $100,000,000 is spent each year on medication for its treatment and prevention. The term diarrhea is defined as the passage of loose or liquid stools at an increased frequency. A stricter definition in the adult population is fecal loss of greater than 300 gm. per day (normal, 100 to 200 gm. per day). The major resultant problem of diarrhea is excess loss of water and electrolytes via the stool. In secretory forms of diarrhea, fluid and electrolyte loss can be substantial.

Pathophysiology

One of the main functions of the gastrointestinal tract is the conservation of water and electrolytes. Oral intake and various secretions into the gut account for the approximately 9 liters received by the duodenum and jejunum each day. Of the amount reaching the duodenum and jejunum, 4 liters is reabsorbed. Sodium and water are passively absorbed, depending upon the amount of osmotic material present, such as disaccharides and starch, which are contained in the chyme. Potassium is also passively absorbed.

Active absorption of sodium occurs in the ileum and colon. Chloride is also actively reabsorbed here and bicarbonate is excreted into the ileal lumen. Passive accumulation of potassium takes place in the colon to maintain ionic equilibrium with fecal concentrations of potassium commonly exceeding two to three times the plasma level. The colon is also extremely efficient in conserving water. Of approximately 1.5 liters of fluid presented there, 90 per cent is reabsorbed.

The mechanisms of diarrhea can be divided into three main categories: osmotic solute load, water and electrolyte transportation abnormalities, and alteration in intestinal motility. More than one etiology may be present at the same time.

Osmotically active substances such as sorbitol and lactulose when ingested are examples of substances producing osmotic diarrhea.

Other examples include the "dumping syndrome," disaccharidase deficiency, celiac sprue, and the use of elemental diets. Through osmosis excess water is drawn into the jejunum. The severity of this type of diarrhea depends upon the capacity of the ileum and colon to absorb the excess fluid. In this form of diarrhea, fluid loss rather than electrolyte depletion is commonly found.

Increased mucosal permeability caused by damage or inflammation of the intestinal mucosa can result in passive secretion of fluid and electrolytes. Examples of this form of diarrhea include inflammatory bowel disease, invasive strains of Shigella, Salmonella, and *Escherichia coli*, laxatives, and enteritis due to radiation. An active secretory process occurs in patients with toxin-producing bacteria, such as *V. cholerae*, Clostridium, and *E. coli*; excessive bile acids; and hormone secreting tumors, such as the pancreatic neoplasm found in the Zollinger-Ellison syndrome.

The exact pathophysiology of the diarrhea induced by motility abnormalities is unclear at the present time. Diarrhea secondary to diabetes, hyperthyroidism, short gut syndrome, and scleroderma is thought to be secondary to muscle function abnormalities of the gastrointestinal tract.

Diagnosis

It is very important to ascertain the severity of the diarrhea in order to develop an appropriate treatment regimen. It is important to know how long the diarrhea has persisted, since some patients claim to have had the problem for many years. Acute and aggressive intervention probably will have minimal effect on the chronic type of diarrhea. The stools should be checked for blood, since diarrhea may be the first sign of colonic cancer. Probably the most important question to ask is whether constipation had been a problem recently. The medical history of the elderly patient with diarrhea should also include questions about the frequency of bowel movements and whether they occur throughout the night. The medication history is important and must include both prescription and nonprescription products. Recent changes in dietary habits or foreign travel should be specifically investigated.

In the physical examination the signs and symptomatology of volume depletion are of paramount importance and include tachycardia, postural hypotension, poor skin turgor, absence of axillary sweat, and elevation of the hematocrit or blood urea nitrogen level. A serum potassium level determination is important to ascertain the degree of diarrhea induced potassium loss. A stool specimen should be examined for blood, fecal leukocytes, ova, parasites, and fat.

The commonest causes of acute diarrhea in the elderly are fecal impactions, bacterial and viral infections, and medications. Encopresis is by far the most frequent occurrence in the nursing home population. Mechanical disimpaction followed by instruction about proper dietary habits and mobility is often all that is needed to correct this form of diarrhea.

Diarrhea Caused by Micro-organisms

With the increased mobility of the world population, much attention has been focused on traveler's diarrhea. This type of diarrhea is very debilitating, since the individual may experience up to 10 to 20 diarrheal episodes a day accompanied by abdominal cramps, chills, fever, nausea, and vomiting. Recent evidence suggests that up to 70 per cent of these cases may be caused by pathogenic strains of *E. coli*. High attack rates are associated with eating salads containing raw vegetables. The number of organisms ingested is the major determinant of infectivity. Gastric acid produces a substantial barrier to enteric infections, and the use of drugs that increase alkalinity, such as antacids and cimetidine, favors the survival of ingested organisms. Avoidance of these drugs and of raw foods and local drinking water should be helpful.

In a double blind controlled study the ingestion of 100 mg. of doxycycline daily led to a reduction of 40 to 55 per cent in the incidence of diarrhea. The protection afforded by this tetracycline derivative seemed to last for at least one week after it was discontinued. The routine use of prophylactic antibiotics always raises the question of development of resistant bacterial strains.

Bismuth subsalicylate (Pepto-Bismol) in a dosage of 60 ml. four times a day has been shown to be effective in the prevention of traveler's diarrhea. Mild constipation and darkening of the stools were the only untoward effects of therapy noted. This drug in a dosage of 30 ml. every half-hour for eight doses is also effective in producing subjective relief of symptoms of diarrhea, nausea, and abdominal cramps, which are frequently seen with traveler's diarrhea. It is possible that the efficacy of this product may be due to the effects of its salicylate content. Fluid and electrolyte replacement remains the most important aspect of therapy in this type of diarrhea.

Giardiasis

Diarrhea caused by *Giardia lamblia* can be treated effectively with quinacrine hydrochloride (Atabrine), 100 mg., or metronidazole (Flagyl), 250 mg., three times daily for seven to 10 days.

Shigellosis

Shigella and salmonella are invasive micro-organisms that characteristically do not produce endotoxins. Invasion of the distal colon and rectum produces urgency, tenesmus, and the passage of blood and mucus. The types of isolated strains of Shigella organisms that require antibiotic therapy have not been established. Ampicillin generally is regarded as the drug of choice if therapy is indicated. Other recommended drugs are a combination of trimethoprim and sulfamethoxazole (Bactrim, Septra) and a single 2.5 gm. dose of tetracycline.

Salmonellosis

Antibiotic therapy is contraindicated in the treatment of salmonellosis unless the typhosa strain is isolated or systemic infection has occurred. Antibiotics not only fail to cure the disease but may also prolong the postconvalescence excretion of the organism. Antimotility drugs should be avoided if diarrhea is caused by invasive organisms. These medications may enhance epithelial penetration and local multiplication of the infecting agent by inhibiting intestinal motility.

Amebiasis

Symptoms of enteral infection caused by the protozoan, *Entamoeba histolytica*, can vary from mild diarrhea to severe dysentery. For treatment of symptomatic intestinal amebiasis, the drug of choice is metronidazole, 750 mg. given three times a day for five to 10 days.

Recently two newly discovered micro-organisms, *Campylobacter fetus* and Yersinia, have been found to be the cause of diarrhea in some elderly patients. For Campylobacter induced diarrhea that is severe, erythromycin, tetracycline, and clindamycin are the drugs of choice. If the patient is septic, an aminoglycoside should be chosen. Central nervous system involvement requires the utilization of chloramphenicol. First line drugs for diarrhea induced by Yersinia include a sulfonamide, trimethoprim-sulfamethoxazole, tetracycline, or chloramphenicol. An aminoglycoside is reserved for cases in which sepsis is evident.

Drug Induced Diarrhea

Almost any drug, including a placebo, can cause diarrhea. For the elderly patient diarrhea is a frequent side effect of colchicine, magnesium hydroxide containing antacids, laxatives, lactulose, guanethidine, quinidine, certain antibiotics, and digitalis preparations. Most diarrhea induced by medications is readily reversible upon discontinuation of the offending drug.

Pseudomembranous enterocolitis has been associated with the use of several antibiotics, including penicillin G, tetracycline, ampicillin, cephalexin, chloramphenicol, trimethoprim-sulfamethoxazole, lincomycin, and clindamycin. Clindamycin has been the antibiotic most frequently implicated, and the incidence ranges from one in 20 to one in 100,000 recipients. The onset of diarrhea may occur up to two weeks after the drug is discontinued. The diagnosis is confirmed by the finding of pseudomembranes composed of mucin, fibrin, white blood cells, and discarded epithelial cells. They are attached to a necrotic mucosal surface of the colon and are seen as exudative white plaques during proctosigmoidoscopy.

As with other forms of acute diarrhea, fluid and electrolyte replacement is essential. The antibiotic that caused the diarrhea should be discontinued. Recent evidence suggests that the causative organism is *Clostridium difficile*, which produces a toxin. The definitive diagnosis is made when the toxin is found in the stool. Stool precautions should be followed meticulously, since this organism can be spread to other patients and attending personnel with resultant production of diarrheal episodes.

Vancomycin in an oral dosage of 250 to 500 mg. four times a day, or cholestyramine resin in a dosage of 4 grams orally four times a day, is considered the pharmacologic treatment of choice. Diphenoxylate and other opiate derivatives have been used without much success and in fact are contraindicated since they may prolong and increase the severity of this form of diarrhea.

Chronic Diarrhea

In all forms of chronic diarrhea it is most important to determine the specific causes of the problem so that definitive therapy can be employed. In addition to increasing the amount of dietary fiber for the management of the irritable bowel syndrome, antidepressants or anticholinergics may also be effective. The administration of cholestyramine resin should be considered in patients with less than 100 cm. of distal ileum in order to bind with unabsorbed bile acids. In elderly patients with ileostomies, the opiates and bismuth compounds can reduce the normal amount of daily ileal excreta.

Treatment

Medical intervention for diarrhea can be divided into three main categories, which include supportive, symptomatic, and specific therapy.

Supportive Therapy

Supportive therapy consists of replacing fluid and electrolyte losses. When intravenous therapy is employed, the solution should be tailored to the specific needs of the patient based on clinical evaluation of the patient and the serum electrolyte levels obtained. Oral replacement therapy can be utilized when the diarrhea is less severe and dehydration is only mild or moderate. If an orally administered solution is utilized, it must contain a carbohydrate to facilitate the absorption of sodium, potassium, and bicarbonate. It is important to recognize the electrolyte content of the various products that are employed today for fluid and electrolyte replacement.

Symptomatic Therapy

Symptomatic therapy involves the use of medications that do not alter the underlying pathophysiology or correct fluid and electrolyte imbalance. These drugs reduce the number of bowel movements or improve the consistency of the stool. Table 6–10 presents the more effective drugs and recommended doses.

Opium Alkaloids. The principal opium alkaloids that affect gastrointestinal smooth muscle function are morphine and codeine. These drugs increase circular smooth muscle tone, which leads to nonpropulsive rhythmic contractions. Also included in this group are tincture of opium and paregoric (camphorated opium tincture). Synthetic antidiarrheal drugs include diphenoxylate and loperamide. To minimize the abuse potential of diphenoxylate, a subtherapeutic dose of 0.025 mg. atropine has been added to Lomotil, the commercial preparation. Loperamide hydrochloride (Imodium) is a synthetic antidiarrheal compound, which is similar in structure to haloperidol, a major tranquilizer. Although loperamide is more costly than generic diphenoxylate, it produces less central nervous system depression, has a more rapid and longer lasting effect, and is probably more effective than diphenoxylate when utilized for chronic diarrhea. The use of opium compounds and synthetic opiates can reduce the inconvenience and discomfort of multiple bowel movements, but their use is associated with the risk of increasing toxicity if a bacterial form of diarrhea is present. These drugs should be avoided in elderly patients with partial bowel obstruction.

Anticholinergic Compounds. Anticholinergic compounds have been frequently employed in antidiarrheal products, but no controlled studies have been documented concerning their effectiveness for this condition. Their only possible benefit is in decreasing intestinal spasm and pain; side effects are a strong deterrent to their use in the elderly.

Adsorbents. Adsorbents such as kaolin, a natural hydrated aluminum silicate clay, and pectin, a polyuronic polymer consisting of purified carbohydrate extracted from citrus fruit or apple pumice, have been used for many years in the management of diarrhea. Kaopectate is a popular proprietary product, which contains 25 per cent kaolin and 1 per cent pectin. The effectiveness of this product is questionable; it may impair the absorption of digoxin.

Anion Exchange Resins. Cholestyramine and colestipol are anion exchange resins, which possess a strong affinity for acidic materials, including bile acids. These drugs have been used in the treatment of antibiotic induced

TABLE 6–10. Antidiarrheal Medications

Category	Product	Average Adult Dosage
Opiates	Tincture of opium (1% morphine)	1.6 to 1.5 ml., p.r.n.
	Paregoric (camphorated opium tincture)	5 ml., p.r.n.
	Codeine	15 mg., q.i.d.
Synthetic opiate derivatives	Diphenoxylate (Lomotil)	5 mg., q.i.d.
	Loperamide (Imodium)	4 mg., initially, followed by 2 mg. p.r.n. up to 16 mg./day
Anticholinergics	Atropine sulfate	0.6 to 1.0 mg. q.i.d.
	Propantheline (Probanthine)	15 mg., q.i.d.
	Tincture of belladonna	0.6 ml., q.i.d.
Absorbents	Kaolin-pectin (Kaopectate)	60 to 120 ml., p.r.n.
Anion exchange resins	Cholestyramine (Questran, Quemid)	4 gm., b.i.d. to q.i.d.
	Colestipol (Colestid)	5 gm., t.i.d.
Lactobacillus	Bacid, Lactinex	4 to 8 capsules/day 1 gram, q.i.d.
Prostaglandin antagonists	Bismuth subsalicylate (Pepto Bismol)	30 ml., q ½ hr. × 8 doses
	Indomethacin (Indocin)	25 mg., q.i.d.

colitis and chronic diarrhea associated with diabetes mellitus, abdominal irradiation, vagotomy, and ileal resection. These drug products must be diluted with a liquid such as fruit juice or added to applesauce and administered at least two hours before meals or other medications, since they complex with fat soluble vitamins and many other medications.

Lactobacillus Acidophilus. Use of *Lactobacillus acidophilus* containing products such as Bacid, Lactinex, and natural yogurt for the treatment of diarrhea has yet to be documented as being effective.

Specific Therapy

Specific therapy is aimed at treating the underlying condition or blocking the cellular mechanism of fluid and electrolyte loss. Examples of this type of therapy include surgery, the discontinuation of diarrhea causing drugs, and the use of an antibiotic such as vancomycin to treat the underlying cause of bacterial diarrhea.

Prostaglandin antagonists such as aspirin and the nonsteroidal anti-inflammatory drugs, including indomethacin and other compounds, such as propranolol, have been shown to be effective in certain types of diarrhea by preventing the activation of adenyl cyclase. Corticosteroids may be effective in diarrhea by increasing sodium-potassium-ATPase activity and thereby initiating an independent absorption process. Bismuth subsalicylate is found in the proprietary product called Pepto-Bismol. Its effectiveness may be primarily due to the salicylate portion of the chemical moiety. Ingestion of 60 ml. of bismuth subsalicylate mixture results in peak plasma salicylate levels of 4 mg. per dl. This level is comparable to that achieved with usual analgesic doses of aspirin. Although the extent of bismuth absorption from the product has not been extensively studied, there is cause for some concern since encephalopathy has been reported with other bismuth compounds in Australia and France. Since the product label does not mention that bismuth subsalicylate contains an aspirin derivative, this product should be avoided in patients taking large daily dosages of salicylates for arthritis, orally administered anticoagulants, uricosurics, or methotrexate. Patients with true aspirin allergy or bleeding disorders should also avoid taking this product.

NAUSEA AND VOMITING

Vomiting is possibly one of the least pleasant experiences of life and can be defined as the forceful expulsion of the gastrointestinal contents through the mouth. Nausea, retching, and vomiting, the three stages of the vomiting act, are not primary pathologic processes but rather are ubiquitous symptoms associated with a wide range of anatomic or pathophysiologic changes. Indeed there exist few areas of medicine in which these manifestations are not seen regularly. Although it unquestionably has protective value, its major medical importance is derived from the number of conditions that may cause or be associated with vomiting.

The etiologic factors associated with nausea and vomiting have been classified into distinct categories and include primary central nervous system disease, metabolic and endocrine disease, chemical and drug induced toxicity, gastrointestinal disease, genitourinary disease, and labyrinthine disease. A more specific listing appears in Table 6–11.[77]

In most instances nausea and vomiting respond to treatment of the underlying disorder, and symptoms usually subside and disappear. However, in certain individuals, most notably the elderly and debilitated, regardless of the etiology, protracted vomiting can lead to life threatening fluid and electrolyte disturbances. The metabolic consequences of vomiting are summarized in Figure 6–3.

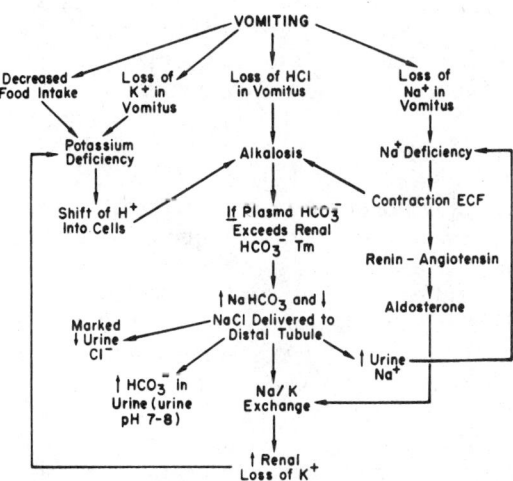

Figure 6–3. Metabolic consequences of vomiting. (From Feldman, M., and Fordtran, J.S. *In* Sleisenger, M.H., and Fordtran, J.S. [Editors]: Gastrointestinal Disease. .Ed. 2. Philadelphia, W.B. Saunders Company, 1978.)

TABLE 6–11. Primary Causes of Nausea and Vomiting*

System or Category	Pathophysiology

Primary central nervous system disease	Elevated intracranial pressure
	Neoplasm
	Infection
	Epilepsy
	Vascular diseases
	  Arteriosclerosis
	  Embolism
	  Vasculitis
	  Migraine
	Psychologic suggestion

Metabolic and endocrine disease	Diabetic ketoacidosis Lactic acidosis Starvation ketosis Hypothyroidism Uremia Adrenal insufficiency

Chemical and drug induced toxicity	Direct effect on chemoreceptor trigger zone
	  Opiates
	  Digitalis glycosides
	  Cancer chemotherapy
	  Radiation sickness
	  Food poisoning
	  Other drug toxicity or withdrawal
	Direct effect on stomach
	  Drug induced gastritis
	  Irradiation enteritis
	  Ethanol toxicity or withdrawal

Gastrointestinal disease	Peptic ulcer
	Reflex esophagitis
	Biliary tract disease
	Hepatic disease
	Gastroenteritis
	Pancreatitis
	Functional disorders
	  Aerophagia
	  Pyloroduodenal spasm
	Mechanical or paralytic obstruction

Genitourinary disease	Endometritis Parametritis Salpingitis Obstructive uropathy Pyelonephritis Renal calculi and stones
Labyrinthine disease	Infection Vascular disturbance Meniere's disease Motion sickness

*Adapted from Mellencamp, E., and Wang, R.I.H.: The patient with nausea. I. Causes. Drug Ther. (Hosp.), 2:62–69, 1977.

Potassium depletion results from a decreased intake of exogenous potassium primarily from food, from loss of potassium ion in the vomitus, and in some individuals from renal potassium wasting. The clinical features of potassium deficiency are muscle weakness, constipation, polydipsia, nocturia, and impaired urinary concentration.

Sodium depletion develops because of loss of sodium in the vomitus and in some instances because of loss of sodium via the kidneys in association with the excretion of bicarbonate. The clinical features of sodium deficiency are hypotension, decreased blood volume, and an increased hematocrit level. Plasma renin and aldosterone levels are elevated, and the creatinine clearance value is reduced.

Alkalosis develops primarily because of the loss of hydrogen ions in the vomitus, but also because of contraction of the extracellular fluid (owing to sodium and chloride depletion) without a concomitant loss of bicarbonate and because of an influx of hydrogen ions into cells caused by potassium depletion. Even though the cause of these fluid and electrolyte disturbances will be obvious if there is a history of vomiting, in many instances in the elderly vigorous replacement therapy has to be undertaken to restore normal acid-base balance.

Vomiting is a complex reflex that is mediated by a "vomiting center" located in the medulla. First described 30 years ago, this center by itself does not carry out the function of vomiting but rather coordinates the activities of other neural structures in its immediate vicinity to produce a complicated patterned response. The vomiting center, as noted in Figure 6–4, receives stimuli from peripheral areas such as the gastric mucosa as well as from areas within the central nervous system itself, in part through the coordination of the chemoreceptor trigger zone also located in the medulla. Stimulation of the chemoreceptor trigger zone, which is the afferent pathway to the vomiting center, is responsible for its activation and may be involved in eliciting nausea and vomiting from a variety of causes. Cardiac glycosides act primarily at this site; the chemoreceptor trigger zone is also important in mediating motion sickness as well as the nausea and vomiting associated with uremia and probably that due to other metabolic disturbances. The efferent pathway is completed by impulses transmitted to the salivary glands and the muscles of the diaphragm, anterior abdominal wall, and upper gastrointestinal tract. The vomiting act itself involves contraction of the diaphragm and abdominal and intercostal muscles with closure of the glottis and elevation of the palate. Efferent nerves to the gastrointestinal tract are of little importance in this coordinated response.

Treatment

Prior to the decision to treat nausea and vomiting, the search for an underlying cause should be undertaken. The use of antiemetics is justified only when vomiting is severe enough to produce significant loss of fluids and electrolytes; when nutritional intake is depressed, especially in cancer patients; when esophageal damage may result from violent retching; or when disruption of surgical suture lines may occur. Therapeutic intervention with antiemetic drugs is acceptable under these circumstances when no alternative therapy exists and the benefits outweigh the risks of adverse reactions or of masking more serious underlying conditions.

Antiemetic drugs may prevent or relieve nausea and vomiting by acting upon the chemoreceptor trigger zone, the cerebral cortex, the vestibular apparatus of the ear, or the vomiting center itself. Ideally the antiemetic chosen should exert its activity at that portion of the reflex arc stimulated by the cause of the vomiting. For example, some drugs are effective in preventing or treating vomiting caused by reflex stimulation of the chemoreceptor trigger zone but are ineffective when the vestibular apparatus is affected directly.

In general, the use of antiemetic drugs for the prevention of nausea and vomiting is more successful than for treatment, especially that caused by motion sickness, radiation, or chemotherapy. Oral dosage forms are most helpful in prevention, and parenteral and suppository forms are most frequently utilized in treatment.

Antiemetic drugs suitable for clinical use fall into four major categories and include anticholinergic drugs, antihistaminic drugs, antidopaminergic drugs, and miscellaneous drugs. This classification is of use primarily as an indicator of expected side effects or adverse reactions rather than therapeutic usefulness, because many drugs that fall into one of these specific categories have little or no efficacy in treating nausea and vomiting. Table 6–12 indicates those drugs that are available, their

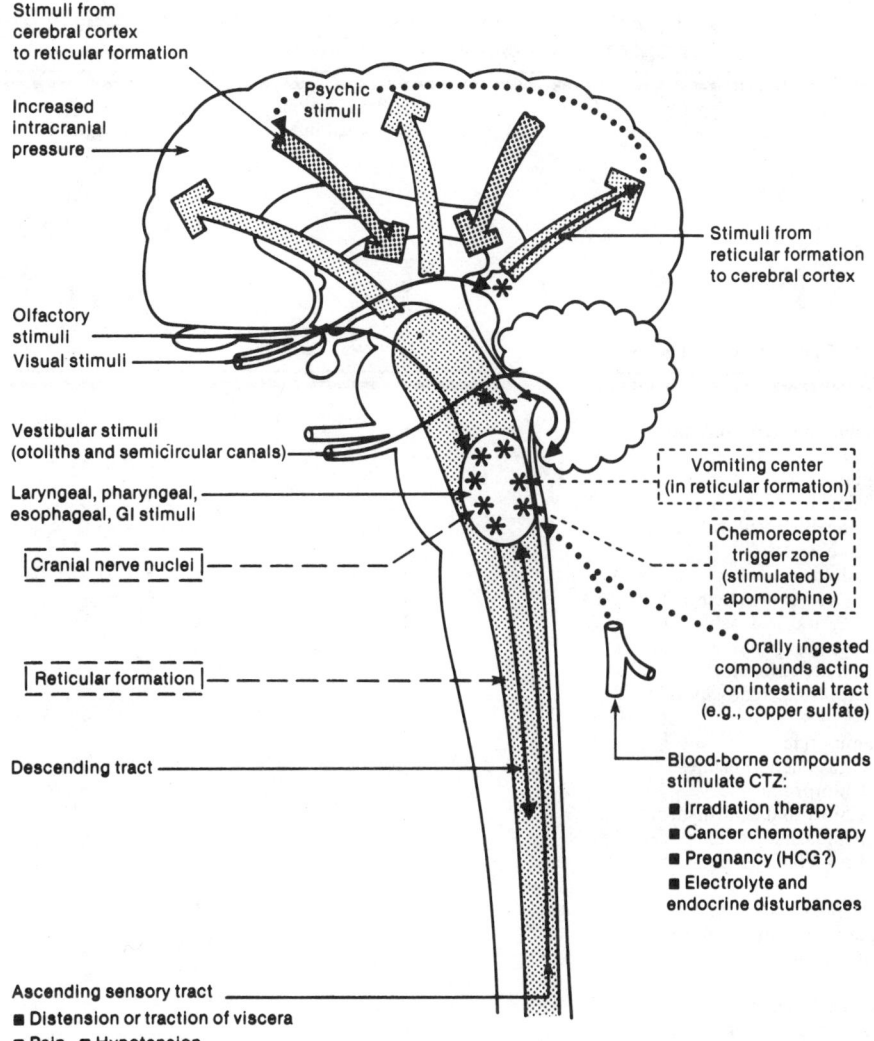

Figure 6-4. The vomiting center responsible for the multifaceted neurologic responses involved in emesis. The center is located in the dorsolateral border of the lateral reticular formation, ventral to the nucleus and tractus solitarius. It receives input from the chemoreceptor trigger zone (CTZ) in the ventral surface of the fourth ventricle, from the cranial nerves, and from the ascending and descending tracts.

dosage forms, and their principal uses in the prevention and treatment of nausea and vomiting of various causes. It should be remembered that treatment should be individualized according to the known effects of the drug and the needs of the patient.

Anticholinergic Drugs

Scopolamine, an anticholinergic drug that appears to act by reducing the excitability of labyrinth receptors and depressing conduction in the vestibular cerebellar pathways, is one of the most effective drugs for the prevention of nausea and vomiting due to motion sickness. However, its use has been limited because of unacceptable side effects, and many clinicians now recommend the use of antihistaminic antiemetics for motion sickness. To minimize the problems of anticholinergic side effects, a skin patch method has been developed for delivering a transdermal dose of scopolamine. When a 2.5 sq. cm. adhesive patch is placed in contact with the skin behind the ear, the drug is released and maintains a level of scopolamine equivalent to an oral dose of 0.2 mg. for 60 to 72 hours. With the exception of the frequent occurrence of dry mouth, no disturbing side

TABLE 6–12. Available Preparations and Principal Uses of Drugs Indicated in Treating Nausea and Vomiting of Various Causes

Drug Classification	Preparations Available				Principal Uses			
	Parenteral	Suppository	Oral	Transdermal*	Vertigo	Motion Sickness	Postoperative Vomiting	Metabolic and Exogenous Toxins, Radiation Sickness, Cytotoxic Drugs
Anticholinergic								
Scopolamine hydrobromide	+		+	+	+	+		
Antihistaminic								
Buclizine hydrochloride			+		±	+		
Cyclizine hydrochloride		+			+	+		
Cyclizine lactate	+				+	+		
Dimenhydrinate	+	+	+		+	+		
Diphenhydramine hydrochloride	+		+		+	+		
Hydroxyzine hydrochloride	+				±	+		
Hydroxyzine pamoate			+		±	+		
Meclizine hydrochloride			+		+	+		
Promethazine hydrochloride	+	+	+		+	+		
Antidopaminergic								
Aliphatic phenothiazines								
Chlorpromazine		+					+	+
Chlorpromazine hydrochloride	+		+				+	+
Promazine hydrochloride	+		+				+	+
Promethazine hydrochloride	+		+				+	+
Piperazine phenothiazines								
Fluphenazine hydrochloride	+		+				+	+
Perphenazine	+		+				+	+
Prochlorperazine		+					+	+
Prochlorperazine edisylate	+		+				+	+
Prochlorperazine maleate			+					
Thiethylperazine maleate	+	+	+				+	+
Butyrophenone								
Haloperidol	+		+				+	+
Metoclopramide	+		+				+	+
Domperidone (investigational)								+
Miscellaneous								
Benzquinamide hydrochloride	+						+	
Diphenidol hydrochloride	+		+		+		+	+
Trimethobenzamide hydrochloride	+	+	+				+	+
Nabilone (investigational)								+
Tetrahydrocannabinol (investigational)								+

*Transdermal application of scopolamine is approved only for the treatment of nausea and vomiting associated with motion sickness in adults.

effects have been reported to result from this low dose. Scopolamine, in conventional dosage forms, has a rapid onset and a short duration of action. Because of this and since repeated doses may have a cumulative effect, scopolamine may be especially useful to prevent nausea and vomiting due to motion sickness of brief duration when only a single small dose is required. Administration of scopolamine in high doses for more than 12 hours is not recommended because of the potential for serious side effects. It is of interest that the antiemetic effect of scopolamine increases only slightly with increased dosage, but side effects increase considerably.

Although combinations of drugs should be used with caution in the elderly, results of controlled studies in volunteers subjected to severe motion indicate that the combination of 0.6 mg. of scopolamine and 25 mg. of promethazine or ephedrine is more effective in preventing nausea and vomiting of vestibular origin than scopolamine alone. This combination is useful primarily for severe motion disturbances or in preventing nausea and vomiting in individuals who are highly susceptible to moderately severe conditions of motion.

Antihistaminic Drugs

Antihistamines, which are thought to affect neural pathways originating in the labyrinth, are effective in preventing nausea and vomiting during episodes of motion sickness. Although promethazine and hydroxyzine are effective in mild to moderate postoperative vomiting, they are less effective than the antidopaminergic drugs and probably should not be used routinely for the treatment of postsurgical nausea and vomiting. Because of their relative safety, they are particularly useful for patients requiring long term therapy and indeed are considered the drugs of choice in preventing and treating vestibular induced vomiting of long duration.

Buclizine, cyclizine, dimenhydrinate, diphenhydramine, hydroxyzine, and promethazine are useful in treating mild to moderate motion sickness; their onset of action is rapid, and their duration of action ranges from four to six hours. Meclizine has a slower onset and a longer duration of action (24 hours) than other antiemetic antihistamines.

Drowsiness is the most common unwanted effect of these drugs, although individual susceptibility to this reaction varies markedly. Anticholinergic side effects can also occur. It is apparent, however, that anticholinergic activity does not correlate with the efficacy of the antihistamines. For example, cyclizine has weak anticholinergic properties but is a useful antiemetic in motion sickness patients.

Although a phenothiazine structurally, promethazine exhibits pronounced antihistaminic activity; it is therefore effective in the prevention and treatment of nausea and vomiting of vestibular origin but has little effect upon vomiting caused by stimulation of the chemoreceptor trigger zone.

The most frequently encountered untoward effect after promethazine administration is sedation. In the usual antiemetic dose promethazine administration rarely results in acute extrapyramidal reactions. However, anticholinergic and antiadrenergic side effects do occur infrequently following oral administration.

Antidopaminergic Drugs

Antidopaminergic drugs, which include many of the phenothiazines and the similarly acting butyrophenone haloperidol, act primarily upon the chemoreceptor trigger zone to combat moderate to severe postoperative vomiting and nausea and vomiting due to radiation therapy or cytotoxic drugs. With the exception of promethazine, these drugs are not useful in preventing nausea and vomiting due to motion sickness.

Phenothiazines. Many of the phenothiazines are available as injectables, as either a tablet or a sustained release capsule, or as a suppository. Although there have not been any controlled comparative studies to determine the most beneficial route of administration, some generalizations can be made. The oral route is the easiest, least expensive, and most practical for long term therapy. However, there have not been any reports indicating an advantage for sustained release capsules when compared to tablets. Therefore, because the former are significantly more expensive, their use cannot be routinely recommended. The parenteral route should be used in emergencies only in patients under direct medical supervision who have nausea, vomiting, or other problems that exclude oral administration.

With regard to the usefulness of rectal preparations of antiemetics, the literature contains few references. The rectum is devoid of villi and therefore has a relatively small surface area for absorption. In addition, a major rate limiting step in the rectal absorptive process is the release of the active constituent from the inert suppository base. The absorption of drugs via the oral route is far superior, and the rectal route of antiemetic administration should be limited to ambulatory patients in whom parenteral administration is not practical and in whom vomiting might interfere with the absorption of the antiemetic given orally.

The phenothiazines that possess antiemetic activity can be classified as either aliphatic or piperazine derivatives. Examples of each of these groups can be found in Table 6-12. Both these groups are approximately equal in antiemetic effect, but they differ substantially in the frequency and severity of the side effects that may occur. Phenothiazines in the piperazine group are less likely to produce autonomic side effects, including postural hypotension, dryness of the mouth, and nasal congestion, than members of the aliphatic group. On the other hand, although extrapyramidal reactions have been reported with the use of all antidopaminergic drugs, presumably in impairing dopaminergic transmission, the incidence of these reactions is greater with phenothiazines of the piperazine group. With long term use of these drugs, extrapyramidal reactions may occur, which include akathisia, dysarthria, dystonia, and parkinson-like symptoms, which are five times more frequent in an aged than in a young population. Tardive dyskinesia, a rare complication of antidopaminergic therapy that appears after prolonged use, is seldom a problem when these drugs are used in treating nausea and vomiting.

Although chlorpromazine is the prototype of the aliphatic phenothiazine compounds, it is regarded as less desirable than some newer compounds because of the greater risk of cholestatic jaundice and leucopenia. Because of the severity of these adverse reactions, especially in the elderly, chlorpromazine should be considered only when vomiting is intractable and cannot be alleviated by other less toxic antiemetics.

Many clinicians regard prochlorperazine, the representative piperazine phenothiazine, to be the antidopaminergic drug of choice for the treatment of nausea and vomiting because of its efficacy and low incidence of side effects. However, the extrapyramidal side effects may render this drug unsuitable for repeated administration, especially in elderly patients. It should be remembered that although these effects are most likely to occur with large doses, signs may appear abruptly in elderly patients taking only moderate doses. The third class of phenothiazines, the piperidine derivatives, is associated with a reduced frequency of extrapyramidal side effects. Unfortunately the occurrence of these side effects has not been separable from antiemetic activity so that representatives of the piperidine class, such as thioridazine, appear to be less effective antiemetics.

Butyrophenones. Although not approved for the treatment of nausea and vomiting, the butyrophenone tranquilizer haloperidol is comparable in efficacy to the piperazine phenothiazines, acting in a similar manner to inhibit impulses at the chemoreceptor trigger zone. It has been administered to alleviate nausea and vomiting following surgery, after radiation therapy, prior to the administration of cytotoxic drugs, and in gastrointestinal disorders. In a recent study haloperidol was shown to be superior to benzquinamide for the control of cis-platin and nitrogen mustard induced emesis, but not for doxorubicin treated patients.[174] Haloperidol, like the phenothiazines, is not effective in the prevention of nausea and vomiting due to motion sickness.

Extrapyramidal reactions associated with haloperidol are similar to those observed following the administration of piperazine phenothiazines but are infrequent or mild at low doses. Because the duration of action of haloperidol may be as long as 24 hours, administration of the drug once or twice daily can alleviate nausea and vomiting without increasing the risk of extrapyramidal reactions in the elderly. Because many elderly patients are uniquely sensitive to the antidopaminergic side effects of haloperidol, a reduced dose of 0.5 to 1.0 mg. is usually advocated. The anticholinergic side effects of haloperidol include blurred or double vision, dryness of the mouth, and nasal congestion and do not occur less frequently than with phenothiazines. However, postural hypotension, which is a common complaint in elderly patients receiving a phenothiazine, appears to occur only rarely with the use of haloperidol. Indeed haloperidol can be used in an extended care facility as an effective antiemetic with minimal side effects.[79]

It should be remembered that the extrapyramidal signs and symptoms that can occur during therapy with all the antiemetic antidopaminergic drugs can be mistaken for central nervous system toxicity due to an unidentified disease responsible for the nausea and vomiting. Therefore, a prompt diagnostic evaluation is of paramount importance. In addition, the sedative effect of these drugs may be potentiated if other central nervous system depressants are administered at the same time. Sedation may be beneficial in some patients (e.g., those with neoplastic disease) but undesirable in others (e.g., those receiving strong analgesics).

Metoclopramide. Two antiemetic drugs, metoclopramide and domperidone, act similarly to the antidopaminergic drugs previously discussed. Both compounds appear to facilitate gastrointestinal motility (but not secretion), which enhances gastric emptying.

Metoclopramide (Reglan) is a chloromethoxy derivative of procainamide having no cardiac, antiarrhythmic, or hemodynamic effects in humans. Pharmacologically it is an antagonist of dopamine, resulting in an excess of cholinergic activity involving gastrointestinal smooth muscle. Metoclopramide causes an increase in lower esophageal contractions, accelerates gastric emptying by increasing both the frequency and amplitude of gastric contractions, and increases smooth muscle contraction and peristalsis in the small intestine. It has little effect on colonic motility and lacks an effect on fluid and electrolyte secretion or absorption in the large intestine.

Metoclopramide is used in single intravenous doses to facilitate radiographic and intubation procedures, including biopsy and endoscopy, by stimulating gastric emptying and small intestinal transit. Metoclopramide's antiemetic effect is believed to be partially mediated by its central antidopaminergic effect. In regard to the small quantity of an administered dose found in the central nervous system, metoclopramide was localized in the area containing the chemoreceptor trigger zone. Its limited central activity is illustrated by its lack of effect in preventing nausea and vomiting due to motion sickness. It has been suggested that the clinically significant antiemetic effect of metoclopramide is due to its increase of gastric motor activity, thereby preventing gastric immobility that precedes vomiting.

Metoclopramide is used in the treatment of nausea and vomiting that occurs with delayed gastric emptying, including dyspepsia, gastroesophageal reflux, gastric and duodenal ulcers, and hiccups.[80] Indeed this drug may be the only antiemetic that modifies the type of visceral stimulation of the vomiting center that can occur in gastrointestinal disorders. It is available as 10 mg. tablets and injection (10 mg. per 2 ml. and 50 mg. per 10 ml).

Although studies have revealed metoclopramide to be approximately equivalent in efficacy to phenothiazine therapy in postoperative vomiting and nausea and vomiting due to radiation therapy, when it has been utilized in chemotherapy induced emesis, conflicting results have been obtained.[81, 82] When metoclopramide was administered to patients receiving regimens containing fluorouracil, no antiemetic effect could be demonstrated.[81] However, in an uncontrolled study of patients receiving cis-platinum therapy, an antiemetic effect was claimed with low dose metoclopramide given orally.[82] Recent clinical trials have established high dose metoclopramide as the preferred treatment in controlling the nausea and vomiting associated with cis-platinum.[175, 176] In these studies the following parameters were critical for maximum efficacy—appropriate dose (2 mg. per kg.), route (intravenous), and schedule (30 minutes before chemotherapy and 1.5, 3.5, 5.5 and 8.5 hours after beginning chemotherapy). With high dose cis-platinum (120 mg. per sq. m.) now being employed, these elements are critical against emesis. Metoclopramide is more likely to benefit patients without previous exposure to chemotherapy than those refractory to standard antiemetics.

At the usual therapeutic dose of 10 mg., adverse reactions to metoclopramide therapy are uncommon. One source noted that, in the elderly, confusion is common with larger doses and recommended 5 mg. for geriatric and debilitated patients.[83] The most common side effects occurring in up to 10 per cent of the patients are drowsiness and lassitude. Extrapyramidal reactions with metoclopramide are much less common than with phenothiazines or haloperidol, but the signs and symptoms produced are the same. The extrapyramidal effects are generally of the dystonic type and usually begin acutely within 36 hours after commencing metoclopramide therapy. The dyskinesias include trismus, torticollis, facial spasms, opisthotonus, and oculogyric crisis. The reactions respond to antiparkinsonian therapy and usually disappear within 24 to 48 hours after stopping metoclopramide therapy. Because metoclopramide can stimulate prolactin release, which in turn may promote growth of breast tissue, it should not be used in patients with breast cancer to suppress nausea and vomiting associated with cytotoxic drug therapy.

A potentially important interaction involves a reduction in the bioavailability of a single cimetidine dose by about 25 per cent following metoclopramide therapy. Additional long term dose studies are needed to determine the clinical impact, if any, of this so-far-unsubstantiated interaction.[177, 178]

Because of its capacity to increase gastric emptying and speed the rate of transit through the small intestine, metoclopramide alters the absorption characteristics of other drugs. Of significance in geriatric patients is the faster absorption of both aspirin and acetaminophen as well as the higher peak blood levels of levodopa when metoclopramide is coadministered. In addition, lower steady state levels of digoxin were found in female patients who also received metoclopramide.

Metoclopramide overdose has resulted in somnolence, disorientation, irritability, agitation, and convulsions. The lowest possible dose should be employed for the control of nausea and vomiting in geriatric and debilitated patients.

Domperidone. Domperidone (motilium), a benzimidazole dopamine antagonist not available commercially in the United States, is being studied for its antiemetic effect. As with metoclopramide, the gastric emptying rate (but not gastric secretion) is significantly enhanced following administration of domperidone.[84] Although it is at an early stage of clinical investigation, the drug has been evaluated in a number of short studies in the treatment of nausea and vomiting of various causes.[85] Of particular importance was the finding that domperidone, when administered rectally for as long as 12 weeks to geriatric patients, was found to be a highly acceptable and effective antiemetic drug. Of great significance was the lack of serious adverse reactions following its use. One case of sudden death has been reported in a patient who received 10 times the manufacturer's recommended dosage, however.[179] The lack of extrapyramidal side effects is the result of the inability of domperidone to cross the blood-brain barrier, even at high doses for prolonged periods of time. In addition, since it does not block dopamine receptors in the basal ganglia and thus cannot interfere with the central action of L-dopa, domperidone could well become the drug of choice in preventing and treating nausea and vomiting caused by this drug.

From the results of these early studies, it is apparent that domperidone is an effective drug in the prophylaxis and therapy of nausea and vomiting of diverse origins. However, more clinical experience is necessary before its claim as an "ideal" antiemetic without extrapyramidal side effects or sedative properties can be validated.

Miscellaneous Antiemetic Drugs

Benzquinamide. Of the miscellaneous antiemetics, benzquinamide appears to be as effective as the dopamine antagonists in the prevention and treatment of postoperative nausea and vomiting, and in fact at the current time this is its only approved indication. Like the phenothiazines, it presumably acts to inhibit stimuli at the chemoreceptor trigger zone. However, unlike the phenothiazines, which tend to lower the blood pressure, benzquinamide has been shown to have a peripheral vascular stimulatory effect, raising both peripheral vascular resistance and intra-arterial pressure without affecting cardiac output, stroke volume, or heart rate.[86] Although no change in arterial blood gas values was recorded in one study of normal volunteers, indicating maintenance of respiratory homeostasis, a study of ventilatory effects in patients who had received benzquinamide after surgery showed an increased respiratory rate in these individuals.[87] These effects, increases in the blood pressure and respiratory rate, are unique among the commercially available antiemetics; thus benzquinamide may be of benefit in patients with central nervous system depression, such as patients who have experienced postoperative hypotension after the anesthetic, those with uremia or ketoacidosis who are likely to experience nausea and vomiting, and those who have received sedative or analgesic drugs. However, the use of this drug in elderly patients with significant hypertension or severe cardiovascular disease should be avoided.

Benzquinamide appears to produce fewer serious adverse effects than the phenothiazines. Drowsiness is noted most frequently; shivering and chills as well as the previously mentioned effects on the cardiovascular system, including a sudden rise in blood pressure and transient cardiac arrhythmias, have also been reported.

Benzquinamide is available only for parenteral use. Since the half-life of benzquinamide in patients with normal liver function is about 40 minutes, the first dose may be repeated in one hour, with subsequent doses administered every three to four hours thereafter for symptomatic treatment.

Although the intramuscular route of administration is considered preferable, benzquinamide can be given intravenously. However, it should be used cautiously, if at all, in elderly patients who are at risk of developing cardiovascular side effects when the drug is given via this route.

Diphenidol. Diphenidol, indicated in the prevention of nausea and vomiting due to motion sickness and other middle and inner ear disorders as well as in the treatment of nausea and vomiting from other causes, appears to have a dual mechanism of action. It acts upon the vestibular apparatus to control vertigo and inhibits the chemoreceptor trigger zone to control nausea and vomiting. Unlike other antiemetics, diphenidol can cause auditory and visual hallucinations and disorientation and confusion at therapeutic doses. These adverse reactions occur in less than 0.5 per cent of the patients, usually within three days after the initiation of therapy, and subside spontaneously within three days after discontinuation of the drug. Diphenidol should not be routinely administered, and its use should be limited to patients who are hospitalized or under close medical supervision. With regard to elderly patients with renal impairment, since approximately 90 per cent of the drug is excreted in the urine, renal dysfunction could cause systemic accumulation with resultant central nervous system toxicity.

Trimethobenzamide. Trimethobenzamide, an antiemetic that has been available commercially for 20 years, is structurally related to the antihistaminic antiemetics but is of little value in the prevention or treatment of nausea and vomiting due to motion sickness. It acts at the chemoreceptor trigger zone to inhibit emetic stimuli and consequently has been promoted for use in alleviating nausea and vomiting due to a wide variety of causes. However, it has been shown to have weak activity, and in a postanesthetic study it appeared to be less efficacious than placebo over a 24 hour postoperative period.[88] In a double blind study of chemotherapy induced nausea and vomiting, the reduction in these symptoms was not considered significant when trimethobenzamide was administered orally at a dose of 200 mg. three times daily.[89] Of note is the lack of side effects attributable to trimethobenzamide administration; at usual doses the incidence of side effects is low. However, with larger doses drowsiness, vertigo, diarrhea, and cutaneous hypersensitivity reactions have been reported. Extrapyramidal reactions or convulsions can also occur, and it appears that elderly or debilitated patients are at greater risk of developing this complication.

Because of its weak antiemetic activity and lack of toxicity at recommended doses, trimethobenzamide may be of use primarily in an ambulatory setting in which the degree of nausea and vomiting is usually less than that encountered in hospitalized patients.

In adults, the usual oral dosage is 250 mg. three or four times daily, but the FDA has recommended that the dose be increased to 400 mg. per capsule in order to achieve the same peak blood levels seen after intramuscular injection of 200 mg. of the drug.[90] It should be remembered that the injectable form of trimethobenzamide is intended for intramuscular administration only. Pain, stinging, burning, redness, and swelling can occur at the injection site. Such effects can be minimized by deep injection into the upper outer quadrant of the gluteal region and by avoiding the loss of solution along the route. The FDA has also proposed that the 200 mg. rectal suppository be removed from the market because of inadequate release of the drug from the suppository base and a consequent lack of therapeutic blood levels.[91] In addition, since the suppositories contain benzocaine in a concentration of 2 per cent, they should not be used in patients known to be sensitive to this or similar local anesthetics. Reformulations of the oral and suppository dosage forms are currently being undertaken by the manufacturer in response to FDA recommendations.

Marijuana and Its Analogues. From the point of view of the patient, nausea and vomiting are perhaps the most difficult symptoms to control in patients with cancer undergoing chemotherapy and often affect compliance, nutrition, and the patient's sense of well-being. The magnitude of this problem is such that for some patients vomiting or retching can occur every few minutes for 12 to 24 hours after chemotherapy has been completed.

The possible role of marijuana and its analogues as useful therapeutic drugs in the treatment of cytotoxic drug induced nausea and vomiting was first raised by anecdotal reports of young cancer patients who found their treatment more tolerable if they smoked marijuana shortly after undergoing chemotherapy. Investigators at the Sidney Farber Center Institute in Boston drew upon these experiences and developed a protocol to test the antiemetic effect of orally administered delta-9-tetrahydrocannabinol (THC), the principal active ingredient of marijuana and its primary mood altering component.[92] Of the 20 patients receiving THC at a dosage of 10 mg. per sq. m., 25 per cent experienced no vomiting, and 45 per cent experienced a substantial reduction in vomiting. In a control group that received a placebo, no reduction in nausea and vomiting was observed. Beneficial effects generally lasted two to three hours, but side effects were common. Although these reactions were largely tolerable, a few patients suffered paranoid ideation, feelings of terror, panic, and visual hallucinations. This study was limited in scope because it primarily involved young patients (median age, 29 years), several of whom were known marijuana users, and it did not involve a control group treated with a standard antiemetic of known therapeutic efficacy.

A more recent study by the same group of investigators compared THC to prochlorperazine in a randomized, double blind, crossover trial.[93] When THC was administered orally at a dosage of 10 mg. per sq. m. three times daily, a satisfactory response was observed in 36 of 79 THC treatment courses as compared to only 16 of 78 treatment courses employing prochlorperazine. All the patients, however, had been chosen after having previously failed to respond to phenothiazine therapy, and once again their average age (32.5 years) was significantly less than the usual age at which cancer occurs.

Another series of studies involving patients with cancer in a relatively young age group showed the oral administration of THC at a dosage of 10 mg. per sq. m. every three hours for a total of five doses to be superior to placebo in preventing nausea and vomiting resulting from high dose methotrexate therapy of osteogenic sarcoma, but not in preventing nausea and vomiting induced by the combination of cyclophosphamide and doxorubicin.[94, 95] The authors circumvented the problem of patients' vomiting their orally administered antiemetics by supplementing them with cigarettes containing THC or placebo. Interestingly, the actual smoking of THC caused nausea and vomiting in some of the patients. Other side effects were transient, sedation being the most common.

Of importance in designing antiemetic therapy for cytotoxic drug induced nausea and vomiting is recognition that different chemotherapeutic drugs can act upon different physiologic pathways to induce these symptoms. The finding that patients receiving cyclophosphamide and doxorubicin were refractory to the antiemetic effects of THC whereas those to whom methotrexate was administered derived a benefit may lend support to this theory. In addition, the factors of age and previous marijuana use are also of significance, not only because of differences in social acceptability and treatment expectations but also because of variability in the absorption, distribution, metabolism, and excretion of this compound. In addition, dysphoric reactions may be acceptable to a previous user, whereas the same reaction in a person who had not been previously exposed to marijuana could be devastating. Since cancer is a disease found with greater frequency in the aged, it is necessary that an antiemetic effect against chemotherapy induced nausea and vomiting be well tolerated in this age group.

With this in mind, investigators at the Mayo Clinic reported the results of a large randomized study comparing the oral administration of 15 mg. of THC, 10 mg. of prochlorperazine, and placebo to older patients (median age, 61 years) receiving methyl CCNU, 5-fluorouracil combination chemotherapy for gastrointestinal malignant disease.[96] These patients were not refractory to phenothiazine therapy, since this was their first course of chemotherapy and none had had previous experience with marijuana. On day 1 the initial dose of antiemetic was given two hours before the patient received chemotherapy. Subsequent doses were administered two hours and eight hours after the initiation of therapy. For the remainder of the study the antiemetic drugs were given three times daily, one-half hour before each meal.

Although both THC and prochlorperazine produced a significant antiemetic effect when compared to placebo, they were about equally effective when compared to each other. With regard to toxicity, however, THC produced significantly more central nervous system side effects than prochlorperazine, which frequently resulted in patients' refusing to continue therapy. From an overall standpoint it was believed that patients treated with THC had a more disagreeable therapeutic experience than those treated with prochlorperazine or even placebo. Similar results were obtained when THC was compared with thiethylperazine in patients with cancer having a mean age of 55 years.[97] Although THC had an antiemetic effect equal to that of thiethylperazine, more than 50 per cent of the THC treated patients had significant central nervous system side effects, including hallucinations and grand mal seizures.

This experience is comparable to a previous report evaluating analgesic effects of similar THC dosage in older adult cancer patients.[98] Single oral doses of 10 and 20 mg. of THC were evaluated for analgesic efficacy as well as toxicity. Significant central nervous system side effects were frequently noted in patients receiving the 20 mg. dose. In addition, 20 per cent of these patients experienced nausea and vomiting. The effects of a 10 mg. dose of THC were relatively mild and of shorter duration. The authors concluded that THC was highly sedating and produced many mental side effects, which in a single 20 mg. dose precluded its therapeutic use. Another disquieting report employing THC at a dosage of 10 mg. per sq. m. three times daily in patients receiving MOPP therapy for Hodgkin's disease indicated a 36 per cent incidence of hallucinations.[99] This increased occurrence of severe central nervous system toxicity may be due to a drug interaction with high doses of prednisone or procarbazine, both of which can cause central nervous system side effects.

A different approach to cannabinoid therapy is to combine phenothiazines with THC. Because phenothiazines antagonize some cannabinoid effects, the combination was proposed to permit administration of higher THC doses while keeping central nervous system toxicity at a tolerable level. A recent report combining THC (7.5 mg. per sq. m.) with prochlorperazine (7.5 mg. per sq. m.) did not achieve a suitable antiemetic effect, but the dose was not as high as originally proposed.[180, 181] More studies are needed to document the antiemetic response to this combination.

A discussion of marijuana and its analogues would not be complete without mention of the synthetic cannabinoids nabilone (Cesamet) and levonantradol. When nabilone was administered orally to patients experiencing severe nausea and vomiting due to cancer chemotherapy, 80 per cent of the patients obtained substantial relief with nabilone as compared to only 32 per cent receiving prochlorperazine.[100] When given a choice between these two drugs for subsequent use as an antiemetic, 75 per cent of the patients preferred nabilone despite the occurrence of annoying side effects, including somnolence, light-headedness, and dry mouth. Despite this fact, the drug was withdrawn for a period of time by the manufacturer because of the development of seizures and the occurrence of some fatalities in laboratory animals treated for prolonged periods with nabilone. Nabilone has been reintroduced for clinical investigation under a new protocol and has been recommended to be placed in Schedule III under the Controlled Substances Act by the FDA Drug Abuse Advisory Committee, even though it appears to have the same abuse potential as THC.

Levonantradol is a synthetic cannabinoid similar to THC in antiemetic activity and toxicity. In a preliminary study 0.1 to 1.5 mg. doses administered intramuscularly every four hours resulted in an overall antiemetic response approaching 90 per cent.[182] Age, size, and prior exposure to marijuana did not appear to influence the antiemetic response. Somnolence and dry mouth were the most commonly encountered side effects. Dysphoria was reported in 16 per cent of the patients.

At the present time the role of marijuana and its analogues in the prevention and treatment of nausea and vomiting due to cytotoxic drug therapy has not been clearly defined. It would appear that differences in patients' sensitivities as a function of age, environment, previous exposure to drugs of the marijuana type, pre-existing psychologic and social factors, and different doses, routes, and frequencies of administration must be resolved before these drugs can be used routinely as antiemetics. Furthermore, some studies indicate that the antiemetic effect varies with the chemotherapeutic drug that is responsible for the vomiting. Therefore, although tetrahydrocannabinol may be clinically useful in alleviating the nausea and vomiting experienced by young patients with cancer, especially those who have not responded to phenothiazine therapy, in the older age group the disadvantages of this therapeutic modality appear to still outweigh its usefulness.

That marijuana and its analogues have great potential as antiemetics in patients of all ages with cancer and that additional clinical research must be undertaken has been recognized by the FDA.[101] On June 26, 1980, the National Cancer Institute proposed to the FDA that marijuana and tetrahydrocannabinol be placed in a special category that would make it available for distribution through selected pharmacies and institutions for use by oncologists and other designated physicians. The proposal was accepted, and at the present time marijuana cigarettes and soft gelatin capsules containing THC are available for investigational use in cancer chemotherapy. Physicians who wish to utilize these drugs investigationally must first obtain a registration for Schedule I controlled substances from the Drug Enforcement Administration and must have an approved investigational new drug application from the Food and Drug Administration. Information regarding the necessary procedures may be obtained from the Research Technology Branch, Division of Research, National Institute of Drug Abuse, Room 9-42, 5600 Fishers Lane, Rockville, Maryland 20857.

Conclusion

Nausea and vomiting are disorders or symptoms of underlying disease with which physicians are frequently confronted. A wide array of drugs may be employed to offer symptomatic relief of these disorders. The etiology of nausea and vomiting and the frequency and severity of the potential side effects of drug therapy should be foremost in the physician's mind as drugs are chosen to manage nausea and vomiting.

ULCERATIVE COLITIS

Ulcerative colitis has been defined as "an acute, subacute, or chronic disease of the colon and rectum of unknown etiology or pathogenesis, with a variable course, unpredictable prognosis, and many local and systemic complications; with rectal bleeding, diarrhea, cramping abdominal pain, fever, anorexia, and weight loss as the principal symptoms; and with proctosigmoidoscopic and x-ray features that are often diagnostic."[102] Because the actual treatment of the condition itself is limited, and because the patient with ulcerative colitis is characterized by a higher than average intelligence and interest in his own condition, the health professional can impart a considerable amount of information about the disease process and the various therapeutic modalities the patient is receiving.

The incidence rate of ulcerative colitis varies from country to country, with ranges of four to seven cases per 100,000 people per year reported.[103-105] Although ulcerative colitis affects all age groups, the highest incidence rates are found in the third to sixth decades of life, with a reported incidence in the latter age group of 80 cases per 100,000 population per year.[106] Patients younger than 20 years account for less than one-fifth of all newly diagnosed cases. However, when the disease does occur in children, the process is more severe than in adults. In elderly patients a typical presentation of the disease can lead to diagnostic difficulty and result in a higher incidence of acute complications, including dilation, perforation, and massive hemorrhage.

Epidemiologic studies have also confirmed the high frequency of this disease among the Jewish population.[107, 108] As many as 10 per cent of the patients with ulcerative colitis have a positive family history of idiopathic inflammatory bowel disease, 10 times the frequency that could be expected if these were random occurrences.[109] Environment does not appear to be a significant factor in the disease's incidence, since nonrelated individuals living with families that are at risk have not shown a greater rate of occurrence than that in the general population.[110] Although a slight predominance of the disease in male children has been reported, it is generally accepted that there is an even distribution of the disease between the sexes.[111, 112]

Although the etiology of ulcerative colitis is not known, there appear to be multiple factors involved. Recently a great deal of emphasis has been placed on reports of immunologic abnormalities in patients with ulcerative colitis. Several groups of investigators have demonstrated the existence of antigen-antibody complexes in this disease.[113, 114] It is not known how they develop, nor is there a correlation of severity of the disease with the titer of antibodies. The deposition of these complexes in blood vessel walls may explain the vascular insufficiency frequently observed in this disease.

Pathophysiology

The lesions of ulcerative colitis usually develop first in the rectum and spread proximally and diffusely. Although the inflammatory process is usually limited to the mucosa of the large intestine, it can and often does extend into the adjacent submucosa. Extensive small intestinal involvement does not occur. However, mild superficial inflammation of the distal portion of the ileum may exist, a condition termed "backwash ileitis." The rectum and left colon are most often involved initially. With subsequent attacks, more and more of the colon becomes affected proximally until eventually the entire colon is involved. The anatomic classification of ulcerative colitis is depicted graphically in Figure 6–5.

The evolution of the lesions in ulcerative colitis is not completely known; some reports indicate that the earliest lesions are microabscesses in the base of colonic crypts. As the microabscesses develop, there is a vascular engorgement of the mucosa and submucosa as

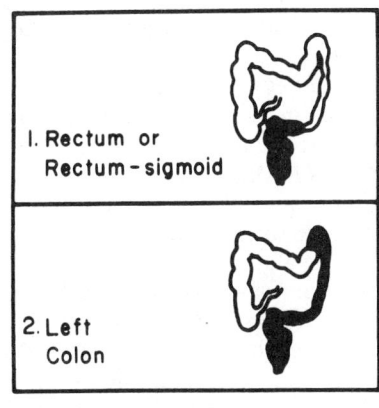
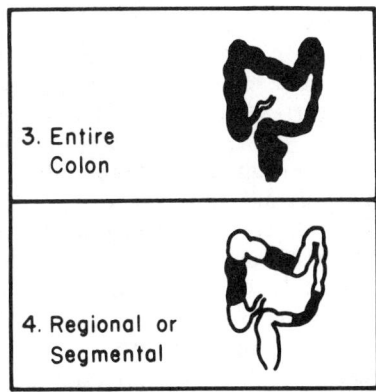

Figure 6–5. Classification of ulcerative colitis according to anatomic type.

well as a significant increase in the number of monocytes and polymorphonuclear leukocytes in the mucosa and at times in the submucosa. The microabscesses in the crypts may coalesce to produce shallow ulcerations of the mucosa, extending down to the muscularis mucosae. Resultant sloughing of the inflamed mucosa produces small ulcerations that enlarge to involve deeper cellular layers and, when adjacent to hanging fragments of the colonic mucosa, result in the formation of pseudopolyps.

Ulceration, vascular engorgement, and the development of granulation tissue result in bleeding and loss of tissue fluids. After this tissue is formed, the wall of the large intestine becomes stiff and rubbery and is reduced to half the normal diameter. In this state it is likely that it becomes less effective in reabsorbing fluid and electrolytes. In severe ulcerative colitis the disease may extend through the muscular and serosal layers of the bowel wall, leading to colonic dilation and toxic megacolon, a complication associated with a high mortality, especially in the elderly.[183]

Within the last several years many reports associating various antibiotics and other drugs with colitis have been published in the medical literature (Table 6–13).[115–118] Antibiotic associated colitis, the most commonly reported type of drug induced colitis, is characterized by diarrhea that begins days to weeks after antibiotic treatment has started. It is associated with dehydration, neutrophilic leukocytosis, and hypoalbuminemia. Polymorphonuclear leukocytes are found in stool samples in which blood is not observed. Plain abdominal roentgenograms may indicate the presence of colitis, and barium enema examination indicates irregularities of the colonic wall. Proctosigmoidoscopy usually shows yellow plaques of pseudomembranes commonly appearing studded about in a congested but otherwise normal mucosa, and biopsy usually provides pathologic confirmation.

Recently it has become clear that the disorder is caused by toxin producing strains of *Clostridium difficile*.[119, 120] This finding has led to two logical but quite different approaches to treatment. The initial therapy with both approaches includes stopping the antibiotic, bowel rest, and vigorous supportive therapy with fluids and electrolytes as well as albumin replacement when necessary.

One form of therapy then is to administer an antibiotic that is active against the suspected pathogen. The drug that has received the greatest attention, orally administered vancomycin in doses of 125 to 500 mg. every six hours, has effected a prompt clinical response, eradication of the toxin, and elimination of the organism.[121, 122]

A second approach uses cholestyramine.[123] Since it was initially thought that bile acid malabsorption might be responsible for antibiotic associated pseudomembranous colitis, this drug was administered to bind these

TABLE 6–13. Drugs Reported to Cause Colitis

Antibiotics	*Antineoplastics*
Chloramphenicol	Fluorouracil
Neomycin	Cyclophosphamide
Penicillin	6-Mercaptopurine
Cephalosporins	
Tetracycline	*Oral Hypoglycemics*
Sulfonamides	Chlorpropamide
Ampicillin	
Lincomycin	*Antirheumatics*
Clindamycin	Phenylbutazone
Sulfamethoxazole-trimethoprim	Gold
Metronidazole	*Other Classes*
	Digitalis glycosides
	Oral contraceptives

acids and thus inhibit secretion of water and electrolytes in the colon. Recent reports now indicate that cholestyramine binds the cytopathic toxin produced by *Colstridium difficile*.[124, 125]

The best treatment of pseudomembranous colitis is prevention. Antibiotics should be administered only for specific indications. Since this drug induced disease may occur when these drugs are used appropriately, early recognition is also important. Diarrhea in a patient who is receiving antibiotics or other drugs listed in Table 6–13 calls for discontinuation of the drug and proctosigmoidoscopic examination. A patient who complains of diarrhea should be questioned about recent antibiotic or other drug exposure. By following these guidelines, the morbidity and mortality of drug induced colitis will be reduced.

Treatment

The goal of therapy in ulcerative colitis is to provide relief from the wide variety of clinical manifestations and complications of the disease, correct deficiency states, maintain nutritional support, and attempt to arrest or reverse the disease process. A reasonable therapeutic plan would be based on the cyclical nature of the disease in most patients and includes the following general principles: early effective management of exacerbations, prolongation of remission, and judicious use of surgery. For the past 25 years the medical management of ulcerative colitis has depended largely on corticosteroids and sulfasalazine.

Corticosteroids. The cornerstone for managing acute attacks and exacerbations of ulcerative colitis is the use of corticosteroids. Depending upon the severity of the disease, these drugs can be administered either rectally, orally, or parenterally to produce rapid improvement in many patients. A favorable response is characterized by a rapid and almost immediate drop in temperature, disappearance of toxemia, increased appetite, gain in weight, a sense of well-being, and, within a few days to a week, a decrease in diarrhea and abdominal discomfort. Changes evident on proctosigmoidoscopic examination appear gradually, and it may be a week to several weeks before improvement is noted. The clinical improvement may be reflected in certain laboratory observations, including a fall in the elevated erythrocyte sedimentation rate, disappearance of blood in the feces, and a restoration of the normal pattern of plasma proteins.

Since the usefulness of topically administered corticosteroids in the treatment of ulcerative colitis was first reported in the 1950's, double blind studies have confirmed their efficacy, and they are now widely used as suppositories, rectal foams, rectal drips, and retention enemas if the disease is mild and limited to the rectum and distal colon. The beneficial effect of topical application is thought to be a result of the local anti-inflammatory effect on the rectal and colonic mucosa, but this is controversial because variable amounts of the topical dose may be absorbed systemically and cause mild adrenal suppression.[126, 127] Since there is no apparent correlation between the therapeutic effects of topically administered corticosteroids and the degree of systemic absorption and adrenal suppression, the steroid having the least capacity for absorption would be preferred. With regard to hydrocortisone, the hemisuccinate is absorbed to a significant degree, and the acetate is absorbed less readily than the alcohol form.

Suppositories containing hydrocortisone acetate are most useful in treating proctosigmoiditis involving the distal portion of the rectum. They can also help those patients with more extensive disease who have urgency and precipitancy of defecation or tenesmus. Proctitis usually responds to the administration of two suppositories daily for four to six weeks.

Foam preparations containing a corticosteroid are easier for a patient to retain than a fluid enema. Although controlled studies have not been undertaken to determine how much of the colon the foams penetrate, there is little doubt of their efficacy in distal colonic disease. The major advantages are marked reduction and rapid relief of tenesmus and better patient compliance due to ease of use.

Retention enemas of hydrocortisone often are administered at bedtime to allow overnight contact with the inflamed mucosa, but a second dose may be retained after a morning bowel movement, particularly in a patient with distal disease who may be susceptible to constipation. Although it was originally believed that 100 ml. of enema fluid spread proximally to cover at least the descending colon, more recent evidence indicates that the correct volume for a given patient may have to be established by adding barium to the enema and studying its spread by roentgenography.[128] If the patient cannot retain enemas because of diarrhea or tenesmus, the topical use of corticosteroids may become possible after the disease process has been controlled with systemic therapy. Once an attack has been under control for two to four weeks, the frequency of administration of retention enemas should be reduced to alternate nights and, if no deterioration occurs in the next two weeks, stopped. Conventional retention enemas probably do not help to maintain remission.

In a recent report, a retention enema of beclomethasone dipropionate was prepared to yield a final concentration of 0.5 mg. per dl. and assessed in patients having exacerbations of distal ulcerative colitis. The clinical and sigmoidoscopic responses after two weeks were similar to that achieved with conventional steroid enemas. However, when adrenocortical function was measured on the morning after the last day of a course of enema therapy, plasma cortisol levels were not suppressed, which is suggestive of a lack of interference with hypothalamic-pituitary-adrenal function. Since other steroid enemas would be expected to inhibit cortisol secretion, the authors indicated that beclomethasone enemas probably could be given regularly over longer periods than conventional steroid enemas.[184]

An alternate approach to the use of retention enemas is the use of slow rectal infusions of corticosteroids. An infusion of methylprednisolone irritates the rectum less and is more readily retained by patients who are liable to incontinence. In addition, there is some evidence that rectal infusions penetrate higher into the colon than do retention enemas.

The beneficial effect of orally administered corticosteroids in treating moderately severe ulcerative colitis has been clearly demonstrated by controlled clinical trials.[129] Administration of 40 to 60 mg. of prednisone or prednisolone frequently brings about improvement or remission in two to four weeks. If there is no response within this period, there is little likelihood of improvement with prolonged oral treatment, and parenterally administered steroids may prove more effective.

Comparison of a single 40 mg. morning dose with doses of 10 mg. four times daily indicates that the use of single daily doses of a corticosteroid in the morning closely parallels the known circadian rhythm of the adrenal gland, causes less adrenal suppression than the same total dose administered throughout the day, is more convenient for the patient, and is therapeutically equivalent. Alternate day steroid therapy has been advocated to reduce side effects, but because many patients with colitis experience symptoms between doses, this form of therapy has not been generally accepted.

When remission is achieved with an initial dosage of 40 mg. per day, tapering to a maintenance dose or complete withdrawal may take only two or three weeks. In some individuals a more gradual reduction and withdrawal may be required to prevent mental depression or relapse. Patients with total colonic involvement may require a continuous maintenance dosage of 10 to 15 mg. daily to prevent a relapse. A steroid retention enema may be added to the regimen to allow for a smoother withdrawal of orally administered steroids in the more resistant cases.

With use of a steroid infusion it should be noted that because of the salt and water retention produced by high doses of hydrocortisone, the use of prednisolone-21-phosphate (having less mineralocorticoid activity) has been advocated.[130] If decisive improvement (i.e., cessation of bloody diarrhea and persistent fever) occurs with five to seven days of this treatment, orally administered corticosteroids can be substituted for the infusion. If, however, the patient fails to respond within several days to parenteral treatment, a decision to perform total proctocolectomy and permanent ileostomy must be seriously considered. Likewise patients who respond only partially to corticosteroid therapy and require relatively large maintenance doses to prevent relapse should be considered for surgical excision of the colon.

The side effects of corticosteroid therapy are numerous and occur frequently. It is important, however, to distinguish the adverse effects of steroid therapy from the complications of ulcerative colitis itself. Electrolyte imbalances (particularly hypokalemia and hypocalcemia with osteoporosis), pathologic fractures, and growth retardation may be caused by the disease but exacerbated by the therapy. On the other hand, if fluid retention, acute psychosis, hypertension, glucose intolerance, seizure disorders, glaucoma, cataracts, or myopathy appears for the first time during steroid therapy, these complications can be attributed to the drug.

Sulfasalazine. Combining in a single molecule both antibacterial and anti-inflammatory activity, sulfasalazine was synthesized almost

40 years ago for the possible treatment of rheumatoid arthritis. Although not effective for that original purpose, the drug was found empirically to be beneficial in treating ulcerative colitis.

When taken orally, the drug is absorbed rapidly but not completely in the upper gastrointestinal tract, and some of the drug re-enters the intestine with bile. The initial step in sulfasalazine metabolism, reductive cleavage of the azo bond, occurs primarily in the colon and is brought about by the activity of intestinal bacteria.[131] Splitting of this bond liberates the two constituents of the molecule, namely, 5-aminosalicylic acid and sulfapyridine. The latter appears to be well absorbed and is detected in blood three to five hours after oral administration, a period of time that is consistent with the transit time of the drug to the site of bacterial activity. Most of the sulfapyridine is excreted with its metabolites in the urine. On the other hand, 5-aminosalicylic acid appears to remain in the colon and is excreted in the feces. Unchanged sulfasalazine is found in the feces; the amount depends upon the transit time and the activity of the intestinal microflora. For example, in a patient with rapid intestinal transit and diarrhea, the excretion of unchanged sulfasalazine in the stool increases. Likewise little is known about the manner in which disease states alter the character of intestinal micro-organisms. Thus, two factors that may vary in ulcerative colitis, namely, the intestinal transit time and the character of intestinal bacteria, may be responsible for significant alterations in the absorption, distribution, and metabolism of sulfasalazine.

Although the mechanism of action of sulfasalazine is not known with certainty, recent evidence indicates that the parent drug may serve merely as a vehicle to deliver the actual therapeutic drug, 5-aminosalicylic acid, to the site of inflammation where it acts to inhibit prostaglandin synthesis.[132, 133] Sulfasalazine has also been reported to counteract fluid and electrolyte loss from the inflamed colon in studies of isolated colonic mucosa.[134] Whether this effect is also due to inhibition of prostaglandin synthesis is unknown at present, but it could contribute to the drug's clinical effectiveness.

Sulfasalazine is generally effective in the treatment of mild to moderate attacks of ulcerative colitis and is administered commonly as the initial therapeutic drug. However, it is not as effective as steroid enemas or the systemic administration of corticosteroids in rapidly inducing remission. Only approximately 30 to 40 per cent of the patients with disease confined to the rectosigmoid attain remission within two weeks after beginning therapy. This is in contrast to the 70 to 90 per cent success rate in inducing remission attributed to corticosteroid administration.

The dosage of sulfasalazine varies according to the age, the severity of the illness, and the tolerance of the patient. Studies of the drug's pharmacokinetics indicate that great individual variations in absorption and metabolism exist, and these may be more significant than the actual dosage in determining the therapeutic as well as the adverse effects at the cellular level.[135]

The usually recommended daily dosage of sulfasalazine varies from 2 to 4 gm. administered in four divided doses after meals and at bedtime. Higher doses of 4 to 8 gm. daily have been employed by some clinicians to treat active and acute disease, but no evidence exists that this is beneficial. In fact higher dosages usually contribute only to increasing adverse reactions to sulfasalazine. By initiating therapy at a low dosage and then increasing the dosage by 0.5 to 1.0 gm. increments every one to two days, the frequency of headache, nausea, and vomiting, which are common side effects of the drug and appear to be dose dependent, is greatly diminished.[136] If slight nausea, headache, or dizziness is encountered, the dosage should be reduced by half, with return to full dosage within three days. In the event of severe nausea and vomiting, therapy should be discontinued for five to seven days and then reinstituted and the dosage gradually increased as tolerated until the appropriate dosage is attained. If improvement is shown, the dosage is maintained until complete remission is achieved as indicated by proctosigmoidoscopic findings. Once remission has occurred, the dosage of sulfasalazine is reduced gradually over several weeks to months to a daily maintenance level. A maintenance dosage of 2 gm. daily appears to be optimal in preventing relapse of the disease.

Although sulfasalazine is used in maintaining remission and preventing recurrences of ulcerative colitis, it is not clear how long use of the drug should be continued. The evidence appears to favor prolonged therapy for more than a year and presumably for many years, until the drug is no longer tolerated or effective.

The clinical use of sulfasalazine is limited by the development of adverse reactions. The most common adverse effects are either gastrointestinal (nausea, vomiting, anorexia, abdominal discomfort), hematologic (hemolytic anemia, leukopenia, agranulocytosis, pancytopenia), or generalized (headaches, vertigo, rash, fever). Side effects, which occur in about 20 per cent of the patients taking the drug, can be further classified as either dose dependent or due to a specific hypersensitivity reaction.

Dose dependent reactions do not correlate with the level of sulfasalazine in the blood, but they do correlate with the level of sulfapyridine; they are more common among slow acetylators than among fast acetylators. In most patients with ulcerative colitis who are rapid acetylators, an optimal dosage schedule of sulfasalazine provides serum sulfapyridine levels of 20 to 40 mcg. per ml. However, genetically slow acetylators require less of the drug to achieve "therapeutic" levels of sulfapyridine in the blood. In these patients, increasing the dosage to more than 4 gm. per day can result in a serum sulfapyridine concentration greater than 50 mcg. per ml., resulting in a marked increase in side effects. Dose dependent reactions are most frequently gastrointestinal. In addition, sulfasalazine may cause hematologic abnormalities that are dose related. Most of these changes are mild, and anemia does not result. However, a recent report indicates that hemolysis should be considered in any patient with ulcerative colitis who is taking sulfasalazine and in whom the loss of blood in the feces or chronic inflammation does not justify the diagnosis of anemia.[137]

The emergence of a previously unreported adverse reaction to sulfasalazine, namely, male infertility, has been documented in four patients.[138] Since the case histories suggested direct toxicity, the authors postulated that a genetically determined acetylator type may have influenced the metabolism of the drug and consequently the occurrence of this side effect. A recent review indicated that this temporary oligospermia with decreased sperm motility and infertility most probably occurred as a consequence of multiple mechanisms. Possible mechanisms include toxic effects on developing spermatozoa, inhibition of folate metabolism, chromium deficiency, and an inhibiting effect on prostaglandins E and F.[185]

Hypersensitivity reactions to sulfasalazine may involve many body tissues including the skin, kidneys, liver, lungs, bone marrow, and blood vessels, thus making a careful search for specific organ involvement in sensitized patients mandatory. Skin rash, occasionally progressing to exfoliative dermatitis, is the most commonly reported hypersensitivity reaction. Hematologic reactions, including bone marrow depression and consequent agranulocytosis as well as autoimmune hemolytic anemia, can also occur. More recently lung disease—in the form of pulmonary infiltrates and eosinophilia, impairment of pulmonary function due to bronchospasm, and fatal fibrosing alveolitis—has been reported. In addition, a lupus-like syndrome with polyarthritis, vasculitis, and antibodies to DNA has been described. Raynaud's phenomenon is an unusual feature of such drug related syndromes and, until a recent report, had not been associated with sulfasalazine therapy.[139] Several case reports have documented severe renal and hepatic toxicity after sulfasalazine therapy.

Although hypersensitivity reactions are rare during sulfasalazine therapy, they can be accompanied by significant morbidity and in some cases mortality. Like most cases of hypersensitivity, the symptoms and signs usually disappear rapidly when sulfasalazine administration is discontinued, but prompt recognition is essential for complete resolution of the adverse reactions.

For those patients who develop a systemic allergic reaction manifested as a rash, an alternative to discontinuation of the drug is desensitization. In a recent report, desensitization to sulfasalazine was initiated with ⅛ tablet (62.5 mg.) per day with subsequent doubling every three to seven days. The protocol was initiated only when the allergic rash had subsided. In all patients, desensitization was started only after the colitis was under control. After desensitization, the underlying disease in all patients improved, and no significant adverse effects were observed with long term administration. The authors concluded that in patients with ulcerative colitis who developed an allergic response to sulfasalazine, desensitization could be easily and safely accomplished with a good long term response.[186]

There have been several reports of drug interactions involving sulfasalazine. Since intestinal bacteria split sulfasalazine, it is possible that antibiotics that decrease the bacterial flora of the colon could affect its metabolism and therapeutic activity. The clinical significance of this interaction has not been determined, but the possibility that the concomitant administration of antibiotics may alter the response of the patient to sulfasalazine should be kept in mind.

Another documented interaction, involving sulfasalazine and iron, results in a decreased blood level of the former due to chelation of ferrous ion by the salicylate moiety of sulfasalazine. However, it has not been determined whether the administration of these two drugs concurrently in any way alters the efficacy of either. In addition, the poor absorption of folic acid frequently noted in patients with ulcerative colitis seems to be further aggravated during therapy with sulfasalazine, and a case of folate deficiency leading to megaloblastic anemia has been reported in a patient taking the drug.[140]

Finally the absorption of digoxin may be impaired by the concomitant administration of sulfasalazine. Although the mechanism of the interaction has not been elucidated, one should consider switching the patient to digitoxin, since similar bioavailability problems have not been reported for this drug.

Other Drug Therapies. Although sulfasalazine and corticosteroids are the mainstays of drug therapy of ulcerative colitis, other approaches to the treatment of this disease have been investigated. A brief description of the more important therapeutic alternatives follows.

Azathioprine. The nonspecific inflammatory bowel diseases, including ulcerative colitis, are among a long list of nonmalignant disorders for which immunosuppressive drugs such as azathioprine have been employed.

In 1972 the first published report of a controlled clinical study involving the use of azathioprine to induce a remission of ulcerative colitis initially treated with prednisolone appeared in the literature.[141] As the corticosteroid dosage was decreased, relapses occurred in 15 of 20 placebo treated patients, but only in nine of 20 patients receiving azathioprine. However, the final report of this study failed to demonstrate any significant benefit when azathioprine was added to a standard corticosteroid regimen in treating ulcerative colitis.[142]

The results of two additional controlled studies of azathioprine in ulcerative colitis have been reported.[143,144] The results of the first study indicated that although the clinical course of the disease did not improve after six months of azathioprine therapy, the drug demonstrated a beneficial effect in permitting a significant reduction of the steroid dosage without apparent worsening of the disease. In the second study, although both drugs reduced clinical symptoms, which resulted in objective improvement of the disease, the degree of benefit was not significantly different in patients treated with either azathioprine or sulfasalazine.

The use of azathioprine in patients with ulcerative colitis requires caution since the drug may suppress host defenses, and these patients are already at risk for many local and systemic problems, including infections. There may be added risk of malignant disease in patients with long standing disease, who already are more vulnerable to carcinoma of the colon. Certainly such therapy must be monitored carefully to ensure that the prospective benefits to the patient exceed the potential short and long term risks.

To sum up the current state of immunosuppressive therapy, the authors of a recent review concluded that azathioprine therapy of ulcerative colitis is unsafe in acute fulminating colitis, inadvisable for permanent maintenance therapy, but conceivably useful as a short term measure in certain patients who are unresponsive or intolerant to accepted doses of steroids and sulfasalazine and unwilling or unable to undergo curative surgery.[145]

Cromolyn Sodium. Since mast cells may be of pathologic significance in ulcerative colitis, several controlled studies have been undertaken to determine the role of cromolyn sodium in this disease. Initially it was thought that treatment of acute disease with cromolyn sodium was therapeutically equal to corticosteroids and sulfasalazine and significantly improved the patients' sense of well-being and the macroscopic and microscopic appearance of the rectal mucosa. However, more recent trials of patients either with active disease or in remission using daily dosages ranging from 800 mg. to 2 gm. showed no benefit when compared with placebo or standard therapeutic modalities.[146,147]

Because cromolyn sodium is absorbed poorly after oral administration, it is possible that the use of a larger oral dose, a longer treatment period, rectal administration, or any combination of these may allow a beneficial therapeutic effect to be demonstrated. Since the only dosage forms of cromolyn sodium commercially available in the United States today are a 20 mg. capsule intended for inhalation only and a solution for nebulizer use only

(20 mg. per 2 ml.), one can conclude readily that the unapproved oral administration of as many as 100 capsules per day would be very expensive and inconvenient and should be postponed until more encouraging results are available.

Vancomycin and Bacitracin. It has been reported that vancomycin may be of benefit in certain individuals with inflammatory bowel disease who have *Clostridium difficile* toxin in their stools during symptomatic relapse of the disease.[148] Four of five patients with ulcerative colitis received vancomycin at oral dosages of 250 to 350 mg. four times daily for varying lengths of time when they failed to improve with intensive corticosteroid therapy. In two patients bloody diarrhea disappeared within three to four days. The other patients improved slowly over a two week period. Disappearance of the toxin was associated with symptomatic improvement in all cases. The authors suggest testing for Clostridium toxin in patients with inflammatory bowel disease uncontrolled with standard medical therapy in order to identify those who might benefit from vancomycin therapy.

Two recent reports indicate that oral doses of bacitracin may be a suitable alternative for treating pseudomembranous colitis and, by implication, patients with inflammatory bowel disease in whom *Clostridium difficile* toxin is present.[149, 150] When it was given orally [25,000 units (500 mg.) dissolved in 10 ml. of water every six hours for seven to 10 days], diarrhea was resolved within 24 to 48 hours and stool cultures in five of the six treated patients became negative.

Bacitracin, like vancomycin, is poorly absorbed from the intestine, thus avoiding the occurrence of systemic toxicity. In addition, it is less expensive, better tasting, and more readily available worldwide than vancomycin. Because relapses have not yet been reported, bacitracin may be especially beneficial in patients who became symptomatic as a result of *Clostridium difficile* overgrowth.

Antidiarrheal and Anticholinergic Drugs. In mild to moderate cases of colitis many clinicians prescribe antidiarrheal drugs such as diphenoxylate and loperamide to decrease the intestinal transit rate. However, it appears that these drugs have their major use when the diarrhea is chronic and arises in the small intestine rather than the colon. Because much of the tenesmus and the passage of blood or mucus in colitis is due to rectal inflammation, it is not surprising that the use of diphenoxylate to reduce bowel frequency in ulcerative colitis has shown little overall therapeutic benefit. Anticholinergic drugs are sometimes used in ulcerative colitis to reduce pain or diarrhea. However, there is no controlled evidence that they reduce the symptoms of the disease. In addition, they may contribute to colonic dilation or mask obstructive symptoms.

Nutritional Supplements. In recent years the importance of nutritional supplementation has been emphasized in patients with moderate to severe ulcerative colitis. By providing a high caloric and protein intake, both oral elemental diets and total parenteral nutrition have been utilized to overcome nutritional deficiencies. Oral elemental diets can supply up to 3,000 calories and 125 gm. of protein per day as amino acids, casein, or egg albumin and are relatively well tolerated by patients with ulcerative colitis. However, since oral elemental diets are hypertonic, it is important to initiate therapy by carefully adjusting the concentrations and volume, or both, in order to prevent gastrointestinal distress and diarrhea caused by a high osmotic load. If a patient cannot tolerate elemental diets because of side effects, parenteral nutrition may be indicated.

A low residue diet is still advocated widely in the treatment of ulcerative colitis, and it is relatively common to find patients following this regimen, even though they have been symptom-free for long periods of time. There is no evidence to suggest that a low residue diet is beneficial other than in relieving symptoms during a relapse of the disease; therefore recommending its continuation during periods of remission is questionable. A low residue diet may prove harmful by aggravating constipation, which is so often a problem when the disease process is limited to the rectum.

Surgery. Historically the first treatment for ulcerative colitis was surgical. Today surgical intervention is indicated only when adequate drug treatment of the disease has failed. Although the need for surgery may become apparent only gradually in a long standing case or may come about with explosive urgency during a severe attack, generally accepted indications for surgery include: failure of a severe attack to respond to drug therapy, perforation of the colon, massive or recurrent severe hemorrhage, toxic megacolon, either recurring, or an initial attack not responding to comprehensive medical measures of three to five days, growth retardation in children whose disease fails to remain under control with steroid therapy, and prevention of subsequent carcinoma in high risk patients. The surgical procedure of choice when disease involvement is diffuse and affects extensive portions of the colon and rectum is a radical excision or panproctocolectomy combined with a permanent ileostomy.

Most patients regain good to excellent general health after panproctocolectomy with ileostomy, but the associated skin problems, the occasional need for surgical revision, problems with ostomy appliances and supplies and the psychologic and aesthetic difficulties that require assistance or simple reassurance indicate that a continued search for better pharmacologic and surgical management is of paramount importance.

Conclusion

The prognosis in any patient suffering from ulcerative colitis is dependent upon a combination of three factors, namely, the age of the patient, the extent of colonic involvement, and, if the disease is active, the severity of the attack. The mortality is highest in patients over the age of 60 years (although life expectancy is considerably reduced, perhaps by as much as 20 years in young patients with ulcerative colitis), those who suffer from severe attacks, and those with extensive disease, involving all or nearly all of the colon and rectum. This knowledge has allowed the development of a much more rational system of management and more precise definition of the respective roles of pharmacologic and surgical treatment.

DRUG INDUCED HEPATITIS

The liver is particularly vulnerable to drug induced injury for a variety of reasons. For orally administered drugs, the portal circulation provides the highest concentration of medication directly to the liver. Owing to its role in the concentration and biotransformation of drug products, the liver is exposed for long periods of time to parent compounds and potentially toxic metabolites. In states of accelerated drug metabolizing activity, enhanced hepatotoxicity can occur if the metabolite is toxic.

The elderly are more apt to experience hepatotoxic reactions because of the large number of medications they ingest and also because the aging liver is more susceptible to the hepatotoxic effects of medication. In elderly patients with jaundice there is a 20 per cent chance that the underlying cause of liver disease is drug induced.[151]

At the present time, it is not possible to predict the patients in whom an insult to the liver will develop as a result of a certain medication. Laboratory testing in animals does not adequately identify the drugs that may be hepatotoxic in humans. In clinical situations in which a drug that is a known hepatotoxin may be required, the benefit of using the product must be weighed against the risk of developing hepatitis. The spectrum of adverse consequences of drugs on the liver spans the entire gamut from mild cholestasis to fulminant hepatitis and death.

Although there are many ways in which to categorize drug induced hepatotoxicity, the type of injury produced in the liver is the most common classification employed. The two major subdivisions in this classification are direct hepatotoxins and idiosyncratic reactions. An "intrinsic" hepatotoxic drug produces hepatotoxicity because of its own molecular structure, has the potential to produce the toxicity in many people, and often has a relatively short and consistent latent period. This characteristic type of reaction is also dose dependent. Drug induced hypersensitivity reactions in the liver can be produced with relatively small doses, cannot be duplicated reliably in laboratory animals, and occur in a small number of patients. Other signs of allergy are often seen, including eosinophilia, skin rash, antibody production, and fever. Some drugs are capable of producing a "mixed" type of hepatotoxicity, which is composed of certain aspects of an intrinsic toxin and a hypersensitivity reaction.

Direct Intrinsic Hepatotoxins

Medications in this category have a direct destructive action on a part of the hepatocyte, such as the plasma membrane or endoplasmic reticulum. As a consequence they distort the metabolism and function of the cell. Carbon tetrachloride is the major agent in this category of hepatotoxins. It produces hepatic necrosis by damaging the endoplasmic reticulum and plasmic membrane. Chloroform is an anesthetic that was abandoned because of its direct hepatotoxic effects.

Indirect Intrinsic Hepatotoxins

Hepatotoxicity induced by drugs in this category interfere with specific metabolic functions, resulting in injury to parenchymal cells or cholestasis. The cytotoxic intrinsic hepatotoxins include ethanol, methotrexate, L-asparaginase, acetaminophen, tetracycline, 6-mercaptopurine, dantrolene sodium, nicotinic acid, and vitamin A. Steatosis (fatty liver) is the most common hepatic lesion associated with the chronic ingestion of ethanol. It is found in 70 to 100 per cent of individuals who drink to excess. Cirrhosis is a well known consequence of alcohol abuse. Methotrexate induced liver disease is related to the frequency of administration. A small daily dose such as that which has been employed in the management of refractory psoriasis is more hepatotoxic than larger doses given at less frequent intervals.[152]

Acetaminophen hepatotoxicity has recently received much attention since this medication is now being used more frequently in suicide attempts. When taken in therapeutic doses, acetaminophen is primarily conjugated with glucuronic acid or sulfate. In overdose situations the parent compound undergoes degradation through a different metabolic route, because the normal routes of biotransformation are saturated. The primary metabolite in this situation is hepatotoxic and requires glutathione for inactivation. Attempts to administer glutathione directly have been unsuccessful because this compound does not penetrate the hepatocyte effectively. N-Acetylcysteine (Mucomyst) is an effective antidote when administered in an oral dose of 140 mg. per kg. initially followed by doses of 70 mg. per kg. every four hours for 17 doses.[153]

Chronic daily ingestion of 100,000 units of vitamin A has resulted in hepatic dysfunction resembling cirrhosis.[154] Large intravenous doses (greater than 2 grams per day) of tetracycline can produce fatal liver disease, but most of these cases have occurred in women in the third trimester of pregnancy.

Indirect hepatotoxins, which produce cholestasis, interfere with bile flow and are not otherwise injurious to liver cells. Rifampin interferes with the excretion of bile and bilirubin transport from the sinusoid into the hepatocyte by competitive inhibition.[155] The C-17 alkylated anabolic steroids, such as testosterone and methandrostenolone (Dianabol), alter the permeability of bile canniculi and enhance back diffusion of the constituents of bile.[156] Chenodeoxycholic acid, a cholesterol gallstone dissolving drug, is converted by intestinal bacteria into lithocholic acid, which can produce hepatic cholestasis. To date, experimental trials with chenodeoxycholic acid have not demonstrated a significant hepatotoxic effect.

Idiosyncratic Drug Induced Hepatotoxicity

Drug induced hypersensitivity reactions that produce hepatic injury usually occur within one to five weeks after the initiation of therapy. The reaction is frequently associated with rash, fever, and eosinophilia. Symptoms usually recur promptly upon rechallenge with a single dose. Hepatic injury may vary from mild cholestatic jaundice, which has been observed with chlorpromazine and erythromycin estolate, to fulminant hepatitis with drugs such as halothane and methyldopa. Fortunately the incidence of the latter form of hepatotoxicity is quite rare.

Intrahepatic cholestasis develops in 0.5 to 1 per cent of the patients taking chlorpromazine. Elderly individuals are much more susceptible to this type of reaction. The estolate salt of erythromycin has caused many cases of cholestatic jaundice. A few cases of a similar type of reaction have been reported with other erythromycin salts. Rifampin and high doses of oxacillin are also capable of inducing cholestatic jaundice.

In addition to hypersensitivity reactions, idiosyncratic hepatotoxicity may result from an underlying metabolic abnormality. It is thought that faulty metabolism may lead to the accumulation of toxic metabolites. The onset of this type of reaction may be variable and can occur many months after the institution of therapy. Upon rechallenge with the suspected drug, days to weeks of continued therapy will be required before signs and symptoms of hepatotoxicity again become evident. Isoniazid and methyldopa are included in this category of medication.

Several drugs are capable of producing a clinical and histologic condition that may be indistinguishable from acute viral hepatitis. Included in this group are methyldopa, phenytoin, isoniazid, nitrofurantoin, and aspirin—drugs to which elderly patients are frequently exposed. As in viral hepatitis, the same drugs can be responsible for the development of chronic active hepatitis.[157-159] Although drug induced chronic active hepatitis is rare, mortality rates range from 10 to 50 per cent.

Patients with underlying collagen vascular disease (especially systemic lupus erythematosus) who are receiving aspirin in a dosage of 2 grams or more per day are at greater risk of developing hepatitis than the normal population.[157] Methyldopa is a widely used antihypertensive drug that has the potential to produce hepatotoxicity, which can be fatal in up to 50 per cent of the patients developing this reaction. Since most cases develop during the first three months of therapy, any patients complaining of flulike symptoms and fever during this time period should be evaluated for drug induced hepatitis. Use of the general anesthetic halothane can result in hepatitis, which occurs at a rate of 1 per 8000 anesthetic administrations. The accompanying mortality rate is approximately 20 per cent. Repeated exposure to halothane increases the risk of developing hepatitis.

Isoniazid is a well known hepatotoxin. In patients older than 50 years of age, the risk of hepatitis is increased to 2.3 per cent.[158] The ingestion of alcohol or rifampin further enhances the hepatotoxic potential of isoniazid.

Long term suppressive therapy for recurrent urinary tract infections with nitrofurantoin has resulted in chronic active hepatitis.[159] Two deaths occurred in patients who continued to take the drug despite the appearance of jaundice. A typical reaction of fever, rash, lymphadenopathy, and hepatomegaly followed by jaundice heralds the onset of phenytoin induced hepatotoxicity. The onset usually occurs after one to five weeks of therapy and is associated with lymphocytosis, eosinophilia, and markedly elevated liver enzyme levels.

Therapy of Drug Induced Hepatitis

When medication is suspected of inducing hepatic injury, it should be stopped immediately and empiric supportive therapy employed. Corticosteroid therapy for severe drug induced hepatotoxicity has been attempted with sporadic success. However, the value of this form of therapy remains to be established in adequately controlled clinical trials.

REFERENCES

1. Kim, S.K., Gerle, R.D., and Rozanski, R.: Cathartic colon. Am. J. Roentgenol., *131*:1079–1081, 1978.
2. Derezin, M.: Laxatives and fecal modifiers. Am. Fam. Phys., *10*:126–128, 1975.
3. Connel, A.M.C.: Variations of bowel habit in two population samples. Br. Med. J., *2*:1095–1099, 1965.
4. Brocklehurst, J.C.: Disorders of the lower bowel in old age. Geriatrics, *35*:47–54, 1980.
5. Hull, C., Greco, R.S., and Brooks, D.L.: Alleviation of constipation in the elderly by dietary fiber supplementation. J. Am. Geriatr. Soc., *27*:410–414, 1980.
6. Smith, R.G., Currie, J.E.J., and Walls, A.D.F.: Whole gut irrigation: a new treatment for constipation. Br. Med. J., *2*:396–397, 1978.
7. Saunders, J.F.: Lactulose syrup assessed in a double-blind study of elderly constipated patients. J. Am. Geriatr. Soc., *26*:236–239, 1978.
8. Sterup, K., and Mosbeck. J.: Trends in the mortality from peptic ulcer in Denmark. Scand. J. Gastroenterol., *8*:49–53, 1973.
9. Puluertaft, C.N.: Comments on the incidence and natural history of gastric and duodenal ulcer. Postgrad. Med. J., *44*:597–602, 1968.
10. Silverstein, F.E.: Peptic ulcer: an overview of diagnosis. Hosp. Pract., *14*:78–87, 1979.
11. Cooke, A.R.: Drugs and gastric damage. Drugs, *11*:36–44, 1976.
12. Cooke, A.R.: Drug damage to the gastroduodenum. *In* Sleisenger, M.H., and Fordtran, J.S. (Editors): Gastrointestinal Disease: Pathophysiology—Diagnosis—Management. Ed. 2. Philadelphia, W.B. Saunders Company, 1978, pp. 809–812.
13. Roverstad, R.A.: The incompetent pyloric sphincter. Bile and mucosal ulceration. Am. J. Dig. Dis., *21*:165–173, 1976.
14. Norgaard, R.P., et al.: Effect of long term anticholinergic therapy on gastric acid secretion, with observations on the serial measurement of peak histalog response. Gastroenterology, *58*:750–755, 1970.
15. Grossman, M.I.: Some minor heresies about vagotomy. Gastroenterology, *67*:1010–1018, 1974.
16. Pearse, A.G.E., Polak, J.M., and Bloom, S.R.: The newer gut hormones: cellular sources, physiology, pathology and clinical aspects. Gastroenterology, *72*:746–761, 1977.
17. Walsh, J.H., et al.: Gastrointestinal hormones in clinical disease: Recent developments. Ann. Intern. Med., *90*:817–828, 1979.
18. Dyck, W.P.: Physiological considerations in peptic ulcer disease. S. Med. J., *72*:252–255, 1979.
19. Doll, R., et al.: Continuous intragastric milk drip in treatment of uncomplicated gastric ulcer. Lancet, *1*:70–73, 1956.
20. Butler, M.L., and Gersh, H.: Antacid vs. placebo in hospitalized gastric ulcer patients: a controlled therapeutic study. Am. J. Dig. Dis., *20*:803–807, 1975.
21. Sturdevant, R.A.L., et al.: Antacid and placebo produced similar pain relief in duodenal ulcer patients. Gastroenterology, *72*:1–5, 1977.
22. Hollander, D., and Harlan, J.: Antacids vs. placebo in peptic ulcer therapy. A controlled double-blind investigation. J.A.M.A., *226*:1181–1185, 1973.
23. Peterson, W.L., et al.: Healing of duodenal ulcer with an antacid regimen. N. Engl. J. Med., *297*:341–345, 1977.
24. Lorber, S.H., Stelzer, F.A., and Mayer, E.M.: Effect of antacid and placebo on pain of duodenal ulcer. Gastroenterology, *74*:1058, 1978.
25. Rune, S.J., and Zachariassen, A.: Acute relief of epigastric pain by antacid in duodenal ulcer patients. Scand. J. Gastroenterol., *15* (Suppl. 58):41–45, 1980.

26. Ippoliti, A.F., et al.: Cimetidine vs. intensive antacid therapy for duodenal ulcer. Gastroenterology, 74:393–395, 1978.
27. Lam, S.K., et al.: Treatment of duodenal ulcer with antacid and sulpiride. A double-blind controlled study. Gastroenterology, 76:315–322, 1979.
28. Isenberg, J.L., et al.: Healing of benign gastric ulcer with low dose antacid and cimetidine. A double-blind randomized placebo controlled trial. N. Engl. J. Med., 308:1319–1324, 1983.
29. Thirty-third annual report on consumer spending—antacids. Drug Topics, 125:68–69, 1981.
30. Drake, D., and Hollander, D.: Neutralizing capacity and cost effectiveness of antacids. Ann. Intern. Med., 94:215–217, 1981.
31. Schneider, R.P., and Roach, A.C.: An antacid tasting: the relative palatability of nineteen liquid antacids. South. Med. J., 69:1312–1313, 1976.
32. Sklar, D., Liang, M.H., and Porta, J.: Antacids' costs, taste and buffering. N. Engl. J. Med., 296:1007, 1977 (letter).
33. Stolinsky, D.C.: Sugar and saccharin content of antacids. N. Engl. J. Med., 305:166–167, 1981 (letter).
34. Personal communication with manufacturer, February 1981.
35. Longstreth, G.F., Go, V.L.W., and Malagelda, J.R.: Postprandial gastric, pancreatic and biliary response to histamine H_2-receptor antagonist in active duodenal ulcer. Gastroenterology, 72:9–13, 1977.
36. Deering, T.B., and Malagelda, J.R.: Comparison of an H_2 receptor antagonist and a neutralizing antacid on postprandial acid delivery into the duodenum in patients with duodenal ulcer. Gastroenterology, 73:11–14, 1977.
37. Brogden, R.N., et al.: Cimetidine: a review of its pharmacological properties and therapeutic efficacy in peptic ulcer disease. Drugs, 15:93–131, 1978.
38. Canavan, J.A.F., and Briggs, J.D.: Cimetidine clearance in renal failure. In Burland, W.L., and Simkins, M.A. (Editors): Cimetidine. Proceedings of the Second International Symposium on Histamine H_2-Receptor Antagonists. Amsterdam, Excerpta Medica, 1977, pp. 75–80.
39. Ma, K.W., et al.: Effects of renal failure on blood levels of cimetidine. Gastroenterology, 74:473–477, 1978.
40. Binder, H.J., et al.: Cimetidine in the treatment of duodenal ulcer: a multicenter double blind study. Gastroenterology, 74:380–388, 1978.
41. Hassan, M., and Sirevs, W.: The factors determining success or failure of cimetidine treatment of peptic ulcer. J. Clin. Gastroenterol., 3:225–229, 1981.
42. Kennedy, T., and Spencer, A.: Cimetidine for recurrent ulcer after vagotomy or gastrectomy: a randomized controlled trial. Br. Med. J., 1:1242–1243, 1978.
43. Finkelstein, W., and Isselbacher, K.J.: Cimetidine. N. Engl. J. Med., 299:992–996, 1978.
44. McCarthy, D.M.: Peptic ulcer: antacids or cimetidine? Hosp. Pract., 14:52–64, 1979.
45. Davis, T.G., Pickett, D.L., and Schlosser, J.H.: Evaluation of a worldwide spontaneous reporting system with cimetidine. J.A.M.A., 243:1912–1914, 1980.
46. McGuigan, J.E.: A consideration of the adverse effects of cimetidine. Gastroenterology, 80:181–192, 1981.
47. Schentag, J.J., et al.: Pharmacokinetics and clinical studies in patients with cimetidine-associated mental confusion. Lancet, 1:177–181, 1977.
48. Taylor, R.H., et al.: Misleading response of malignant gastric ulcers to cimetidine. Lancet, 1:686–688, 1978.
49. Elder, J.B., Ganguli, P.C., and Gillespie, I.E.: Cimetidine and gastric cancer. Lancet, 1:1005–1006, 1979.
50. Englert, E., et al.: Cimetidine, antacid and hospitalization in the treatment of benign gastric ulcer. Gastroenterology, 74:416–425, 1978.
51. Almy, T.P., and Howell, D.A.: Diverticular disease of the colon. N. Engl. J. Med., 302:324–331, 1980.
52. Heller, S.N., and Hackler, L.R.: Changes in the crude fiber content of the American diet. Am. J. Clin. Nutr., 32:1510–1514, 1978.
53. Rogers, A.I.: Colonic diverticular disease. Sommerville, New York, Hoechst-Roussel Pharmaceuticals Inc., 1975, pp. 1–20.
54. Ueidenheimer, M.C., Corman, M.L., and Coller, J.A.: Diverticular disease of the colon. Geriatrics, 29:77–83, 1974.
55. Meyers, M.A., et al.: Pathogenesis of diverticulitis complicating granulomatous colitis. Gastroenterology, 74:24–31, 1978.
56. Eastwood, M.A., et al: Comparison of bran, ispaghula and lactulose on colon function in diverticular disease. Gut, 19:1144–1147, 1978.
57. Hyland, J.M.P., and Taylor, I.: Does a high fibre diet prevent the complications of diverticular disease? Br. J. Surg., 67:77–79, 1980.
58. Dwyer, J.T., et al.: Dietary fiber and fiber supplements in the therapy of gastrointestinal disorders. Am. J. Hosp. Pharm., 35:278–287, 1978.
59. Stephen, A.M., and Cummings, J.H.: Water-holding by dietary fibre in vitro and its relationship to faecal output in man. Gut, 20:722–729, 1979.
60. Painter, N.S., Almeida, A.Z., and Colebourne, K.W.: Unprocessed bran in treatment of diverticular disease of the colon. Br. Med. J., 2:137–140, 1972.
61. Daniel, O., Basu, P.K., and Al-Samarrae, H.M.: Use of glucagon in the treatment of acute diverticulitis. Br. Med. J., 3:720–722, 1974.
62. Brogden, R.N., et al.: Metronidazole in anerobic infections: a review of its activity, pharmacokinetics and therapeutic use. Drugs, 16:387–417, 1978.
63. Karran, S., and Lane, R.H.S.: Calculous disease and cholecystitis. In Wright, R., et al. (Editors): Liver and Biliary Disease. Philadelphia, W.B. Saunders Company, 1979, pp. 1191–1218.
64. Hermann, R.E.: Biliary disease. Drug Ther., 5:36–49, 1980.
65. Glenn, F.: Silent gallstones. Ann. Surg., 193:251–252, 1981.
66. Coronary Drug Project Research Group: Gallbladder disease as a side effect of drugs influencing lipid metabolism. N. Engl. J. Med., 296:1185–1190, 1977.
67. Danzinger, R.G., et al.: Dissolution of cholesterol gallstones by chenodeoxycholic acid. N. Engl. J. Med., 286:1–8, 1972.
68. Shoenfeld, L.J.: Update: chenodeoxycholic acid and gallstones. J.A.M.A., 245:2378–2384, 1981.
69. Maton, P.N., Murphy, G.M., and Dowling, R.H.: Ursodeoxycholic acid treatment of gallstones. Lancet, 2:1297–1301, 1977.
70. Dowling, R.H., Hoffman, A.F., and Barbara, L.: Workshop on Ursodeoxycholic Acid. Baltimore, University Park Press, 1979, pp. 1–88.
71. Joiner, K.A., and Gorbach, S.L.: Acute septic

complications in gastrointestinal emergencies. Clin. Gastroenterol., *10*:93–106, 1981.
72. Swenson, R.M.: Cholecystitis and Cholangitis. *In* Mandell, G.L., Douglas, R.G., Bennett, J.E. (Editors): Principles and Practice of Infectious Diseases, New York, John Wiley & Sons, Inc., 1979, pp. 644–649.
73. Chow, A.W.: Intraabdominal sepsis. *In* Yoshikawa, T.I., Chow, A.W., and Guze, L.B. (Editors): Infectious Diseases—Diagnosis and Management. Boston, Houghton Mifflin Professional Publishers, 1980, pp. 141–154.
74. Girard, R.M., and Legros, G.: Retained and recurrent bile duct stones. Ann. Surg., *193*:150–154, 1981.
75. Thistle, J.L., et al.: Mono-octonoin. A dissolution agent for retained cholesterol bile duct stones: physical properties and clinical application. Gastroenterology, *78*:1016–1022, 1980.
77. Mellencamp, E., and Wang, R.I.H.: The patient with nausea. I. Causes. Drug Ther. (Hosp.), *2*:62–69, 1977.
78. Feldman, M., and Fordtran, J.S.: Vomiting. *In* Sleisenger, M.H., and Fordtran, J.S. (Editors): Gastrointestinal Disease. Ed. 2. Philadelphia, W.B. Saunders Company, 1978, pp. 200–216.
79. Mellencamp, E., and Wang, R.I.H.: The patient with nausea. III. Cancer, pregnancy, or surgery. Drug Ther., *2*:47–58, 1977.
80. Greenberger, N.J., Arvanitakis, C., and Hurwitz, A.: Metoclopramide. *In* Drug Treatment of Gastrointestinal Disorders. Monographs in Clinical Pharmacology. Edinburgh, Churchill, Livingstone, 1979, Vol 3, pp. 30–33.
81. Ward, H.W.C.: Metoclopramide and prochlorperazine in radiation sickness. Br. J. Clin. Pharmacol., *2*:52, 1975.
82. Frytak, S., and Moertel, C.G.: Management of nausea and vomiting in the cancer patient. J.A.M.A., *245*:393–396, 1981.
83. O'Malley, K., Judge, T.G., and Crooks, J.: Geriatric clinical pharmacology and therapeutics. *In* Avery, G.S. (Editor): Drug Treatment. Ed. 2. New York, ADIS Press, 1980, pp. 158–181.
84. Van Nueten, J.M., et al.: Inhibition of dopamine receptors in the stomach: an explanation of the gastrokinetic properties of domperidone. Life Sci., *23*:453–458, 1978.
85. Reyntjens, A.: Domperidone as an anti-emetic; summary of research reports. Postgrad. Med. J., 55 (Suppl. 1):50–54, 1979.
86. Kingston, R.S., et al.: Cardiovascular effects of benzquinamide in man. Acta Anesth. Scand., *19*:187–192, 1975.
87. Mull, J.D., and Smith, T.C.: Comparison of the ventilatory effects of two antiemetics, benzquinamide and prochlorperazine. Anesthesiology, *40*:581, 1974.
88. Purkis, I.E.: The action of thiethylperazine, a new antiemetic compared with perphenazine, trimethobenzamide and a placebo in the suppression of postanesthetic nausea and vomiting. Can. Anesth. Soc. J., *12*:595–607, 1965.
89. Moertel, C.G., Reitemeier, R.J., and Gage, R.P.: A controlled clinical evaluation of antiemetic drugs. J.A.M.A., *186*:116–118, 1963.
90. Trimethobenzamide hydrochloride injection and capsules. Fed. Reg., *44*:2017, 1979.
91. Trimethobenzamide hydrochloride suppositories. Fed. Reg., *44*:2021, 1979.
92. Sallan, S.E., Zinberg, N.E., and Frei, E., III: Antiemetic effects of delta-9-tetrahydrocannabinol in patients receiving cancer chemotherapy. N. Engl. J. Med., *293*:795–797, 1979.
93. Sallan, S.E., et al.: Antiemetics in patients receiving chemotherapy for cancer. N. Engl. J. Med., *302*:135–138, 1980.
94. Chang, A.E., et al.: Delta-9-tetrahydrocannabinol as an antiemetic in cancer patients receiving high-dose methotrexate: a prospective, randomized evaluation. Ann. Intern. Med., *91*:819–824, 1979.
95. Chang, A.E., et al.: A prospective evaluation of delta-9-tetrahydrocannabinol as an antiemetic in patients receiving adriamycin and cytoxan chemotherapy. Cancer, 1981.
96. Frytak, S., et al.: Delta-9-tetrahydrocannabinol as an antiemetic for patients receiving cancer chemotherapy: a comparison with prochlorperazine and a placebo. Ann. Intern. Med., *91*:825–830, 1979.
97. Colls, B.M., et al.: The antiemetic activity of tetrahydrocannabinol vs metoclopramide and thiethylperazine in patients undergoing cancer chemotherapy. N.Z. Med. J., *91*:449–451, 1980.
98. Noyes, R., Brunk, S.F., and Avery, D.H.: The analgesic properties of delta-9-tetrahydrocannabinol and codeine. Clin. Pharmacol. Ther., *18*:84–89, 1975.
99. Kluin-Neleman, J.C., et al.: Delta-9-tetrahydrocannabinol (THC) as an antiemetic in patients treated with cancer chemotherapy: a double-blind cross-over trial against placebo. Vet. Hum. Toxicol., *21*:338–340, 1979.
100. Herman, T.S., et al.: Superiority of nabilone over prochlorperazine as an antiemetic in patients receiving cancer chemotherapy. N. Engl. J. Med., *300*:1295–1297, 1979.
101. Bernstein, J.G.: Marijuana—new potential, new problems. Drug Ther., *10*:38–48, 1980.
102. Roth, J.L.A.: Ulcerative colitis. *In* Bockus, H.L. (Editor): Gastroenterology. Ed. 3. Philadelphia, W.B. Saunders Company, 1976, pp. 645–749.
103. Bonnevie, O., Riis, P., and Anthonisen, P.: An epidemiological study of ulcerative colitis in Copenhagen County. Scand. J. Gastroenterol., *3*:432–438, 1968.
104. Monk, M., et al.: An epidemiological study of ulcerative colitis and regional enteritis among adults in Baltimore. I. Hospital incidence and prevalence, 1960–1965. Gastroenterology, *53*:198–210, 1967.
105. Evans, J.G., and Acheson, E.D.: An epidemiological study of ulcerative colitis and regional enteritis in the Oxford area. Gut, *6*:311–314, 1965.
106. Ament, M.E.: Inflammatory disease of the colon, ulcerative colitis and Crohn's colitis. J. Pediatr., *86*:322–334, 1975.
107. Acheson, E.D.: Distribution of ulcerative colitis and regional enteritis in United States veterans with particular reference to the Jewish religion. Gut, *1*:261–293, 1960.
108. Achesen, E.D., and Nefzger, M.D.: Ulcerative colitis in the United States Army in 1944. Epidemiology: comparison between patients and controls. Gastroenterology, *44*:7–19, 1963.
109. Farmer, R.G., Michner, W.W., and Mortimer, E.A.: Studies of family history among patients with inflammatory bowel disease. Clin. Gastroenterol., *9*:271–278, 1980.
110. Almy, T.P., and Sherlock, P.: Genetic aspects of

ulcerative colitis and regional enteritis. Gastroenterology, 51:757–763, 1966.
111. Davidson, M., Bloom, A.A., and Lunger, M.M.: Chronic ulcerative colitis of childhood. J. Pediatr., 67:471–490, 1965.
112. Michener, W.M.: Ulcerative colitis in children; problems in management. Pediatr. Clin. N. Am., 14:159–173, 1967.
113. Doe, W.F., Booth, C.C., and Brown, D.L.: Evidence for complement-binding immune complexes in adult coeliac disease, Crohn's disease and ulcerative colitis. Lancet, 1:402–403, 1973.
114. Jewell, D.P., and MacLennan, I.C.M.: Circulating immune complexes in inflammatory bowel disease. Clin. Exp. Immunol., 14:219–226, 1979.
115. Bartlett, J.G.: Antibiotic associated pseudomembranous colitis. Rev. Infec. Dis., 1:530–539, 1979.
116. Keighly, M.R.B.: Antibiotic associated pseudomembranous colitis—pathogenesis and management. Drugs, 20:49–56, 1980.
117. Silva, J., Jr., and Fekety, R.: Clostridia and antimicrobial enterocolitis. Am. Rev. Med., 31:327–333, 1981.
118. Pierce, P.F., Jr., et al.: Antibiotic associated pseudomembranous colitis. An epidemiological investigation of a cluster of cases. J. Infect. Dis., 145:269–274, 1982.
119. Bartlett, J.G., et al.: Antibiotic-associated pseudomembranous colitis due to toxin-producing clostridia. N. Engl. J. Med., 298:531–534, 1978.
120. Bartlett, J.G., et al.: Role of *Clostridium difficile* in antibiotic-associated pseudomembranous colitis. Gastroenterology, 75:778–782, 1978.
121. Tedesco, F., et al.: Oral vancomycin for antibiotic-associated pseudomembranous colitis. Lancet, 2:226–228, 1978.
122. Keighley, M.R.B., et al.: Randomized control trial of vancomycin for pseudomembranous colitis and postoperative diarrhea. Br. Med. J., 2:1667–1669, 1978.
123. Burbige, E.J., and Milligan, F.D.: Pseudomembranous colitis-association with antibiotics and therapy with cholestyramine. J.A.M.A., 231:1157–1158, 1975.
124. Kreutzer, E.W., and Milligan, F.D.: Treatment of antibiotic-associated pseudomembranous colitis with cholestyramine resin. Johns Hopkins Med. J., 143:67–72, 1978.
125. Humphrey, C.D., et al.: Partial purification of a toxin found in hamsters with antibiotic-associated colitis. Gastroenterology, 76:468–476, 1979.
126. Farmer, R.G., and Schumacher, O.P.: Treatment of ulcerative colitis with hydrocortisone enemas—comparison of absorption and clinical response. Am. J. Gastroenterol., 54:229–236, 1970.
127. Farmer, R.G., and Schumacher, O.P.: Treatment of ulcerative colitis with hydrocortisone enemas: relationship of hydrocortisone absorption, adrenal suppression and clinical response. Dis. Colon Rectum, 13:355–361, 1970.
128. Swarbrick, E.T., Loose, H., and Lennard-Jones, J.E.: Enema volume as an important factor in successful topical corticosteroid treatment of colitis. Proc. Roy. Soc. Med., 67:753–754, 1974.
129. Wall, A.J.: The use of glucocorticoids in intestinal disease. Med. Clin. N. Am., 57:1271–1276, 1973.
130. Truelove, S.C., and Jewell, D.P.: Intensive intravenous regimen for severe attacks of ulcerative colitis. Lancet, 1:1067–1070, 1974.
131. Peppercorn, M.A., and Goldman, P.: The role of intestinal bacteria in the metabolism of salicylazosulfapyridine. J. Pharmacol. Exp. Ther., 181:550–562, 1972.
132. Klotz, U., et al.: Therapeutic efficacy of sulfasalazine and its metabolites in patients with ulcerative colitis and Crohn's disease. N. Engl. J. Med., 303:1499–1502, 1980.
133. Van Hees, P.A.M., Bakker, J.H., and Van Tongeren, J.H.M.: Effect of Sulphapyridine, 5-aminosalicylic acid and placebo in patients with idiopathic proctitis: study to determine the active therapeutic component of sulphasalazine. Gut, 21:632–635, 1980.
134. Harris, J., Archampong, E.O., and Clark, C.G.: The effect of salazopyrine on water and electrolyte transport in the human colon measured in vivo and in vitro. Gut, 13:855, 1971.
135. Schroder, H., and Cambell, D.E.S.: Absorption metabolism and excretion of salicylazosulfapyridine in man. Clin. Pharmacol. Ther., 13:539–551, 1972.
136. Das, K.M., et al.: Adverse reactions during salicylazosulfapyridine therapy and the relation with drug metabolism and acetylator phenotype. N. Engl. J. Med., 289:491–495, 1973.
137. Van Hees, P.A., et al.: Hemolysis during salicylazosulfapyridine therapy. Am. J. Gastroenterol., 70:501–505, 1979.
138. Levi, A.J., et al.: Male infertility due to sulphasalazine. Lancet, 2:276–278, 1979.
139. Reid, J., et al.: Raynaud's phenomenon induced by sulphasalizine. Postgrad. Med. J., 56:106–107, 1980.
140. Schneider, R.E., and Beeley, L.: Megaloblastic anemia associated with sulphasalazine treatment. Br. Med. J., 2:1638–1639, 1977.
141. Jewell, D.P., and Truelove, S.C.: Azathioprine in ulcerative colitis: an interim report on a controlled therapeutic trial. Br. Med. J., 1:709–712, 1972.
142. Jewell, D.P., and Truelove, S.C.: Azathioprine in ulcerative colitis: final report on a controlled therapeutic trial. Br. Med. J., 4:627–630, 1974.
143. Rosenberg, J.L., et al.: A controlled trial of azathioprine in the management of chronic ulcerative colitis. Gastroenterology, 69:96–99, 1975.
144. Caprilli, R., Carratu, T., and Babbini, M.: A double-blind comparison of the effectiveness of azathioprine and sulfasalazine in idiopathic proctocolitis: preliminary report. Am. J. Dig. Dis., 20:115–120, 1975.
145. Sacher, D.B., and Present, D.H.: Immunotherapy in inflammatory bowel disease. Med. Clin. N. Am., 62:173–183, 1978.
146. Dronfield, M.W., and Langman, M.J.S.: Comparative trial of sulphasalazine and oral sodium cromoglycate in the maintenance of remission in ulcerative colitis. Gut, 18:A973, 1977.
147. Willoughby, C.P., et al.: Comparison of disodium cromoglycate and sulphasalazine as maintenance therapy for ulcerative colitis. Lancet, 1:119–122, 1979.
148. LaMont, J.T., and Trinka, Y.M.: Therapeutic implications of *Clostridium difficile* toxin during relapse of chronic inflammatory bowel disease. Lancet, 1:381–383, 1980.
149. Finch, R.G., et al.: Relapse of pseudomembranous colitis after vancomycin therapy. Lancet, 2:1076–1077, 1980.
150. Chang, T.W., et al.: Bacitracin treatment of antibiotic-associated colitis and diarrhea caused by *Clos-*

tridium difficile toxin. Gastroenterology, *78*:1584–1586, 1980.
151. Eastwood, H.O.H.: Causes of jaundice in the elderly: a survey of diagnosis and investigation. Geront. Clin., *13*:69–81, 1971.
152. Podurgiel, B.J., et al.: Liver injury associated with methotrexate therapy for psoriasis. Mayo Clin. Proc., *48*:787–792, 1973.
153. Rumack, B.H., and Peterson, R.G.: Acetaminophen overdosage: incidence, diagnosis and management in 416 patients. Pediatrics, *62* (Suppl):898–903, 1978.
154. Russell, R.M., et al.: Hepatic injury from hypervitaminosis A resulting in portal hypertension and ascites. N. Engl. J. Med., *291*:435–440, 1974.
155. Pessayre, D., et al.: Isoniazid-rifampin fulminant hepatitis: a possible consequence of the enhancement of isoniazid hepatotoxicity by enzyme induction. Gastroenterology, *72*:284–289, 1977.
156. Rosenoer, B.M., and Tornay, A.S.: Drugs and the liver. Med. Clin. N. Am., *63*:405–412, 1979.
157. Seaman, W.E., Ishak, K.G., and Plotz, P.H.: Aspirin-induced hepatotoxicity in patients with systemic lupus erythematosus. Ann. Intern. Med., *80*:1–8, 1974.
158. Kopanoff, D.E., Snider, D.E., and Caras, G.J.: Isoniazid-related hepatitis: U.S. Public Health Service cooperative surveillance study. Am. Rev. Resp. Dis., *17*:191–201, 1978.
159. Sharp, J.R., Ishak, K.G., and Zimmerman, H.J.: Chronic active hepatitis and severe hepatic necrosis associated with nitrofurantoin. Ann. Intern. Med., *92*:14–19, 1980.
160. Moshel, M.G., Spitaels, J.M., and Kahn, F.: Short- and long-term studies of duodenal ulcer with sucralfate. J. Clin. Gastroenterol., *3* (Suppl. 2): 159–161, 1981.
161. Adams, G.D., et al.: Cimetidine or propantheline combined with antacid therapy for short-term treatment of duodenal ulcer. Dig. Dis. Sci., *27*:388–393, 1982.
162. Colin-Jones, D.G., et al.: Cimetidine and gastric cancer: preliminary report from post-marketing surveillance study. Br. Med. J., *285*:1311–1313, 1982.
163. Freston, J.W.: Cimetidine II. Adverse reactions and patterns of use. Am. Int. Med., *97*:728–734, 1982.
164. Somogyi, A., and Gualer, R.: Drug interactions with cimetidine. Clin. Pharmacokinet., *7*:23–41, 1982.
165. Berner, B.D., et al.: Ranitidine—a new H_2 receptor antagonist. Clin. Pharm., *1*:499–509, 1982.
166. Patwardhan, R.V., et al.: Cimetidine spares the glucuronidation of larazepam and oxazepam. Gastroenterology, *79*:912–916, 1980.
167. Feelay, J., Wilkinson, G.R., and Wood, A.J.: Reduction of liver blood flow and propranolol metabolism by cimetidine. N. Engl. J. Med., *304*:692–695, 1981.
168. Jensen, R.T., et al.: Cimetidine-induced impotence and breast changes in patients with gastric hypersecretory states. N. Engl. J. Med., *308*:883–887, 1983.
169. Danilewitz, M., Tim, L.O., and Hirschowitz, B.: Ranitidine suppression of gastric hypersecretion resistant to cimetidine. N. Engl. J. Med., *306*:20–22, 1982.
170. Bories, P., et al.: Use of ranitidine without mental confusion in patient with renal failure. Lancet, *2*:755, 1980.
171. Feeley, J., and Guy, E.: Ranitidine also reduces liver blood flow. Lancet, 169, Jan. 16, 1982.
172. Heagerty, A.M., and Castledon, C.M.: Failure of ranitidine to interact with propranolol. Br. Med. J., *248*:1304, 1982.
173. Colin-Jones, D.G., et al.: Post-marketing surveillance of the safety of cimetidine: 12 month mortality report. Br. Med. J., *286*:1713–1716, 1983.
174. Neidhart, J.A., et al.: Specific antiemetics for specific cancer chemotherapeutic agents. Cancer, *47*:1439–1443, 1981.
175. Gralla, R.J., et al.: Antiemetic efficacy of high dose metoclopramide-randomized trials with placebo and prochlorperazine in patients with chemotherapy induced nausea and vomiting. N. Engl. J. Med., *305*:905–909, 1981.
176. Strum, S.B., et al.: Intravenous metoclopramide. An effective antiemetic in cancer chemotherapy. J.A.M.A., *247*:2683–2686, 1982.
177. Gugler, R., Brand, M., and Somogyi, A.: Impaired cimetidine absorption due to antacids and metoclopramide. Eur. J. Clin. Pharmacol., *20*:225–228, 1981.
178. Kanto, J., et al.: The effect of metoclopramide and propantheline on the gastrointestinal absorption of cimetidine. Br. J. Clin. Pharmacol., *11*:629–632, 1981.
179. Joss, R.A., et al.: Sudden death in a cancer patient on high dose domperidone. Lancet, *1*:1019, 1982.
180. Homesley, H.D., et al.: Failure of delta-9-tetrohydrocannabinol and prochlorperazine to control chemotherapy induced nausea and vomiting. Proc. Am. Soc. Clin. Oncol., *1*:62, 1982.
181. Garb, S.: Cannabinoids in the management of severe nausea and vomiting from cancer chemotherapy. J. Clin. Pharmacol., *21*:575–595, 1981.
182. Cronin, C.M., et al.: Antiemetic effect of intramuscular levonantradol in patients receiving anti-cancer chemotherapy, J. Clin. Pharmacol., *21*:435–505, 1981.
183. Carr, N., and Schofield, P.F.: Inflammatory bowel disease in the elderly. Br. J. Surg., *69*:223–225, 1982.
184. Cimana, C.R., et al.: Beclomethasone dipropionate enemas for treating inflammatory bowel disease without producing Cushing's syndrome or hypothalamic-pituitary-adrenal suppression. Lancet, *1*:579–583, 1982.
185. Kirsher, J.B., and Shorter, R.G.: Recent developments in "nonspecific" inflammatory bowel disease. N. Engl. J. Med., *306*:775–785, 1982.
186. Korelitz, B.I., et al.: Desensitization to sulfasalazine in allergic patients: an important therapeutic modality. Gastroenterology, *82*:1104, 1982.
187. Anon.: Ranitidine (Zantac). Med. Letter, *24*:111–113, 1982.

CHAPTER 7

INFECTIOUS DISEASES IN THE ELDERLY

Harry A. Gallis

Infectious illnesses account for a significant number of acute and chronic medical problems in the elderly. In the individual who is already compromised by one or more chronic debilitating diseases, infection may be seen with increased frequency and may result in the patient's demise. In some instances this may be the welcome terminal event; however, frequently infection may interrupt an otherwise useful and happy existence. The judicious use of antimicrobial drugs therefore is a necessary part of the geriatrician's therapeutic tools. This chapter discusses some of the effects of aging on the pharmacokinetics of antimicrobial drugs, the general indications for the use of certain drugs, and aspects of the presentation and treatment of infections as they apply to the elderly individual.

THE USE OF ANTIMICROBIAL DRUGS IN THE ELDERLY

The pharmacokinetics of several classes of drugs have been studied in elderly individuals; however, the information available about antibiotics is certainly not comprehensive. Several generalizations may be made with regard to the absorption, distribution, metabolism, and excretion of antibiotics (see also Chapter 2).

There are no known significant alterations in the rate or extent of gastrointestinal absorption of antimicrobial drugs in the elderly, even in the presence of achlorhydria. Changes in body composition, such as an increase in the proportion of body fat, which normally occurs in the elderly, could theoretically lead to the accumulation of lipid soluble drugs or lead to excessive levels of drugs that are not lipid soluble. There are no known clinical implications of these phenomena. The normal decrease in serum albumin levels with age does not appreciably alter the distribution or metabolism of such drugs as benzylpenicillin or sulfadiazine. Decreased regional blood flow secondary to vascular disease or congestive heart failure could have a significant effect on the metabolism of drugs by the liver or on renal excretion of drugs and their metabolites.

Although there have been no significant studies of age related changes in the hepatic metabolism of antibiotics, there are extensive data relating to renal excretion. It is well known that renal function, as measured by the glomerular filtration rate (GFR) and the renal blood flow, decreases with age. For instance, the average creatinine clearance rate normally decreases from 123 to 65 ml. per min. or less from age 20 to 95. This may be predicted by the formula, $GFR = 153 - 0.96 \times age$. Numerous disease processes may accelerate the loss of renal function. In addition, renal blood flow normally decreases by approximately 50 per cent over the same span. Other useful formulas for calculating the creatinine clearance that take the serum creatinine level into account are as follows:

1. Creatinine clearance (female value = 90% of male value)* $= \dfrac{98 - (0.8\,[\text{age in years} - 20])}{\text{Serum creatinine level (mg./dl.)}}$

2. Creatinine clearance (female value = 90% of male value)* $= \dfrac{98 - 16\left(\dfrac{\text{age} - 20}{20}\right)}{\text{Serum creatinine level (mg./dl.)}}$

3. Creatinine clearance (female value = 85% of male value)* $= \dfrac{140 - \text{age}}{\text{Serum creatinine level (mg./dl.)}}$

4. Creatinine clearance* $= \dfrac{24\text{ hour urine creatinine level (mg.)} \times 100}{\text{Serum creatinine level (mg./dl.)} \times 1440}$

5. Creatinine clearance* $= \dfrac{\text{Wt.(kg.)} \times (140 - \text{age in years})}{\text{Serum creatinine level (mg./dl.)} \times 72}$

TABLE 7–1. Classification of Renal Impairment by Creatinine Clearance

	Creatinine Clearance (ml./min.)
Mild impairment	40-70
Moderate impairment	20-40
Severe impairment	5-20
Anuria	< 5

The nomogram shown in Figure 7–1 is useful for rapidly evaluating endogenous creatinine clearance.

Renal impairment is usually classified as shown in Table 7–1.

Thus, in the elderly individual with a normal serum creatinine value, there may be a significant decrease in the glomerular filtration rate, since creatinine production decreases with age and declining muscle mass. This information indicates that drugs excreted primarily by the kidney should not be administered to the elderly without some estimation of renal function and appropriate modification of dosage, especially when considering nephrotoxic and ototoxic antibiotics such as the aminoglycosides.

Table 7–2 presents a compilation of selected pharmacokinetic and dosage information relevant to treating infectious diseases in the elderly. The prescriber should be alert to proper dosing in view of the pharmacokinetic characteristics of each drug and the problems unique to each patient. Specific guidelines for the administration of each antibiotic are presented under the review of each class of drugs. Table 7–3 presents a compilation of some of

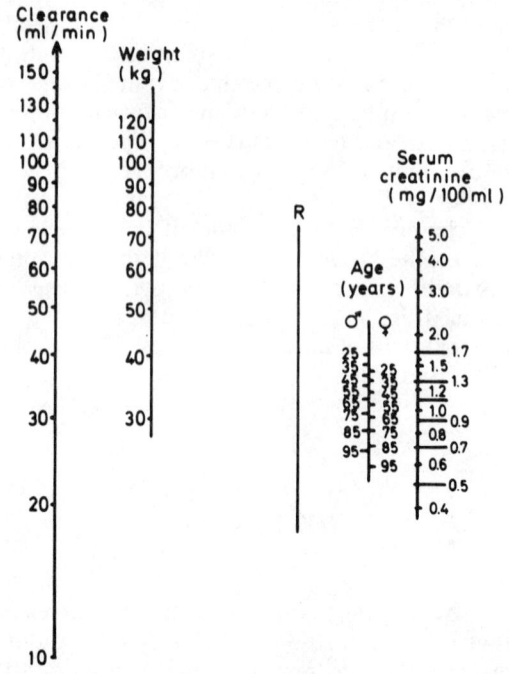

Figure 7–1. Nomogram for rapid evaluation of endogenous creatinine clearance. With a ruler, join weight to age, keeping the ruler at the crossing point of the line marked R. Then move the right hand side of the ruler to the appropriate serum creatinine value and read the creatinine clearance value from the left side of the nomogram. (From Siersback-Nielson, K., et al.: Rapid evaluation of creatinine clearance. Lancet, 1:1133, 1971.)

*Creatinine clearance values in ml. per min. per 1.73 sq. m. of body surface area.

TABLE 7–2. Selected Pharmacokinetic and Dosage Information for Antibiotics

Drug	Oral	Intra-muscular	Intra-venous	Normal $T_{1/2}$ (Hours)	Normal Dosing Interval (Hours)	Primary Route of Excretion	Adjustment for Renal Failure	Usual Daily Dosage
Penicillin G	+	+	+	0.5	4–8	Renal	↓ Dose	Varies
Penicillin V	+	–	–	0.5	6	Renal	↑ Interval, ↓ dose	1–2 gm.
Methicillin	–	+	+	0.5	4	Renal	↑ Interval	8–12 gm.
Nafcillin	+	+	+	0.5	4–6	Hepatic	None	8–12 gm.
Oxacillin	+	+	+	0.4	4–6	Renal	None	8–12 gm.
Cloxacillin	+	–	–	0.5	6	Hepatic	None	1–2 gm.
Dicloxacillin	+	–	–	0.5–0.9	6	Renal	None	1–2 gm.
Ampicillin	+	+	+	1.5	6	Renal	↑ Interval	1–12 gm.
Amoxicillin	+	–	–	0.9–2.3	8	Renal	↑ Interval	1–2 gm.
Carbenicillin	+	+	+	1.5	4	Renal	↓ Dose, ↑ interval	20–30 gm.
Ticarcillin	–	+	+	1.0–1.5	4–6	Renal	↓ Dose, ↑ interval	15–20 gm.
Bacampicillin	+	–	–	—	12	Renal	↑ Interval	0.8–1.6 gm.
Mezlocillin	–	+	+	1.0	4–6	Renal	↓ Dose, ↑ interval	Varies (no more than 24 gm./day)
Piperacillin	–	+	+	1.0	4–6	Renal	↓ Dose, ↑ interval	Varies (no more than 24 gm./day)
Azlocillin	–	–	+	1.0	4–6	Renal	↓ Dose, ↑ interval	Varies (no more than 24 gm./day)
Tetracycline	+	+	+	7–11	6	Renal, hepatic	↓ Dose, ↑ interval	1–2 gm.
Oxytetracycline	+	–	+	9	6–12	Renal, hepatic	↓ Dose, ↑ interval	1–2 gm.
Doxycycline	+	–	+	14–25	12–24	Renal, hepatic	None	100–200 mg.
Minocycline	+	–	+	12–15	12	Renal, hepatic	↓ Dose	100–200 mg.
Methacycline	+	–	–	6–10	6	Renal, hepatic	↓ Dose	600 mg.
Demeclocycline	+	–	–	6–10	6	Renal, hepatic	↓ Dose	600 mg.
Chloramphenicol	+	+	+	1.6–3.3	6	Renal (metabolites)	None	2–6 gm.
Erythromycin	+	–	+	1.2–2.6	6	Hepatic	None	1–2 gm.
Lincomycin	+	+	+	4–5	6	Hepatic	↓ Dose	1–2 gm.
Clindamycin	+	+	+	2.0–2.5	6	Hepatic	None	1.2–2.4 gm.
Vancomycin	–	–	+	6–8	6	Renal	↑ Interval	2 gm.
Gentamicin	–	+	+	2	8	Renal	↑ Interval	3–5 mg./kg.
Tobramycin	–	+	+	2.5	8	Renal	↑ Interval	3–5 mg./kg.
Kanamycin	–	+	+	2.0–3.0	8–12	Renal	↑ Interval	15 mg./kg.
Amikacin	–	+	+	2.0–2.5	8–12	Renal	↑ Interval	15 mg./kg.
Streptomycin	–	+	–	2.5	12	Renal	↑ Interval	15–30 mg./kg.
Netilmicin	–	+	+	2.0–2.5	8–12	Renal	↓ Dose, ↑ interval	3–4 mg./kg.
Cefoperazone	–	+	+	1.6–2.1	12	Hepatic, Renal	↓ Dose	2–4 gm.
Cephalothin	–	+	+	0.5–0.9	6	Renal	↓ Dose	6–12 gm.
Cephapirin	–	+	+	0.3–0.6	6	Renal	Minimal	4–8 gm.
Cephradine	+	+	+	0.8–2.0	6	Renal	↓ Dose, ↑ interval	4–8 gm.
Cefazolin	–	+	+	1.5–2.2	8	Renal	↓ Dose, ↑ interval	2–4 gm.
Cefoxitin	–	+	+	0.7–1.0	6–8	Renal	↓ Dose, ↑ interval	4–8 gm.
Cefamandole	–	+	+	0.5–1.0	4–6	Renal	↓ Dose, ↑ interval	4–8 gm.
Cephalexin	+	+	–	0.5–1.2	6	Renal	Minimal	1–2 gm.
Cefaclor	+	+	–	0.6–1.0	8	Renal	Minimal	1.5–2.0 gm.
Cefadroxil	+	–	–	1.1–1.4	8–12	Renal	↑ Interval	1.0–1.5 gm.
Cefotaxime	–	+	+	1.0	6–8	Renal	↓ Dose	6–12 gm.
Moxalactam	–	+	+	1.8–2.0	8–12	Renal	↓ Dose, ↑ interval	4–12 gm.
Amphotericin B	–	–	+	12–24	24	Renal?	None	0.3–0.5 mg./kg.
Flucytosine	+	–	–	6	6	Renal	↓ Dose	75–150 mg./kg.
Miconazole	–	–	+	20–24	6 8	Hepatic	None	1.2–3.6 gm.
Isoniazid	+	+	+	1.5–3.0	24	Hepatic	None	5–10 mg./kg.
Ethambutol	+	–	–	8	24	Renal	↓ Dose	15 mg./kg.
Rifampin	+	–	–	3	24	Hepatic	None	600 mg.

TABLE 7-3. Selected Adverse Drug Interactions with Antimicrobial Drugs

Penicillins			
Ampicillin	Allopurinol[1]—increased incidence of skin rash		
Carbenicillin, Ticarcillin	Aminoglycosides[1]—decreased aminoglycoside activity in renal failure		
Cephalosporins			
Cephalothin	Aminoglycosides[1]—increased nephrotoxicity		
Cefamandole Cefoperazone Cefaclor Moxalactam	Alcohol-disulfiram-like effect		
Aminoglycosides	Cephaloridine,[2] cephalothin,[2] polymyxins[2]—increased nephrotoxicity Ethacrynic acid[2]—increased ototoxicity Curare-like drugs[2]—neuromuscular blockade Carbenicillin, ticarcillin[1]—decreased aminoglycoside activity		
Neomycin (oral)	Digoxin, penicillin V[3]—decreased digoxin and penicillin levels Warfarin[4]—increased anticoagulant effect		
Chloramphenicol	Warfarin[5]—increased anticoagulant effect Orally administered hypoglycemics[5]—increased hypoglycemia Phenytoin[5]—increased phenytoin toxicity Barbiturates[6]—decreased chloramphenicol levels		
Tetracyclines	Antacids, iron, kaolin, pectin, bismuth[3]—decreased tetracycline levels Barbiturates, carbamazepine[5]—decreased tetracycline activity Methoxyflurane[1]—increased nephrotoxicity		
Clindamycin, lincomycin	Kaolin-pectin[3]—decreased peak level		
Rifampin	Warfarin,[6] orally administered contraceptives,[7] corticosteroids,[6] tolbutamide[6]—decreased anticoagulation, contraceptive, corticosteroid, and hypoglycemic effects, respectively		
Isoniazid	Alcohol[1]—increased hepatotoxicity Aluminum antacids[3]—decreased isoniazid effect Phenytoin[5]—increased phenytoin effect Disulfiram[8]—psychosis, ataxia		
Aminosalicylic acid	Probenecid[9]—increased PAS toxicity Diphenhydramine[3]—decreased PAS effect		
Amphotericin B	Digitalis[10]—digitalis toxicity		
Griseofulvin	Warfarin[6]—decreased anticoagulant effect		
Nalidixic acid	Warfarin[11]—increased anticoagulant effect		
Sulfonamides	Warfarin[11]—increased anticoagulant effect Phenytoin[11]—increased phenytoin toxicity Orally administered hypoglycemics[1]—increased hypoglycemia Methotrexate[11]—increased methotrexate toxicity		
Polymyxins	Aminoglycosides[2]—increased nephrotoxicity Curare-like drugs[2]—neuromuscular blockade		

Mechanisms:
[1] Unknown.
[2] Additive effect.
[3] Inhibition of absorption.
[4] Decreased vitamin K synthesis.
[5] Inhibition of microsomal enzymes.
[6] Induction of microsomal enzymes.
[7] Increased metabolism.
[8] Altered disulfiram metabolism.
[9] Decreased renal excretion.
[10] Hypokalemia.
[11] Displacement from binding sites.

the more commonly occurring and clinically significant drug-drug interactions seen with antimicrobial drugs.

ANTIMICROBIAL DRUGS

The following sections deal with the major groups of antibiotics. For more detailed information the reader is directed to textbooks that deal solely with antibiotics and the therapy of specific infectious diseases.[1-3] This chapter attempts to deal primarily with the properties of these drugs that pertain in particular to the elderly.

Penicillins

Classically the penicillins have been of greatest use in the treatment of infections due to gram positive organisms (staphylococci, streptococci, pneumococcus, and clostridia) and in gonorrhea, syphilis, and meningococcal disease. Clinical modifications (semisynthetic penicillins) have extended the spectrum to include penicillinase producing staphylococci, gram negative enteric organisms, Pseudomonas, Hemophilus, and Bacteroides.

The penicillins may be divided into two large groups, the natural penicillins and the semisynthetic penicillins. The most important natural penicillins are penicillin G, penicillin V (phenoxymethyl), and benzathine penicillin. The semisynthetics include ampicillin, amoxicillin, bacampicillin, carbenicillin, ticarcillin, mezlocillin, piperacillin, azlocillin, and the penicillinase resistant penicillins (methicillin, nafcillin, oxacillin, cloxacillin, and dicloxacillin). Table 7-4 lists selected characteristics of the penicillins.

Penicillin G is unstable at low pH levels, and thus a majority of the drug is destroyed by gastric acid when it is administered orally. Approximately 15 per cent is absorbed, resulting in peaks of approximately 0.6 µg. per ml. after a 250 mg. (400,000 units) dose. The more acid stable penicillins are therefore preferred for oral use. Intramuscular doses generally result in 10-fold higher blood levels than orally administered penicillin G, while the procaine salt delays absorption from muscle and produces more prolonged blood levels (peaks at two hours with low levels at 24 hours). The benzathine salt, which is poorly soluble in water, produces very low but extremely prolonged (three to four weeks) blood levels after a single intramuscular injection. Penicillin V is acid stable and produces serum peaks of 1.5 to 2.0 µg. per ml. following a 250 mg. oral dose. The potassium salt is better absorbed than the sodium salt. Penicillin G derivatives and penicillin V are primarily used in the treatment of infections caused by streptococci, pneumococci, meningococci, spirochetes, and anaerobes (excluding *Bacteroides fragilis*). Penicillin G is more active against gonococci and meningococci than is penicillin V.

The semisynthetic penicillins include the penicillinase resistant group (methicillin, nafcillin, cloxacillin, dicloxacillin, and oxacillin), the aminopenicillins (ampicillin, bacampicillin, amoxicillin), and the anti-pseudomonas penicillins (carbenicillin, indanylcarbenicillin, mezlocillin, piperacillin, azlocillin, and ticarcillin). The penicillinase resistant drugs are used primarily in the treatment of staphylococcal infections (80 per cent of *Staph. aureus* organisms produce penicillinase). The aminopenicillins are particularly useful against Hemophilus, gonococci, some gram negative organisms (*E. coli, Proteus mirabilis,* Salmonella, Shigella), and enterococci. The anti-pseudomonas penicillins have particular activity against many strains of *Pseudomonas aeruginosa, E. coli,* and Proteus but particularly Pseudomonas, especially when the penicillin is combined with an aminoglycoside. As in all other infections, the final choice of penicillins should be determined by the organism isolated and the in vitro sensitivity pattern when applicable (Table 7-5).

The penicillins are generally nontoxic drugs, except in the circumstances of allergies, prolonged therapy, and high dose therapy. Allergic manifestations include immediate hypersensitivity (anaphylaxis with bronchospasm, urticaria, angioedema, shock) and delayed reactions (other rashes, serum sick-

TABLE 7-4. Selected Characteristics of the Penicillins*

	Penicillinase Resistant	Acid Stable	% Protein Bound
Penicillin G	No	No	60
Acid stable			
Penicillin V	No	Yes	80
Penicillinase resistant			
Methicillin	Yes	No	40
Nafcillin	Yes	Yes	90
Oxacillin	Yes	Yes	90
Cloxacillin	Yes	Yes	93–95
Dicloxacillin	Yes	Yes	96
Ampicillins			
Ampicillin	No	Yes	20
Hetacillin	No	Yes	20
Bacampicillin	No	Yes	20
Amoxicillin	No	Yes	20
Cyclacillin	No	Yes	20
Extended spectrum			
Carbenicillin	No	Yes†	50
Ticarcillin	No	No	45
Mezlocillin	No	No	16–42
Piperacillin	No	No	16

*Reprinted with permission from Facts and Comparisons, 1983, p. 328.
†Indanyl derivative.

TABLE 7-5. Spectrum of Action of Penicillins

Penicillin G	Streptococci, pneumococcus, meningococcus, gonococcus, spirochetes, Listeria, anaerobes (except *Bacteroides fragilis*)
Penicillin V	Streptococci (except enterococcus), pneumococcus
Ampicillin, Bacampicillin, Amoxicillin	Same as penicillin G, in addition to Salmonella, Shigella, Hemophilus, *Proteus mirabilis,* and some *E. coli*
Methicillin Nafcillin, Oxacillin	Penicillinase producing staphylococci, streptococci (except enterococcus), pneumococcus
Azlocillin, Carbenicillin, Mezlocillin, Piperacillin, Ticarcillin	All penicillin G sensitive organisms, in addition to *Proteus mirabilis* and some *E. coli,* Pseudomonas, Enterobacter, Serratia, and *B. fragilis*

TABLE 7-6. General Guidelines for Modification of Antibiotic Dosing in Renal Failure

Dosing greatly altered—drug levels should be monitored
   Aminoglycosides, vancomycin, flucytosine

Dosing moderately altered—drug toxicities low, use nomograms when available
   Cephalosporins
      Minimal dose reduction—cephalothin, cefoperazone, cephapirin, cephalexin, cefaclor
      Moderate dose reduction—cefamandole, cefazolin, cefoxitin, cephradine, cefadroxil, cefotaxime and moxalactam
   Penicillins
      Minimal dose reduction—ampicillin, amoxicillin, methicillin, oxacillin
      Moderate dose reduction—penicillin G, carbenicillin, ticarcillin, mezlocillin, piperacillin, azlocillin
   Miscellaneous
      Doxycycline, minocycline, ethambutol, trimethoprim-sulfamethoxazole and other sulfonamides

No alterations necessary
   Amphotericin B, miconazole
   Isoniazid, rifampin
   Chloramphenicol, clindamycin, erythromycin
   Cloxacillin, dicloxacillin, oxacillin, nafcillin

Avoid with glomerular filtration rate less than 25 ml./min.
   Nitrofurantoin, methenamine mandelate, nalidixic acid, tetracyclines (except doxycycline), sulfonamides

---

ness, erythema nodosum). Interstitial nephritis and Coombs positive hemolytic anemia may occur during prolonged high dose therapy. Evidence of neurotoxicity (confusion, hyperreflexia, muscle irritability, myoclonus, seizures, and coma) may be seen after rapid infusions or excessively high doses, especially in the setting of meningitis (with increased central nervous system permeability). Reversible bone marrow suppression with pancytopenia also may be observed. Platelet dysfunction may be induced by carbenicillin, as well as hypokalemic alkalosis secondary to chelation of potassium and hydrogen during excretion.

The natural penicillins are excreted primarily by the kidney, 10 per cent by glomerular filtration and 90 per cent by tubular secretion; the latter may be inhibited by probenecid. Table 7-6 provides some general guidelines for modifying antibiotic doses in renal failure. Carbenicillin, ticarcillin, mezlocillin, piperacillin, and azlocillin should be given in decreased doses in renal insufficiency (Table 7-7), and doses of penicillin G and ampicillin should be modified only in severe renal insufficiency (glomerular filtration rate less than 10 ml. per min.), i.e., maximal daily doses of 10 million units and 2 to 4 g., respectively. Dosages of oxacillin, cloxacillin, dicloxacillin, and nafcillin, which are metabolized primarily by the liver, do not require modification in severe renal insufficiency. The dosing interval for methicillin, however, should be doubled under these circumstances.

Other considerations in the elderly are the sodium and potassium content of the various penicillins, which may aggravate congestive heart failure or hyperkalemia in the patient with diabetes or renal failure. Carbenicillin contains 5.28 mEq. of sodium per gram and ticarcillin, 5.2 mEq. of sodium per gram; mezlocillin, 1.85 mEq. per gram; piperacillin, 1.98 mEq. per gram; oxacillin, nafcillin, methicillin, and ampicillin, approximately 3 mEq. per gram; and sodium penicillin G, approximately 2 mEq. per million units. The potassium salt of penicillin G contains 1.7 mEq. of potassium and 0.3 mEq. of sodium per million units. Carbenicillin and ticarcillin may produce

TABLE 7-7. Dosage Guidelines for Use of Mezlocillin, Piperacillin, Azlocillin, Ticarcillin, and Carbenicillin in Adults with Impaired Renal Function*

Mezlocillin

Creatinine Clearance (ml./min.)	Urinary Tract Infection		Serious Systemic Infection
	Uncomplicated	*Complicated*	
>30		Usual recommended dosage	
10–30	1.5 gm. every 8 hours	1.5 gm. every 6 hours	3 gm. every 8 hours
<10	1.5 gm. every 8 hours	1.5 gm. every 8 hours	2 gm. every 8 hours

Piperacillin

Creatinine Clearance (ml./min.)	Urinary Tract Infection		Serious Systemic Infection
	Uncomplicated	*Complicated*	
>40		No adjustment	
20–40	No adjustment	9 gm./day (3 gm. every 8 hours)	12 gm./day (4 gm. every 8 hours)
<20	6 gm./day (3 gm. every 12 hours)	6 gm./day (3 gm. every 12 hours)	8 gm./day (4 gm. every 12 hours)
Patient on hemodialysis	Hemodialysis removes 30 to 50% of piperacillin in 4 hours; 1 gm. additional dose should be administered following each dialysis period		6 gm./day (2 gm. every 8 hours)

Azlocillin

Creatinine Clearance (ml./min.)	Half-life (hours)	Urinary Tract Infection		Serious Systemic Infection
		Uncomplicated	*Complicated*	
>80	1		Usual recommended dose	
30–79	2			
10–30	4	1.5 gm. every 12 hours	1.5 gm. every 8 hours	2 gm. every 8 hours
<10	6	1.5 gm. every 12 hours	2.0 gm. every 12 hours	3 gm. every 12 hours

Ticarcillin

The half-life of ticarcillin in patients with renal failure is approximately 13 hours. The initial loading dose should be 3 gm. IV followed by IV doses as indicated below:

Creatinine Clearance (ml./min.)	IV Dose and Frequency
>60	3 gm. every 4 hours
30–60	2 gm. every 4 hours
10–30	2 gm. every 8 hours
<10	2 gm. every 12 hours
<10 with hepatic dysfunction	2 gm. every 24 hours

Carbenicillin

The serum half-life of carbenicillin in severe renal insufficiency is approximately 12 hours. Dosages of 2 gm. IV every 8 to 12 hours usually yield serum levels of approximately 100 mcg./ml. and few adverse effects.

*Reprinted with permission from Facts and Comparisons, 1983, pp. 336g, j. l. r.

hypokalemia through the binding of potassium during excretion by the kidney.

Serious hypersensitivity reactions have been reported. Anaphylactic reactions are more probable following parenteral administration. Less severe manifestations of hypersensitivity involve the skin and mucous membranes. Dermal allergic symptoms generally respond well to antihistamines, corticosteroids (topical or systemic administration), and discontinuation of the penicillin. For more severe allergic reactions, emergency measures may require the use of epinephrine, aminophylline, oxygen, intravenously administered steroids, and airway management. Ampicillin rashes are seen with increased frequency in patients with renal insufficiency and are correlated with a significant increase in peak levels.

High doses of penicillin G, ticarcillin, carbenicillin, and the extended spectrum penicillins (azlocillin, mezlocillin, piperacillin) may cause bleeding disorders through decreased platelet aggregation and decreased thrombus formation. Patients with renal impairment, in whom excretion of these drugs is delayed, should be observed closely for signs of an increased bleeding tendency and decreased platelet aggregation. Upon withdrawal of the drug, bleeding abnormalities revert to normal.

Gastrointestinal side effects may be associated with oral use and include glossitis, stomatitis, sore mouth, black tongue, altered taste, diarrhea, flatulence, nausea, and vomiting. Rarely a patient may manifest transient elevations of the SGOT, SGPT, and LDH levels.

Hematologic toxicity may occur rarely as anemia, hemolytic anemia, thrombocytopenia, eosinophilia, leukopenia, neutropenia, and agranulocytosis. These reactions are believed to be allergic in origin and are usually reversible upon discontinuation of the penicillin.

Neurotoxicity may occur with very high serum levels. Symptoms of neurotoxicity may include lethargy, depression, combativeness, hallucinations, anxiety, confusion, asterixis, and seizures. These symptoms may be hard to differentiate in the elderly. Headache and dizziness have also been reported.

Other side effects include oral, vaginal, or rectal moniliasis, fever, pain at the injection site, deep vein thrombosis, and thrombophlebitis after intravenous administration. Interstitial nephritis is rare and most often is associated with high doses of methicillin.

Probenecid blocks the renal tubular secretion of the penicillins and may prolong the duration of penicillin activity. Carbenicillin, ticarcillin, mezlocillin, piperacillin, and azlocillin may be synergistic with the aminoglycoside antibiotics in the treatment of Pseudomonas infections. Ampicillin may cause false positive urine glucose results with Clinitest.

For relatively minor infections (impetigo, pharyngitis, furunculosis, cellulitis, some pneumonias, gonorrhea, and urinary tract infections), the penicillins may be given orally and should be given on an empty stomach. Penicillin V and amoxicillin are generally the best absorbed drugs. For more serious infections, such as endocarditis, meningitis, and septicemias, treatment should be given intramuscularly or intravenously. Penicillin G, ampicillin, methicillin, and carbenicillin produce the highest cerebrospinal fluid levels in patients with meningitis (15 to 40 per cent of serum levels). Therapy should be guided by the etiologic agent and sensitivity testing, as well as cost considerations in some instances.

Table 7–8, which includes 10 beta-lactam antibiotics (five penicillins and five cephalosporins), indicates the relative wholesale cost of antimicrobials often used to treat serious infections. The cost of these drugs, when marked up, is substantial and is increased by the charges made for intravenous fluid vehicles, administration sets, and, in some instances, infusion pumps. Often the expensive beta-lactam antibiotics offer no therapeutic advantage over much less expensive penicillins and cephalosporins that have been used suc-

TABLE 7–8. Cost to the Pharmacy for One Day of Therapy with Each of 10 Beta-lactam Antibiotics*

Drug	Cost per Gram ($)	Daily Dose (g)†	Cost ($)/Day of Therapy
Cefazolin	6.00	3	18.00
Cephalothin	5.00	4	20.00
Cefamandole	6.00	6	36.00
Cefoxitin	7.00	6	42.00
Ticarcillin	3.00	18	54.00
Carbenicillin	2.00	30	60.00
Mezlocillin	4.00	16	64.00
Piperacillin	4.00	16	64.00
Cefotaxime	11.00	6	66.00
Moxalactam	12.00	6	72.00

*Cost estimate is based on average wholesale price (McKesson Econofiche Price Data, February 1982).

†Based on a representative medium range dose of each antibiotic.

cessfully for years. The physician must guard against subordinating acquired knowledge and clinical experience to Madison Avenue marketing tactics.

Cephalosporins

The cephalosporins comprise a large group of broad spectrum antibiotics that are closely related to the penicillins.[4-7] These antibiotics are effective against gram positive (staphylococci, streptococci, and pneumococci) and many gram negative organisms (*E. coli*, Klebsiella, *Proteus mirabilis*). Newer derivatives show increased activity against Enterobacter, indole positive Proteus, Hemophilus (cefamandole), Serratia, and *Bacteroides fragilis* (cefoxitin, cefoperazone). They are effective in the treatment of pneumonias, soft tissue infections, peritonitis, endocarditis, septicemias, osteomyelitis, and urinary tract infections due to susceptible organisms. With the exception of moxalactam they are not effective in meningitis (poor cerebrospinal fluid penetration). These antibiotics are resistant to staphylococcal penicillinase and thus represent excellent second line drugs in some penicillin allergic patients, but they should be avoided or used with care in patients with a history of immediate hypersensitivity. In addition, because of their broad spectrum of activity, bactericidal action, and low toxicity, these drugs have been favored by surgeons for prophylaxis when those regimens are indicated.

There are numerous preparations of these drugs that can be administered intramuscularly, intravenously, or orally (see Table 7–2). The prototype drug, cephalothin, has been used in the broadest group of infections. It has an excellent record of low toxicity (except perhaps in combination with aminoglycosides) and efficacy. Disadvantages include a short half-life and a moderate incidence of phlebitis. Cefazolin has the advantages of higher blood levels, a longer half-life, and intramuscular administration. The newer drugs, cefamandole, cefotaxime, moxalactam, cefoperazone, and cefoxitin, have the advantage of a broader spectrum. There are several oral preparations (cephalexin, cephradine, cefaclor, cefadroxil) that variously have the advantage of good patient tolerance, good serum levels, and less frequent dosing (cefaclor, cefadroxil).

Peak serum levels after 500 mg. doses of the orally administered drugs range from 5 to 10 µg. per ml., and the parenterally administered drugs produce levels of 10 to 100 µg. per ml. with similar doses. These drugs are excreted primarily unchanged by renal tubular secretion, similar to penicillin G. Alterations in dosage in renal failure vary from drug to drug (see Tables 7–2 and 7–6). In general, cephalothin and cefoperazone require the least adjustment and cefazolin the most.

Doses of parenteral cephalosporins in renal failure are variable. With cephradine the usual adult dosage is 2.0 to 4.0 gm. per day in equally divided doses four times daily. With renal impairment the loading dose is 750 mg. and the maintenance dose is 500 mg. every six to 12 hours if the creatinine clearance is more than 20 ml. per min., every 12 to 24 hours if the clearance is 15 to 19 ml. per min., every 24 to 40 hours if the clearance is 10 to 14 ml. per min., every 40 to 50 hours if the clearance is 5 to 9 ml. per min., and every 50 to 70 hours if the clearance is less than 5 ml. per min.

With cephapirin the usual parenteral dosage is 500 mg. to 1.0 gm. every four to six hours. Patients with reduced renal function of moderate severity or a serum creatinine level above 5 mg. per dl. should be treated with 7.5 to 15 mg. per kg. every 12 hours.

The usual adult dosage of cephalothin is 500 mg. to 1.0 gm. every four to six hours. Life threatening infections may require up to 12 gm. daily. When renal function is impaired, an intravenous loading dose of 1.0 to 2.0 gm. may be given, with the maintenance dose determined by the severity of the infection, the susceptibility of the organism, and the degree of renal dysfunction. The maximal maintenance dosage of cephalothin is 2.0 gm. every six hours if the creatinine clearance is 50 to 80 ml. per min., 1.5 gm. every six hours if the clearance is 25 to 50 ml. per min., 1.0 gm. every six hours if the clearance is 10 to 25 ml. per min., 0.5 gm. every six hours if the clearance is 2 to 10 ml. per min., and 0.5 gm. every eight hours if the clearance is less than 2.0 ml. per min.

The usual daily dosage of cefazolin to treat moderate to severe infections is 500 mg. to 1.0 gm. given three to four times daily. Occasionally 12 gm. per day may be necessary. Cefazolin is not readily excreted in patients with impaired renal function. After a 500 mg. loading dose, renally impaired patients should receive cefazolin on the following basis: If the creatinine clearance is 40 to 70 ml. per min., administer 250 to 500 mg. (mild to moderate infection) and 500 to 1250 mg. (severe infection) every 12 hours; if the clearance is 20 to 40 ml. per min., administer 125 to 250 mg. (mild to moderate infection) and 250 to 600 mg. (severe infection) every 12 hours; if the clearance is 5 to 20 ml. per min., administer 75 to 150 mg. (mild to moderate infection) and 150 to 400 mg. (severe infection) every 24 hours; if the clearance is less than 5.0 ml. per min., administer 37.5 to 75 mg. (mild to moderate infection) and 75 to 200 mg. (severe infection) every 24 hours.

The usual dosage range for cefamandole is 500 mg. to 1.0 gm. three to six times daily. In life threatening infections, dosages up to 2.0 gm. every four hours may be required. When renal function is impaired, a loading dose of 1.0 to 2.0 gm. may be administered, and the following maintenance dosage schedule should be followed: If the creatinine clearance is greater than 80 ml. per min., administer 1.0 to 2.0 gm. every six hours (mild to moderate infection) and 2.0 gm. every four hours (severe infection); if the clearance is 50 to 80 ml. per min., administer 0.75 to 1.5 gm. every six hours (mild to moderate infection) and 1.5 gm. every four hours or 2.0 gm. every six hours (severe infection); if the clearance is 25 to 50 ml. per min., administer 0.75 to 1.5 gm. every eight hours (mild to moderate infection) and 1.5 gm. every six hours or 2.0 gm. every eight hours (severe infection); if the clearance is 10 to 25 ml. per min., administer 0.5 to 1.0 gm. every eight hours (mild to moderate infection) and 1.0 gm. every six hours or 1.25 gm. every eight hours (severe infection); if the clearance is 2 to 10 ml. per min., administer 0.5 to 0.75 gm. every 12 hours (mild to moderate infection) or 0.67 gm. every eight hours or 1.0 gm. every 12 hours (severe infection); if the clearance is less than 2.0 ml. per min., administer 0.25 to 0.5 gm. every 12 hours (mild to moderate infection) and 0.5 gm. every eight hours or 0.75 gm. every 12 hours (severe infection).

A dual mechanism of excretion (hepatic and renal) enables cefoperazone to be administered in usual doses to patients with hepatic or renal impairment. If renal as well as hepatic failure exists, serum levels should be monitored. The usual adult dosage is 1.0 to 2.0 gm. every 12 hours. In severe infections the daily dosage may be increased to 6 to 12 gm. per day.

The usual adult dosage range for cefoxitin is 1.0 to 2.0 gm. three to four times daily. In patients with impaired renal function an initial loading dose of 1.0 to 2.0 gm. may be given. The following maintenance dosage schedule should be followed in patients with impaired renal function: If the creatinine clearance is 30 to 50 ml. per min., administer 1.0 to 2.0 gm. every eight to 12 hours; if the clearance is 10 to 29 ml. per min., administer 1.0 to 2.0 gm. every 12 to 24 hours; if the clearance is 5 to 9 ml. per min., administer 0.5 to 1.0 gm. every 12 to 24 hours; if the clearance is less than 5.0 ml. per min., administer 0.5 to 1.0 gm. every 24 to 48 hours.

The usual adult dosage range for cefotaxime is 1.0 gm. three to four times daily. The maximal daily dosage should not exceed 12 gm. In patients in whom the creatinine clearance value is less than 20 ml. per min. per 1.73 sq. m., the dosage should be reduced by 50 per cent.

The usual adult dosage range for moxalactam is 2 to 6 gm. daily in divided doses every eight hours. In renal dysfunction a loading dose of 1.0 to 2.0 gm. may be administered. The following maintenance dosage schedule should be followed in patients with impaired renal function: If the creatinine clearance is 50 to 80 ml. per min., administer 0.5 to 3.0 gm. every eight hours; if the clearance is 25 to 50 ml. per min., administer 0.25 to 3.0 gm. every 12 hours; if the clearance is 2 to 25 ml. per min., administer 0.25 to 1.0 gm. every eight hours; if the clearance is less than 2.0 ml. per min., administer 0.25 to 1.0 gm. every 12 to 24 hours.

Adverse reactions to the cephalosporins include hypersensitivity (skin rashes and anaphylaxis). Allergic reactions may be seen in 5 to 10 per cent of known penicillin allergic patients. Controversy exists as to whether this represents true cross allergenicity. Positive Coombs test results are frequently observed, but hemolytic anemia is rare. Reversible granulocytopenia occurs rarely. Gastrointestinal symptoms such as nausea and diarrhea may be seen with orally administered drugs. Phlebitis with intravenous infusion is a common problem with cephalosporins. Cefazolin produces the least pain on intramuscular injection. Hypoprothrombinemia with moxalactam and cefamandole have been reported.

A boxed warning has been added to the labeling of moxalactam, which states that moxalactam may interfere with hemostasis by three different mechanisms—hypoprothrombinemia, platelet dysfunction, and, rarely, immune mediated thrombocytopenia. Bleeding can be associated with these induced abnormalities. A total of 2.5 per cent of clinical trial patients treated for four days or more experienced a bleeding event, most of which were serious.

Bleeding associated with hypoprothrombinemia can be prevented by the use of vitamin K. It is recommended that patients who receive moxalactam be given 10 mg. of vitamin K per week prophylactically. The inhibition of platelet function, which may be accompanied by a prolonged bleeding time, is dose dependent and generally can be avoided by limiting the dosage to 4 gm. per day. It is recommended that the bleeding time be monitored in patients with normal renal function who receive more than 4 gm. of moxalactam per day for more than three days. All patients with significantly impaired renal function should have appropriate dosage reduction and should be monitored periodically with bleeding times. If the bleeding time becomes unduly prolonged, moxalactam should be discontinued.

If bleeding occurs and the prothrombin time is prolonged, vitamin K should be given. Fresh frozen plasma, packed red cells, and platelet concentrates may be required. Moxalactam should be discontinued if bleeding is due to platelet dysfunction.

Bleeding during moxalactam therapy may also be related to complications of underlying diseases (i.e., sepsis, malignant disease, renal and hepatic dysfunction). Hepatic and renal dysfunction, poor alimentation, thrombocytopenia, and the concomitant use of high doses of heparin (more than 20,000 units per day), orally administered anticoagulants, and other drugs that affect hemostasis (e.g., aspirin) are factors that may increase the risk of bleeding during moxalactam therapy.

As with the penicillins, probenecid administered concurrently with cephalosporins inhibits the renal tubular secretion of the cephalosporins. Concurrent use of drugs with nephrotoxic potential, such as the aminoglycosides, may potentiate the probability of nephrotoxicity when administered with cephalosporins. This potential interaction is not a contraindication to the use of this excellent combination with its synergistic bactericidal capability; renal function does need to be monitored closely, however. If alcoholic beverages are consumed concurrently with cefamandole or moxalactam, a disulfiram-like reaction may occur. The cephalosporins may yield false positive urine glucose reactions with Clinitest tablets but not with the enzymatic tests, such as Clinistix and Tes-Tape.

Aminoglycosides

Aminoglycoside antibiotics (streptomycin, neomycin, kanamycin, gentamicin, tobramycin, netilmicin, amikacin) are an extraordinarily useful and important class of bactericidal drugs with a broad spectrum of activity against gram negative bacteria. As a single group of drugs, they have the greatest activity against the gram negative enteric organisms and *Pseudomonas aeruginosa*. They also possess a certain degree of activity against staphylococci and *Streptococcus faecalis*. Streptomycin, kanamycin, and amikacin are also active against *Mycobacterium tuberculosis* and some of the atypical mycobacteria.

For the treatment of systemic infections, these drugs must be given intramuscularly or intravenously. Table 7–9 presents selected characteristics and dosage guidelines for the use of the aminoglycosides. In patients with normal renal function, streptomycin, kanamycin, and amikacin are given in dosages of 15 mg. per kg. per day in divided doses. Streptomycin may be given in single doses of 500 to 1000 mg. intramuscularly in tuberculous infections and in divided doses in endocarditis. This drug may be poorly tolerated in the elderly (vestibulotoxicity). Kanamycin and amikacin may be given in two or three daily doses of 7.5 or 5 mg. per kg., respectively, producing peak levels of 15 to 30 μg. per ml. Gentamicin and tobramycin, on the other hand, are given at eight hour intervals in doses of 1.0 to 1.5 mg. per kg. with maximal dosages of 3 to 5 mg. per kg. per day. Serum levels of 4 to 8 μg. per ml. are generally produced.

All aminoglycosides are excreted primarily unchanged by glomerular filtration, and thus the dosage level must be radically altered in renal failure. When possible, serum levels should be monitored when prolonged therapy, high dose therapy, or use in patients with abnormal renal function is contemplated. Aminoglycosides do not penetrate into the spinal fluid or into the eye to any significant degree. If such infections are to be treated, intrathecal or subconjunctival doses of the drug must be given.

In contrast to most groups of antibiotics, these drugs have very narrow toxic to thera-

TABLE 7-9. Selected Characteristics and Dosage Guidelines for the Aminoglycosides*

	Half-life (hr.)		Therapeutic Serum Levels (mcg./ml.)	Toxic Serum Levels (mcg./ml.)		Dose (mg./kg./day)
	Normal	Anephric		Peak[1]	Trough[2]	Normal Ccr
Streptomycin	2–3	27	25	>50	>5	15–25
Kanamycin	2–2.5	40–96	8–16	>35	>10	15
Gentamicin	1.2–5.0	21–70	4–10	>12	>2	3–5
Tobramycin	1.0–2.0	27–70	4–8	>12	>2	3–5
Amikacin	0.8–2.8	28–87	8–16	>35	>10	15
Netilmicin	2–2.5	32–52	0.5–10	>16	>4	3.0–6.5

*Reprinted with permission from Facts and Comparisons, 1983.
[1] Measured 1 hour after administration.
[2] Measured immediately prior to next dose.

peutic ratios; i.e., toxicity may be observed at or just above the therapeutic levels. With amikacin and kanamycin, toxicity is less likely with peak levels less than 30 μg. per ml. and troughs below 10 μg. per ml. For tobramycin and gentamicin, peaks of less than 10 and troughs of less than 2 mg. per ml. are optimal. Loading and maintenance doses of amikacin, gentamicin, kanamycin, and tobramycin may be predicted by nomograms such as the one proposed by Sarubbi and Hull, which takes into account lean body weight and calculated or measured creatinine clearance (Fig. 7–2).[8] Accuracy in dosing should be confirmed by serum levels. The serum creatinine level should be monitored at 48 and 72 hour intervals or daily if renal function is changing.

The major toxic effects are renal (tubular necrosis), otic (tinnitus, high frequency hearing loss, deafness, and vertigo), and hematologic (reversible granulocytopenia). Hypersensitivity reactions such as skin rashes are rare. Nephrotoxicity may be potentiated by hypotension, dehydration, or combined use with cephalothin or potentially nephrotoxic antibiotics, such as colistin, vancomycin, or other aminoglycosides. Ototoxicity is potentiated by the simultaneous administration of ethacrynic acid or high doses of furosemide. Audiograms should be monitored if high dose or long term therapy is contemplated. The complaint of tinnitus may precede serious ototoxicity.

Rapid intravenous administration (less than five minutes) may produce a curare-like neuromuscular blockade with respiratory arrest. This may be prevented by slower administration and reversed by calcium or neostigmine. Carbenicillin, when used simultaneously, may inactivate aminoglycosides in vivo, thus decreasing serum levels. This phenomenon is probably of importance only in the patient with renal insufficiency. Oral doses of neomycin used in gut sterilization may result in low levels of absorption, which may lead to serious toxicity. Because of its extreme nephrotoxicity, this drug may not be used parenterally and should not be used to irrigate soft tissue spaces because significant absorption may occur. It is safe to use, however, as a bladder irrigant.

In the elderly, less toxic classes of drugs such as cephalosporins or broad spectrum penicillins should be used whenever possible when sensitivity tests indicate efficacy in the treatment of gram negative infections. In serious infections, aminoglycosides used in combination with an appropriate cephalosporin or penicillin may allow lower doses of both drugs, thus minimizing toxicity while producing a synergy in bactericidal activity.

Erythromycin

Erythromycin is the major member of the macrolide family of antibiotics. This drug has a broad spectrum of activity, is bacteriostatic at normal therapeutic levels, and is used primarily for infections due to gram positive bacteria and other organisms causing pneumonia.[9] Erythromycin may be used in pneumonia or bronchitis due to staphylococci, pneumococci, streptococci, mycoplasma, and Legionnaire's bacillus. It is also effective in nonserious staphylococcal and group A streptococcal soft tissue infections and may also be used in the treatment of diphtheria, gonorrhea, and syphilis in the penicillin allergic patient.

Erythromycin may be given orally or in-

Figure 7–2. Guidelines for calculating loading and maintenance doses of four frequently prescribed aminoglycosides. (From Sarubbi, F.A., and Hull, H.J.: Amikacin serum concentrations; prediction of levels and dosage guidelines. Ann. Intern. Med., 89:612–618, 1978.)

1. Select loading dose in mg./kg. (ideal weight) to provide peak serum levels in range listed below for desired aminoglycoside:

Aminoglycoside	Usual Loading Doses	Expected Peak Serum Levels
Tobramycin, Gentamicin	1.5 to 2.0 mg./kg.	4 to 10 µg./ml.
Amikacin, Kanamycin	5.0 to 7.5 mg./kg.	15 to 30 µg./ml.

2. Select maintenance dose (as percentage of chosen loading dose) to continue peak serum levels indicated above according to desired dosing interval and the patient's corrected creatinine clearance.*

		Percentage of Loading Dose Required for Dosage Interval Selected		
C(c)cr (ml./min.)‡	Half-life (hr.)†	8 hr. (Percentage)	12 hr. (Percentage)	24 hr. (Percentage)
90	3.1	84	—	—
80	3.4	80	91	—
70	3.9	76	88	—
60	4.5	71	84	—
50	5.3	65	79	—
40	6.5	57	72	92
30	8.4	48	63	86
25	9.9	43	57	81
20	11.9	37	50	75
17	13.6	33	46	70
15	15.1	31	42	67
12	17.9	27	37	61
10	20.4	24	34	56
7	25.9	19	28	47
5	31.5	16	23	41
2	46.8	11	16	30
0	69.3	8	11	21

*Calculate corrected creatinine clearance C(c)cr as:
 C(c)cr male = 140 − age/serum creatinine.
 C(c)cr female = 0.85 × C(c)cr male.
†Alternatively, one-half of the chosen loading dose may be given at an interval approximately equal to the estimated half-life.
‡Dosing for patients with reduced renal function should be assisted by measured serum levels.

travenously; however, pain is generally produced by intramuscular injection. There are four different types of oral preparations, the free base and acid stable salts and esters, including estolate, ethylsuccinate, and stearate. Erythromycin base is acid labile and must be delivered to the duodenum for absorption. Enteric coated preparations of erythromycin base are therefore the preferred form of the drug. Hepatotoxicity of the estolate and ethylsuccinate preparations and variable absorption of the stearate in the presence of food decrease the appeal of these preparations. Erythromycin is excreted primarily in the active form in bile. Less than 10 per cent of the drug is excreted by the kidney. Therefore, for average dosing no modification is necessary in renal failure. Serum levels should be monitored if erythromycin is used in patients with severe liver disease. Erythromycin is well distributed in most bony tissues but is generally not useful in meningitis.

Erythromycin free base should be taken on an empty stomach at least one hour before or two hours after meals with a full glass of water to maximize absorption. Peak serum levels after oral doses of 250 mg. range from approximately 0.7 to 1.5 µg. per ml. Peak levels after intravenous injection (500 mg. of erythromycin lactobionate) range from 10 to 15 µg. per ml. Intravenous injections should be given over 15 minutes in at least 50 ml. of sterile water to decrease local pain and phlebitis.

The major side effects of oral doses of erythromycin are gastrointestinal (nausea, cramping, vomiting, and diarrhea). Pseudomembranous colitis has occurred rarely. Many individuals are unable to tolerate 500 mg. oral doses. Phlebitis occurs frequently with intravenous preparations. Cholestatic hepatitis has been reported with the estolate and rarely with the ethylsuccinate derivatives. If this adverse effect occurs, it usually is seen after one to two weeks of therapy. Reversible hearing loss has been observed with high doses administered intravenously, especially in patients with abnormal renal function. Some orally administered erythromycin preparations contain tartrazine, which may cause allergic reactions in susceptible individuals.

Dosage and product strengths are expressed as erythromycin base equivalents. Because of absorption and biotransformation differences, however, 400 mg. of the ethylsuccinate ester is required to achieve serum levels comparable to 250 mg. of the base, stearate, or estolate. The usual adult oral dosage for soft tissue infections is 250 mg. (400 mg. of ethylsuccinate) every six hours. The dosage may be increased up to 4.0 gm. per day according to the nature and severity of the infection. The intravenous administration of erythromycin is recommended when oral administration is not feasible or the severity of the infection requires immediate high and predictable blood levels. Continuous intravenous infusion is preferable to intermittent infusion. Administration of erythromycin by intravenous push is not recommended owing to the irritant properties of the drug.

Clindamycin and Lincomycin

These drugs are related in spectrum of activity to erythromycin but have the added advantage of excellent activity against anaerobic bacteria. Because of the side effect of colitis, these drugs should be reserved in general for serious infections. They may be used in the treatment of gram positive infections in the penicillin allergic patient; however, clindamycin is relatively ineffective in the treatment of staphylococcal endocarditis. Clindamycin is an excellent drug for the treatment of many anaerobic infections of the skin, soft tissues, and abdominal cavity, especially when *Bacteroides fragilis* is isolated. Lincomycin and clindamycin do not readily diffuse into the cerebrospinal fluid and therefore are not useful in the treatment of meningitis.

Clindamycin is better absorbed from the gastrointestinal tract and is more active than lincomycin and therefore is the preferred drug. Levels achieved after oral administration are not greatly altered by food. Clindamycin phosphate may be administered intravenously or intramuscularly in doses of 300 to 600 mg. every six hours. The usual adult oral dosage is 150 to 300 mg. every six hours. Clindamycin is metabolized primarily by the liver and excreted via the bile, although the half-life may be prolonged in severe renal failure. Dosages should be decreased in patients with moderate to severe concomitant renal and hepatic disease (Tables 7–2, 7–6). Peak levels after oral doses are in the 2 to 4 μg. per ml. range, and parenteral doses may produce peaks of 5 to 10 μg. per ml.

The major adverse reactions are cutaneous (urticaria, maculopapular rash, morbilliform-like rash, erythema multiforme [rare]), and gastrointestinal (hepatitis, colitis, and diarrhea). If a hypersensitivity reaction occurs, the drug should be discontinued. Persistence of diarrhea, cramps, fever, or bloody stools warrant discontinuation of the drug and proctoscopic examination. These side effects occur with increased frequency with the oral preparation and may be seen with increased frequency in the elderly. Pseudomembranous colitis may occur and is diagnosed by the findings of whitish plaques or inflammatory changes on proctoscopic examination or by *C. difficile* toxin assay. This colitis is caused by overgrowth in the colon by toxin producing *Clostridium difficile*. Mild cases of colitis may respond to drug discontinuation alone. Moderate to severe cases should be treated by discontinuation of clindamycin and administration of oral doses of vancomycin, 125 to 500 mg. four times daily, along with fluid, electrolyte, and protein supplementation. Antiperistaltic drugs should not be used to control the diarrhea.

Tetracyclines

The tetracyclines (tetracycline, oxytetracycline, methacycline, doxycycline, demeclocycline, and minocycline) compose a group of bacteriostatic drugs that have seen widespread use because of their relative lack of toxicity and broad spectrum of activity. Tetracyclines may be used as the primary drugs in brucellosis, rickettsial, chlamydial, and mycoplasmal infections, cholera, relapsing fever, and minor venereal diseases. They are also used in a variety of urinary, respiratory, and intra-abdominal infections, depending upon the causative agents. Tetracyclines also have a wide spectrum of activity against many anaerobic bacteria (e.g., Bacteroides, Fusobacterium, and Actinomyces).

The tetracyclines are generally administered orally or intravenously. With the exception of doxycycline, which may be administered with meals, tetracyclines should be given one hour before or two hours after meals to maximize absorption. Absorption is decreased by cations, such as aluminum or calcium, found in antacids. Doxycycline is best given with or after meals to decrease gastric irritation and nausea (absorption is not impaired). Intravenous dosages of tetracyclines should be limited to 2 gm. per day or 200 mg. of doxycycline. These drugs are concentrated in the liver and bile and, with the exception of doxycycline and minocycline, are excreted primarily unchanged in the urine. Appropriate dosage adjustments must be made in patients with impaired renal function. Doxycycline and minocycline are excreted primarily by nonrenal routes. Doxycycline and minocycline are highly lipid soluble and readily penetrate the cerebrospinal fluid, eye, and prostate. Tetracycline and demeclocycline are of intermediate lipid solubility.

The major side effects and toxic effects are hypersensitivity (skin rashes, fever, and photosensitivity), gastrointestinal (anorexia, nausea, vomiting, stomatitis, glossitis, monilial overgrowth, and diarrhea), renal (catabolism, acidosis, azotemia, renal tubular acidosis, and a Fanconi-like syndrome, especially with outdated drug), and vestibular (nausea, vomiting, dizziness, vertigo, and ataxia, primarily with minocycline). Tetracyclines may directly stimulate the growth of Candida and result in the production of thrush, esophagitis, or vaginitis. Reference should be made to Table 7-2 for dosage guidelines.

Chloramphenicol

Chloramphenicol is a broad spectrum bacteriostatic drug.[10] Currently it is a drug of choice for serious *Hemophilus influenzae* infections, typhoid fever, and brain abscess (in combination with penicillin). It also may be used in the treatment of rickettsial infections, infections due to *Bacteroides fragilis,* and meningitis due to gram negative rods. It is the second choice to penicillins in pneumococcal and meningococcal meningitis.

Chloramphenicol may be given intravenously or orally (in the individual with normal gastrointestinal motility) with similar peak levels. The usual total daily dosage is 30 to 50 mg. per kg. in the adult, given in four divided doses, and this should yield a serum concentration in the therapeutic range (5 to 20 mcg. per ml.). Because of delayed absorption, the drug should not be given intramuscularly. This antibiotic penetrates well into all body fluids. Levels 30 to 50 per cent of serum levels are achieved in the cerebrospinal fluid, even in the absence of inflamed meninges. Ninety per cent of the drug is metabolized by the liver to a reduced form or to the glucuronide, and these inactive metabolites are excreted by the kidney. Approximately 10 per cent is excreted unaltered. The simultaneous administration of barbiturates, with resultant stimulation of hepatic microsomal enzymes, may result in decreased blood levels of chloramphenicol because of more rapid metabolism. Conversely, chloramphenicol may inhibit microsomal enzyme activity, resulting in inhibition of the metabolism of other drugs, such as phenytoin, tolbutamide, chlorpropamide, cyclophosphamide, and coumadin, leading to an enhanced response and possible toxic reactions from these agents.

The most severe side effect of chloramphenicol is bone marrow suppression. This usually results in a reversible anemia, and occasionally thrombocytopenia and leucopenia. Irreversible idiosyncratic aplastic anemia may occur in approximately 1:25,000 to 1:40,000 of the patients. The reversible bone marrow suppression may occur with increased frequency in the elderly or in malnourished individuals. The drug should be discontinued upon the appearance of reticulocytopenia, leukopenia, thrombocytopenia, or anemia. The irreversible type of marrow depression may occur weeks or months after therapy. An encephalopathy characterized by headache, nightmares, hallucinations, confusion, and lethargy may be seen with excessive dosages (6 to 8 gm. per day). Adverse gastrointestinal effects (nausea, vomiting, glossitis, stomatitis, diarrhea, and enterocolitis) occur rarely. Hypersensitivity reactions are rare.

Chloramphenicol should not be used in trivial infections or in situations in which an equally effective drug can be employed. When its use is indicated, blood counts should be monitored every three to four days. Mild decreases in the hemoglobin level may be followed cautiously. Hemolysis may occur in individuals with the Mediterranean type of glucose-6-phosphate dehydrogenase deficiency, but generally does not occur in the milder form seen in blacks. Courses of therapy longer than two to three weeks are seldom indicated. The patient should be encouraged to notify the physician if fever, sore throat, tiredness, or unusual bleeding or bruising is noted.

Sulfonamides and Trimethoprim

The first widely effective antibacterial drug to be used clinically was a sulfonamide. Ever since the introduction of prontosil in 1935, these drugs have been used for therapy or prophylaxis in a wide variety of infectious illnesses. In many of these indications their use has been supplanted or supplemented by newer, more effective drugs. The most current uses are in the treatment of urinary tract infections due to susceptible gram negative bacteria, chancroid, Chlamydia, Nocardia, and sensitive meningococci. Combinations containing a sulfonamide and trimethoprim are effective against a large percentage of gram negative organisms, organisms causing chronic bronchitis, chronic prostatitis, and otitis media, and *Pneumocystis carinii*. The combination of sulfadiazine and pyrimethamine is effective in toxoplasmosis, and sulfadoxine with pyrimethamine (Fansidar) is useful in chloroquine resistant malaria.

Sulfonamides and the various combinations are well absorbed and are usually given orally, although parenteral combination preparations of sulfamethoxazole and trimethoprim may be required in the management of severe or complicated urinary tract infections, chronic bronchitis due to susceptible strains of *H. influenzae* and *S. pneumoniae*, enteritis caused by susceptible strains of *S. flexneri* and *S. sonnei*, and for the treatment of *P. carinii* pneumonitis.

The usual dosage for urinary tract infections is 2 to 4 gm. of sulfisoxazole, sulfamethoxazole, or sulfadiazine. In addition, a 2 to 4 gm. loading dose is usually used to initiate therapy. For the treatment of systemic infections such as nocardiosis, blood levels of 10 to 20 mg. per 100 ml. should be achieved. Steady state levels are reached after 48 to 72 hours. Virtually all the drugs are absorbed from the gastrointestinal tract, but food may delay absorption. Sulfonamides are partially acetylated by the liver. The acetylated form and the free drug are excreted by glomerular filtration and tubular secretion. The urinary solubility of sulfonamides is pH dependent. To prevent the possibility of crystalluria, the patient should be encouraged to drink large volumes of liquid when consuming the soluble sulfonamides. Alkalinization of the urine by the concomitant administration of bicarbonate is recommended if the less soluble sulfonamides (sulfadiazine, sulfapyridine, sulfamerazine) are utilized. Sulfonamides penetrate well into the cerebrospinal fluid, aqueous humor, other tissues, and saliva. Trimethoprim penetrates well into prostatic tissues, sputum, bile, aqueous humor, cerebrospinal fluid, and vaginal secretions.

Sulfonamides must be used in reduced doses in renal insufficiency and should be avoided with creatinine clearances less than 20 ml. per min. (Table 7-6). Trimethoprim, however, is excreted into the urine in sufficient concentrations to inhibit most urinary pathogens, even in renal failure. The usual dosage of trimethoprim may be used unless the creatinine clearance is below 25 ml. per min. Below this level, a maximum of two tablets daily is given (usual dose, two tablets twice daily). The recommended dosage for the treatment of *Pneumocystis carinii* pneumonia is 12 to 16 tablets daily in divided doses.

The major side effects of sulfonamides are hypersensitivity (skin rash, photosensitivity, urticaria, pruritus, serum sickness, anaphylaxis, and Stevens-Johnson syndrome), blood dyscrasias (aplastic anemia, hemolytic anemia, granulocytopenia, thrombocytopenia), and renal damage secondary to crystalluria. Other adverse effects from the sulfonamides may include nausea, diarrhea, abdominal pain, anorexia, headache, ataxia, drug fever, chills, and malaise. The toxic effects of trimethoprim are gastrointestinal (nausea, vomiting, diarrhea, stomatitis), renal (a fall in creatinine excretion), hematologic (anemia, granulocytopenia, and thrombocytopenia—the latter may be enhanced in the elderly patient being given diuretics for heart failure), and hypersensitivity disorders (skin rashes in approximately 3 per cent of the patients, rare Stevens-Johnson syndrome, or toxic epidermal necrolysis).

Urinary Anti-infectives

The major drugs in this class (other than the sulfonamides and trimethoprim) are nalidixic acid, cinoxacin, nitrofurantoin, and methenamine mandelate. All these drugs are administered orally and are used primarily in patients with recurrent urinary infections not associated with bacteremia. Nitrofurantoin, methenamine mandelate, and trimethoprim may be used as prophylactic suppressive drugs in the prevention of recurrent urinary tract infection.

Nalidixic acid is effective against most urinary gram negative pathogens except for Pseudomonas species. The drug is well absorbed when given orally. A majority is metabolized by the liver, and only a small amount of the active drug is excreted into the urine. Nalidixic acid is administered in doses of 1 gm. four times daily. There are no guidelines for the reduction of doses in renal failure; however, active drug in significant concentration appears in the urine even in severe renal failure. The major adverse reactions are gastrointestinal disorder (nausea), hypersensitivity (pruritus, urticaria, exfoliation, and bullous photosensitivity reactions), and neurologic disorders (visual disturbances, tremor, headache, dizziness, toxic psychosis with confusion and hallucinations). The major use of this drug should be in the treatment of recurrent urinary tract infections in the penicillin-sulfonamide allergic patient and perhaps in azotemia. If it is used in suboptimal dosages, resistance may develop rather quickly.

Nitrofurantoin is active primarily against *Streptococcus faecalis* and *E. coli,* and it has variable activity against other gram negative urinary pathogens. The macrocrystalline form is well absorbed and may produce less nausea than the crystalline form. Significant serum levels are not achieved and active drug is rapidly excreted into the urine. The usual adult dosage is 50 to 100 mg. four times daily. A single nightly dose of 50 to 100 mg. may be effective in prophylaxis against recurrent urinary infections because there is little propensity for resistant strains to develop. When the creatinine clearance falls below 40 to 50 ml. per min., less drug is excreted into the urine and toxic serum levels may occur. Therefore, the drug is contraindicated in renal insufficiency and should be used with extreme caution in the elderly. The major side effects are gastrointestinal disorders (nausea, vomiting, hepatitis) and hypersensitivity (skin rash, fever, eosinophilia) and neurologic (peripheral neuritis—ascending motor and sensory neuropathy—more common in the elderly and in renal insufficiency), pulmonary (acute pneumonitis with cough, fever, dyspnea, and eosinophilia, subacute pneumonitis, and chronic pneumonitis with pulmonary fibrosis), and hematologic disorders (hemolysis in glucose-6-phosphate dehydrogenase deficiency).

Methenamine mandelate and methenamine hippurate are orally administered urinary antiseptics that combine mandelic or hippuric acid with methenamine. These drugs are well absorbed and are excreted into the urine where the only significant antibacterial effect is observed. This is secondary to the hydrolysis of methenamine to formaldehyde at an acid pH. Formaldehyde is usually generated after one to two hours at levels of 30 to 60 mg. per ml., at which it is active against all species of bacteria. Significant formaldehyde is not formed at alkaline pH levels, in the presence of infection due to urease positive bacteria such as Proteus, and with indwelling Foley catheters. The major indications for these drugs are in prophylaxis against recurrent infections (1.0 gm. twice daily for methenamine hippurate and 1.0 gm. four times daily for methenamine mandelate). The concomitant administration of acidifying drugs is not necessary. The major adverse reactions are gastrointestinal (nausea, vomiting) and allergic (pruritus, urticaria, skin rash).

Cinoxacin is structurally related to nalidixic acid and is indicated for the treatment of initial and recurrent urinary tract infections in adults caused by *E. coli, P. mirabilis, P. vulgaris, Klebsiella pneumoniae,* and other Klebsiella species and Enterobacter species. Cinoxacin is comparable in effectiveness to nalidixic acid, nitrofurantoin, and trimethoprim-sulfamethoxazole. Advantages over nalidixic acid appear to be cinoxacin's higher urinary levels and a twice daily dosage regimen, which may facilitate compliance.

Moreover, cinoxacin has a lower incidence of side effects than nalidixic acid. Adverse effects include gastrointestinal effects (nausea [3 per cent], anorexia, vomiting, diarrhea, abdominal cramps), hypersensitivity reactions (rash, urticaria, pruritus, edema), and central nervous system effects (headache and dizziness). Bacterial resistance to cinoxacin appears to be less than that seen with the use of nalidixic acid.

The usual adult dosage of cinoxacin is 1.0 gm. daily. It may be administered in four divided doses, although a twice daily regimen is equally effective. Therapy should continue for seven to 14 days. Cinoxacin may be administered with food. Cinoxacin is eliminated primarily by the kidneys, and therefore lower doses should be employed in patients with reduced renal function. If the creatinine decrease is greater than 80 ml. per min., the adult dosage is 500 mg. twice daily. The dosage should be reduced to 250 mg. three times daily if the creatinine clearance is between 50 and 80 ml. per min., to 250 mg. twice daily if the clearance is 20 to 49 ml. per min., and to 250 mg. daily if the clearance is less than 20 ml. per min. Cinoxacin should not be administered in anuric patients.

Vancomycin

Vancomycin is a cell wall active bactericidal antibiotic, which is effective only against gram positive bacteria. Its major uses are in the treatment of serious infections caused by susceptible stains of *Staphylococcus aureus* and *epidermidis,* streptococci (including enterococci and pneumococci), and *Clostridium difficile* (treatment of antibiotic induced colitis).

This drug is available as a powder for oral solution and in an intravenous form and is usually administered to adults in total daily dosages of 30 mg. per kg. (500 mg. intravenously every six hours). Oral doses are typically used in the treatment of pseudomembranous colitis. Vancomycin is also used occasionally in preoperative prophylactic regimens for colon surgery and in gut sterilization in cancer chemotherapy patients. Absorption from the gastrointestinal tract is negligible. Vancomycin may be used in septicemias, pneumonias, or endocarditis caused by *Staph. aureus, Staph. epidermidis, Strep. pyogenes, Strep. pneumoniae* (especially penicillin resistant strains), and *Strep. faecalis* (enterococcus). Vancomycin is one of the drugs of choice in the treatment of these infections in penicillin allergic patients.

Approximately 80 per cent of injected vancomycin is excreted unchanged by the kidneys. Significant metabolism does not occur. It is well distributed in all body fluids with the exception of the meninges (except in the presence of inflammation) and the eye. In the presence of nearly total renal failure, 1.0 gm. doses may be administered every seven to 10 days; this drug is not removed by dialysis. In cases of less severe renal failure, serum levels should be used to monitor dosing and toxicity (attempting peak levels of 20 to 25 µg. per ml. and troughs of 5 µg. per ml.). Sensitive organisms may be inhibited by less than 2 µg. per ml.

The major toxic effects are auditory (tinnitus, mild deafness). The drug should be avoided, if possible, in patients with hearing loss. Deafness may be preceded by tinnitus. The elderly are more susceptible to auditory damage. Nephrotoxicity was suspected by some authors but probably does not occur to any significant degree. Allergic reactions with eosinophilia and urticaria may also occur. Phlebitis and fever occur rarely. A histamine release-like reaction may be seen with the rapid infusion of 500 to 1000 mg. doses. Therefore, vancomycin should be diluted into 100 to 200 ml. of 5 per cent dextrose solution or 0.9 per cent sodium chloride and administered over 20 to 30 minutes. Vancomycin administration with the concurrent use of other neurotoxic or nephrotoxic drugs (e.g., aminoglycosides, cephaloridine, paromomycin, polymyxin B, and colistin) should be avoided if possible.

Antituberculous Drugs

Isoniazid is the cornerstone of antituberculous therapy. Unless hypersensitivity or hepatotoxicity occurs, all treatment regimens should include this bactericidal drug. Although isoniazid resistance has increased in some areas of the world, such as Southeast Asia and the Western United States, the nationwide incidence of primary resistance is only 3 to 5 per cent. Even "sensitive" populations of *M. tuberculosis* contain a few resistant organisms; therefore, all regimens should contain at least two drugs to prevent emergence of resistance and drug failure. The usual dosage is 5 to 10 mg. per kg. per day as a single dose, higher dosages being reserved for patients with serious disease. The dosage should be decreased in severe hepatic or renal failure to 150 to 200 mg. per day.

Minimal to moderately advanced pulmonary tuberculosis should be treated with two drugs. The primary choices at this time are ethambutol and rifampin. The cure rates with either drug in combination with isoniazid are nearly identical; however, more rapid culture conversion occurs with rifampin. This is important when short term regimens (less than one year) are contemplated. In areas where high incidences of isoniazid resistance occur, triple drug regimens containing isoniazid, ethambutol, and rifampin should be used until sensitivity data are available. Because of increased streptomycin ototoxicity in the elderly, this drug should be reserved or should be administered in reduced dosages.

Isoniazid is metabolized primarily by acetylation in the liver, and approximately 40 per cent is excreted unchanged. Active drug and metabolites are excreted by the renal route. About 50 per cent of a dose of isoniazid is acetylated by the liver. There are two populations of acetylators, "slow" and "rapid." Hepatotoxicity is seen more often in rapid acetylators, because hepatotoxicity appears to be related to the acetylated metabolite (although controversy exists), whereas neurotoxicity occurs more frequently in slow acetylators owing to the higher blood levels of isoniazid. Significant hepatotoxicity occurs in approximately 2 to 3 per cent of individuals over the age of 50 and is potentiated by alcohol use. Hepatitis resulting from isoniazid is characterized primarily by anorexia and nausea, with hepatic enzyme elevations similar to those seen with infectious hepatitis (primarily transaminases).

There is controversy over the routine monitoring of liver function tests; however, the high risk patient, such as the elderly individual with pre-existing liver disease, especially the alcoholic, should be monitored every one to two months. Hepatotoxicity may occur at any point during therapy. Neurotoxicity may occur in individuals taking more than 5 mg. per kg. per day and may be prevented or minimized by the daily administration of 50 mg. of pyridoxine (vitamin B_6) without any decrease in antituberculous activity. Peripheral neuropathy is usually preceded by paresthesias of the feet and hands. Other neurotoxic adverse effects, which are uncommon at conventional doses, are optic neuritis, convulsions, memory impairment, and toxic psychosis. Fever, arthritis, systemic lupus-like syndromes with positive antinuclear antibody reactions, skin rashes, nausea, and epigastric distress are the most common side effects. Isoniazid may decrease the metabolism of phenytoin, and it may be necessary to adjust the phenytoin dosage downward.

Ethambutol is administered as a single daily dose of approximately 25 mg. per kg. After two months this is reduced to 15 mg. per kg. per day. Patients undergoing dialysis and those with creatinine clearance values less than 10 ml. per min. should receive 5 mg. per kg. per day; 10 mg. per kg. per day should be given in patients with creatinine clearances up to 25 ml. per min. The primary toxic effects include neurologic disorders (peripheral neuropathy, optic neuritis, decreased visual acuity), hypersensitivity (skin rash, pruritus, arthralgias), and hyperuricemia. Visual acuity and color vision should be monitored at one to two month intervals when daily dosages of 25 mg. per kg. are used.

Rifampin is given as a single daily dose of 600 mg. The average peak blood level is 7 μg. per ml., although the range is wide. This drug is metabolized by the liver; therefore, dosages need not be altered in renal insufficiency. The major side effect of rifampin is hepatotoxicity, seen with increased frequency in the elderly and in individuals with liver disease, especially alcoholics. Increased hepatotoxicity may also occur when it is given in combination with isoniazid. Asymptomatic transaminase elevations may occur and remit early in therapy without changes in dosage or discontinuation of the drug, which may be continued cautiously. Patients receiving rifampin and other hepatotoxic drugs should be monitored closely. Rifampin may produce a broad depression in cell mediated immunity and may falsely depress cutaneous tuberculin reactions. Acute renal failure or an influenza-like syndrome occasionally may be seen in patients given intermittent rifampin therapy; therefore, the drug should be readministered cautiously. Immune thrombocytopenia, gastrointestinal upset, and skin rashes may also occur. Rifampin causes an orange discoloration of virtually all body fluids. It also stimulates microsomal enzymes, thus enhancing the metabolism and decreasing the effectiveness of tolbutamide, orally administered contraceptives, corticosteroids, warfarin, and methadone.

Streptomycin was the first clinically effective antituberculous drug and is still useful as a second or third line drug. Increased vestibular toxicity may be seen in the elderly, and dosages should be reduced, as for kanamycin and amikacin, in renal insufficiency (Table 7-6). The usual dosage is 15 mg. per kg. per day in patients with normal renal function, with a maximal dosage of 1.0 gm. per day. In the elderly, poor tolerance may preclude doses greater than 500 mg. per day.

Data relating to the alternative antituberculous drugs (para-aminosalicylic acid, cycloserine, pyrazinamide, ethionamide, and capreomycin) may be obtained from standard references. Because of significant gastrointestinal, hepatic, and renal toxicity, these drugs are unlikely to be well tolerated in the elderly; therefore, they should be reserved for problems of drug resistance and atypical infection.

Antifungal Drugs

In contrast to the antibacterial drugs, with an extremely large number available, the physician's choice of antifungal drugs is limited. Several generalizations may be made with regard to antifungal therapy. The deep or invasive fungi are usually treated with amphotericin B and occasionally with miconazole or flucytosine. Dermatophyte infections are usually treated with griseofulvin or topical preparations of miconazole or clotrimazole. Invasive candidiasis is usually treated with amphotericin B, but clotrimazole, miconazole, or nystatin may be used topically.

Amphotericin B is the most important and broadest spectrum drug of this class. It is the drug of choice for invasive infection, specifically candidiasis, cryptococcosis, blastomycosis, coccidioidomycosis, aspergillosis, mucormycosis, histoplasmosis, and sporotrichosis. Amphotericin B should be used primarily for the treatment of patients with progressive and potentially fatal fungal infections. It should not be used to treat cases of suspected fungal disease. This drug is usually given intravenously, although it may be instilled locally (intrathecally, intra-articularly, intraperitoneally, or into the urinary bladder) under certain circumstances. The route of metabolism is unclear. Initial intravenous doses are not generally modified in cases of renal insufficiency. Amphotericin B is slowly excreted by the kidney. The cumulative urinary output over a seven day period amounts to about 40 per cent of the drug infused. With intravenous doses of 0.5 to 1.0 mg. per kg. per day, peak levels of 1.5 to 2.0 mg. per ml. are achieved. Levels exceeding the minimal inhibitory concentrations of most fungi are maintained for 24 to 48 hours because of the long half-life of amphotericin B (approximately 24 hours); hence, alternate day therapy may be used in non-life threatening circumstances. The drug does not penetrate the meninges in significant concentrations, and infections in the orbit, bone, and central nervous system respond variably. Occasionally amphotericin B must be instilled intrathecally or intracisternally (coccidioidal and cryptococcal meningitis) in doses of 0.2 to 0.5 mg.

The toxic effects of this drug have made many a physician blanch to think of its use; however, serious toxicity that would prevent administration is rare.[11] The most frequent side effects are nausea, vomiting, anorexia, fever, myalgia, arthralgia, epigastric pain, hypokalemia, pain at the injection site, chills, and headaches. Occasionally hypotension, arrhythmias, blood dyscrasias, and hearing loss are observed. Phlebitis is generally not a problem if intravenous sites are rotated every 24 to 48 hours. The major toxic effect is a predictable and potentially severe decrease in renal function that must be carefully titrated. Renal function tests should be performed at least weekly. If the blood urea nitrogen value exceeds 40 mg. per 100 ml. or the serum creatinine value exceeds 3.0 mg. per 100 ml., the drug should be discontinued or the dose reduced markedly until renal function has improved. The drug also may induce anemia and renal tubular acidosis.

Unless the infection is immediately life threatening, amphotericin B should be given by slow intravenous infusion over six hours at a concentration of 0.1 mg. per ml. in gradually increasing dosages (0.1, 0.2, 0.3 mg. per kg. per day, and so on) until the desired dosage level (0.3 to 0.5 mg. per kg. per day or 0.6 to 1.0 mg. per kg. every other day) is achieved. One milligram test doses can be bypassed by beginning the first infusion slowly. The drug is supplied in a powder that achieves a colloidal dispersion in dextrose and water. It is incompatible with electrolyte containing solutions and forms precipitates. It should be mixed in an appropriate volume of 5 per cent dextrose in water. Prepared solutions should be protected from light and unused portions discarded after 24 hours at room temperature or seven days under refrigeration. If side effects do not occur, the infusion may be given over one to two hours. Premedication with aspirin, Benadryl, Thorazine, hydrocortisone acetate, or meperidine is useful in selected patients who experience side effects.

The daily dosage and the total cumulative dose of amphotericin B depend upon the type of infection. Candida infections are generally the most sensitive, frequently responding to daily dosages of 5 to 10 mg. or total dosages of less than 100 mg. On the other hand, coccidioidomycosis may require months to years of therapy with total dosages of 4 to 8 gm. (occasionally resulting in significant permanent renal damage). Amphotericin B may be used in combination with flucytosine (see subsequent paragraphs) in the treatment of cryptococcal meningitis; however, the toxic effects of both drugs must be carefully monitored.

Flucytosine (5-fluorocytosine, Ancobon) is an orally administered, fluorinated analogue of cytosine. The drug is transported into the fungal cell by cytosine permease and is deaminated to form 5-fluorouracil. However, low levels of 5-fluorouracil may be found in the blood of patients receiving this drug, which may account for occasional cases of bone marrow suppression. Flucytosine has a rather narrow spectrum of activity and is used primarily to treat infections due to Candida species, Torulopsis, Cryptococcus, and the organisms causing chromomycoses. Minimal benefit has been observed in some cases of aspergillosis. The remainder of the pathogenic fungi are virtually totally resistant.

Flucytosine is administered orally four times daily at six hour intervals in a total daily dosage of 75 to 200 mg. per kg. With maximal doses, peak levels of 50 to 100 μg. per ml. are observed. Minimal therapeutic serum concentrations are 25 to 50 μg. per ml.; toxicity generally occurs at levels above 100 μg. per ml. Absorption from the gastrointestinal tract is excellent, and virtually all the drug (90 per cent) is excreted by glomerular filtration unchanged in the urine. Flucytosine penetrates well into all body fluids, including the cerebrospinal fluid (50 to 100 per cent of serum levels in the presence of meningitis) and the aqueous humor. Significant protein binding probably does not occur. Flucytosine should be administered at a decreased dosage in patients with renal insufficiency. One method of approximating the dosing interval is to multiply 6 (the usual interval) by the serum creatinine level to arrive at a new dosing interval for the administration of a dose of 37.5 mg. Because of the potential for toxicity in the patient with impaired renal function or inadequate bone marrow function, serum levels of flucytosine should be measured when possible. Baseline hematologic, hepatic, and renal function tests are useful.

The major toxic effects of flucytosine are gastrointestinal (nausea, vomiting, diarrhea), hematologic (granulocytopenia, thrombocytopenia, rare aplastic anemia), and hepatic disorders (elevated transaminase levels) and skin rash. The gastrointestinal reactions may be alleviated by administration of the drug after meals or by dividing each dose over a 30 to 60 minute period. Bone marrow suppression is more commonly seen in patients receiving other cytotoxic drugs and in the setting of decreased renal function, especially in the patient receiving amphotericin B concomitantly who develops gradual nephrotoxicity. Bone marrow toxicity is seen frequently with peak levels greater than 100 μg. per ml. (and possibly in patients with measurable levels of 5-fluorouracil). With careful monitoring, flucytosine may be given to patients with liver disease.

Candida endophthalmitis and cryptococcal meningitis are frequently treated with the combination of amphotericin B (0.3 mg. per kg. per day) and flucytosine (75 to 150 mg. per kg. per day). Although this combination appears to be more effective, at least in the latter setting, increased bone marrow toxicity may be observed. Hence, patients should undergo careful monitoring of blood counts and the serum creatinine level twice weekly. Flucytosine levels should be monitored, especially when high doses are used.

The imidazole drugs (clotrimazole, miconazole, and ketoconazole) have a wide range of activity, similar to that of amphotericin B. They appear to act by damaging the plasma membrane. Clotrimazole is useful topically in the treatment of candidiasis and other superficial mycoses. Miconazole is also an excellent drug for topical use, which may also be given intravenously or intrathecally when amphotericin B cannot be used or has failed to yield benefit. Ketoconazole is a new oral drug that is extremely active in candidiasis and dermatophyte infections.

Clotrimazole is given orally as 0.5 gm. tablets, as vaginal tablets (100 mg.), or topically in a 1 per cent cream. Significant blood levels of this drug decline over one to two weeks owing to the induction of hepatic microsomal enzymes, thus decreasing its usefulness as a drug for systemic infections.

Miconazole is given intravenously in doses of 200 to 600 mg. over a period of 30 to 60 minutes every eight hours. The preferred diluent is 0.9 per cent sodium chloride or 5 per cent dextrose in water. Miconazole may also be administered intrathecally (20 mg. per dose, undiluted) as an adjunct to the intravenous treatment of fungal meningitis. A 2 per cent cream is also available for topical use.

Ketoconazole has a broad spectrum of antifungal activity, and the oral dosage form is indicated for use in the treatment of candidiasis, chronic mucocutaneous candidiasis (possibly the therapy of choice), oral thrush, candiduria, coccidioidomycosis, histoplasmosis, chromomycosis, and paracoccidioidomycosis. Ketoconazole has a broader spectrum of activity than flucytosine and may prove to be a better drug than griseofulvin for treating dermatophytic infections. Ketoconazole is well tolerated, with nausea and vomiting occurring in about 3 per cent of the patients, pruritus in 1.5 per cent, and abdominal pain in 1.2 per cent.

Ketoconazole requires acidity for dissolution and absorption; therefore, ketoconazole administration should be separated from the administration of antacids, anticholinergics, and H_2 receptor blockers (cimetidine, ranitidine) by at least two hours. Elderly patients with achlorhydria may be required to dissolve a ketoconazole tablet in 4.0 ml. of an aqueous solution of 0.2 N hydrochloric acid, add this mixture to a glass of water, and then ingest the liquid. Ketoconazole may be administered as a single daily dose in the dosage range of 200 to 600 mg. daily.

The imidazole drugs generally undergo hepatic metabolism and are excreted primarily in the bile. No dosage alterations are necessary in cases of renal failure. The major toxic effects with all three imidazoles are hematologic (anemia) and gastrointestinal (nausea, vomiting) disorders and skin rashes or pruritus.

Griseofulvin is an orally administered antifungal drug that is useful only in dermatophyte infections. Its exact mechanism of action is unknown, but it may perturb DNA replication. The drug is given orally in doses of 500 mg. one to three times daily. Absorption is enhanced by fatty meals. It is metabolized by the liver and is given in unchanged doses in renal failure.

The major uses of griseofulvin are in the treatment of tinea capitis (six to eight weeks), tinea corporis (three to four weeks), and onychomycoses (six to 24 months). Topically applied drugs are frequently combined with oral doses of griseofulvin in the treatment of tinea corporis. The major toxic effects are gastrointestinal disorders (nausea, diarrhea), rashes, photosensitivity, and headache.

IMMUNIZATION IN THE ELDERLY

This section does not attempt to deal with immunization practices in general; the major issues to be discussed are those that deal with maintenance of immunity and the prevention of respiratory illnesses in the elderly. An immunization history should be a part of the initial evaluation in all elderly individuals. In general the childhood illnesses such as measles, mumps, rubella, varicella, polio, and pertussis may be ignored, for most individuals over the age of 65 are immune. In the next few decades, however, this situation may change as the prevalence of these diseases decreases in the general population, thus decreasing the chance of natural exposure and acquired immunity.

Tetanus and Diphtheria. Every adult should be immunized against tetanus and diphtheria. Any individual who has never been immunized should receive a primary series of tetanus-diphtheria toxoid. This should be given as 0.5 ml. intramuscular injections every two months for three doses, followed by a booster at one year and every 10 years thereafter. For individuals who are certain of having been immunized, a booster should be given every 10 years. In the case of tetanus, 250 to 500 units of tetanus immune globulin should be given with a tetanus-diphtheria booster for dirty wounds in individuals who have not received booster doses or who have not been immunized for more than five years. The mortality from tetanus in individuals over the age of 70 is greater than 60 per cent—three to four times that in younger adults and children—thus emphasizing the need for the maintenance of immunity. In many instances the source of tetanus is not identified; however, presumably disease could occur secondary to a decubitus ulcer or an occult diverticular abscess.

Influenza. The current recommendations for influenza vaccination include all individuals over the age of 65 and high risk patients of all ages with chronic illnesses such as heart disease, diabetes, immunosuppression, malignancy, chronic obstructive pulmonary disease, and renal failure. Patients undergoing chemotherapy for malignancy should not receive vaccine simultaneously with chemotherapy as a poor antibody response may occur. Since vaccines are killed virus products, the major reactions are local tenderness or fever. The only contraindication to these vaccines is allergy to eggs. Vaccine should be administered yearly two to three months prior to expected epidemic periods using the strain of virus predicted to be prevalent in a particular season.

Polyvalent Pneumococcal Polysaccharide Vaccine. Geriatric patients and the same high risk group just noted probably should receive polyvalent pneumococcal polysaccharide vaccine. In addition, asplenic individuals should also be vaccinated (because of the increased risk of overwhelming pneumococcemia in this setting). The antibody response rate may be diminished in individuals being given heavy immunosuppression therapy, and responses are poor in hypogammaglobulinemia. The vaccine contains 50 µg. of polysaccharide from the 14 most prevalent strains. Immunity probably lasts at least five years. The vaccine should not be administered more frequently than every three years because more severe local reactions may occur. The major side effects are local tenderness and swelling.

DIAGNOSIS AND MANAGEMENT OF INFECTION IN THE ELDERLY

Respiratory Tract Infections

Respiratory tract infections are among the most common causes of illness in all age groups. The types of infections vary at different ages; e.g., otitis media, mastoiditis, and pharyngitis are more common in children, and lower respiratory infections are more prevalent in the elderly and other adults.

Acute Sinusitis. Acute sinusitis may arise as a complication of an upper respiratory viral infection. Facial pain, purulent drainage, fever, and poor opacification of the sinuses by transillumination all suggest bacterial sinusitis. The most common infecting agents are *H. influenzae and S. pneumoniae*, with occasional cases due to mixed bacteria, anaerobes, *S. pyogenes, and Staph. aureus*. The usual antibiotic regimens include amoxicillin, 500 mg. four times daily, trimethoprim-sulfamethoxazole, two tablets twice daily, or cefaclor, 500 mg. three times daily. Erythromycin, 250 to 500 mg. four times daily, or a tetracycline derivative may also be used. Antihistamines should be avoided in order to prevent drying of secretions. Nosedrops as decongestants are effective in reducing edema and allowing drainage. Saline nasal irrigation may also be helpful. Sinus puncture and drainage are occasionally necessary. Complications include osteomyelitis of the frontal bone, meningitis, and brain abscess.

Acute Bronchitis. Acute bronchitis may be associated with or complicate the common cold or influenza. Frequently this is purely a consequence of viral infection, but it occasionally may be secondary to bacterial superinfection, suggested by the persistence of cough, fever, and purulent secretions.

Similar exacerbations of bronchitis may be seen in the patient with chronic obstructive pulmonary disease. Although controversy exists about antibiotic therapy and its long term benefits, symptoms in acute exacerbations may be shortened by short courses of orally administered antibiotics similar to those just mentioned in the section on sinusitis.

Influenza. Influenza is an acute, usually epidemic, upper and lower respiratory tract infection associated with fever, cough, and myalgias. Epidemics usually occur during the winter months, with peaks in January through March, and are associated with increased respiratory mortality, especially in the elderly.

There are three types of influenza viruses, A, B, and C. The latter is usually associated only with common cold symptoms. Types A and B undergo frequent antigenic variation; hence, new strains are commonly encountered. Increased mortality may be seen in individuals with underlying cardiac and pulmonary diseases.

The incidence of influenza may be decreased by immunization. In the United States, vaccines containing the predicted prevailing strain of virus are usually available in September of each year. All individuals over 65 years of age and those with underlying cardiorespiratory illnesses or other risk factors should be vaccinated at least one month and preferably two to three months in advance of the anticipated epidemic. A 70 to 80 per cent efficacy rate can be anticipated. Unvaccinated high risk individuals may be partially protected by the use of amantidine, 100 mg. twice daily. Amantidine appears to prevent the entry of virus into cells and cell to cell transmission of virus. For this reason, marginal benefit may also be obtained in the treatment of patients already ill with influenza.

Patients with influenza may require hospitalization with oxygen supplementation. Hypoxemia is a frequent finding, even in younger individuals. Because influenza virus produces necrosis of tracheobronchial epithelial cells, bacterial superinfection may occur. This is seen later in the course of a viral infection or after a period of transient improvement. Increased fever and productive cough associated with leucocytosis frequently accompany superinfection. The most important bacterial pathogens are *S. aureus, S. pneumoniae,* and *H. influenzae.* Antibiotic therapy should be based upon Gram staining and cultures of purulent secretions. Primary influenzal pneumonia is uncommon.

Pneumonia. Pneumonia is one of the most common serious infectious problems in the elderly. Pulmonary infections are frequently encountered in geriatric patients who die in the hospital. There are many predisposing factors to pneumonia that are frequently found in the elderly; these include heart failure, altered mental status or coma secondary to cerebrovascular disease, chronic pulmonary disease, and diabetes. Although the pneumococcus still is the most common cause of sporadic bacterial pneumonia, staphylococci and gram negative organisms are seen more frequently in individuals with underlying diseases or hospitalized patients. In addition, various forms of aspiration pneumonia (acid gastric contents, foreign bodies, upper airway or oral flora, mineral oil) may be encountered. Mycoplasmal and viral pneumonias may be encountered occasionally. Recurrent pneumonia, especially in the same location, should raise the suspicion of partial bronchial obstruction secondary to a tumor or foreign body. Chronic pneumonia may be due to many etiologies; however, one should think of an indolent mycotic infection, tuberculosis, neoplasm, vasculitis, and drug reactions. Pneumonia may be complicated by lung abscess, pleural effusion or empyema, and seeding of other organs with subsequent meningitis, endocarditis, or pericarditis.

As in many other situations, the presenting symptoms and signs in the elderly may be minimal or nonspecific. The usual signs of chills, fever, cough, pleuritic chest pain, and sputum production may be absent. A rise in the pulse and respiratory rates, decreased appetite, and increased confusion may be the only signs and symptoms. Because of decreased cooperation, the physical examination may be unrewarding. The chest x-ray view may be difficult to obtain or may not show an infiltrate early in the infection. When possible, sputum and blood cultures should be obtained. A Gram stain of the sputum may be of value to the experienced observer. Endotracheal suction or transtracheal aspiration may be required to obtain a sputum specimen for Gram staining and culture.

Treatment. The treatment depends upon the severity of the illness. The patient may require hospitalization for optimal therapy. Parenteral treatment should be given when possible, at least initially. In the less seriously ill patient without significant underlying diseases, treatment may be given at home or in the nursing home setting. If there are no complicating factors, the patient should be treated for pneumococcal infection (penicillin, erythromycin, or cephalosporin). The usual treatment for pneumococcal pneumonia is procaine penicillin, 600,000 to 1.2 million units intramuscularly two to three times daily, or penicillin V, 500 mg. given orally four times daily. Erythromycin, cephalexin, and cefaclor, 500 mg. orally three to four times daily, are good alternatives and have the advantage of staphylococcal coverage. With the exception of gram negative organisms, erythromycin probably provides the best spectrum of any drug against the usual causes of pneumonia (pneumococcus, staphylococci, other streptococci, Mycoplasma, and Legionnaire's bacillus). When Hemophilus is suspected as a result of Gram staining or culture, therapy should include ampicillin, cefaclor, chloramphenicol, or trimethoprim-sulfamethoxazole. Pneumonia caused by a gram negative organism should be treated with a broad spectrum cephalosporin (cefoxitin, cefotaxime, or cefamandole), an aminoglycoside, or an extended spectrum penicillin (mezlocillin, piperacillin, or azlocillin) until sensitivity data are obtained. In the seriously ill patient in whom the diagnosis is unclear, treatment with an aminoglycoside in addition to a penicillin or cephalosporin may be warranted in view of the risks of superinfections in such circumstances.

In the patient who does not respond favorably in three to five days, complicating features should be sought (e.g., metastatic infection, pleural effusion, empyema, drug reaction, bronchial obstruction, or unsuspected pathogens). Bronchoscopy, thoracentesis, and physical therapy occasionally may be required for diagnosis and treatment.

Tuberculosis

Tuberculosis has been a decreasing problem in the United States over the last 20 to 30 years. At the present time, however, the greatest risk is in the population over 45. The decline in the younger population is no doubt secondary to effective chemotherapy and public health programs that have made it possible to identify the tuberculosis infected individual and bring an end to person to person transmission. This has decreased the likelihood that a susceptible individual will encounter tuberculosis in his lifetime. By contrast, the individual over age 65 had a 60 to 80 per cent probability of acquiring primary disease during childhood or young adulthood. These individuals represent the largest reservoir of potential cases.

Tuberculosis is caused by *Mycobacterium tuberculosis* (rarely *M. bovis*). Similar infections are occasionally encountered that are due to *M. kansasii* or *M. intracellulare*. *M. tuberculosis* is an obligate aerobic respiratory pathogen of man and other primates. The organism is transmitted by respiratory droplets from individuals with pulmonary infection, reaches the terminal bronchi, and initiates a pneumonic process during which silent dissemination may occur to any organ in the body. In the majority of cases this primary infection resolves and organisms become sequestered in various body sites where they may remain dormant for decades. During this period of time the skin test to tuberculin becomes positive. Clinically apparent disease may recur in any body site, particularly the apices of the lungs, the kidneys, the meninges, or bone, or it may present in a disseminated (miliary) form, which is usually secondary to rupture of infectious material into an artery, vein, or lymphatic vessel.

Symptoms. The usual symptoms of pulmonary disease are cough, low grade fever, night sweats, weight loss, and general debility. Disseminated disease may present as a fever of undetermined origin, or it may be unsuspected in the setting of other chronic illness. Tuberculous meningitis usually presents with symptoms of subacute meningitis over a period of several days to weeks. Tuberculosis should be suspected in the case of any infectious or inflammatory process in which an organism is not isolated from body fluids that appear to be purulent.

Because of the nonspecific nature of many of the symptoms of tuberculosis, the illness may be unsuspected for weeks to months in elderly individuals with coexisting disease. The risks are probably greater in diabetes, silicosis, postgastrectomy, malignant disease, underlying diseases that impair cell mediated immunity, corticosteroid therapy, malnutrition, and alcoholism. The unusual presentations such as mass lesions, pleural effusion, pericarditis, lower lobe involvement, nodules, and subtle miliary disease may result in delays in diagnosis. Anergy to intermediate PPD may be present in 10 to 20 per cent of elderly patients with active disease. Some of these patients have positive reactions to second strength PPD.

Diagnosis. The diagnosis of pulmonary disease should be made by staining and culturing concentrated specimens of sputum or body fluids and tissues. Several specimens should be obtained and reviewed by experienced observers. The diagnosis of tuberculous pleuritis or pericarditis usually requires pleural or pericardial tissue. Acid fast stains usually yield negative results with pleural, pericardial, and cerebrospinal fluids, and positive cultures may not be reported for four to six weeks. Therefore, in certain settings therapy must be based upon clinical suspicion. Six to eight urine cultures may be required to confirm the diagnosis of renal tuberculosis. The histologic findings in biopsy materials, such as pleura, pericardium, liver, lymph nodes, and pulmonary tissue, may help make an early diagnosis.

Treatment. It is generally accepted that younger individuals (less than 35 years of age) with a positive intermediate PPD reaction or a recent conversion from negative to positive should be given isoniazid for one year in order to decrease the likelihood of clinical disease during the remainder of the patient's life span. Because of the increase in abnormal liver enzyme values and clinical hepatitis in individuals over 45, routine prophylaxis is not recommended in the elderly. The presence of several risk factors, however, may alter this decision in certain circumstances.

Mild to moderate cavitary tuberculosis should be treated with two antituberculosis drugs, such as isoniazid and ethambutol. More extensive pulmonary infections and renal, osseous, and central nervous system tuberculosis are usually treated with three-drug regimens, such as isoniazid, ethambutol, and rifampin. The latter drug is generally better tolerated in the elderly than streptomycin. A possible increased risk of hepatitis with isoniazid-rifampin regimens requires careful monitoring of liver function tests during therapy. Rapid increases in transaminase levels may require cessation of isoniazid and substitution of alternate regimens. Asymptomatic elevations of enzyme levels (less than three times normal) may be observed with frequent careful follow-up.

In the more debilitated patient with fever and anorexia, low dosage corticosteroid therapy (10 to 15 mg. of prednisone per day) in addition to antituberculous drugs may improve the appetite, decrease fever, and provide an anabolic effect. This dosage should be tapered and discontinued over a three to six week period. In patients with extensive pulmonary involvement, supplemental oxygen may be required.

Patients with nonrespiratory disease are generally not contagious. Careful evaluation of family contacts, especially young children, should be undertaken in conjunction with the pediatrician and local health department. The number of contacts in the nursing home setting may be extensive, for patients may go undiagnosed for several weeks. This requires frequent PPD testing of individuals involved in the intimate care of elderly or otherwise debilitated patients.

Meningitis and Other Central Nervous System Infections

Meningitis refers to inflammation and infection of the leptomeninges. Other central nervous system infections may differ in the locale of the infection (brain abscess, epidural abscess, subdural empyema) or the presentation (encephalitis). The three major categories of meningitis are bacterial, fungal, and viral ("aseptic"). Rare infections may be seen secondary to protozoa (ameba, Toxoplasma) and parasites. The most common etiologic bacteria are the pneumococcus and Meningococcus, less common isolates including gram negative rods and *M. tuberculosis*. The most common forms of fungal meningitis are cryptococcal, coccidioidal, and histoplasmal. These vary in frequency with geographic locales. Viral meningitis is most frequently caused by enteroviruses (such as coxsackie, ECHO, and polio) and mumps and lymphocytic choriomeningitis viruses. Sporadic viral encephalitis is most frequently due to *Herpes simplex,* whereas epidemics of encephalitis are frequently due to arboviruses.

The infecting agents most frequently gain access to the central nervous system through the circulation; however, occasionally local extension may occur through the cribriform plate, sinuses, middle ear, or mastoids or as a result of a neurosurgical procedure, trauma, or malignant disease of the central nervous system. Bacterial meningitis in the elderly is frequently associated with an underlying disorder (e.g., following neurosurgery, central nervous system trauma, diabetes, decubitus ulcers, or immunosuppression). In these settings unusual organisms such as staphylococci, Listeria, and gram negative organisms should be suspected. Brain abscess may be seen more frequently in the patient with endocarditis, lung abscess, otitis, sinusitis, mastoiditis, or central nervous system trauma. Epidural or subdural abscesses may be secondary to trauma, operative procedures, or septicemia or may arise in the setting of subdural hematoma.

Diagnosis. The most common symptoms of meningitis are fever, headache, stiff neck, and alterations in the state of consciousness. In the elderly, however, these symptoms may not be easily discerned from the patient's underlying state. Nevertheless confusion, stupor, headache, and nuchal rigidity are usually present. Aseptic meningitis may be associated only with fever and severe headache, with less depression of mental status, unless this is aggravated by the height of the fever. Fungal or tuberculous meningitis may have a presentation of weeks to months, fever and headache being the most common symptoms.

The suspicion of meningitis should be confirmed immediately by lumbar puncture. This may be difficult in the elderly because of deformities of the spine, and neurologic or neurosurgical assistance may be required. Bacterial meningitis is usually associated with several hundred to several thousand polymorphs per milliliter of cerebrospinal fluid, with elevated protein and depressed glucose levels. Viral infections usually show a lymphocytic pleocytosis with normal glucose and slightly elevated protein levels. Patients with fungal and tuberculous meningitis frequently have low glucose and elevated protein levels and either a lymphocytic or polymorphonuclear pleocytosis. Gram staining, culture, and special procedures for the identification of bacterial or fungal antigens should also be performed.

Treatment. The initial treatment should be based on a Gram stain of the cerebrospinal fluid and the clinical setting. In sporadic meningitis without associated illness, the organism is usually a pneumococcus or meningococcus. Disease caused by these organisms should be treated with penicillin G or chloramphenicol (for penicillin allergic patients). The penicillin dose (15 to 20 × 10^6 units) should be decreased in renal insufficiency and the drug should be infused over 30 to 60 minutes to prevent seizures. Staphylococcal infections should be treated with nafcillin or an equivalent drug. Infections with gram negative organisms should be treated with carbenicillin, chloramphenicol, moxalactam, or cefotaxime, as indicated by the sensitivity pattern. Carbenicillin penetrates the meninges to approximately 15 per cent of serum levels, while chloramphenicol reaches levels 30 to 50 per cent of serum levels, even in the absence of inflammation. Resistance may develop during therapy with chloramphenicol. The intrathecal administration of aminoglycosides (administered by intraventricular reservoir) may be considered in this setting. Moxalactam and cefotaxime have emerged as the drugs of choice to treat infections caused by gram negative rods, however. In contrast to other cephalosporins, these antibiotics penetrate the meninges in concentrations of 5 to 15 mcg. per ml., which generally exceeds the MIC's of most gram negative rods. Patients should be treated with 2.0 to 3.0 gm. administered intravenously every six to eight hours.

Tuberculous meningitis should be treated with isoniazid, rifampin, and ethambutol, all of which cross the meninges in inflammation. Fungal meningitis is usually treated by the intravenous or intrathecal administration of amphotericin B. Flucytosine may be used in candidal or cryptococcal meningitis, usually in combination with amphotericin B. The only form of viral encephalitis that responds to therapy is *Herpes simplex* induced encephalitis. This is treated with adenine arabinoside (Vidarabine), 15 μg. per kg. per day for 10 days by constant infusion over 12 to 24 hours per day. Biopsy of brain tissue is usually required to make this diagnosis.

A brain abscess is treated with penicillin and chloramphenicol. Surgery is usually performed once the abscess has localized. The treatment of epidural abscess depends upon the infecting agent. Otitic or sinus related abscesses in adults should be treated with a penicillinase resistant penicillin in addition to chloramphenicol.

Urinary Tract Infection

Disorders of the urinary tract increase with age. Urinary tract infections are the second most common cause of febrile illness in people over 65, second only to respiratory infections. Urinary tract disorders include the gradual decline in glomerular filtration rate that accompanies normal aging, which may be accelerated by diabetes, atherosclerosis, or hypertension. In addition, various neurologic diseases may lead to incontinence or urinary retention, frequently necessitating the placement of urinary catheters. Prostatitic hypertrophy and carcinoma of the bladder and prostrate may result in obstructive uropathy.

The most frequent causes of urinary tract infections are enteric gram negative bacilli (*Escherichia coli* in women and *Proteus mirabilis* in men and in nephrolithiasis) and *Streptococcus faecalis* (enterococcus). Occasionally *Staphylococcus aureus* may be seen. *Candida albicans* and *Torulopsis glabrata*—yeast species—are frequently seen in patients with indwelling catheters and in those who have had previous antibiotic therapy; these infections also occur more frequently in patients with diabetes.

The majority of urinary infections result from perineal and urethral colonization with resultant retrograde infection via the urethra. The most important normal defense mechanism in the prevention of urinary tract infection is the complete emptying of the bladder. Ureteral reflux, residual urine secondary to partial obstruction or neurogenic bladder, and foreign bodies such as stones may result in the retention of small or large amounts of infected urine. Similarly, indwelling bladder catheters inevitably become infected in time, even with proper care. Infection may occur periurethrally or through the catheter lumen if a sterile closed system is not maintained. The collecting system should always be kept below the level of the bladder, and urine should not be allowed to run back into the bladder. If the catheter must be disconnected to change the bag, this should be done with sterile technique. A new catheter should be inserted every three to four weeks in patients requiring catheters for prolonged periods in order to prevent obstruction of the lumen. Hematogenous seeding of the urinary tract is an uncommon occurrence but may be seen in patients with disseminated infections (especially *Staphylococcus aureus*).

The majority of urinary infections in the elderly are asymptomatic. In the community, 15 to 20 per cent of women over the age of 65 are bacteriuric; this incidence may increase to 50 per cent in the ninth decade. Incidences in men are approximately half those for women. The prevalence of bacteriuria increases in hospitalized patients, in the chronically ill, and in hypertensive patients.

Diagnosis. The first symptoms of urinary tract infections may be dramatic (e.g., the development of fever, hypotension, and the full blown picture of gram negative septicemia), or there may be the typical presentation of dysuria, frequency, and hematuria with or without high fever and flank pain (indications of upper tract involvement). Symptomatic urinary tract infection may be the first harbinger of structural abnormality of the urinary tract (e.g., urinary retention in the patient with prostatism). More serious complications may be seen in the presence of obstructive uropathy or diabetes (e.g., papillary necrosis, perinephric abscess, or renal carbuncle).

Urinary tract infection may be suspected because of abnormal results on urinalysis (pyuria, hematuria, bacteriuria) or the presence of symptoms already described. The absolute diagnosis is confirmed by culture (standard techniques or various urine culture screening kits may be used). The greatest accuracy (95 per cent) results when a catheterized specimen or suprapubic aspirate is obtained. A single positive clean-catch midstream urine specimen yields an 85 per cent reliability in women. The isolation of the same organism in two consecutive clean-catch specimens in colony counts of more than 100,000 organisms per ml. is as reliable as the results with a catheterized specimen. Urine may also be aspirated aseptically through the tubing of an indwelling catheter. The integrity of the closed system should not be disrupted nor should urine be obtained from the collecting bag.

Treatment. Controversy exists over the treatment of asymptomatic bacteriuria. Since the prevalence is so high in many elderly populations, it is hardly cost-effective or warranted to identify and treat the entire bacteriuric population, especially since the likelihood of recurrence is high. The most important factor that governs an adverse outcome and complications in the patient with urinary tract infection is the presence of obstruction. Relief of any obstruction to urinary flow is of the utmost importance. This may require an indwelling catheter or intermittent catheterization in the patient with a neurogenic bladder, paraplegia, or altered mental status, or surgical management of bladder neck obstruction or nephrolithiasis.

The treatment of uncomplicated infection should involve the use of the most benign antimicrobial drug for seven to 10 days. A more prolonged course of therapy (two to four weeks) may be required in the patient with upper tract involvement (pyelonephritis). Such drugs as sulfonamides (1.0 gm. four times daily), trimethoprim-sulfamethoxazole (two tablets twice daily), ampicillin (500 mg. four times daily), amoxicillin (500 mg. three times daily), cephalexin (500 mg. four times daily), or nitrofurantoin (100 mg. twice daily) may be used. If necessary, aminoglycosides may be used with care. In the patient with moderate to severe renal insufficiency, the safest drugs are the penicillin and cephalosporin derivatives in reduced dosage as indicated by the level of renal function. Rashes and vaginitis may occur with many of these drugs. Ampicillin rashes are seen more frequently in patients with reduced renal function. The prolonged use of nitrofurantoin in such patients results in a higher incidence of neurotoxicity.

Complicated or septicemic infections should be treated parenterally with antibiotics (ampicillin, a cephalosporin, an aminoglycoside), depending upon culture data and the history. The patient with chronic urinary tract infection who has had previous therapy probably should receive an aminoglycoside, at least until antimicrobial sensitivity data are available. Then a less toxic drug should be used if possible. In the nursing home setting many of these drugs may be given intramuscularly if intravenous therapy is not possible. The cephalosporin best tolerated by the intramuscular route is cefazolin. The initial or loading dose of an aminoglycoside need not be factored for renal function; therefore, the patient with an abnormal filtration rate will have adequate blood levels for several hours until renal function data are available. These patients are frequently dehydrated, and vigorous fluid therapy must be administered with careful monitoring of the cardiovascular status.

In younger women, recurrent episodes of cystitis may be prevented by the prophylactic use of antibiotics, such as trimethroprim administered in a single nightly dose. This may prove useful in selected elderly patients. Chronic antibiotic suppression in the patient with an indwelling catheter is controversial. Since all such patients are ultimately infected, prophylaxis frequently is directed at resistant organisms. The most important aspect in long term catheter drainage is the prevention of obstruction. Therefore, the catheter should be changed at frequent intervals (three to four weeks) to prevent the formation of concretions.

Several maxims are important in the use of catheters. Closed sterile systems should always be used (unless one opts for intermittent self-catheterization). The bags should be kept well drained and below the level of the bladder. The perineal area should be cleansed with soap and water twice daily. Catheters should not be irrigated unless obstruction is suspected. If urine is flowing freely and the entire tubing is not filled with urine, the catheter is probably not obstructed. If sediment and grit are adhering to the sides of the tubing, the catheter may be becoming obstructed. Careful records should be kept in areas where there are patients who need catheters for long periods in order to monitor obstructive and infectious problems. If infection occurs in a patient in whom short term drainage is being used, antibiotics may be useful in suppressing the growth of organisms; however, in long term cases, therapy is usually directed at resistant organisms.

Vaginitis

Atrophic vaginitis (estrogen depletion) is a frequent finding in elderly women. Candida (monilial) vaginitis may be a complication of diabetes or the use of broad spectrum antibiotics or corticosteroids. Trichomonas vaginitis is usually sexually transmitted and thus is seen more frequently in sexually promiscuous populations.

Estrogen lack results in atrophy of the normal vaginal mucosa. These changes respond rapidly to topical or systemic estrogen therapy. Candida vaginitis may be secondary to an alteration of normal flora with overgrowth of yeasts or possibly to increased glucose content in patients with diabetes. Tetracyclines directly stimulate the growth of Candida, in addition to suppressing other flora, and frequently induce candidiasis.

The most frequent symptoms are vaginal discharge, pruritus, dyspareunia, and urinary frequency or urgency. Candida vaginitis is usually associated with a thick whitish or cheesy discharge, whereas Trichomonas infections produce a more frothy exudate.

A vaginal examination should be performed to assess the presence or absence of a discharge, atrophic changes, or fissures. A wet smear should be made of any discharge in a search for Trichomonas. If the result with this preparation is negative, the coverslip may be removed and the specimen then stained with Gram stain, which will easily demonstrate gram positive Candida yeast forms if they are present.

Symptomatic atrophic vaginitis may be treated with topically applied estrogen creams for intermittent short courses as necessary. Endometrial carcinoma may occur with increased frequency with prolonged topical or systemic estrogen therapy. Candida vaginitis is treated with vaginal suppositories or tablets containing nystatin (mycostatin), clotrimazole (Lotrimin), or miconazole (Micatin) for 10 to 14 days. Control of diabetes, if present, is also helpful. Trichomonas infections are treated with metronidazole (Flagyl), 250 mg. three times daily for 10 days. Sexual partners should be treated concomitantly.

Prostatitis

Prostatitis is most frequently caused by enteric gram negative organisms, enterococci, and staphylococci. Acute bacterial prostatitis may occur secondary to ascending urethral infection; however, the pathogenesis of many infections is unknown. In the elderly, new infection may occur secondary to instrumentation of the genitourinary tract or after prostatic surgery. Seeding of the prostate gland frequently occurs in the patient with an indwelling urethral catheter.

The symptoms of acute prostatitis include fever, chills, perineal or back pain, and symptoms of urinary tract infection. The prostate gland is swollen and very tender. By contrast, chronic prostatitis may produce no symptoms, although low back pain, perineal pain, and dysuria may occur. Local pain and tenderness may not be present. The major difficulties may arise from recurrent seeding of the urinary tract, with resultant infection.

Acute prostatitis is usually associated with a positive urine culture. Prostatic massage should be avoided because bacteremia may be induced. Chronic prostatitis may be diagnosed by culture of prostatic secretions or by culture of the urine before and after prostatic massage. Ejaculate cultures are probably most accurate.

Acute bacterial prostatitis should be treated, as for any urinary tract infection, with an antibiotic to which the infecting agent is sensitive. Because of the acute inflammatory response, good tissue levels are achieved with most antibiotics. In severe infections, urinary retention may occur and a suprapubic catheter may be required. Chronic prostatitis is more difficult to eradicate because of poor antibiotic penetration. The best tissue levels result with erythromycin and trimethoprim-sulfamethoxazole. Erythromycin, however, is effective only against gram positive bacteria. Trimethoprim-sulfamethoxazole should be used for approximately three months. If relapse occurs, long term half-dose suppression may be employed.

Bone and Joint Infections

Infectious Arthritis

Infectious arthritis has always been most common among children and adolescents. In the last two decades, however, an increasing number of cases have been seen in the elderly.

The most frequent causative organism in the elderly is *Staphylococcus aureus*. Less frequently infections may be caused by various streptococci, *Mycobacterium tuberculosis*, and gram negative bacilli. Infection in young adults is frequently caused by *Neisseria gonorrhoeae* and in children by *Hemophilus influenzae;* however, these organisms are seldom isolated in septic arthritis in the elderly. In addition to pyogenic arthritis, a postinfectious nonsuppurative arthropathy may be seen two to three weeks after gastroenteritis caused by Salmonella, Shigella, or Yersinia. Also the prodrome of hepatitis B may include a diffuse symmetrical polyarthritis resembling rheumatoid arthritis.

Unless the joint is infected as a result of trauma or intra-articular injections, septic arthritis is due to the hematogenous spread of bacteria. The arthritis of hepatitis B is mediated by immune complex deposition. The postdiarrheal arthropathies associated with Salmonella, Shigella, and Yersinia are seen more frequently in individuals possessing the histocompatibility antigen HLA-B27. Patients with rheumatoid arthritis, osteoarthritis, diabetes mellitus, or hematologic malignant disease, or those being treated with corticosteroids, are more prone to septic arthritis.

Diagnosis. The usual symptoms and signs of septic arthritis are fever, pain, swelling, redness, and effusion in the involved joint or joints. Frequently, in the elderly, however, the symptoms are less acute, and the infection may occur in joints previously involved by rheumatoid arthritis or osteoarthritis. Monoarticular involvement of the knee or hip is the most common presentation in adults and in the elderly. Chronic oligoarticular arthropathies with joint destruction should suggest a tuberculous or fungal etiology. Leucocytosis, anemia, and an elevated erythrocyte sedimentation rate are the most frequent abnormalities detected in laboratory tests. The diagnosis is made by joint aspiration, which usually reveals purulent fluid (leucocyte count greater than 50,000 to 100,000 with a predominance of polymorphonuclear leucocytes). Smears of joint fluid for bacteria, mycobacteria, and fungi, as well as appropriate cultures, will confirm the diagnosis. Occasionally in the more chronic forms synovial biopsy is necessary. Patients with rheumatoid arthritis, especially those taking corticosteroids and those with bacteremia, are more likely to have multiple joints involved. Simultaneous adjacent bone involvement (osteomyelitis) is much less common in adults than in children younger than one year of age. Destruction of the articular cartilage may occur if definitive treatment is delayed.

Treatment. Once the diagnosis is made, treatment should be begun on the basis of either a Gram stain or culture results. If results of Gram staining are negative, empiric therapy should be begun with a semisynthetic penicillinase resistant penicillin (e.g., oxacillin) or a cephalosporin (in the penicillin allergic patient). The initial dosage of oxacillin should be 50 mg. per kg. given in divided doses intravenously if the infection is localized, or 100 to 150 mg. per kg. if blood cultures are positive. Aminoglycosides may be required in gram negative infections. Localized septic arthritis may be treated with oral doses of drugs appropriate to the infecting organism once the patient has been stabilized. If possible, serum levels should be monitored to insure absorption. Since all antibiotics except the polymyxins penetrate well into joints, the intraarticular administration of antibiotics is not usually required unless polymyxins are used (e.g., occasionally required for Pseudomonas infections). Surgical drainage should be performed in most instances because repeated needle aspiration may not adequately reach all areas of the affected joints. Therapy should be continued for two to four weeks. If the infection is associated with other foci of infection, as in endocarditis, four to six weeks of therapy may be necessary. Tuberculous arthritis should be treated with isoniazid, 5 to 10 mg. per kg. per day, and ethambutol, 15 mg. per kg. per day, for 18 to 24 months. Fungal arthritis should be treated with a drug appropriate for the infecting organism. If amphotericin B is to be used, especially for sporotrichosis or coccidioidomycosis, a total dosage of more than 2.0 grams is usually required over a six to 12 week period.

If treatment is initiated before the articular cartilage is destroyed, full return of function may be expected. Because of the limited blood supply, late therapy of septic arthritis of the hip may result in avascular necrosis. Degenerative arthritis and decreased range of motion may complicate a poor result. In the elderly it is not uncommon for limitation of motion to persist, even though the joint may not be severely damaged.

Total joint replacement is a frequently used modality in the treatment of various forms of arthritis, especially in the elderly. The incidence of early or late infection of a prosthesis varies from series to series; however, the average ranges from 1.5 to 2.0 per cent. Even with the prophylactic use of appropriate antibiotics at the time of insertion, these devices may become infected. The usual infecting organisms are *Staphylococcus aureus, Staphylococcus epidermidis,* and gram negative bacilli. These infections may respond to surgical débridement, suction drainage, and appropriate antibiotics, with preservation of the prosthesis. Aminoglycosides are frequently required for gram negative organisms, and monitoring of renal and auditory function is necessary. Occasionally long term suppressive oral treatment with antibiotics may preserve a prosthesis. Bone involvement and loosening of the prosthesis usually require removal of the device, resulting in loss of function or fusion of the affected joint. Occasionally a new prosthesis may be inserted, and some authors (mostly European) recommend the use of antibiotic impregnated acrylic cement.

Osteomyelitis

Although virtually any bone in the body may become infected, osteomyelitis in the elderly usually occurs in the distal lower extremity in patients with vascular disease or diabetes mellitus. Decubitus ulcers may lead to infection of underlying bones, and urinary infections may be associated with vertebral osteomyelitis.

Any bacterial or fungal pathogen may cause osteomyelitis. Septicemic infections are frequently caused by staphylococci and enteric gram negative rods. Nonsepticemic infections frequently occur secondary to trauma or to overlying contiguous foci of infection. Therefore, these infections are frequently due to a mixed flora, including staphylococci, enteric gram negative organisms, streptococci, and anaerobes.

Osteomyelitis occurs following bacteremia (which is frequently inapparent) or trauma, or it may be a result of contiguous infection, such as chronic ulcers secondary to peripheral vascular disease or decubitus ulcers. Osteomyelitis associated with urinary tract infections may be seen secondary to asymptomatic bacteriuria or prostatitis and frequently involves the dorsal or lumbar spine. Presumably these infections arise as a result of retrograde infection through the vertebral venous system. Tuberculous osteomyelitis may occur in any bone in the body secondary to activation of quiescent granulomatous foci within the bone marrow.

Diagnosis. Symptoms of acute hematogenous osteomyelitis include high fever, chills, and local pain in the involved area. Chronic osteomyelitis is frequently associated only with a draining sinus or local tenderness. The only laboratory findings may be anemia and an elevated sedimentation rate. The acute form is usually associated with and diagnosed by positive blood cultures. Periosteal elevation and new bone formation are the cardinal radiographic findings. Radionuclide bone scans are frequently positive before changes are visible on x-ray examination. Tomography may be required to adequately visualize vertebral osteomyelitis. Bone biopsy and débridement may be required to make an etiologic diagnosis. Anaerobic cultures should be used when there is vascular insufficiency, diabetes, or decubitus ulcers. Tuberculosis should be considered when routine cultures are negative or the patient has a history of tuberculosis.

Treatment. Acute hematogenous osteomyelitis is usually treated with high parenteral doses of an appropriate antibiotic (as outlined under septic arthritis). Chronic osteomyelitis may require surgical débridement for both diagnosis and treatment. Therapy should be designed to cover all organisms isolated from deep within the bone and may need to be continued for four to six months, frequently using such drugs as oxacillin, 4 to 6 gm. orally, with probenicid. Surgical removal of affected bone or amputation of part of an extremity is frequently required in patients with diabetes or vascular insufficiency.

Skin Infections

Cutaneous problems are relatively frequent in the elderly. Infections of the skin may occur with greater ease because of age related thinning and dryness. Other illnesses, such as diabetes, peripheral venous or arterial insufficiency, congestive heart failure and peripheral edema, and malignant disease, may make the skin unusually susceptible to breakdown. General debility frequently results in decubitus ulcers. Nonetheless many cutaneous infections occur in normal skin (furuncles, cellulitis, or impetigo) or following trauma from cuts, burns, bites, or surgery.

Impetigo. Impetigo is usually a group A beta streptococcal disease, which may become secondarily colonized by *Staphylococcus aureus*. It usually begins with erythema, which progresses to vesicopustule formation and the development of an amber crust. More prominent bullous lesions suggest a primary staphylococcal etiology. Streptococcal impetigo may occasionally progress to the formation of indurated lesions (ecthyma) with heaped up erythematous borders, usually on the lower extremity, with or without lymphangitis and systemic toxicity. The majority of these infections may be treated with orally administered antibiotics—penicillin V or erythromycin for streptococci and dicloxacillin or erythromycin for staphylococci (250 to 500 mg. four times daily).

Furunculosis. Furunculosis is a deep abscess-like infection, frequently arising from an infected hair follicle. It may progress to a carbuncle (an aggregate of furuncles). Furuncles may occur as isolated or multiple lesions; they may be idiopathic or secondary to an underlying illness, such as diabetes. They are usually caused by *Staphylococcus aureus* and occasionally by gram negative organisms, especially in patients with other illnesses. Staphylococcal infections should be treated with either dicloxacillin, oxacillin, or erythromycin (250 to 500 mg. orally four times a day). Warm soaks and drainage may assist in the healing of larger lesions.

Cellulitis and Erysipelas. Cellulitis and erysipelas are characterized by erythema, induration, and tenderness of the involved skin. Erysipelas occurs most frequently on the face. It differs from cellulitis in that the border between involved and uninvolved skin is very sharply demarcated. Erysipelas is almost exclusively a group A beta streptococcal infection and should be treated with penicillin V or erythromycin, 250 to 500 mg. orally four times a day. More seriously ill patients should be hospitalized and treated with procaine penicillin G, 600,000 units intramuscularly every 12 hours. Cellulitis may arise secondary to trauma, a furuncle, or a surgical incision. The most common etiologic agents are staphylococci and streptococci. Blood and local tissue cultures should be performed, and the patient should receive broad streptococcal-staphylococcal coverage. Drainage or pus should be Gram stained when available. In hospitalized patients gram negative enteric organisms are frequently responsible. Patients with peripheral vascular disease or diabetes may develop infections with a variety of aerobic and anaerobic organisms, such as anaerobic synergistic cellulitis or gangrene, clostridial cellulitis, or clostridial myonecrosis (gas gangrene). These infections require more sophisticated anaerobic culture techniques and vigorous surgical débridement. Antimicrobial therapy for these more serious infections should include clostridial (10 to 20 million units of penicillin G), anaerobic (clindamycin, 1.2 to 2.4 gm. per day) and enteric coverage (gentamicin or tobramycin, 3 to 5 mg. per kg. per day).

Decubitus Ulcers. Decubitus ulcers arise secondary to prolonged pressure, usually in the chronically debilitated individual who is incapable of spontaneous movement. They may be prevented by vigorous nursing care, including frequent turning, good skin hygiene, and alternating pressure mattresses or water beds. Once decubitus ulcers occur, they may become superinfected with a variety of bacteria, usually staphylococci, streptococci, enteric organisms, or anaerobes. The infection may extend into underlying muscle or bone and may result in septicemia. For larger lesions, vigorous surgical débridement and skin grafting are often necessary. Antimicrobial therapy should be tailored to the organisms isolated from cultures, as noted in the previous section.

Herpes Zoster. Herpes zoster is a viral infection of the peripheral nerves. It arises as a result of reactivation of latent varicella virus from sensory ganglia. It is seen with increased frequency in the elderly and in illnesses that alter cell mediated immunity (Hodgkin's disease, other lymphomas, corticosteroid therapy, other types of immunosuppression, radiation therapy). The patient with herpes zoster frequently presents with pain, and many times he has not noticed the cutaneous eruption or it has not occurred. Patients occasionally have undergone unnecessary abdominal surgery prior to the eruption of herpes zoster on the abdomen.

The rash is characterized by vesicles on an erythematous base in a dermatomal distribution. In the immunocompromised patient, cutaneous and visceral dissemination may occur. The rash usually lasts one to two weeks and is associated with varying degrees of pain. Postherpetic neuralgia may occur in 30 to 40 per cent of elderly individuals and occurs more frequently after involvement of the trigeminal nerve. Pain should be well controlled, avoiding addictive drugs. Prednisone (1 mg. per kg. per day) is frequently helpful in the prevention of postherpetic neuralgia. The dosage should be tapered rapidly over one to two weeks. Topical analgesia with benzocaine containing lotions is frequently effective. Secondary infection occasionally may occur. Postherpetic neuralgia is frequently helped by phenytoin, the combination of amitriptyline and prolixin, or chlorprothixene.

Intravascular Infections

The following definitions are necessary as an introduction to the discussion of septicemia: *Bacteremia* refers to invasion of the blood by bacteria and may or may not produce any symptoms. *Septicemia* is bacteremia with signs and symptoms such as chills, fever, or hypotension. *Septic shock* is a constellation of signs and symptoms such as hyperventilation, hypotension, confusion, fever (or hypothermia), and oliguria, which if untreated may progress to organ failure and death; this may be caused by gram positive or gram negative bacteria.

Any bacterial pathogen may invade the blood. In the elderly the most common organisms are staphylococci, pneumococci, and gram negative enteric bacilli. Bacteria may enter the blood from any focus of infection. The infection may be occult, such as a diverticular abscess or gingival infection, or a more apparent source such as pneumonia, urinary tract infection, or a decubitus ulcer may be responsible. The signs of septicemia may resolve with appropriate therapy, or the disease may progress rapidly to irreversible shock and death. The final outcome is usually dependent upon the underlying condition of the patient. Gram negative septic shock frequently results in peripheral vasodilation, hypotension, tachycardia, and decreased cardiac output, which may progress to peripheral vasoconstriction, confusion, coma, oliguria, and failure of other organ systems. This is thought to be due to release of various toxic bacterial products.

The usual symptoms of septicemia are chills and fever. These may evolve into the picture of septic shock, or the septicemia may be arrested by rapid intervention with appropriate treatment. In the elderly, hypothermia or confusion may be the only sign. Septicemias frequently arise from the urinary, pulmonary, and gastrointestinal tracts. Knowledge of the patient's medical history may help in predicting the site of origin. If therapy is delayed owing to failure to make an early diagnosis, or if the bacteremia is massive, shock with hypotension, oliguria, disseminated intravascular coagulation, congestive heart failure, and respiratory failure may ensue. Cutaneous manifestations of sepsis such as petechiae, ecthyma gangrenosum, or peripheral infarction may support the diagnosis. In addition to the physical findings and a high index of suspicion, the diagnosis should be confirmed with blood, urine, and sputum cultures when indicated.

Septicemic urinary and pulmonary infections may be treated only with appropriate antibiotics and intravenous fluids when indicated. Correction of underlying conditions, such as urinary retention, obstructed urinary catheter, cholecystitis, or abscess, should be undertaken as rapidly as possible. When early signs of shock exist, hospitalization is indicated, and the patient's intravascular volume status and urinary output should be monitored. Fluid management should be vigorous and should include normal saline or protein plasma expanders. Care should be taken not to produce excessive volume expansion, and a Swan-Ganz catheter may be required. Broad spectrum antibiotics should be administered parenterally (e.g., penicillinase resistant penicillin, extended spectrum penicillin, or a cephalosporin alone or in combination with an aminoglycoside). Because of rapid changes in renal function and possible acute renal failure, the dosage of aminoglycosides should be limited when feasible. Frequently a single aminoglycoside loading dose of 2 mg. per kg. in a patient with impaired renal function suffices until a more definitive etiologic diagnosis is made. The site of origin of the infection should be vigorously sought and treated. Surgical management of many infections may be necessary and should not be delayed if such a management approach is feasible.

Endocarditis

The term infective endocarditis encompasses a broad group of infectious complications of cardiovascular disease. This replaces the older term, "subacute bacterial endocarditis," to include all presentations (acute, subacute) and etiologies (bacterial, fungal). In addition, one may include infection of the endothelial surface of veins, arteries, arteriovenous fistulas, prosthetic grafts, and prosthetic heart valves.

Almost every bacterial and fungal pathogen is capable of initiating infection of an endothelial surface. Prosthetic device infections are most likely to be due to fungi or unusual bacteria. The most common organisms are still streptococci ("viridans" group, pneumococcus, enterococcus) and staphylococci *(S. aureus and S. epidermidis)*. Gram negative organisms and fungi account for less than 10 per cent of all cases.

Naturally occurring infective endocarditis is secondary to a transient bacteremia or fungemia. Infection of a prosthetic device may occur through this mechanism or through contamination of the endocardial surface of a prosthetic device during a surgical procedure. In addition, prosthetic devices are more susceptible to infection following bacteremia, as are previously damaged heart valves (e.g., rheumatic heart disease, congenital or sclerotic valvular heart disease, prolapsing mitral valve). Abnormalities associated with increased turbulence are at highest risk.

Experimental models indicate that infection is initiated at sites of endothelial damage induced either by turbulence or a foreign body, such as an intracardiac catheter. In addition, by unknown mechanisms, virulent organisms such as staphylococci, pneumococci, or gonococci may initiate infection on previously normal heart valves. A platelet-fibrin thrombus may occur at the initial site followed by the attachment of micro-organisms. Microcolonies subsequently enlarge, and more fibrin is deposited to form vegetations. These friable collections are apt to become dislodged and produce arterial emboli to the brain, kidneys, spleen, or coronary arteries, resulting in septic or bland infarcts. Further damage to the endocardial or valvular surface may result in mycotic aneurysms or worsening valvular insufficiency. Organisms such as gram negative rods *(Escherichia coli, Klebsiella pneumoniae)*, which are killed by the action of antibodies and complement, are less likely to survive in the blood and hence are less common infective agents.

Diagnosis. Depending on the virulence of the infecting organism, the symptoms of endocarditis may be insidious ("subacute") or fulminant ("acute"). The typical case is characterized by fever, which may be low grade, sweats, weight loss, weakness, fatigability, arthralgias, complications of infarcts, and skin lesions, such as petechiae, Osler's nodes, and splinter hemorrhages. Acute bacterial endocarditis may be associated with the more sudden onset of chills, fever, and congestive heart failure. Historically some patients recall having undergone a procedure associated with transient bacteremia, such as a dental extraction or genitourinary instrumentation. Endocarditis is also frequently seen in intravenous drug users and patients undergoing hemodialysis.

The physical examination usually shows signs of heart disease (new murmurs, congenital lesions, prosthetic valve), fever, skin lesions of mucosal surfaces and the distal extremities, and splenomegaly. The laboratory evaluation may show anemia, an elevated sedimentation rate, gross or microscopic hematuria, pyuria, proteinuria, elevated gamma globulin levels, and evidence of renal dysfunction. Blood cultures are positive in 85 to 90 per cent of patients. "Culture negative" endocarditis may be due to fastidious organisms or fungi; the latter should be suspected with increased frequency in patients with prosthetic heart valves.

If the diagnosis of endocarditis is entertained, four to six blood cultures should be obtained over a 24 to 72 hour period. If the illness is more fulminant, cultures should be performed over a one to two hour period and immediate empiric therapy should be begun. Anaerobic culture media should be used, as should special supplements for some fastidious organisms when cultures are negative. Arterial cultures are possibly of value in fungal endocarditis. Consultation with the microbiologist should be obtained for assistance in isolation, identification, and antibiotic sensitivity testing of organisms.

The percentage of elderly individuals noted in reports of endocarditis has increased during the last 20 years. The prevalence of patients with underlying rheumatic heart disease is decreasing, but increasing numbers with aortic valve deformity, arteriosclerosis, and mitral valve prolapse are encountered. Owing to the nonspecific nature of the symptoms of endocarditis (such as fatigue, weight loss, anorexia, low grade fever, congestive heart failure), this illness is likely to be overlooked in the elderly. This is complicated by the observation that fever is less likely to be prominent in this age group. Murmurs may be absent in as many as 30 per cent of the patients. In one series of cases of endocarditis in the elderly, endocarditis was suspected in only 40 per cent of the patients. The mortality rate is also higher in the elderly (over 60 per cent in individuals over 70 years of age). *Staphylococcus aureus* is the most common pathogen in the elderly patient with endocarditis. A high index of suspicion is appropriate in the elderly individual who presents with a nonspecific illness associated with fever. For example, fever with a recent cerebrovascular accident is a classic presentation of endocarditis, which may go undiagnosed. In addition, patients with bacteremias or endocarditis secondary to *Streptococcus bovis*, a nonenterococcal group D Streptococcus, frquently have underlying colon disease (carcinoma, diverticular disease).

Treatment. Antibiotics are the cornerstone of treatment in infective endocarditis. If at all possible, attempts should be made to isolate and characterize the infecting agent.

Antimicrobial therapy should be initiated on the basis of the apparent infecting agent and altered on the basis of sensitivity testing. Endocarditis should be treated with bactericidal drugs when possible (penicillins, cephalosporins, vancomycin) because bacteriostatic drugs (tetracyclines, sulfonamides, chloramphenicol) usually fail. Some organisms (enterococci) require the addition of a second drug, such as an aminoglycoside, in order to achieve a synergistic effect. Because of decreased renal function in the elderly, these regimens may produce more toxicity.

Infections caused by *Staphylococcus aureus* should be treated with a semisynthetic penicillinase resistant drug, such as oxacillin or nafcillin or cephalothin. In the penicillin allergic patient, vancomycin is the drug of choice, although a cephalosporin may be used with caution in the patient with a history of delayed reactions. *Staphylococcus epidermidis* is resistant to oxacillin or nafcillin more frequently than *Staph. aureus*. A cephalosporin or vancomycin may be required. Experimental regimens that include rifampin and gentamicin are being evaluated in patients with resistant *Staph. epidermidis* infections. Therapy should be continued for six weeks.

Viridans streptococci are usually exquisitely sensitive to penicillin G, except perhaps in patients taking penicillin prophylactically for rheumatic heart disease or infections that develop during antibiotic therapy. Penicillin G given alone for four weeks or in combination with streptomycin for the first two weeks is usually curative. Vancomycin, cephalosporins, erythromycin, or clindamycin may be used in the penicillin allergic patient. Infections due to *S. faecalis* (enterococcus) do not usually respond to penicillin alone. Combination regimens of high dose penicillin and an aminoglycoside for four to six weeks are required. Vancomycin is the drug of choice in enterococcal infections in the penicillin allergic individual. Infections caused by pneumococci or beta-hemolytic streptococci should be treated for four weeks with penicillin G.

Infections due to miscellaneous organisms should be treated according to sensitivity data. Hemophilus infections usually require combinations of ampicillin and chloramphenicol or aminoglycoside. Gram negative rod infections may require ampicillin, cephalosporins, or an extended spectrum penicillin (carbenicillin, ticarcillin, azlocillin, mezlocillin, piperacillin) in combination with gentamicin, tobramycin, or amikacin or trimethoprim-sulfamethoxazole in combination with surgery. Fungal infections generally require surgery in combination with amphotericin B and occasionally flucytosine.

The patient with congestive heart failure (especially in the setting of aortic regurgitation) may require immediate operative intervention with valve replacement. Prosthetic device infections usually require surgical débridement or replacement if a cure is to be achieved. These special decisions should be made in consultation with the cardiologist, infectious disease specialist, and thoracic surgeon.

Infections in the Compromised Host

There are many processes that alter host resistance to infections. These range from subtle defects in the performance of phagocytic cells, as is seen in diabetes mellitus and renal failure, to the profound absence of granulocytes produced by cancer chemotherapy. In addition, decreases in lymphocyte function occur with advancing age. Certain infections such as herpes zoster and lower respiratory illnesses are seen with increased frequency in the elderly. The incidence of tuberculosis is highest in the elderly; however, this may represent a higher proportion of cases of subclinical tuberculosis contracted during childhood. The elderly are at greater risk of death during influenza epidemics and following bacteremia. The reasons for the adverse outcome of infections in the elderly are frequently unclear, but they probably represent subtle combinations of many factors.

There are several common associations between certain diseases and specific types of infections. When the physician is aware of the patient's underlying problems, he may frequently predict the type of infection encountered. Some of these common associations are included in Table 7–10. Infectious complications of selected conditions frequently encountered in the elderly are included in Table 7–11.

Because of the possibility of opportunistic infection in the seriously ill patient, antimicrobial therapy should be given as soon as possible. Once appropriate cultures have been obtained, broad spectrum antibiotics should be given. The choice should be individualized on the basis of the type of infection and any previously available data regarding infection and underlying disease. When no clues are available, a cephalosporin, such as cefazolin or cefamandole, and an aminoglycoside (or carbenicillin) should be given intravenously. These combinations provide coverage for most gram positive infections (staphylococci, streptococci, and pneumococci) and gram negative infections (enteric organisms and Pseudomonas). When specific organisms are isolated, the spectrum should be narrowed in order to reduce the risk of superinfection. In gram negative infections the granulocytopenic patient (less than 500 to 1000 polymorphonuclear leucocytes) should receive two drugs that are active against the infecting organism (e.g., cephalosporin with aminoglycoside, cephalosporin with carbenicillin, or carbenicillin with aminoglycoside).

TABLE 7–10. Common Associations Between Diseases and Infections

Diabetes mellitus	*Staphylococcus aureus*, Candida, Torulopsis
	Group B Streptococcus, mucormycosis
Hodgkin's disease	Herpes zoster, tuberculosis, cryptococcosis
Chronic lymphocytic leukemia	Pneumococcus, Klebsiella
Multiple myeloma	Pneumococcus, Klebsiella
Acute leukemias, granulocytopenia	Enteric gram negative organisms, Pseudomonas, staphylococci, Aspergillus, Mucor, Pneumocystis

TABLE 7–11. Infectious Complications of Diseases of the Elderly

Peripheral vascular disease	Cellulitis, gangrene, osteomyelitis
Diabetes mellitus	Urinary tract infection, vaginitis, balanitis, mucormycosis, as above in vascular disease
Prostatic hypertrophy	Urinary tract infection
Congestive heart failure	Pneumonia
Valvular heart disease	Bacterial endocarditis
Cerebrovascular disease	Aspiration pneumonia, decubitus ulcers, urinary tract infection

Fever of Undetermined Origin

The term fever of undetermined origin should be distinguished from the clinical syndrome of acute febrile illness. The former refers to illnesses that are more indolent and cryptic and generally includes patients with temperatures of 101° F. (38.3° C.) or greater for more than three weeks who have undergone an initial screening evaluation for relatively obvious problems. Acute febrile illnesses are much more common and are usually infectious. By contrast, only one-third of the patients with fever of undetermined origin have an infectious illness.

The most common etiologies encountered in patients with fever of undetermined origin are infectious, neoplastic, and inflammatory. The more common infectious illnesses are intra-abdominal disease (liver, gallbladder), endocarditis, and tuberculosis. Neoplastic diseases such as lymphoma, nephrocarcinoma, and metastatic tumors to the liver frequently cause fever. Vasculitic illnesses frequently are found in the inflammatory category (systemic lupus erythematosus, polyarteritis nodosa, giant cell arteritis). Miscellaneous disorders such as pulmonary embolism or drug fever are occasionally encountered. An etiology may never be found in 5 to 15 per cent of cases.

The mechanism of fever production in infectious illness is generally thought to be secondary to pyrogen release from microorganisms and leucocytes. Fever secondary to inflammatory and neoplastic diseases is poorly understood. It is generally stated that fevers of undetermined origin are frequently due to unusual presentations of common diseases rather than to exotic problems.

The symptoms are extremely varied, depending upon the etiology. In general, however, the patient does not show the "textbook" picture of the disease in question, for otherwise the diagnosis would not be in question. Patients with ultimately serious disease generally appear chronically or acutely ill, have lost weight, have persistent fever, and may show further evidence of malnutrition on laboratory testing (anemia and hypoalbuminemia). The sedimentation rate may be greatly raised in many types of illness.

Every patient with fever of undetermined origin should have a thorough medical history (travel, occupation, animal exposure, drug ingestion, exposure to toxins or infectious disease) and a careful physical examination, which should be repeated at frequent intervals. A systematic approach to laboratory testing should be considered (complete blood count, urinalysis, erythrocyte sedimentation rate, blood chemistries, antibody titers to appropriate infecting agents, urine and blood cultures, and chest x-ray examination) with follow-up of any leads. Further investigation such as gallbladder, gastrointestinal, and genitourinary contrast studies, abdominal computed tomographic scan, bone marrow examination, and liver biopsy as indicated may be undertaken. Abdominal exploration may be indicated in selected patients.

An excellent review of the problem of fever of undetermined origin in the elderly has been published by Esposito and Gleckman.[12] They reviewed the data relating to 111 patients between the ages of 65 and 86. Infection was present in 36 per cent, malignant disease in 24 per cent, connective tissue disease in 26 per cent, miscellaneous illnesses in 9 per cent, and no ultimate diagnosis in 5 per cent. In general, the elderly patient with fever of undetermined origin is more likely to have a serious illness than a younger individual. Diseases such as systemic lupus, Still's disease, and atrial myxoma were not encountered in this group of patients.

Vague complaints such as abdominal discomfort, headache, and muscle stiffness and a history of urinary tract infection should be noted and repeated examinations should be performed. It should be noted that mild anemia and elevation of the sedimentation rate may be seen normally in the elderly. The alkaline phosphatase level may be elevated in Paget's disease, and hence an elevated value may not represent a hepatic abnormality. Slight but stable elevations in rheumatoid factor levels may also be seen in 30 per cent of healthy elderly individuals. Giant cell arteritis is an extremely important illness in this population and may present with polymyalgia rheumatica, headache, or visual disturbances. Temporal artery biopsy is required to make a definite diagnosis. Among the infectious illnesses, abdominal abscess, hepatobiliary disease, endocarditis, and tuberculosis are the most common.

Infection of Vascular Grafts and Pacemakers

Infection around pacemaker wires or battery pockets is relatively uncommon (less than

2 per cent of all pacemakers). Endocarditis occurs under these circumstances even less commonly (0.2 per cent). Infections around pacemaker wires are usually associated with bacteremia and generally occur shortly after placement of the device. These infections are usually caused by *Staph. aureus.* Pacemaker pocket infections are generally more indolent, and although they may also be caused by *Staph. aureus,* they are frequently associated with less pathogenic skin flora, such as *Staph. epidermidis* and diphtheroids. These infections must be treated by the systemic administration of antibiotics, removal of the infected device, and insertion of a new pacemaker under antibiotic cover. Since most pacemaker infections occur at the time of insertion, subsequent prophylaxis against endocarditis is not necessary.

The incidence of vascular graft infections is similar to that of pacemaker infections. The majority of infections of inguinal and lower extremity grafts occur within two months after placement, but most abdominal aortic graft infections occur after one year. Infections may occur in the perioperative period or may be secondary to infection in local contiguous tissues or bacteremias. The most common infecting agents are *Staph. aureus, Staph. epidermidis,* and gram negative enteric bacilli. Infections should be treated with antibiotics appropriate to the infecting agent (doses similar to those for endocarditis) for four to six weeks. Surgery is usually required when the infection involves suture lines or in the presence of bleeding, pseudoaneurysm formation, or thrombosis.

REFERENCES

1. Kucers, A., and Bennett, N.M.: The Use of Antibiotics. Philadelphia, J.B. Lippincott Company, 1979.
2. Garrod, L.P., et al.: Antibiotic and Chemotherapy. New York, Churchill Livingstone, 1981.
3. Mandell, G.L., et al.: Principles and Practice of Infectious Diseases. New York, John Wiley & Sons, Inc., 1979.
4. LeFroch, J.L., et al.: Cefoxitin therapy in aerobic, anaerobic, and mixed aerobic-anaerobic infections. Drug Intel. Clin. Pharm. *16:*306, 1982.
5. Cunha, B.A., and Ristuccia, A.M.: Third generation cephalosporins. Med. Clin. N. Am., *66:*283, 1982.
6. Dudley, M.N., and Barriere, S.L.: Cefotaxime: microbiology, pharmacology and clinical use. Clin. Pharm., *1:*114, 1982.
7. Reed, M.D., et al.: Evaluation of moxalactam. Clin. Pharm., *1:*124, 1982.
8. Sarubbi, F.A., and Hull, J.H.: Amikacin serum concentrations: prediction of levels and dosage guidelines. Ann. Intern. Med., *89:*612, 1978.
9. Meade, R.H.: Antimicrobial spectrum pharmacology, and the use of erythromycin derivatives. Am. J. Hosp. Pharm., *36:*1185, 1979.
10. Powell, D.A., and Nahata, M.C.: Chloramphenicol: new perspectives of an old drug. Drug Intel. Clin. Pharm., *16:*295, 1982.
11. Maddux, M.S., and Barriere, S.L.: A review of complications of amphotericin B therapy: recommendations for precautions and management. Drug Intel. Clin. Pharm., *14:*177, 1980.
12. Esposito, A.L., and Gleckman, R.A.: Fever of unknown origin in the elderly. J. Am. Geriatr. Soc., *26:*498, 1978.

CHAPTER 8

BONE AND JOINT DISORDERS

Ronald P. Evens and David W. Hawkins

This chapter is devoted to four joint and bone disorders, or arthritides, that commonly occur in the elderly: osteoarthritis, rheumatoid arthritis, ankylosing spondylitis, and gouty arthritis. Hyperuricemia is reviewed as it relates to gout and as it occurs alone in the elderly. In each of the four rheumatologic diseases, the joint is the focus of the degenerative process, with local cartilage and bone disruption as prominent features. The symptom complex is usually nonspecific, including painful joints with possible tenderness and swelling and compromised range of motion of the joints. Almost every person over 60 years of age manifests some signs or symptoms of joint disease, and significant involvement is reported to occur in 28 to 87 per cent.[1-5] Osteoarthritis is the most common process, with incidences as high as 80 to 90 per cent in the elderly (based on x-ray evidence).[2] Rheumatoid arthritis ranks second, with an incidence of over 50 per cent in the elderly.[3] These diseases can first become symptomatic during an arthritic patient's later years, but they usually develop during middle age and progress into the older age period of life. Since these diseases are chronic, lifelong problems, their cumulative incidence explains their nearly universal prevalence in elderly patients.

The content of this chapter includes the pathophysiologic features of these four arthritides, that is, their prevalence, diagnosis, clinical presentation, pathology, and progression. Table 8–1 summarizes their major distinguishing components. Second, general pharmacotherapeutic principles are discussed that are applicable to all the arthritides. Third, each antirheumatic and anti-inflammatory drug is reviewed in depth within its pharmacotherapeutic class. Fourth, some specific pharmacotherapeutic guidelines are noted for each disease process. The unique features of gout and hyperuricemia among the arthritides necessitate relatively more discussion in the latter section.

PATHOPHYSIOLOGY

The arthritides are slowly progressive articular diseases in terms of both pathologic involvement and clinical presentation. Such progression from an early onset leads to the middle to late stages of osteoarthritis and ankylosing spondylitis that usually are manifested in the elderly. By contrast, rheumatoid arthritis and gout can occur initially in young or old patients. In the aged, the clinical presentation of rheumatoid arthritis can be differentiated further between the type of disease starting at a young age and persisting into old age versus a late developing disease in old age. Table 8–1 presents an overview of the major clinical features of each disease.

Osteoarthritis

Degenerative joint disease is another common name for osteoarthritis.[2,6-9] Its onset is

TABLE 8–1. Clinical Features of the Arthritides*

Parameter	Osteoarthritis	Rheumatoid Arthritis	Ankylosing Spondylitis	Gout
Age at diagnosis	40–60	20–60	15–30	20–60
Sex	> 45 yr., F > M < 45 yr., M > F	F > M	M >> F	M > F
Joint pain	1+ to 4+	1+ to 4+	1+ to 4+	1+ to 4+
Joint swelling	0 to 2+	2+ to 4+	0 to 2+	2+ to 4+
Morning stiffness	1+ to 2+	1+ to 4+	1+ to 2+	WNL
Joint sites (major)	DIP, knee, hip, MTP, CMC, spine	PIP, cervical spine, cricoarytenoid, knee, ankle	Iliosacral, lumbar and cervical spine, costovertebral, hip, shoulder, knee	MTP, tarsal
Erythrocyte sedimentation rate	WNL	High	High	WNL/high
Rheumatoid factor	5–10%	80%	WNL	WNL
Latex fixation	WNL	High	WNL	WNL
X-ray	Osteophytes, sclerosis, joint space loss	Joint space loss, erosion, ankylosis	Joint space wide, erosion, sclerosis, syndesmophytes, whiskering, eburnation	Tophi, lateral erosion
Synovial fluid				
Appearance	Transparent	Cloudy	Transparent	Cloudy, urate crystals
WBC	1000–3000	RA cells	1,000–50,000	10,000–12,000
Complement	WNL	Low	High	High
Nodules	Heberden, Bouchard	Subcutaneous	—	Tophi
Antigen	—	—	HLA-B27	—
Systemic disease	—	Fatigue, weakness, anemia, pleuritis, vasculitis, neuropathy	Anemia, fatigue, fever, iritis	Hyperuricemia, Nephropathy, Nephrolithiasis

*RA, rheumatoid arthritis cells.
Symptom scale—0 (none) to 4+ (severe).
CMC, carpometacarpal
DIP, distal interphalangeal
MTP, metatarsophalangeal
PIP, proximal interphalangeal
WNL, within normal limits.

usually during the middle years of life, and its incidence is age related, such that about 85 to 100 per cent of people over 70 years old develop this type of arthritis. The prevalence based on sex is not striking for all patients with osteoarthritis, but women outnumber men above the age of 45, and the converse is true below 45 years.

The sites of involvement are the diarthrodial joints, especially the weight bearing ones, usually in a bilateral fashion. The commonly afflicted joints are the knee, distal interphalangeal, first carpometacarpal, and proximal interphalangeal joints, hips, spine (especially lumbar and cervical areas), and foot (primarily the metatarsophalangeal joint).

Osteoarthritis historically has been considered to be related to chronic "wear and tear" of bone and joints, but its etiology is unknown. Possible contributory factors in its pathogenesis include biochemical abnormalities, an abnormal repair process, destructive enzymes, physical stress, and aging. The integrity of the matrix of articular cartilage changes as a result of a smaller polysaccharide content (glycosaminoglycans), particularly chondroitin sulfate. In regenerating cartilage, chondrocytes proliferate and synthesize new matrix, but the cartilage becomes fibrous. Synovial enzymes are postulated to break down cartilage, e.g., collagenase, cathepsin (the chondrocytes' lysosomal enzyme), hydrolase, and hyaluronidase. Chronic physical trauma facilitates cartilage destruction. Excessive use of a joint can lead to osteoarthritis, which is commonly observed in athletes (e.g., football—knee; baseball—shoulder, elbow; soccer—ankle, foot, knee; boxing—hands; bicycling—patella). Aging causes cartilage to change, with a reduction in collagen proteins and alterations in mucopolysaccharides. Genetic factors have not been correlated with disease activity.

Pathologic abnormalities principally involve articular cartilage and subchondral bone. Also inflammation can be associated with osteoarthritis, but the extent of synovitis is variable. Degeneration of cartilage occurs in a stepwise fashion, first early softening and yellowing, then fissuring, flaking, and fibrillation, and finally erosion with denudation of bone. Subchondral bone becomes sclerotic and eburnated. Bony prominences (osteophytes) develop as a result of exudation of cancellous bone at the joint margin, particularly where ligaments or the articular capsule attach to bone. Especially in women, articular cartilage hypertrophies commonly at the distal interphalangeal joints to form the typical Heberden nodes, and sometimes at the proximal interphalangeal joints to form Bouchard's nodes.

The prominent complaint of patients is pain with exercise and possibly at rest or at night. The onset is insidious. Tenderness and swelling of bones and cartilage can occur at the joints. Joint stiffness is localized at the involved joints and has a shorter duration than in rheumatoid arthritis, that is, about 30 minutes versus over one hour. The limitation in the range of motion of afflicted joints gradually progresses, leading to disability. Extraarticular disease generally is not found. Laboratory parameters are usually within normal limits and include such tests of rheumatoid disease as the erythrocyte sedimentation rate, latex fixation, and rheumatoid factor. Synovial fluid is generally normal, but knee effusions have occurred. Roentgenographic examinations reveal loss of joint space, calcifications in joint margins (osteophytes), and sclerosis of subchondral bone. These x-ray changes generally lag behind the appearance of severe clinical manifestations. Nodules, especially Heberden's nodes, classically develop, as already noted.

Rheumatoid Arthritis

Rheumatoid arthritis is a polyarthritis of the diarthrodial joints, characterized as a progressive, symmetric, highly inflammatory, immunologic, and potentially crippling disease.[10–14] The disease pattern is slowly progressive and episodic with spontaneous remissions and relapses. The rate of progression, severity of acute attacks, and duration of remissions and relapses vary quite widely between subjects. The peak onset occurs at about 35 to 45 years of age, but it can start at any time from the fifteenth to the sixtieth year of life and beyond. The disease occurs in about 13 per cent of the general population, with an increasing rate of occurrence with age, such that 30 to 50 per cent or more of the elderly manifest symptoms. The sex ratio favors women somewhat over men (2:1 to 3:1). Rheumatoid arthritis involves many peripheral joints and has manifold systemic components. Synovitis of joints is typically bilateral in distribution and includes the proximal and distal interphalangeal and metacarpophalangeal joints in the hands, the wrists, cervical spine, feet (metatarsophalangeal joints), and the cricoarytenoid joint in the neck. Other large joints like the knee, ankle, elbow, and shoulder are also involved but less frequently.

Chronic synovitis is the basic inflammatory abnormality in rheumatoid arthritis. An immunologic mechanism has been well outlined, with a likely lysosomal enzyme component and a possible initial infectious contribution. The proposed pathogenesis involves an initial antigenic stimulus, possibly infectious in origin, for the synthesis of immunoglobulins (IgG antibodies) and rheumatoid factor by plasma cells in the synovium or synovial fluid. Complement is bound to the immunologic aggregates, and neutrophils are attracted to the articular area. Immune complexes are ingested by the neutrophils, forming rheumatoid arthritis (RA) cells in the synovium. Lysosomal enzymes, such as acid hydrolases and cathepsin D, are released by the neutrophils, in addition to other inflammatory mediators, such as prostaglandins, to produce an inflammatory reaction. Other enzymes, including acid mucopolysaccharides and collagenase, possibly are involved in cellular destruction. The synovium becomes edematous and chronically infiltrated with neutrophils and lymphocytes. Lymphoid nodules may form. The synovial lining hypertrophies, especially at its attachment near the articular cartilage. Granulation tissue (pannus) forms, extends over the cartilage surface, destroys the cartilage, and eventually erodes subchondral bone. Bone and cartilage are lost, fibrous or bony connections form between bones (ankylosis), and tendons and ligaments weaken, leading to unstable joints with compromised mobility and subluxation.

The prominent symptoms and signs of rheumatoid arthritis are painful, swollen, and tender joints with significant morning stiffness (over one hour) and several systemic complications.[10–14] The diagnosis and assessment of rheumatoid arthritis is quite subjective but has been standardized by the American Rheumatism Association with 11 criteria: morning stiffness, pain or tenderness on motion, swelling in one joint, swelling in a second joint, symmetrical soft tissue swelling, subcutaneous nodules, x-ray changes, positive test for rheumatoid factor, poor mucin precipitation in the synovial fluid, and histologic changes in the synovium or nodules.[15] The first five criteria should persist for six weeks. Five or more criteria are required for a "definite" diagnosis, and three to four constitute "probable" disease. Similar, but more restrictive, criteria have also been recommended ("New York criteria") which include three painful joint groups in the limbs; swelling, limited motion, subluxation, or ankylosis in three joint groups in the hands, wrist, or foot; x-ray evidence of joint erosions; and a positive test for rheumatoid factor.[12] Also, other connective tissue inflammatory diseases must be ruled out to justify a diagnosis of rheumatoid arthritis, including systemic lupus erythematosus, scleroderma, dermatomyositis, gout, rheumatic fever, Reiter's syndrome, and the shoulder-hand syndrome. Laboratory signs of rheumatoid arthritis are common, particularly those of an immunologic type; rheumatoid factor with a titer over 1:160 or latex fixation also with a titer over 1:160 or C reactive protein determinations are usually positive. The erythrocyte sedimentation rate is usually significantly elevated. X-ray evidence of rheumatoid arthritis is detectable in more advanced disease, with joint space narrowing, erosions in margins of joints, bony ankylosis, and juxta-articular osteoporosis.

Extra-articular manifestations are very common in rheumatoid arthritis. Subcutaneous nodules form in about 25 per cent of the patients at several trauma points, like the forearm, olecran bursa, and Achilles tendon. Lung complications include pleuritis, pneumonitis, and granulomas. Neurologic disease occurs, primarily entrapment peripheral neuropathies like the carpal tunnel syndrome, and also sensory polyneuropathies, both related to subluxation of joints in the wrist and spine. Mild to moderate anemia commonly occurs. Systemic vasculitis produces digital arteritis, leg ulcers, and fever, another common general manifestation. Other possible, but uncommon, complications include pericarditis, scleritis, splenomegaly, and myopathy.

The presentation of rheumatoid arthritis in the elderly patient, 50 to 70 years of age or older, was studied in the late 1960's by several rheumatology groups.[16–22] Generally, late onset rheumatoid arthritis is more benign in course than the early adult onset type, even though pain, stiffness, and swelling routinely involve at least two joints, and hematologic parameters are almost universally and significantly elevated (e.g., erythrocyte sedimentation rate, 90 per cent positive with 50 per cent over 60 mm. per hour; latex fixation, 50 to 90 per cent positive; and rheumatoid factor, 40 to 50 per cent positive). Deformities and subluxations are rare; this would be expected, since the duration of the disease is short, limiting its progression. Subcutaneous nodules occur half as often or less frequently. Sites for joint involvement are similar that is, the proximal interphalangeal, metacarpophalangeal, and metatarsophalangeal joints and the wrists, but with more knee and shoulder involvement.

Ankylosing Spondylitis

Spondylarthritis and Marie-Strümpell disease are other names for this chronic, yet episodic, inflammatory disease predominantly involving the axial skeleton.[23–29] In a representative report, ankylosing spondylitis accounted for 1.6 per cent of 15,000 cases of rheumatic disease in a Scottish clinic over a 23 year period.[23] Men vastly outnumber women (8:1 to 10:1) as victims of this form of arthritis. Its onset is usually earlier in life (15 to 40 years of age) than that of the other arthritides. Progression is quite gradual and often extends insidiously into the later period of life, when deformity and disability become significant. The primary sites for the development of synovitis and damage are the iliosacral joints, the lumbosacral vertebrae (especially the apophyseal joints), and the costovertebral joints. The large peripheral joints are inflamed in at least one-third of the patients with ankylosing spondylitis, primarily the hips, shoulders, and knees and, less commonly, the ankles, heels, and manubrosternal joints.

The erosive synovitis usually starts in the sacroiliac joints at one or both sides of the skeleton and the lumbosacral spine, especially where ligaments attach to bone.[24-29] Mononuclear cells infiltrate the synovium, the synovial membrane proliferates, and granulation tissue forms and invades subchondral bone (osteitis). Erosion of bone occurs particularly at the sacroiliac joints and anterior vertebrae (spondylitis), with sclerosis developing. Ossification of multiple soft tissue structures is a hallmark feature of ankylosing spondylitis. Bony ankylosis (osseous connections between bones) or syndesmophytes form between adjacent vertebrae at the sites of previous anuli fibrosi. Spinal ligaments and tendons calcify, forming whiskers of bony material. Fusion of bones across the joint space occurs at the sacroiliac joint and the vertebrae, eventually producing spinal rigidity and a "bamboo" spine. Asymmetric peripheral joints also develop synovitis and calcifications. This familial disease has a significant genetic etiologic factor, since in 95 per cent or more of the patients with ankylosing spondylitis, serum specimens are positive for the HLA-B27 antigen.

Low back pain with or without morning stiffness is the early complaint in about 75 per cent of the afflicted young adults; it is intermittent, sometimes nocturnal, slowly progressive, and relieved by exercise. Sacroiliac tenderness is a cardinal manifestation. The arthropathy gradually extends up the spine and encompasses adjacent joints. The lumbar spine is flattened, with loss of the normal curve (lordosis). Back pain is relieved by bending over, leading to kyphosis. The cervical spine is eventually involved, with excess curvature developing. Costovertebral involvement is common, limits chest expansion, and results in dyspnea, since the patient avoids the pain associated with deep breathing. Laboratory signs include a high erythrocyte sedimentation rate in over 80 per cent of the patients with ankylosing spondylitis, a mild anemia, and a positive HLA-B27 antigen titer. X-ray examination shows sacroiliac erosions, widening of margins, subchondral sclerosis, and joint fusion. Spinal deformities include syndesmophytes and whiskering in previous soft tissue areas. Osteoporosis is observed in vertebral bodies and the sacroiliac areas adjacent to joints.

General systemic complaints are common, with fatigue, a daily fluctuating fever, and anorexia, but are less frequent than in rheumatoid arthritis. Extra-articular complications are common, predominantly iritis, which occurs in 25 to 40 per cent of the patients with ankylosing spondylitis and is frequently unilateral. Aortic insufficiency and pulmonary fibrosis are the other long term, late sequelae. Compression radiculitis or cauda equina develops late in the disease, causing sensory and motor disturbances in the extremities.

The diagnostic criteria for ankylosing spondylitis have been developed recently at an international conference in Rome.[28,29] They include low back pain for over three months unrelieved by rest, pain and stiffness in the thorax, chest expansion limitation, a reduction in lumbar spinal motion, iritis, and x-ray evidence of sacroiliitis and syndesmophytes.

Gout

Hyperuricemia and gout occur in individuals who have some abnormality in either the production or elimination of uric acid, or both.[30-37] Men are affected 10 times more often than women; the mean age of onset of gout is 47 years. Gout is a disease manifested by acute attacks of arthritis, nephrolithiasis, gouty nephropathy, and aggregated deposits of sodium urate (tophi) occurring in cartilage, tendons, and synovial membranes. These pathologic events are more likely to occur when hyperuricemia is present, but they may occur when serum urate levels are below the saturation point.

Acute attacks of gouty arthritis are characterized by a rapid onset of excruciating pain, swelling, and inflammation. The attack is typically monoarticular at first, most often affecting the first metatarsophalangeal joint; then, in order of frequency, the sites of involvement are the insteps, ankles, heels, knees, wrists, fingers, and elbows.

The American Rheumatism Association has developed classification criteria for the diagnosis of gout.[30,31] A definite diagnosis requires the identification of uric acid crystals in the synovial fluid of an afflicted joint or tophus formation. In the absence of these definite signs, a suggestive diagnosis requires presence of six of 12 clinical, laboratory, or x-ray parameters. These include more than one attack of acute arthritis, maximal inflammation developing within one day, a monoarthritic attack, redness observed over the joints, a swollen and painful first metatarsophalangeal joint, a unilateral attack involving the first metatarsophalangeal joint, a unilateral tarsal joint attack, a suspected tophus, hyperuricemia, asymmetric joint swelling on x-ray examination, subcortical cysts without erosion visible on x-ray films, and a negative synovial fluid culture.

The development of crystal-induced inflammation in gout first involves the precipitation of urate crystals in synovial fluid. Then a number of chemical mediators cause vasodilation, increase vascular permeability, and stimulate chemotactic activity of polymorphonuclear leukocytes. Phagocytosis of urate crystals by the leukocytes results in rapid lysis of cells and a discharge of proteolytic enzymes into the cytoplasm. The inflammatory reaction that ensues lasts three to 14 days if left untreated. Articular destruction occurs with repeated attacks. Although acute attacks of gouty arthritis may occur without apparent provocation, a number of conditions under the right circumstances may precipitate an attack. These include stress, trauma, surgery, rapid lowering of the serum uric acid level by ingestion of uric acid lowering drugs, and ingestion of certain drugs known to elevate the serum uric acid level (e.g., thiazide diuretics).

Nephrolithiasis occurs in 10 to 25 per cent of the patients with gout. It also occurs in hyperuricemic patients with no history of gout. Factors predisposing individuals to uric acid nephrolithiasis include excessive urinary excretion of uric acid, an acidic urine, and a highly concentrated urine. The stones that form are of three types: pure uric acid stones, mixed uric acid–calcium oxalate stones, and calcium oxalate stones. Uric acid has a pK_a of 5.5. Therefore, when the urine is acidic, uric acid exists primarily in the un-ionized, less soluble form. When an acidic urine is saturated with uric acid, stones precipitate out spontaneously. In patients with uric acid nephrolithiasis, the urinary pH is typically less than 6.0 and frequently less than 5.5.

There are two types of gouty nephropathy. First, the formation of uric acid crystals in the collecting tubules or ureter is related to acute hyperuricaciduria. The blockage of urine flow leads to acute renal failure. Second, chronic deposition of urate crystals can occur in the renal parenchyma, but this is a rare complication of gout, even with hyperuricemia. Microtophi may form with a surrounding giant cell inflammatory reaction. A decrease in the kidney's capacity to concentrate urine and the presence of proteinuria may be the earliest pathophysiologic disturbances. Hypertension and nephrosclerosis are common sequelae, and chronic renal insufficiency could ultimately result.

Tophi are uncommon in the general population of gouty subjects and are a late complication of hyperuricemia. The most common site of tophaceous deposits in patients with recurrent acute gouty arthritis is at the base of the great toe (the metatarsophalangeal joint). However, visible tophi may also occur in the ear lobes, olecran bursa, ankles, heels, knees, wrists, and hands. Eventually even the hips, shoulders, and spine may be affected. In addition to causing obvious deformities, tophi may damage surrounding soft tissue, cause joint destruction and pain, and even lead to nerve compression syndromes, including the carpal tunnel syndrome.

Hyperuricemia

Hyperuricemia may be an asymptomatic condition with an increased serum uric acid level as the only apparent abnormality.[31,33–35] Hyperuricemia can be defined biochemically as a serum urate concentration of 7.5 mg. per dl. or higher. In man, uric acid is the end product of the degradation of purines. It serves no known physiologic purpose and therefore is regarded as a waste product. The miscible pool of uric acid amounts to about 1200 mg. The size of the urate pool may increase up to 18,000 to 31,000 mg. in individuals with gout. The purines from which uric acid is produced originate from three sources—dietary purines, the conversion of tissue nucleic acid to purine nucleotides, and the de novo synthesis of purine bases. All purines enter a common metabolic pathway, which leads to the production of either nucleic acid or uric acid. When purine metabolism is normal, the average man produces about 600 to 800 mg. of uric acid each day. A 24 hour urine collection can be used for diagnosis, a value above 800 mg. of uric acid indicating overproduction. Some clinicians employ a morning (e.g., 10 A.M.) spot urine test and calculate a uric acid excretion ratio, but the clinical utility of this method requires confirmation.[31]

Excessive uric acid may occur as a consequence of the increased breakdown of tissue nucleic acids associated with myeloproliferative and lymphoproliferative disorders. Dietary purines play an insignificant role in the generation of hyperuricemia in the absence of a derangement in purine metabolism or elimination. Along the metabolic pathway, several enzyme systems regulate the direction of purine metabolism. An abnormality in any of these regulatory systems could result in an overproduction of uric acid. To date, only two enzyme defects of purine metabolism are known to cause an overproduction of uric acid, namely, phosphoribosyl pyrophosphate (PRPP) synthetase and hypoxanthineguanine phosphoribosyl transferase (HG-PRT). The defect associated with PRPP synthetase results in an increased intracellular concentration of PRPP. The build-up of PRPP accelerates the rate of urine biosynthesis de novo and, consequently, the production of uric acid. HG-PRT is responsible for the conversion of guanine to guanylic acid and hypoxanthine to inosinic acid. These two conversions require PRPP as the cosubstrate and are important in reutilization reactions involved in the synthesis of nucleic acids. A deficiency in the HG-PRT enzyme would lead to an increased metabolism of guanine and hypoxanthine to uric acid and more PRPP to interact with glutamine in the first step of the purine pathway. A partial deficiency of the enzyme may be responsible for marked hyperuricemia in otherwise normal healthy individuals.

Hyperuricemia does not occur as long as a balance exists between uric acid production and elimination. Uric acid is eliminated in two ways. Most of the uric acid produced each day is excreted in the urine. About 200 mg. is eliminated through the gastrointestinal tract after being enzymatically degraded by colonic bacteria. In the presence of renal failure, the elimination of uric acid through the gastrointestinal tract increases several times. A decline in the urinary excretion of uric acid leads to hyperuricemia and an increased miscible pool of sodium urate. This situation may arise if any of the components involved in the renal metabolism of uric acid is altered. Almost all the urate in plasma is freely filtered across the glomerulus. Following glomerular filtration, urate undergoes passive tubular reabsorption, active tubular secretion, and then passive tubular reabsorption again. In the initial part of the proximal tubule, 98 to 100 per cent of the filtered urate is reabsorbed back into the blood. Therefore, the final concentration of uric acid in the urine is largely dependent upon the efficiency ratio of active tubular secretion to postsecretory reabsorption. Hyperuricemic individuals who excrete less than 600 mg. of uric acid per 24 hours may be defined as relative underexcretors of uric acid.

GENERAL PHARMACOTHERAPEUTIC PRINCIPLES

The goals of therapy in the arthritides are relief of pain, reduction of inflammation, maintenance or restoration of joint function, and prevention of deformities of joints.[38-45] The expected result is full control of rheumatic symptoms in at least 70 per cent of the patients with drugs and physical therapy.

Assessment of the disease response to therapy is limited by the subjective nature of the manifestations of rheumatic disease.[46,47] However, these symptoms can be scaled to provide a measure of the extent of drug activity; e.g., a 10 cm. visual analogue pain scale allows the patient to rank pain from none to worst, before and after therapy, in order to calculate the degree of pain relief. Also a composite of symptoms, e.g., an articular index, is quite useful in determining the scope of disease modification. When each symptom in the composite is similarly decreased in intensity, the usefulness of the assessment of drug efficacy is increased.

Monitoring parameters are divided into four categories: symptoms, functional capacity, bone and synovial fluid signs, and hematologic status. Symptomatic grading includes pain relief, morning stiffness (timed), swelling (ring size), and analgesic intake. Functional capacity is quantified by grip strength (pressures), range of motion of joints (degrees of change), onset of fatigue (timed), and walking distance (timed/length). Bone is assessed by x-ray examination and biopsy with histologic examinations. Joint fluid is examined by biochemical analysis and microscopic evaluation. The hematologic status is assessed by measuring the erythrocyte sedimentation rate, rheumatoid factor, latex fixation, and C reactive proteins—primarily an immunologic assessment.

Levels of Therapy for Arthritides

Four levels of therapy with many steps are employed to achieve the aforementioned goals. These steps are outlined in Table 8–2 and reviewed in the subsequent commentary.

The first level of treatment involves general physical measures to improve joint function and pharmacologic intervention to control the early mild symptoms. Both these measures constitute the basic therapy continued throughout the course of a rheumatic disease. Physical therapy is based on the premise of a proper balance of joint immobilization through rest or splinting to prevent further trauma to an inflamed joint and exercise to maintain joint function and muscle strength.

In addition, the arthritic patient is frequently very anxious and disturbed about the crippling potential of his disease, and requires a major effort in regard to patient counseling. Clinicians should minimize the emotional stress by explaining fully the disease pathology and the likely gradual control that will follow sequential chemotherapy. The patient's energies should be channeled toward self-control of the arthritis through physical therapy and compliance with long term drug therapy. Initial drug therapy is intended primarily to control pain, which is the most common early sign of rheumatic disease and frequently occurs alone in the initial stages. Nonsteroidal anti-inflammatory drugs are usually employed at lower analgesic doses, e.g., aspirin, 2 to 4 gm. per day, and ibuprofen, 800 to 1800 mg. per day.[48,49] Other analgesics, like acetaminophen or propoxyphene, possess no anti-inflammatory activity but are recommended as adjunctive therapy to control pain without inflammation.[2,7,43,44,48] However, some clinicians do not use such analgesics because of their limited activity in inflammatory diseases like the arthritides.[45]

At the second level of therapy, control of inflammation is the main objective, halting synovitis, the primary pathologic abnormality of rheumatic disease that is responsible for many of the patient's symptomatic complaints and acute physical disabilities. Nonsteroidal anti-inflammatory drugs are the drugs of first choice at anti-inflammatory doses commensurate with the progressing pathologic process. The 20 commercially available drugs are similar in pharmacologic, therapeutic, and toxicologic actions.

Aspirin remains the preferred drug among the nonsteroidal anti-inflammatory drugs, since all these drugs have equal efficacy, and the cost of aspirin is far below that of the alternatives. Intolerance to aspirin is a common phenomenon, which warrants a change to another nonsteroidal anti-inflammatory drug. Continued daily therapy should be employed even during quiescent periods between rheumatic exacerbations. Nocturnal pain and major morning stiffness require additional night-time dosing with these drugs. Indomethacin and phenylbutazone are the most toxic nonsteroidal anti-inflammatory drugs without established superiority for the control of disease activity. Both these reasons relegate them to the last alternative among the available nonsteroidal anti-inflammatory drugs. If single arthritic joints are acutely inflamed in an asymmetric pattern, do not respond to nonsteroidal anti-inflammatory drugs, and impair mobility, the intra-articular administration of corticosteroids is begun at this level of therapy.

When the rheumatic disease is not sufficiently controlled by nonsteroidal anti-inflammatory drugs, the more powerful and

TABLE 8–2. Levels of Therapy for Arthritides

First level	Baseline program
	1. Physical therapy
	   a. Rest
	   b. Exercise
	   c. Splinting
	2. Patient education and counseling
	3. Analgesia
	   a. Pain without inflammation—analgesics
	   b. Pain with inflammation—nonsteroidal anti-inflammatory drugs

Second level	Inflammatory control
	1. Nonsteroidal anti-inflammatory drugs
	   a. Chronic daily dosage
	   b. Night-time dosage
	2. Intra-articular doses of corticosteroids

Third level	Disease modifying drugs* 1. Gold 2. Penicillamine 3. Antimalarial drugs
Fourth level	Immunosuppressive therapy* 1. Corticosteroids (oral route) 2. Cytotoxic drugs

*These drugs are used primarily in rheumatoid arthritis.

more toxic disease modifying drugs are prescribed to control the inflammatory process, avoid serious articular damage, and possibly arrest or slow progression of the disease. Gold compounds are still considered the drugs of choice in this third level. Penicillamine is becoming popular as an alternative to gold because of the convenience of oral administration, with similar efficacy and adverse effects. Cross toxicity between gold and penicillamine can occur occasionally in an individual patient. Chloroquine is employed if toxicity to gold and penicillamine is unacceptable. Its ocular side effects account for its ranking third. Nonsteroidal anti-inflammatory drugs, usually at full dosages, and physical therapy are continued throughout any acute treatment period with these disease modifying drugs.

When severe rheumatic disease does not respond to both nonsteroidal anti-inflammatory drugs and gold or penicillamine, and the possibility of serious disability also exists, immunosuppressive therapy with corticosteroids, azathioprine, or cyclophosphamide is instituted to hold the inflammation in check. The cytotoxic drugs can even interrupt disease progression. The many serious side effects of these drugs restrict their use to the last stage of treatment.

Individualization of Therapy

The arthritides are slowly progressive, lifelong diseases characterized by spontaneous exacerbations and remissions occurring at variable intervals and for variable durations. This significant interpatient variation necessitates the optimizing of disease control on an individual patient basis within the levels of therapy just discussed. A series of specific pharmacotherapeutic principles forms the basis for this individualization:[38-48]

1. Monitoring parameters should be quantifiable in order to determine a definitive response to therapy.

2. The placebo response to drug therapy can account for a significant percentage and degree of pain relief—as high as 50 per cent or more.

3. The majority of patients usually have similar responses to all the nonsteroidal anti-inflammatory drugs, but one patient can respond quite differently to one category of drugs than to another (e.g., aspirin versus ibuprofen versus sulindac). Therefore, several nonsteroidal anti-inflammatory drugs can be tried in a serial fashion in an effort to produce the most beneficial results in a particular subject.

4. The level of disease activity at any time (e.g., number, severity, or duration of symptoms) should influence the initial dosage selection and the rate of dosage increase to achieve an optimal response commensurate with the extent of the disease.

5. The overall disease pattern helps in determining the aggressiveness of antirheumatic therapy in regard to both drug and dosage selection. As the disease pattern changes, the drug dosage should be adjusted accordingly.

6. Concomitant diseases should be considered in drug selection in order to avoid exacerbation with the antirheumatic drugs (e.g., ulcer disease, renal failure, and hypertension).

7. A careful history of past drug exposures and their outcomes helps in making future drug selections and in minimizing the potential for drug toxicity.

8. Less toxic drugs should be used first to minimize adverse effects. For the oral therapies, gastric intolerance can be minimized by dosing with meals. Cross allergenicity among the nonsteroidal anti-inflammatory drugs is a common phenomenon and warrants caution when changing drugs for this reason.

9. Antirheumatic drugs are prescribed first as single drugs in a serial fashion to find the most effective drug prior to using combination therapy.

10. Before changing drug therapy, the duration of treatment for each antirheumatic drug is adapted to that drug's onset of peak action (e.g., about one to four weeks for nonsteroidal anti-inflammatory drugs and at least three to six months for the disease modifying drugs).

11. The cost of drug therapy is a valid consideration to provide the least expensive, yet most effective, treatment.

12. Failure in rheumatic disease improvement with drug therapy requires the assessment of dose, frequency, and compliance before changing to a new therapy.

The elderly patient potentially can respond to drug therapy for arthritis in a different manner from that in younger adults.[1,3-5] Multiple diseases involving nonarticular organ systems are very likely to afflict an elderly patient and can influence drug or dosage decisions. The following diseases can increase the incidence or severity of side effects of antirheumatic drugs: peptic ulcer disease, chronic constipation, cerebrovascular insufficiency, renal failure, cardiovascular disease, peripheral vascular disease, and thromboembolic disease. Also the aged patient has an increased chance of sustaining bone injuries, which is related to physical deterioration and osteoporosis. Such injuries directly produce or complicate bone and joint disease. Many old patients live alone and suffer psychologic isolation—both increasing inactivity and losses in functional capacity, decreasing their expectation for improvement, and leading to noncompliance. Patient education and physical therapy therefore become even more important measures to maximize disease control.

Nondrug Treatment Measures

Along with drug therapy to control inflammation, physical therapy is a major component of treatment throughout the course of all the arthritides, especially in the elderly.[2,7,12,14,22,26,27,29,45] A balanced physical therapy program involves rest and the use of splinting, exercise, heat, and assistive devices.[2,22,50,51] Alternating periods of rest and exercise ideally minimize joint trauma and maximize function. Fatigue is a common complaint, particularly in rheumatoid arthritis and ankylosing spondylitis, and these patients require adequate rest.[52,53] Extended nights of restful sleep and daytime naps or full rest periods can prevent fatigue and improve the overall activity level. When an acute flare-up of joint inflammation occurs, complete bed rest is encouraged to immobilize the joint and limit joint trauma. However, at least 10 hours of sleep with a morning and an afternoon rest period (one to two hours) should suffice to significantly reduce pain, stiffness, and swelling. Rest for an inflamed joint is achieved with splinting, which accomplishes three goals—the relief of pain, the localized reduction of specific joint stress, and the prevention of contracture deformities.[50,51,54] Splints are most commonly employed for the wrist, knee, and neck. For example, the wrist splint covers and immobilizes the hand, wrist, and distal forearm with a contoured device, but the fingers are free to move, resulting in a rested, yet functional, hand. A back brace restores spinal column alignment and prevents deformity when spinal arthritis is a problem.

Exercises are necessary to maintain muscle strength and joint flexibility. Postural training is a key element in preventing spinal deformities in ankylosing spondylitis. The patient is instructed to sit and stand erect and to avoid bending. The legs should be kept extended while the patient is sitting and sleeping to prevent contractures at the knee. Joint mobility is aided through range of motion exercises, with controlled flexion and extension at afflicted joints. Resistive exercises, such as isometric exercises, help to strengthen muscles and are particularly useful for bedridden patients. Active exercise includes sports that require extension of the extremities, like walking, swimming, and tennis, which help prevent joint deformities. A major caution in regard to exercises is their avoidance during an acute flare-up in order to reduce the chance of joint trauma.

Thermotherapy provides symptomatic relief of pain and possibly inflammation. A warm tub bath (e.g., 102° F. [39° C.]) is the most common technique, and hot packs can be useful for single joints. Assistive devices can reduce stress on chronically inflamed weight bearing joints (e.g., a cane or even crutches in severe cases for the hips and knee, a firm mattress for the spine and hips, and thin head pillows for the spine). Gentle massage helps to reduce stiffness and muscle spasm. Occupational therapy can create a work-play plan to minimize fatigue. Good nutrition is a part of an overall program to provide and maintain energy and muscle strength.

ANTIRHEUMATIC–ANTIGOUT DRUG THERAPY

The number of antirheumatic drugs has increased to over 30 products, adding both useful alternatives for and confusion to the pharmacotherapeutic management of the arthritides. In general, the geriatric patient with rheumatic disease responds to drug therapy like other adults except for the previously noted special considerations. Table 8–3 lists the drugs by pharmacologic-chemical categories and also presents their dosage ranges, based on clinical trials. The discussion that follows concerns the efficacy, dosage, pharmacokinetics, and side effects of each drug.

TABLE 8–3. Antirheumatic and Antigout Drugs

Drug	Usual Daily Dosage Range	Formulations*
Salicylates		
Aspirin	3.9–5.1 gm.	325 mg. T
		650 mg. T
Sodium salicylate	3.9–5.1 gm.	325 mg. T
		650 mg. T.
Choline salicylate (Arthropan)	5.2–7.0 gm.	870 mg. per 5 ml. L
Choline magnesium salicylate (Trilisate)	4.5–6.0 gm.	650 mg. T
Magnesium salicylate (Magan, Mobidin)	3.9–5.1 gm.	545 mg. T
		600 mg. T
Salsalate (Disalcid)	3–4 gm.	750 mg. T
		500 mg. T
Diflunisal (Dolobid)	0.5–1.5 gm.	250 mg. T.
		500 mg. T
Buffered aspirin (Bufferin, Ascriptin)	3.9–5.1 gm.	325 mg. T
		650 mg. T
Phenylproprionic acids		
Benoxaprofen (Oraflex)—limited availability	0.4–1.0 gm.	400 mg. T
		600 mg. T
Fenoprofen (Nalfon)	1200–3200 mg.	200 mg. C
		300 mg. C
		600 mg. T
Ibuprofen (Motrin, Rufen)	1200–3600 mg.	300 mg. T
		400 mg. T
		600 mg. T
Naproxen (Naproxyn, Anaprox)	500–1000 mg.	250 mg. T
		375 mg. T
		500 mg. T
Indole-Indenes		
Indomethacin (Indocin)	75–150 mg.	25 mg. C
		50 mg. C
		75 mg. TR
Tolmetin sodium (Tolectin)	1200–1600 mg.	200 mg. T
		400 mg. C
Sulindac (Clinoril)	300–400 mg.	150 mg. T
		200 mg. T
Pyrazolones		
Oxyphenbutazone (Tandearil, Oxalid)	200–400 mg.	100 mg. T
Phenylbutazone (Butazolidin, Azolid)	200–400 mg.	100 mg. T
		100 mg. C
Phenylanthranilic acid		
Mefenamic acid (Ponstel)	750–1000 mg.	250 mg. C
Meclofenamic acid (Meclomen)	200–400 mg.	50 mg. C
		100 mg. C
Oxicam		
Piroxicam (Feldene)	20 mg.	10 mg. C
		20 mg. C
Gold salts		
Aurothioglucose (Solganal)	50 mg. (weekly)	50 mg. per ml. I
Aurothiomalate (Myochrysine)	50 mg. (weekly)	10 mg. per ml. I
		25 mg. per ml. I
		50 mg. per ml. I
Penicillamine (Cuprimine)	250–750 mg.	125 mg. C
		250 mg. C

(Table continued on page 288)

TABLE 8–3. (Continued)

Drug	Usual Daily Dosage Range	Formulations*
Antimalarial drugs		
Chloroquine phosphate (Aralen)	250 mg.	500 mg. T
Hydroxychloroquine sulfate (Plaquenil)	200–600 mg.	200 mg. T
Corticosteroid		
Oral, systemic, e.g., prednisone	8–12 mg.	1 and 5 mg. T
Intra-articular, e.g., prednisolone TBA	2–20 mg. (monthly)	20 mg. per ml. I
Cytotoxic drugs		
Cyclophosphamide (Cytoxan)	75–150 mg.	25 mg. T 50 mg. T
Azathioprine (Imuran)	75–150 mg.	50 mg. T
Uricosuric drugs		
Probenecid (Benemid)	1000–2000 mg.	500 mg. T
Sulfinpyrazone (Anturane)	200–500 mg.	200 mg. C 100 mg. T
Antigout drugs		
Colchicine	0.6–1.8 mg.	1.0 mg. per 2 ml. I 0.6 mg. T
Allopurinol (Zyloprim)	300 mg.	100 mg. T 300 mg. T

*C, capsule. I, injection. L, liquid. T, tablet. TR, timed release capsule.

Salicylates

Aspirin has been the drug of choice for antirheumatic therapy for over 25 years and has been in use for over 100 years.[55–60] About a 50 per cent response rate is observed with aspirin alone (3 to 6 gm. per day) for the control of pain, swelling, joint immobility, and morning stiffness. The onset of anti-inflammatory drug action begins after about one to two weeks, and up to four weeks may be required for a maximal effect on the synovitis. The mechanism of action of all nonsteroidal anti-inflammatory drugs is interference with the enzyme cyclo-oxygenase, which is essential for the production of prostaglandins. Hence, the amplification of the inflammatory process by these mediators is blunted.[13,61]

Aspirin absorption is characteristically complete and rapid, with a peak concentration within one-half hour.[59] The generally accepted, although not definitively established, therapeutic blood level range is 20 to 30 mg. per dl. for salicylates.[59,62–64] Steady state serum levels are achieved equally well with buffered and enteric coated aspirin formulations, but some enteric coated products are characterized by poor bioavailability.[65,66] Aspirin metabolism involves five pathways, two of which are saturated at antirheumatic doses, with the result that small dosage changes produce large increments in plasma levels.[64] A sixfold increase is produced in the plasma half-life, from two to four hours up to 15 to 30 hours, and also in blood levels following a dosage change from 1.5 to 3.0 gm. per day.[59] The standard dosage is 3 to 6 gm. per day, and the dose frequency historically has been four to six times a day. A two to three times a day dose regimen is reasonable for use with enteric coated tablets, since the half-life is quite long at antirheumatic doses and gastric intolerance is not likely with the coated tablet formulation.

The major side effects of aspirin involve the gastrointestinal, hematologic, and otologic systems.[55,58,59] Gastric intolerance with nausea, dyspepsia, heartburn, anorexia, and gastritis occurs in over 30 per cent of arthritic patients. Fecal blood loss is usually occult, in an amount of 4 to 12 ml. per day. Gastric mucosal changes include ulcers, erosion, and erythema, which are shown to occur frequently with long term antirheumatic therapy.[67,68] Enteric coating reduces the gastric irritation of aspirin to a minimal degree, but buffered products cause erosive changes equal to those of plain aspirin in frequency and severity.[68,69] The bleeding time is prolonged at least two- to threefold and persists for the life span of the altered platelets (about one week) following even low aspirin doses, e.g., 325 mg. daily.[70,71] Hepatotoxic reactions are characterized by slight to marked elevations in liver enzyme levels, according to several trials and case reports, and are reversible.[72] Hypersensitivity or allergic reactions with aspirin are manifested in two ways: skin lesions with urticaria or angioedema, and respiratory distress with bronchospasm, rhinorrhea, and lacrimation.[73]

Concurrent use of salicylates with orally administered anticoagulants may lead to marked potentiation of the anticoagulant's effect as a result of plasma protein displacement by salicylates. The risk of gastrointestinal ulceration is increased when salicylates are given with steroids, phenylbutazone, oxyphenbutazone, or alcohol. Salicylates antagonize the uricosuric effect of probenecid and sulfinpyrazone. Aspirin may inhibit the diuretic action of spironolactone.

Six other salicylates or salicylate derivatives are available for clinical use: sodium salicylate, choline salicylate, choline magnesium salicylate, magnesium salicylate, salsalate, and diflunisal. Although sodium salicylate is probably as effective as the other nonsteroidal anti-inflammatory drugs, such as indomethacin, the substantial sodium content (about 31 mEq. per 5 gm. dose) limits its clinical utility.[74] Choline salicylate (Arthropan) has a bioavailability similar to that of aspirin with more rapid absorption.[75-82] Its solution formulation is a unique feature, but its bad taste decreases its usefulness. Magnesium salicylate is marketed without published documentation of comparative efficacy or toxicity.

Choline Magnesium Salicylate. Choline magnesium salicylate (Trilisate) is actually a combination of two salicylate salts (choline and magnesium). Its half-life changes with its dose, just like aspirin, and is approximately 18 hours at antirheumatic dosages, e.g., above 3 gm. per day.[83] The dosing frequency guideline is twice daily administration. Its salicylate levels and efficacy equal those of aspirin, with similar improvement in joint signs and morning stiffness.[84,85] Although the scope of side effects of choline magnesium salicylate mimics that of aspirin, the frequency is much less, e.g., tinnitus in 5 per cent and gastrointestinal pain and nausea in 6 per cent.[85] Fecal blood loss is negligible.[86] Choline magnesium salicylate has the two advantages of twice a day dosing and lower toxicity, but its cost is much greater than that of aspirin.

Salsalate. Salsalate (Disalcid) is a disalicylate hydrolyzed in vivo to salicylate. Steady state levels of salsalate are about the same as those of aspirin, although absorption is a little slower.[87-89] Its anti-inflammatory activity mimics that of aspirin, and comparable relief of joint pain and inflammation occurs in rheumatoid arthritis, osteoarthritis, and other musculoskeletal diseases.[87-93] The dosing range is somewhat less than that of aspirin, since the salt form delivers more salicylate per gram, that is, 3 versus 3.6 gm. Gastrointestinal intolerance and tinnitus with salsalate can occur with frequency and severity similar to, but usually lower than, that of aspirin.[91-93] Gastric hyperemia and erosion and blood loss are inconsequential.[94-96]

Diflunisal. Diflunisal (Dolobid) is a derivative of salicylic acid with analgesic, anti-inflammatory, and fever reducing properties. It is thought that diflunisal exerts its analgesic and anti-inflammatory effects by inhibiting prostaglandin synthetase.

Diflunisal is well absorbed orally. The plasma half-life of diflunisal is eight to 12 hours, thus making a twice daily dosing regimen possible. The drug is excreted almost exclusively in the urine as two soluble glucuronides. Diflunisal is approximately 99 per cent bound to plasma protein.

Although diflunisal has less effect on platelet function and bleeding time than aspirin, high doses may have a substantial clinical effect on platelet function. The adverse effects seen most commonly are gastrointestinal (nausea, dyspepsia, gastrointestinal pain, and diarrhea—3 to 9 per cent), central nervous system (headache—3 to 9 per cent), and allergic reactions (rash—3 to 9 per cent). Because diflunisal is so highly bound to plasma protein (99 per cent), concurrent therapy with other highly bound drugs (e.g., coumarin anticoagulants, phenytoin, propranolol) may lead to an exaggerated response to one of the drugs. Patients with a history of peptic ulcer disease should be monitored very closely while they are receiving diflunisal.

In treating mild to moderate pain, the initial adult dose of diflunisal should be 1000 mg., followed by 500 mg. every 12 hours. Some patients may require 500 mg. every eight hours. This dose range is comparable in analgesic effectiveness to that of 650 mg. of aspirin,

650 mg. of acetaminophen, and 650 mg. of acetaminophen with 100 mg. of propoxyphene napsylate. In treating osteoarthritis, the suggested dosage range is 500 to 1000 mg. daily in two divided doses. Maintenance dosages higher than 1500 mg. daily are not recommended.

Phenylpropionic Acids

Four drugs are currently available for their antirheumatic action—fenoprofen (Nalfon), ibuprofen (Motrin), naproxen (Naprosyn), and benoxaprofen (Oraflex). The pharmacologic and toxicologic profiles of these nonsteroidal anti-inflammatory drugs are almost the same,[97] although benoxaprofen has a greater potential for causing serious liver damage, and its use is highly restricted. The biopharmaceutical and pharmacokinetic properties of these drugs are nearly identical in terms of absorption (80 to 90 per cent), protein binding (95 to 99 per cent), and hepatic metabolism (90 to 93 per cent),[98-104] but the half-life of naproxen (14 hours) and benoxaprofen (25 to 32 hours) is great when compared to both ibuprofen (two hours) and fenoprofen (two to three hours). Therefore, a once daily dosing schedule is used for benoxaprofen and a twice daily schedule for naproxen; ibuprofen and fenoprofen are usually given four times a day. However, a twice daily schedule for the latter two is possible because of more sustained tissue levels (e.g., synovial fluid) and the slow changes in the inflammatory process.[105] The dosage ranges from 400 mg. to 1.0 gm. per day for benoxaprofen, 1200 to 2400 mg. per day for fenoprofen, 1200 mg. to 3600 mg. per day for ibuprofen, and 500 to 1000 mg. per day for naproxen. Drug interactions with food, aspirin, and antacids delay and decrease absorption of these nonsteroidal anti-inflammatory drugs by 16 to 46 per cent, but the clinical significance of these interactions has not been established.[98-104,106]

The efficacies of the phenylpropionic acids are the same as those of aspirin for the treatment of rheumatoid arthritis.[107-119] Osteoarthritis is also similarly controlled by all the nonsteroidal anti-inflammatory drugs.[120-126] For acute gouty arthritis, naproxen, ibuprofen, and fenoprofen have been successfully employed and are equal in activity to that of indomethacin and phenylbutazone, according to initial reports.[127-129] The dosing scheme for acute gout differs from that of the other arthritides in that high initial dosages are employed for one to three days, dosage tapering being correlated with control of the acute attack. For example, when fenoprofen was given in doses of 800 mg. every six hours for one day and then tapered as needed, 94 per cent of the patients had a good to excellent response.[109] Steroid doses can be lowered when a nonsteroidal anti-inflammatory drug like naproxen is used for arthritis.[130]

Side effects with the phenylpropionic acids involve the gastrointestinal and other systems. The frequency and severity of occult blood loss, nausea, dyspepsia, and gastric erosion (about half as often) are much lower than with aspirin.[67,131-135] Patients with a history of peptic ulcer disease have received naproxen without clinical consequence in almost all cases.[135] However, gastrointestinal hemorrhage has been associated with each nonsteroidal anti-inflammatory drug.[136] Tinnitus occurs infrequently.[112-119] Benoxaprofen produces a very high incidence of sun-related adverse effects and onycholysis. Benoxaprofen has also been implicated in the causation of a few cases of severe, and even fatal, liver disease. Recent case reports implicate benoxaprofen in renal and cardiovascular reactions (e.g., salt and water retention, nephrotic syndrome, exacerbation of hypertension). Allergic reactions, both urticarial and bronchospastic, show 75 to 100 per cent cross allergy between aspirin and these nonsteroidal anti-inflammatory drugs.[73] Bleeding times during phenylpropionic acid use are generally prolonged to a clinically insignificant degree, with inhibition of platelet aggregation to variable degrees.[137-139]

Patients should be advised of the following while taking one of the phenylpropionic acids: (1) avoid aspirin while taking this medication; (2) if gastrointestinal upset occurs, take with food or antacids; (3) full therapeutic effects may not be seen for one to two weeks; (4) notify the physician if gastric upset, skin rash, itching, visual disturbances, weight gain, edema, black stools, or persistent headaches occur.

Indole and Indenes

Three drugs make up this category of the nonsteroidal anti-inflammatory drugs. Indomethacin is the prototype, and tolmetin (Tolectin) and sulindac (Clinoril) are structural analogues. The bioavailability for all three drugs is rapid (peak levels within one to three hours) and is complete (over 90 per cent).[140-146] Protein binding is at or above 90 per cent for each drug. Elimination primarily involves hepatic biotransformation with renal and fecal excretion of metabolites. The half-lives vary significantly among the indole-indenes and are one hour for tolmetin, six to seven hours for indomethacin, and seven hours for sulindac.[140-146] Sulindac is considered a pro-drug and is metabolized to an active species, a sulfide, that has an 18 hour half-life that accounts for most, if not all, of sulindac's anti-inflammatory activity.

The efficacy of indomethacin in rheumatoid arthritis has been described as good to excellent in 62 per cent and good or very good in 86 per cent of the patients in uncontrolled trials.[147,148] The typical dosage is 75 to 150 mg. per day in three divided doses. For the treatment of gout, indomethacin has produced complete resolution of acute gout within 24 to 72 hours in 81 per cent of the patients in five trials.[149-153] A decreasing dosing scheme is used for gout therapy, e.g., a 75 mg. dose, then 25 to 50 mg. every six hours for two days, and then 25 to 50 mg. every eight hours. The comparative effectiveness of indomethacin in rheumatoid arthritis, osteoarthritis, ankylosing spondylitis, and gout is considered about equal to that of all the nonsteroidal anti-inflammatory drugs.[122,124-126,154-162] Nighttime dosing with indomethacin (75 to 100 mg.) is employed for the control of nocturnal pain and major morning stiffness as an adjunctive treatment to daily nonsteroidal anti-inflammatory drug therapy.[163,164] The antirheumatic activity of tolmetin is rated as similar to that of other nonsteroidal anti-inflammatory drugs (e.g., aspirin, ibuprofen, and phenylbutazone) for the treatment of rheumatoid arthritis and osteoarthritis at dosages of about 1200 to 1600 mg. daily in three to four divided doses.[165-174]

Sulindac also possesses analgesic, antiinflammatory, and antipyretic properties.[143] Broad antirheumatic activity has been shown for sulindac in comparison to other nonsteroidal anti-inflammatory drugs in the treatment of rheumatoid arthritis, osteoarthritis, ankylosing spondylitis, and gout.[175-182] Dosages are 150 to 200 mg. on a twice daily schedule. Night-time dosing of sulindac (200 mg.) has been successfully used for the control of nocturnal pain and morning stiffness.[183]

The toxicity profile for the indole-indenes includes significant gastrointestinal and neurologic reactions. Indomethacin produces the most frequent and most severe effects, which usually occur within the first two days of therapy.[141] Up to 50 per cent of the patients experience side effects, and they are dose related, e.g., a 36 per cent rate below a 150 mg. dose and 60 to 70 per cent at 150 to 200 mg.[147,184] Gastrointestinal symptoms are common and include nausea (>10 per cent), diarrhea (10 per cent), abdominal pain (3 per cent), and ulcers (2 per cent).[147,184] Occult blood loss is less severe than with aspirin.[185] Central nervous system problems are quite common, particularly headache (25 per cent) and vertigo or dizziness (15 per cent), with occasional cases of depression, psychosis, and hallucinations.[147] Tolmetin is less toxic than indomethacin and produces fewer reactions than aspirin and phenylbutazone.[168-170] Typical gastrointestinal reactions occur in about 25 per cent of the patients. Other adverse effects include anorexia, flatulence, urticaria, peptic ulcer, anxiety, mental confusion, syncope, and paresthesias. Water retention and hypertension are infrequent, but significant, potential problems.[167,172] Sulindac toxicity occurs in about 25 per cent of the patients and is generally less severe than aspirin toxicity.[143] The common gastrointestinal effects are nausea, abdominal pain, and constipation, but gastric erosion and blood loss are minimal.[144,174,186,187] Dry mouth is a frequent complaint.[175] Neurologic problems are common—dizziness, drowsiness, tiredness, and headache.[143,175] The bleeding time has been reported to be both normal and moderately elevated.[143,188]

Pyrazolones

Phenylbutazone and its active metabolite, oxyphenbutazone, compose this class of nonsteroidal anti-inflammatory drugs. Plasma levels of phenylbutazone increase in a nonlinear fashion with dosage increases. Higher doses provide greater relief than lower doses, although the clinical response does not correlate directly with plasma levels.[189-191] Protein binding is approximately 98 per cent.[41] The half-life is 37 to 76 hours.[192] Biotransformation of phenylbutazone occurs in the liver, and several metabolites result, including oxyphenbutazone.[41]

The efficacy of phenylbutazone is consistently about equal to that of the other nonsteroidal anti-inflammatory drugs, without proven advantage in rheumatoid arthritis, osteoarthritis, ankylosing spondylitis, and gout.[120,123,157–161,170,174,180,181,193–195] The standard dosage is 100 to 400 mg. daily in three or four divided doses. For acute gout the initial dosages are high—200 mg. three or four times a day—in order to achieve a rapid response in two to three days; then the dosage is tapered. The pharmacotherapeutic actions of oxyphenbutazone and phenylbutazone are almost identical.[196]

The side effects of the pyrazolones are less frequent than those with indomethacin.[159,160] However, the more serious blood dyscrasias restrict their use as a last choice among the nonsteroidal anti-inflammatory drugs. Phenylbutazone and oxyphenbutazone cause gastrointestinal irritation (nausea, pain, stomatitis, and ulceration) in approximately 6 per cent of the patients.[196,197] Edema has been reported in 3 to 9 per cent of the patients.[123,174,197] Bone marrow suppression occurs infrequently (one in 80,000 to 150,000 patient months of treatment), but the possible leukopenia, pancytopenia, thrombocytopenia, agranulocytosis, or aplastic anemia can be life threatening. Aplastic anemia occurs more often in the elderly than in young adults and typically after at least three months of therapy. Agranulocytosis occurs within three months after therapy is begun in younger subjects. Although serial blood counts are recommended, the spontaneity and insidiousness of the blood dyscrasias reduce their screening value. Other adverse effects that have been reported include urticaria, arthralgia, drug fever, anaphylactic shock, serum sickness, pruritus, headache, drowsiness, lethargy, mental confusion, hyperglycemia, tinnitus, and blurred vision. Patients should be instructed to contact their physician if sore throat, mouth sores, chills, fever, unusual bleeding or bruising, blurred vision, unusual weight gain, or skin rash occurs.

Phenylanthranilic Acids

Mefenamic acid (Ponstel) is the older product in this category and meclofenamate sodium (Meclomen), the newer one. The analgesic and anti-inflammatory activities of mefenamic acid are similar to those of aspirin in the arthritides.[38,41,42] The dosage is 250 mg. on a three to four times a day schedule. Meclofenamate has also exhibited efficacy in the control of rheumatoid arthritis, osteoarthritis, ankylosing spondylitis, and gout.[198–204] A dosage of 200 to 400 mg. per day is employed, which is divided into four equal doses.

The side effects of these two drugs commonly involve the gastrointestinal and neurologic systems and significantly limit their clinical utility. Mefenamic acid produces dyspepsia in 33 per cent and diarrhea in 10 to 15 per cent of the patients. Maculopapular rashes, headache, dizziness, and drowsiness also occur.[38,41,42] Meclofenamate frequently causes gastrointestinal reactions, a 40 to 90 per cent incidence, including nausea, abdominal pain, diarrhea, pyrosis, anorexia, constipation, and flatulence.[198–206] These adverse effects commonly have been moderate to severe. Cessation of administration of the drug is usually necessary in over one-third of the patients, necessitated particularly by diarrhea. Tolerance to the side effects usually does not develop during long term use.[205] Therefore, the prominent gastrointestinal side effects of mefenamic acid and meclofenamate, without added efficacy, give these two drugs a secondary status among the nonsteroidal anti-inflammatory drugs.

Oxicams

Piroxicam (Feldene) is the first of a new class of nonsteroidal anti-inflammatory drugs known as the oxicams. It compares favorably with the other nonsteroidal anti-inflammatory drugs in its efficacy in the treatment of arthritic conditions. Its effect appears to be related to its capacity to inhibit prostaglandinbiosynthesis.

Owing to its extended half-life (approximately 50 hours) piroxicam may be given once daily. Peak anti-inflammatory effects are usually observed after one week of therapy. Gastrointestinal intolerance is the most commonly reported adverse effect, although the incidence appears to be lower than with aspirin and several other nonsteroidal anti-inflammatory drugs. The elderly appear to be more susceptible to gastrointestinal blood loss secondary to therapy with piroxicam.

Piroxicam may be taken with gold salts or corticosteroids. Whether a steroid sparing effect occurs is not yet known. Piroxicam should not be given with aspirin, for the combination does not appear to increase effectiveness and may predispose to adverse gastrointestinal effects. It has been suggested that piroxicam may have an extended action in positively affecting the underlying arthritic disease process. There are no published data objectively supporting this claim at this time.

In the treatment of rheumatoid and osteoarthritis, the initial and maintenance dosage should be 20 mg. administered once daily. Because of the long half-life there is a progressive increase in the response over several days. Higher than recommended doses do not increase effectiveness but do increase the possibility of adverse effects.

Gold Salts

Although parenteral gold therapy has been used to treat rheumatoid arthritis for 50 years, its efficacy and safety were first established by controlled study in 1960 and then confirmed in numerous clinical trials and discussed in reviews.[207-225] Gold is indicated for chronic active progressive disease that fails to respond to nonsteroidal anti-inflammatory drugs or for acute attacks in patients with high rheumatoid factor titers.[225] Articular erosion can be prevented, and disease progression can be arrested. A favorable response is seen in about 75 per cent of gold treated patients; that is, disease control is realized in 50 per cent and a remission occurs in about 20 to 25 per cent.[226] Long term therapy over several years has resulted in a high 70 per cent remission rate in patients who can tolerate the side effects.[217,218] Gold treatment early in the course of the disease has a more favorable effect in terms of changes visible on x-ray examination than late onset therapy.[216] A six to 12 month trial should be planned, since the onset of a therapeutic effect is very slow, usually two to six months.[213,215] Furthermore, a remission may not even occur until over 12 months of therapy have elapsed.[218] Treatment may continue for an indefinite period following a clinical response, as long as toxic effects are tolerable.

Parenteral administration of gold is started with a 10 mg. test dose to check for excessive acute toxicity.[224,225] At one week an injection of 25 mg. is given. Then the induction period employs a weekly 50 mg. intramuscular dose until 1 gm. has been administered. Higher doses, e.g., 150 mg. per week, provide no additional benefit and produce only more toxicity.[215] The patient's response to gold therapy during the induction period dictates subsequent prescribing. If no response is noted, gold is discontinued. If a partial response is demonstrated, gold is reordered on a weekly schedule until a response is achieved within a one to two year period. Once remission is achieved, the interval between gold injections is extended to a biweekly schedule, and if possible eventually to a once a month frequency, for as long as disease control is sustained. Work continues in the development of an effective oral dosage form for gold.

The pharmacokinetic profile of gold has been studied.[224-228] One 60 mg. dose of aurothiomalate produces a peak blood level of about 700 mcg. per dl. within two to eight hours. A 50 mg. dose at three to four week intervals results in a steady state gold level of 100 ± 25 mcg. per dl. In general, serum levels do not directly correlate with beneficial or toxic effects.[229,230] Gold is widely distributed to tissues, even though there is a great amount of protein binding to serum albumin (92 per cent).[231] High tissue concentrations are found in the liver, skin, kidneys, bone, eyes, and reticuloendothelial system. Gold is deposited in synovial tissue at a concentration one-half of the serum level. Excretion is a very slow process, related to persistent tissue storage; the half-life is at least one week and low blood levels persist for many months.[231-233] Excretion occurs through the kidneys (70 per cent) and liver (30 per cent).

Gold toxicity commonly and seriously limits its clinical use in the treatment of the arthritides.[223-225,234] Reactions are dose related, e.g., 18 per cent at 25 mg. per week and 40 per cent at 100 mg. per week. Mucocutaneous reactions are the most common problems, with a 15 to 30 per cent incidence. A metallic taste is also noted. Pruritus is an almost universal complaint when skin rash develops, and the dermatitis usually progresses to scaly erythematous lesions on the hands and face. However, any type of skin rash is possible, e.g., urticaria, maculopapules, vesicles, or purpura. Stomatitis and eosinophilia occur frequently with the rash. The skin lesions regress within two to three weeks upon discontinuation of gold therapy. Exfoliative dermatitis is a potential life threatening sequela, and thus gold should be discontinued when a rash develops. Retreatment is possible without reaction at a later date at a lower dose. Gold dermatitis may also involve a nitritoid reaction related to the vehicle used. The oil preparation of aurothioglucose produces fewer local vasomotor skin reactions than the aqueous preparation of aurothiomalate.[235,236]

Kidney toxicity is manifested as proteinuria in 3 to 17 per cent of the patients taking gold.[223-225] The nephrotic syndrome may develop in a small number of patients. Hematopoietic toxicity is caused by bone marrow suppression and includes thrombocytopenia, granulocytopenia, and aplastic anemia. Eosinophilia occurs commonly (5 to 40 per cent). Ocular chrysiasis develops at cumulative doses above 1 gram and is reversible.[237] Other ophthalmic reactions include cataracts, corneal ulceration, and retinopathies. Unusual gastrointestinal reactions such as colitis and hepatitis have been observed.

Penicillamine

The chelating drug, penicillamine (Cuprimine), possesses anti-inflammatory activity and can slow the progression of arthritis.[238,239] Its status as an antirheumatic drug is becoming equal to that of gold with regard to efficacy, and it has the convenience of oral dosing.[219,240] About 50 to 70 per cent of the patients with rheumatoid arthritis experience significant clinical improvement with penicillamine.[241-251] Patients who have failed to benefit from gold therapy may respond to penicillamine therapy and vice versa.[219,251] The onset of response begins after six weeks of treatment, and maximal disease control is achieved within three to six months. Corticosteroid doses in steroid dependent arthritic patients can be reduced with penicillamine. The dosing of penicillamine is presently undergoing a downward revision to a maximum of 1 gm. per day.[239,250-253] The "go low, go slow" dosing scheme employs 250 mg. dosage increments and long intervals between dose changes, that is, one to three months, in order to reduce toxicity. Daily dosages of less than 600 mg. have been shown to be similar in efficacy to high doses of over 1 gram per day.[251] However, some patients may require more than 1 gram per day for optimal disease control.[250,254]

Penicillamine toxicity is similar in scope to that of gold; it occurs equally often or more frequently, necessitates discontinuation of the drug as often or less often, and is dose related.[219,239,240] The overall incidence of all adverse reactions is 50 to 60 per cent at dosages of 500 to 1250 mg. per day. Skin rashes occur in 12 to 44 per cent of the patients.[241,250] Pruritus is a typical finding, accompanied by maculopapular or morbilliform eruptions, all of which occur within the first month of treatment.[239] A late rash presents after months of therapy as red scaly lesions on the trunk. Loss of taste is also a problem in 12 to 20 per cent of the patients. Nausea, vomiting, anorexia, and dyspepsia occur frequently. Stomatitis occurs in 1 to 10 per cent of the cases. Renal toxicity with proteinuria occurs in 5 to 20 per cent of the cases and is likely related to the size of the daily dosage.[255,256] Blood dyscrasias primarily involve the platelets; thrombocytopenia has been observed in 3 to 27 per cent of penicillamine treated patients.[254,255] Neutropenia has occurred in less than 5 per cent, and aplastic anemia is a rare phenomenon. The low dose scheme is being assessed in an effort to reduce toxicity, and the toxicity figures cited may be revised to lower frequencies. However, two low dose studies have demonstrated that such reactions are still common.[241,254] Other rare and serious adverse reactions include myasthenia gravis, Goodpasture's syndrome, and arteritis.[257-259]

Antimalarial Drugs

Chloroquine and hydroxychloroquine form this category of disease modifying drugs.[260] They are indicated in progressive articular disease when nonsteroidal anti-inflammatory drugs are inadequate for disease control and toxicity is unacceptable with gold or penicillamine.[252,261] The efficacy of chloroquine equals that of gold and azathioprine for improving the articular index, reducing morning stiffness, and increasing grip strength.[263,264] The onset of response is slow and gradual, usually six to 12 weeks, and maximal drug action may require six months. The dosages are usually 250 mg. daily for chloroquine and 200 to 400 mg. per day for hydroxychloroquine.

Ocular abnormalities create the major restriction for antimalarial drug use in arthritis.[260,261,264-266] These drugs concentrate in the eyes to a degree 100-fold higher than in the blood because of drug binding to melanin. Visual dysfunction occurs in 18 to 46 per cent of the patients taking antimalarial drugs.[260] Diplopia and loss of accommodation are reversible problems. Asymptomatic corneal opacities are commonly found. Retinopathy is the most clinically significant dose related ocular reaction and results in blurred vision, night blindness, and scotomas. Blindness is a possible sequela. Fundoscopic examination reveals hyperpigmentation, especially around the macula. As the drug accumulates, the incidence of retinopathy increases; thus 600 mg. is recommended as the maximal total cumulative dose. Neurologic side effects include irritability, nervousness, nightmares, vertigo, tinnitus, nystagmus, headache, dizziness, and neuromyopathy. Adverse gastrointestinal effects include anorexia, vomiting, diarrhea, and nausea. Skin reactions include hyperpigmentation, lichenoid patches, adverse exfoliative dermatitis, alopecia, pruritus, and a wide spectrum of skin eruptions. Adverse hematologic effects are rare and include aplastic anemia, agranulocytosis, leukopenia, thrombocytopenia, and hemolysis in glucose-6-phosphate dehydrogenase deficient patients.

Corticosteroids

Because of the great number of serious side effects, oral corticosteroid therapy is indicated only for the treatment of very resistant arthritic disease that is unresponsive to nonsteroidal anti-inflammatory drugs and the disease modifying drugs.[267,268] Severe attacks of arthritis in multiple joints can be controlled by a short course of oral doses of steroids, such as 20 to 60 mg. of prednisone per day for a few days. Small doses (e.g., 5 to 12 mg. of prednisone daily) can be administered on a long term basis. A single morning dose minimizes suppression of normal diurnal adrenal secretion.[269,270] Bedtime dosing of steroids has been tried successfully in a few patients.[271] Alternate day dosing is generally ineffective for rheumatic disease. Adrenocorticotrophic hormone is used for recalcitrant gouty arthritis in a dose of 40 units three or four times a day for a few days during attacks.[31,32]

The following brief list summarizes the manifold potential toxic effects associated with systemic corticosteroid use:[272,273]

1. Endocrine—adrenal suppression, hyperglycemia, Cushing's syndrome.
2. Musculoskeletal—osteoporosis, myopathy, aseptic necrosis of bone.
3. Cardiovascular—salt and water retention, hypokalemia, hypertension.
4. Ocular—glaucoma, posterior subcapsular cataracts.
5. Skin—acne, bruises.
6. Neurologic—euphoria, dysphoria, dependence.
7. Gastrointestinal—gastritis.
8. Hematologic—leukocytosis, lymphopenia.
9. Infections—viral, fungal, and bacterial.

The elderly patient with arthritis frequently has coexisting diseases (e.g., osteoporosis, cataracts, hypertension, and infections) or is debilitated, either of which potentially can increase the frequency and severity of these adverse reactions.

The intra-articular administration of corticosteroids is indicated for asymmetric monoarticular arthritis, when mobility is restricted, or when deformity is present in any of the four arthritides.[268,274] Their adjunctive use is reasonable for single acutely inflamed joints and acute tenosynovitis or bursitis while the disease modifying drugs like gold are slowly taking affect. The response is rapid; swelling and pain are greatly reduced within 24 hours after an injection. The suspension formulations of the corticosteroids provide a long duration of action, usually two to four weeks, with single injections. The major products are triamcinolone acetonide, prednisolone tebutate, and hydrocortisone tebutate. The dose is adjusted to the joint size.

The administration of corticosteroids by the intra-articular route requires caution. The physical activity of the specific joint must be limited for 48 hours following an injection to avoid joint damage as a result of premature excessive mobilization. The injection procedure involves the adjunctive use of a local anesthetic to control pain from the procedure, aseptic technique, the withdrawal of excess fluid, and flushing of the needle to prevent crystal deposition in the synovial membranes. The interval between injections should be no less than four weeks—usually eight weeks—to minimize joint destruction. The prominent complications include septic arthritis, crystalline synovitis, cutaneous atrophy, and destructive arthropathy. Proper intra-articular administration of steroids as noted will avoid significant toxicity in the majority of patients, even in those receiving many injections over several years.[275]

Cytotoxic Drugs

Cyclophosphamide (Cytoxan) and azathioprine (Imuran) can arrest the progress of arthritic disease, prevent joint destruction, and effect partial or complete remission in 67 to over 90 per cent of moderately to severely ill patients.[276-280] Corticosteroid doses may be reduced by 50 per cent or completely withdrawn when cytotoxic drugs are used. The indications for their use include a life threatening or crippling disease, reversible synovitis, the failure of conventional treatment, the absence of infection or a blood cell abnormality, and the capability for close follow-up. The onset of action is gradual, starting after six weeks, with a maximal effect at three to four months, or longer. Dosages for both drugs have ranged from 1.0 to 2.5 mg. per kg. per day, but low doses of 1 mg. per kg. per day provide disease control similar in degree to that with high doses in most patients.[279,280]

The toxicity of the cytotoxic drugs prevents their routine prescription for arthritis.[279,281] Blood dyscrasias are dose related, reversible, and delayed in onset. Both cyclophosphamide and azathioprine produce leukopenia at normal doses in 20 to 90 per cent and 4 to 39 per cent of the patients, respectively. Thrombocytopenia occurs less frequently with both drugs. Gastrointestinal intolerance is also very common with both drugs—a 5 to 90 per cent incidence of nausea, vomiting, pain, and diarrhea. Skin rashes occur during cytotoxic therapy, and reversible alopecia is a frequent complication with cyclophosphamide. Infections pose a significant threat because of immunosuppression; they are frequently nonbacterial and involve fungi, viruses, and protozoa. Azathioprine produces hepatotoxicity in a small percentage of patients. Cyclophosphamide may cause sterility with azoospermia in men (up to 100 per cent) and amenorrhea and ovarian suppression in women (up to 20 per cent). Cystitis is commonly caused by a cyclophosphamide metabolite in the urine, and its clinical presentation ranges from mucosal irritation to overt hemorrhage. Adjunctive procedures are necessary and will minimize this toxic effect. These include the avoidance of bedtime dosing, emptying the bladder before retiring and regularly during the day, and hydrating adequately.

Uricosuric Drugs

Probenecid (Benemid) and sulfinpyrazone (Anturane) compose this category of drugs employed for the maintenance therapy of gout and hyperuricemia. Both produce a manifold increase in the excretion of uric acid by preventing renal tubular reabsorption or tubular secretion at the proximal renal tubules.[32,33,282-284] About 75 to 80 per cent of the patients with tophaceous gout and hyperuricemia can be successfully controlled, with a sustained reduction in the serum uric acid level and significant clinical improvement.[33,282] However, although the uric acid level is almost always reduced, some patients may not experience cessation of acute attacks of gout during this treatment.[285] In cases of moderate to severe renal failure, these two drugs are generally ineffective. Salicylates interfere with their uricosuric activity.

Therapy with both probenecid and sulfinpyrazone is initiated at low doses for gout in order to minimize excessive uricosuria and possible renal crystallization and also to reduce the chance of precipitating an acute attack of gout. The starting dosage is 0.5 to 1.0 gm. per day for probenecid and 100 to 200 mg. per day for sulfinpyrazone, both on a twice daily divided dose schedule.[32,35,37,282] Typical maintenance doses are 1.0 to 2.0 gm. per day on a twice daily regimen and 200 to 400 mg. per day in three to four divided doses, respectively. Both drugs are well absorbed upon oral administration, achieve peak serum levels within one to two hours, are highly protein bound (90 per cent for probenecid and 98 per cent for sulfinpyrazone), and are partially metabolized and excreted in the kidney.[33,282] The half-life for probenecid is about six to 12 hours and two to four hours for sulfinpyrazone.[37,282,286,287]

The first side effect of concern is the precipitation of an acute gout attack during the initial six to 12 months of preventive uricosuric therapy, which can occur in 10 to 20 per cent of the patients with gout.[33,282] Frequently colchicine is prescribed concomitantly at low daily doses (0.5 mg.) as a prophylactic measure to avoid this problem. Crystallization of uric acid in the kidney is another potential major reaction during initiation of uricosuric therapy, which is minimized by adequate hydration and possibly aided by urine alkalinization. Both probenecid and sulfinpyrazone produce gastrointestinal disturbances (e.g., nausea) and hypersensitivity reactions (e.g., rashes and drug fever) at a low to moderate frequency.[33,37,280] For example, probenecid has produced gastric effects in 1 to 3 per cent and allergic problems in 1.5 to 5 per cent of the patients.[33,37,288] Side effects necessitate cessation of drug therapy in 2 to 5 per cent of the patients who are treated with probenecid.[37]

Antigout Drugs

Colchicine and allopurinol (Zyloprim) are both employed for long term gout control, but only colchicine can arrest an acute attack. Colchicine possesses a unique anti-inflammatory action in suppressing leukocyte chemotaxis and possibly phagocytosis.[289,290] Intracellular microtubular proteins are bound by colchicine; then the tubules disaggregate, changing cell structure, inhibiting cell function, and decreasing cell movement.

An acute gouty arthritic attack is rapidly controlled within a few hours or up to 48 hours in 75 to 100 per cent of the patients receiving colchicine therapy orally or parenterally.[32,282] Early therapy within 12 hours after the onset of an attack usually permits rapid and complete disease control, but a delay in treatment for 24 hours decreases the response. For an acute attack a loading dose regimen is instituted for colchicine; a dose of 0.5 to 1 mg. is given at intervals of every one to two hours until a response is achieved, intolerable side effects occur, or the maximal total dosage is achieved (about 8 mg.).[32,33,289] The usual total dosage is 4 to 6 mg., but it varies greatly from patient to patient and between attacks in one patient. Parenteral therapy provides an alternative route, causing less gastric toxicity and possibly producing a more rapid response.[289-291] A 1 to 3 mg. dose is mixed in 20 ml. of normal saline and given slowly over several minutes into an established intravenous line. Meticulous administration avoids extravasation and potential tissue necrosis and also sclerosis of the veins. One or two further doses may be repeated at six to 12 hour intervals. Long term prophylactic therapy can follow, in a 0.5 to 1.5 mg. dose, depending on the clinical history of gout (attack frequency and severity).[289,291] A marked reduction in attack frequency is realized in about 90 per cent of the gouty arthritic patients receiving maintenance therapy with colchicine.

Colchicine is rapidly taken up by a wide variety of cells, especially leukocytes. After oral administration the serum half-life is only 20 to 30 minutes, and the volume of distribution is very large (2.19 L. per kg.).[289,292] Leukocytes actually concentrate colchicine and very slowly release the drug, which is still measurable in the urine over one week after treatment. Biliary excretion is a major route of elimination.

The toxicity of colchicine primarily limits its use. During initial oral therapy, 25 to 80 per cent of the patients experience gastrointestinal reactions, particularly diarrhea, and also nausea, vomiting, and cramps.[288,289] Long term oral therapy results in many fewer abdominal complaints. Alopecia and allergic reactions have occurred infrequently.[287,290] Overdoses with colchicine are extremely toxic.[289,293,294] Severe abdominal effects occur first, with vomiting, diarrhea, and cramping. Electrolyte disturbances and dehydration result. Toxic hepatitis is observed, with elevations of liver enzyme levels. Cardiovascular problems include severe hypotension, renal failure, and shock. Blood dyscrasias reported in decreasing order of severity include aplastic anemia, agranulocytosis, and thrombocytopenia. Other adverse effects rarely reported include peripheral neuritis, myopathy, purpura, loss of hair, azoospermia, seizures, coma, and death.

Allopurinol is the hypouricemic drug that inhibits the enzyme xanthine oxidase, preventing the formation of uric acid from the precursors, xanthine and hypoxanthine, in the purine metabolic pathway.[32,33,37,282,295] Normalization of uric acid levels can be achieved in almost all patients with gout regardless of whether overproduction or underexcretion is the problem.[296,297] Complete control of gouty attacks has been observed in 60 to 100 per cent of allopurinol treated patients.[298,299] The reduction in the uric acid level begins within 24 to 48 hours and is maximal at one to two weeks. Control of gouty attacks occurs within a few months. Allopurinol should be continued indefinitely, since drug withdrawal causes a return of acute gouty attacks.

The common dosage is 200 to 400 mg. per day, but in resistant cases up to 1 gm. per day may be required.[32,33,37,282,296-299] The initial dosage is usually 100 mg. per day. Colchicine (0.5 mg. per 100 mg. of allopurinol) is used concomitantly to avoid precipitating acute attacks during the initial treatment period with allopurinol. Single daily doses of allopurinol are equally as effective as a twice daily regimen.[282,297] Allopurinol's half-life is only two to three hours, but its active metabolite, oxipurinol, has a 28 hour half-life, allowing a once daily treatment.

Acute arthritis poses an untoward threat in up to 10 per cent of the patients with gout during initial allopurinol therapy, but is readily controlled by colchicine.[33] Side effects occur in up to 10 to 20 per cent of the patients receiving allopurinol, but in one report reactions were observed only in about 3.5 per cent.[288] Gastrointestinal and allergic reactions (skin rash or fever) are the most common.[33,37,282] Alopecia has been observed.[33,289] Toxic epidermal necrolysis and exfoliative dermatitis have been reported.[288,300] Several other severe toxic reactions may occur rarely, e.g., leukopenia, thrombocytopenia, hepatitis, and vasculitis.[282]

SPECIFIC THERAPEUTIC GUIDELINES

For the three arthritides—osteoarthritis, rheumatoid arthritis, and ankylosing spondylitis—the initial drug therapy involves a prescription of nonsteroidal anti-inflammatory drug for the control of pain and inflammation. The majority of patients respond to such therapy within a few weeks, with control of signs and symptoms of synovitis, improvement in joint mobility, and an increase in the general well-being. Guidelines for the use of nonsteroidal anti-inflammatory drugs are generally the same for each rheumatic disease and are described in detail in the previous commentary. The efficacy and toxicity of the individual drugs also have been addressed. As each drug is employed, appropriate monitoring for the specific toxicity profile of that drug is required, including the potential for additive toxicity when two drugs are prescribed concomitantly. The most important specific guideline is individualization of therapy to the patient's disease needs and his responses to therapy.

Physical therapy and general measures have been described for the arthritides in a collective fashion as baseline therapy. Specific joint immobilization with splinting provides much needed rest for single inflamed joints in all four arthritides. However, specific maneuvers are necessary and should be amplified for individual diseases. Osteoarthritis frequently involves the hip and knee joints. Besides a proper balance of rest, splinting, and exercise, assistive physical therapy by using a cane for walking can reduce stress and pain at these major joints and improve mobility.[2] Local heat therapy or hot baths particularly can help reduce the muscle spasms that complicate the degenerative joint changes of osteoarthritis. Ankylosing spondylitis requires several specific physical measures to slow or minimize back deformities.[24-27,29] The use of back braces and hard mattresses, less bending, and postural training aid in keeping the spine in a more normal straight position. Breathing exercises, such as blowing up balloons, can help to maintain chest expansion and reduce restrictions associated with costovertebral involvement in ankylosing spondylitis.

Orthopedic surgery is most commonly used for the late stages of osteoarthritis when joint damage has occurred.[2,7] The four possible procedures include synovectomy, osteotomy, arthrodesis, and prosthetic replacement. Persistent synovitis with synovial membrane destruction, significantly impaired mobility, and poor drug responsiveness are the indications for a synovectomy. Osteophytes are removed from joints when they are a source of pain and inflammation. Arthrodesis is seldom used any longer because of loss of patient mobility and the availability of other superior procedures. Hip replacement with a methacrylate prosthesis is useful in severe osteoarthritis to manage joint deformity and return mobility to a joint. Function can be restored and pain is relieved in the majority of severely ill patients. Patients with knee prostheses do not respond as well. Ankylosing spondylitis can require surgery; wedge osteotomy can reduce the flexion deformity of the spine.

Suppressive therapy with gold, penicillamine, and antimalarial or immunosuppressive drugs, as well as corticosteroids, should be employed for moderate to severe rheumatoid arthritis as described in the earlier discussion. However, their efficacy in ankylosing spondylitis is generally characterized as poor, is controversial, and is inadequately documented, pro or con. For example, penicillamine was briefly described as being completely ineffective in two reports, but it also has been noted to cause significant clinical improvement in two reports.[301-304] As for osteoarthritis, most reviews do not even discuss the role of disease suppression therapy.[6,7] Huskisson further generalizes that the risk is likely not worth the unestablished benefit.[8] Nonsteroidal anti-inflammatory drugs usually suffice for symptom control in osteoarthritis; however, the disease continues to progress.[3] Corticosteroids are recommended for intra-articular use in all four arthritides for the treatment of a single joint that is inflamed. However, oral therapy is generally restricted to very recalcitrant cases of rheumatoid or gouty arthritis.

Acute gout historically has been and still is treated with colchicine, the most effective modality; but its frequent and severe gastrointestinal toxicity necessitates a continued search for new treatments. The elderly can be more susceptible to its gastrointestinal side effects, and they commonly have poor veins, precluding the intravenous use of colchicine. Nonsteroidal anti-inflammatory drugs are quite effective substitutes, indomethacin and phenylbutazone having established efficacy. Since major side effects remain a problem with these two nonsteroidal anti-inflammatory drugs, fenoprofen, ibuprofen, and naproxen have been successfully tried and are becoming alternatives with the least toxicity and similar efficacy.[32] The course of therapy for acute gouty arthritis lasts from only a few days to about eight to 10 days, with the use of decreasing doses.

For the prevention of acute gouty nephrolithiasis and during long term prophylactic therapy, adjunctive therapy is recommended. First, adequate hydration requires ingestion of 2 to 3 liters of fluid per day, especially in cases of excessive uric acid excretion. Also alkalinizing drugs are intended to make the urine less acid (pH about 6.0 to 6.5) but not alkaline, and to improve uric acid solubility (about 85 per cent at this pH). Sodium bicarbonate can be used in a 2 to 6 gm. dosage per day in three to four equally divided doses. However, the significant sodium load must be considered, particularly in the elderly, who frequently have coexisting cardiovascular disease. Shohl's citric acid and sodium citrate solution is an alternate urinary alkalinizer given in a dosage of 20 to 60 ml. per day. Acetazolamide, an inhibitor of carbonic anhydrase, also can be employed in a 250 mg. dose at bedtime to avoid an acid urine in the morning. Finally, dietary control is generally encouraged to modify, although not eliminate, purine intake, especially from high content items like sardines, anchovies, sweetbreads, beer, liver, kidney, yeast, and herring. The drug of choice is allopurinol to reduce serum and urine uric acid concentrations.

Prophylactic therapy for gouty arthritis with or without hyperuricemia involves colchicine, allopurinol, probenecid, or sulfinpyrazone. The withholding of therapy is prudent if the acute attack is mild, is the first one, and is accompanied only by a normal or minimally elevated uric acid level in the serum and urine. Some patients may never have another attack, or it may not recur for many years. Low dose colchicine therapy (0.5 to 1.5 mg. per day) is indicated for long term preventive therapy in gouty arthritis without tophi and elevated uric acid levels. If the prodrome of an acute attack is experienced, a couple of extra doses should abort the attack. Treatment is continued for several years, and then a long symptom-free period warrants a trial of cessation of drug administration.

For gout and mild hyperuricemia, uricosuric therapy with probenecid or sulfinpyrazone is indicated to reduce the serum uric acid level to about 6 mg. per dl., as long as renal function is normal and no renal calculi exist. Allopurinol is recommended for tophaceous gout and gout with renal failure and in instances of very high levels of uric acid excretion (over 1 gm. per day), a history of renal calculi, prior cytotoxic therapy, inefficacy of uricosuric drugs, or overproduction of uric acid. The initial doses of probenecid, sulfinpyrazone, and allopurinol are kept low to avoid uric acid deposition in the kidneys and to minimize the risk of precipitating acute gout. Concomitant colchicine administration is employed to prevent the latter complication. Hydration and urinary alkalinization are used to avoid renal uric acid deposition.

CONCLUSION

The pharmacotherapeutic management of the arthritides involves a series of maneuvers with a wide selection of drugs over a protracted period of time. The foregoing discussion includes the major pathophysiologic features of each disease, general pharmacotherapeutic guidelines, and especially key factual information for each drug alternative, so that informed decisions can be made by the physician in managing the elderly patient with an arthritic disease.

REFERENCES

1. Cohen, D.B., Witwer, M.W., and Schmid, F.R.: Arthritis in the aged. I.M.J., *140*:187, 1971.
2. Bienenstock, H., and Fernando, K.R.: Arthritis in the elderly: an overview. Med. Clin. N. Am., *60*:1173, 1976.
3. Kolodny, A.L., and Klipper, A.R.: Bone and joint diseases in the elderly. Hosp. Pract., *11*:91, 1976.
4. Mowat, A.G.: Drug treatment of arthritis in the elderly. Age Ageing, *8*(Suppl.):14, 1979.
5. McBeath, A.A.: Family practice and problems of aging. Postgrad. Med., *57*:171, 1975.
6. Lee, P., et al.: The etiology and pathogenesis of osteoarthrosis: a review. Semin. Arthritis Rheum., *3*:189, 1974.
7. Moskowitz, R.W.: Management of osteoarthritis. Hosp. Pract., *14*:75, 1979.
8. Huskisson, E.C.: Osteoarthritis Changing concepts in pathogenesis and treatment. Postgrad. Med., *65*:97, 1979.
9. Peyron, J.G.: Epidemiologic and etiologic approach of osteoarthritis. Semin. Arthritis Rheum., *8*:288, 1979.
10. Rodman, G.P., McEwen, C., and Wallace, S.L.: Primer on the rheumatic diseases. J.A.M.A., *224*(Suppl. 5):25, 1973.

11. Johnson, J.S., et al.: Rheumatoid arthritis, 1970–1972. Ann. Intern. Med., 78:937, 1973.
12. Sack, K.E., and Rosenthal, S.H.: Rheumatoid arthritis: an overview. Tex. Med., 72:45, 1976.
13. Weissman, G.: Rheumatoid arthritis: how the nonsteroidal anti-inflammatory agents work. Med. Times, 104:64, 1976.
14. Williams, R.C., Jr.: Rheumatoid arthritis. Hosp. Pract., 14:57, 1979.
15. Ropes, M.W., et al.: 1958 revision of diagnostic criteria for rheumatoid arthritis. Bull. Rheum. Dis., 9:175, 1958.
16. Adler, E.: Rheumatoid arthritis in old age. Ir. J. Med. Sci., 2:607, 1966.
17. Brown, J.W., and Sones, D.A.: The onset of rheumatoid arthritis in the aged. J. Am. Geriatr. Soc., 15:873, 1967.
18. Moesmann, G.: Subacute rheumatoid arthritis in old age. I. Acta Rheum. Scand., 14:14, 1968.
19. Moesmann, G.: Clinical features in subacute rheumatoid arthritis in old age. Acta Rheum. Scand., 14:285, 1968.
20. Nastro, L.J.: Aggressive management of rheumatoid arthritis in the elderly. J. Am. Geriatr. Soc., 18:63, 1970.
21. Ehrlich, G.E., Katz, W.A., and Cohen, S.H.: Rheumatoid arthritis in the aged. Geriatrics, 25:103, 1970.
22. Ditunno, J., and Erlich, G.E.: Care and training of elderly patients with rheumatoid arthritis. Geriatrics, 25:164, 1970.
23. Sinclair, R.J.G.: Treatment of rheumatic disorders with special reference to ankylosing spondylitis. Proc. R. Soc. Med., 64:1031, 1971.
24. Neustadt, D.H.: Ankylosing spondylitis. Postgrad. Med., 61:124, 1977.
25. Engleman, E.G., and Engleman, E.P.: Ankylosing spondylitis. Recent advances in diagnosis and treatment. Med. Clin. N. Am., 61:347, 1977.
26. Calabro, J.J.: Early diagnosis and management of ankylosing spondylitis. Med. Times, 105:80, 1977.
27. Smythe, H.: Therapy of the spondyloarthropathies. Clin. Orthop., 143:94, 1979.
28. Forouzesh, S., and Bluestone, R.: The clinical spectrum of ankylosing spondylitis. Clin. Orthop., 143:53, 1979.
29. Doherty, S.M., and Yates, D.A.H.: Ankylosing spondylitis. Practitioner, 224:35, 1980.
30. Wallace, S.L., Robinson, H., and Masi, A.T.: Preliminary criteria for the classification of the acute arthritis of primary gout. Arthritis Rheum., 20:395, 1977.
31. Gall, E.P.: Hyperuricemia and gout. Postgrad. Med., 65:163, 1979.
32. Gordon, G.V., and Schumacher, H.R.: Management of gout. Am. Fam. Physician, 19:91, 1979.
33. Mangani, R.J.: Drug therapy reviews: pathogenesis and clinical management of hyperuricemia and gout. Am. J. Hosp. Pharm., 36:497, 1979.
34. Boss, G.R., and Seegmiller, J.E.: Hyperuricemia and gout: classification, complication and management. N. Engl. J. Med., 300:1459, 1979.
35. Klinenberg, J.R.: Hyperuricemia and gout. Med. Clin. N. Am., 61:299, 1977.
36. Fox, I.H., and Kelley, W.N.: Management of gout. J.A.M.A., 242:361, 1979.
37. Talbott, J.H.: Drug treatment of gout. Clin. Rheum. Dis., 5:657, 1979.
38. Constable, T.J., et al.: Drug treatment of rheumatoid arthritis. Lancet, 1:1176, 1975.
39. Smyth, C.J., and Bravo, F.J.: Antirheumatic drugs: clinical pharmacology and therapeutic aspects. Drugs, 10:394, 1975.
40. Hart, F.D.: Which antirheumatic drug? Drugs, 11:451, 1976.
41. Brooks, P.M., and Buchanan, W.W.: Current management of rheumatoid arthritis. Recent Adv. Rheum., 1:33, 1976.
42. Huskisson, E.C.: Anti-inflammatory drugs. Semin. Arthritis Rheum., 7:1, 1977.
43. Evens, R.P.: Antirheumatic agents. Am. J. Hosp. Pharm., 36:622, 1979.
44. Huskisson, E.C.: Routine drug treatment of rheumatoid arthritis and other rheumatic diseases. Clin. Rheum. Dis., 5:697, 1979.
45. Jacobs, R.P.: Update on the treatment of rheumatoid arthritis. Primary Care, 6:483, 1979.
46. Lee, P., et al.: Evaluation of analgesic action and efficacy of antirheumatic drugs. J. Rheumatol., 3:283, 1976.
47. Lee, P., and Dick, W.C.: The assessment of disease activity and drug evaluation in rheumatoid arthritis. Recent Adv. Rheum., 1:1, 1976.
48. Huskisson, E.C.: Simple analgesics for arthritis. Br. Med. J., 4:196, 1974.
49. Winter, L., Jr., Bass, E., Recant, B., and Cahaly, J.F.: Analgesic activity of ibuprofen (Motrin) in postoperative oral surgical pain. Oral Surg., 45:159, 1978.
50. Sinaki, M.: Role of physical medicine and rehabilitation in the care of rheumatoid arthritic patients. Minn. Med., 62:358, 1979.
51. Jenkins, D.G.: The rehabilitation of the arthritic patient. Practitioner, 224:73, 1980.
52. Smith, R.D., and Polley, H.F.: Rest therapy for rheumatoid arthritis. Mayo Clin. Proc., 53:141, 1978.
53. Smith, R.D.: Bed rest at home for rheumatoid arthritis. Arthritis Rheum., 23:263, 1980.
54. Ehrlich, G.E.: Splinting for arthritis. Med. Times, 96:485, 1968.
55. Buchanan, W.W., Rooney, P.J., and Rennie, J.A.N.: Aspirin and the salicylates. Clin. Rheum. Dis., 5:499, 1979.
56. Fremont-Smith, K., and Bayles, T.B.: Salicylate therapy in rheumatoid arthritis. J.A.M.A., 192:1133, 1965.
57. Calabro, J.J., and Paulus, H.E.: Anti-inflammatory effects of acetylsalicylic acid in rheumatoid arthritis. Clin. Orthop., 71:124, 1970.
58. Bayles, T.B.: Salicylate therapy in rheumatoid arthritis. Med. Clin. N. Am., 52:703, 1968.
59. Kozin, F.: Aspirin therapy in the rheumatic disease. Wis. Med. J., 75:S126, 1976.
60. Maclagen, T.J.: Treatment of acute rheumatism by sialicin and salicylic acid. Lancet, 1:342, 1876.
61. Nickander, R., McMahon, F.G., and Ridolfo, A.S.: Nonsteroidal anti-inflammatory agents. Ann. Rev. Pharmacol. Tox., 19:469, 1979.
62. Smiley, J.D.: Rheumatoid arthritis. Postgrad. Med., 58:17, 1975.
63. Rubin, A., et al.: Interactions of aspirin with nonsteroidal anti-inflammatory drugs in man. Arthritis Rheum., 16:635, 1973.
64. Levy, G., and Giacomini, K.M.: Rational aspirin dosage regimens. Clin. Pharmacol. Ther., 23:247, 1978.
65. Canada, A.T., Little, A.H., and Creighton, E.L.: The bioavailability of enteric-coated acetylsalicylic

acid: a comparison with buffered ASA in rheumatoid arthritis. Part ii. Curr. Ther. Res., *19*:554, 1976.
66. Canada, A.T., and Little, A.H.: The bioavailability of enteric-coated acetylsalicylic acid: a comparative study in rheumatoid arthritis. Part i. Curr. Ther. Res., *18*:727, 1975.
67. Pemberton, R.E., and Strand, L.J.: A review of upper gastrointestinal effects of the newer non-steroidal anti-inflammatory agents. Dig. Dis. Sci., *24*:53, 1979.
68. Silvoso, G.R., et al.: Incidence of gastric lesions in patients with rheumatic disease on chronic aspirin therapy. Ann. Intern. Med., *91*:517, 1979.
69. Lanza, F.L., Royer, G.L., Jr., and Nelson, R.S.: Endoscopic evaluation of the effects of aspirin, buffered aspirin, and enteric-coated aspirin on gastric and duodenal mucosa. N. Engl. J. Med., *303*:136, 1980.
70. Sutor, A.H., Bowie, E.J.M., and Owen, C.A., Jr.: Effect of aspirin, sodium salicylate and acetaminophen on bleeding. Mayo Clin. Proc., *46*:178, 1971.
71. O'Brien, J.R.: Effects of anti-inflammatory agents on platelets. Lancet, *1*:894, 1968.
72. Kanada, S.A., Kolling, E.M., and Hindin, B.I.: Aspirin hepatotoxicity. Am. J. Hosp. Pharm., *35*:330, 1978.
73. Szczeklik, A., Gryglewski, R.J., and Czerniawska-Mysik, G.: Clinical patterns of hypersensitivity to nonsteroidal anti-inflammatory drugs and their pathogenesis. J. Allergy Clin. Immunol., *60*:276, 1977.
74. Dick, C., et al.: Effect of anti-inflammatory drug therapy on clearance of 133Xe from knee joints of patients with rheumatoid arthritis. Br. Med. J., *3*:278, 1969.
75. Broh-Kahn, R.H.: Choline salicylate: a new, effective and well-tolerated analgesic anti-inflammatory and antipyretic agent. Int. Rec. Med. Gen. Pract. Clin., *173*:217, 1960.
76. Wolf, J., and Aboody, R.: Choline salicylate: a new and more rapidly absorbed drug for salicylate therapy. Int. Rec. Med. Gen. Pract. Clin., *173*:234, 1960.
77. Leary, J.F.: Preliminary pharmacological comparison of choline salicylate with acetylsalicylic acid. Int. Rec. Med. Gen. Pract. Clin., *173*:259, 1960.
78. Nevinny, D., and Gowans, J.D.C.: Observations on the usefulness of a new liquid salicylate in arthritis. Int. Rec. Med. Gen. Pract. Clin., *173*:242, 1960.
79. Thomas, R.P.: Comparative evaluation of the effectiveness of choline salicylate in various types of arthritis. Am. Pract., *11*:305, 1960.
80. Scully, F.J.: Choline salicylate: an effective, well tolerated drug for treatment of rheumatic diseases. South. Med. J., *53*:12, 1960.
81. Brooke, J.W.: Preliminary observations concerning the use of choline salicylate in various types of arthritis. Am. Pract., *11*:305, 1960.
82. Everett, A.D.: Choline salicylate for arthritic and rheumatic pain (letter). Lancet, *2*:316, 1961.
83. Cohen, A., Thomas, G.F., and Cohen, E.B.: Serum concentration safety and tolerance of oral doses of choline magnesium trisalicylate. Curr. Ther. Res., *23*:358, 1978.
84. Cohen, A.: A comparative blood salicylate study of two salicylate tablet formulations utilizing normal volunteers. Curr. Ther. Res., *23*:772, 1978.
85. Lechner, B.J., and Blechman, W.J.: Double comparison—Trilisate T.M. tablets vs. aspirin. Florida Fam. Physician, *28*:51, 1978.
86. Cohen, A., and Garber, H.E.: Comparison of choline magnesium trisalicylate and acetylsalicylic acid in relation to fecal blood loss. Curr. Ther. Res., *23*:187, 1978.
87. Harthon, L., and Hedstrom, M.: Hydrolysis of salicylic acid in human blood and acetylsalicylic acid. Acta Pharmacol. Tox., *29*:155, 1971.
88. Nordvist, P., Harthon, J.F.G., and Karlsson, R.: Metabolic kinetics of salicylsalicylic acid, aspirin, and sodium-salicylate in man. Nord. Med., *74*:1074, 1965.
89. Liyanage, S.P., and Tambar, P.K.: Comparative study of salsalate and aspirin in osteoarthrosis of the hip or knee. Curr. Med. Res. Opin., *5*:450, 1978.
90. Aberg, G., and Larsson, K.S.: Pharmacological properties and some antirheumatic salicylates. Acta Pharmacol. Tox., *28*:249, 1970.
91. Singleton, P.T., Jr.: Salsalate: its role in the management of rheumatic disease. Clin. Ther., *3*:80, 1980.
92. Deodhar, S.D., et al.: A short-term comparative trial of salsalate and indomethacin in rheumatoid arthritis. Curr. Med. Res. Opin., *5*:185, 1977.
93. Regalado, R.G.: The use of salsalate for control of long-term musculoskeletal pain: an open, noncomparative assessment. Curr. Med. Res. Opin., *5*:454, 1978.
94. Edmar, D.: Effects of salicylates on the gastric mucosa as revealed by roentgen examination and the gastrocamera. Acta Radiol. (Diagn.), *11*:57, 1971.
95. Leonards, J.R.: Absence of gastrointestinal bleeding following administration of salicylsalicylic acid. J. Lab. Clin. Med., *74*:911, 1969.
96. Thune, S.: Gastrointestinal bleeding and salicylates. Nord. Med., *79*:352, 1971.
97. Baum, J.: When to prescribe nonsteroidal anti-inflammatory drugs. Geriatrics, *84*:51, 1979.
98. Rubin, A., et al.: A profile of the physiological disposition and gastrointestinal effects of fenoprofen in man. Curr. Med. Res. Opin., *2*:529, 1974.
99. Gruber, C.M.: Clinical pharmacology of fenoprofen: a review. J. Rheumatol., *3*(Suppl. 2):8, 1976.
100. Kaiser, D.G., and Vangiessen, G.J.: GLC determination of ibuprofen in plasma. J. Pharm. Sci., *63*:219, 1974.
101. Davies, E.F., and Avery, G.S.: Ibuprofen: a review of its pharmacological properties and therapeutic efficacy in rheumatic disorders. Drugs, *2*:416, 1971.
102. Davis, L.J.: Ibuprofen. Drug Intell. Clin. Pharm., *9*:501, 1975.
103. Runkel, R., et al.: Naproxen—metabolism, excretion, and comparative pharmacokinetics. Scand. J. Rheumatol., Suppl. 2:29, 1973.
104. Segre, E.J.: Naproxen metabolism in man. J. Clin. Pharmacol., *15*:316, 1975.
105. Glass, R.C., and Swannell, A.J.: Concentrations of ibuprofen in serum and synovial fluid from patients with arthritis. Proc. Br. Pharm. Soc., September 1978, p. 453P.
106. Segre, E., et al.: Interaction of naproxen and aspirin in the rotund man. Scand. J. Rheumatol., Suppl. 2:37, 1973.
107. Reynolds, P.M.G., and Whorwell, P.J.: A single blind crossover comparison of fenoprofen, ibuprofen, and naproxen in rheumatoid arthritis. Curr. Med. Res. Opin., *2*:461, 1974.
108. Huskisson, E.C., et al.: Four new anti-inflammatory

drugs: responses and variations. Br. Med. J., *1:*1048, 1976.
109. Lewis, J.R.: New rheumatic agents: fenoprofen calcium (Nalfon), naproxen (Naproxyn), and tolmetin sodium (Tolectin). J.A.M.A., *237:*1260, 1977.
110. Huskisson, E.C., et al.: Treatment of rheumatoid arthritis with fenoprofen: comparison with aspirin. Br. Med. J., *1:*176, 1974.
111. Zuckner, J., and Auclair, R.J.: Fenoprofen calcium therapy in rheumatoid arthritis. J. Rheumatol., *3*(Suppl. 2):18, 1976.
112. Gum, O.B.: Fenoprofen in rheumatoid arthritis: a controlled crossover multicenter study. J. Rheumatol., *3*(Suppl. 2):26, 1976.
113. Sigler, J.W., Ridolfo, A.S., and Bluhm, G.B.: Comparison of benefit to risk ratios of aspirin and fenoprofen: controlled multicenter study in rheumatoid arthritis. J. Rheumatol., *3*(Suppl. 2):49, 1976.
114. Dornan, J., and Reynolds, W.J.: Comparison of ibuprofen and acetylsalicylic acid in treatment of rheumatoid arthritis. Can. Med. Assoc. J., *110:*1370, 1974.
115. Brooks, C.D., et al.: Aspirin and ibuprofen in the treatment of rheumatoid arthritis. Rheumatol. Phys. Med., *10*(Suppl):9, 1970.
116. Blechman, W.J., et al.: Ibuprofen or aspirin in rheumatoid arthritis therapy. J.A.M.A., *233:*336, 1975.
117. Diamond, H., et al.: A multicenter double-blind crossover comparison study of naproxen and aspirin in patients with rheumatoid arthritis. Scand. J. Rheumatol., Suppl. 2:171, 1973.
118. Hill, H.F.H., et al.: Naproxen: a new nonhormonal anti-inflammatory agent. Ann. Rheum. Dis., *33:*12, 1974.
119. Alexander, S.J.: Clinical experience with naproxen in rheumatoid arthritis. Arch. Intern. Med., *135:*1429, 1975.
120. Wojtulewski, J.A.: Fenoprofen in the treatment of osteoarthritis. Curr. Med. Res. Opin., *2:*551, 1974.
121. McMahon, F.J., Jain, A., and Onel, A.: Controlled evaluation of fenoprofen in geriatric patients with osteoarthritis. J. Rheumatol., *3*(Suppl. 2):76, 1976.
122. Royer, G.L., Jr., et al.: A six month double-blind trial of ibuprofen and indomethacin in osteoarthritis. Curr. Ther. Res. Opin., *17:*234, 1975.
123. Moxley, T.E., et al.: Ibuprofen versus buffered phenylbutazone in the treatment of osteoarthritis. J. Am. Geriatr. Soc., *23:*343, 1975.
124. Clarke, A.K., et al.: A double-blind comparison of naproxen against indomethacin in osteoarthritis. Arzneimittelforsch., *25:*302, 1975.
125. Barnes, C.G., et al.: A double-blind comparison of naproxen with indomethacin in osteoarthritis. J. Clin. Pharmacol., *15:*347, 1975.
126. Cochrane, G.M.: A double blind comparison of naproxen with indomethacin in osteoarthritis. Scand. J. Rheumatol., Suppl. 2:89, 1973.
127. Wilkins, R.F., Case, J.B., and Huix, F.J.: The treatment of acute gout with naproxen. J. Clin. Pharmacol., *15:*363, 1975.
128. Schweitz, M.C., Nashel, D.J., and Alepa, F.P.: Ibuprofen in the treatment of acute gouty arthritis. J.A.M.A., *239:*34, 1978.
129. Wanasukapunt, S.: Effect of fenoprofen calcium on acute gouty arthritis. Arthritis Rheum., *19:*933, 1976.
130. Flores, J.J.B., and Rojas, S.V.: Naproxen: corticosteroid-sparing effect in rheumatoid arthritis. J. Clin. Pharmacol., *15:*373, 1975.
131. Loebl, D.H., et al.: Gastrointestinal blood loss: effect of aspirin, fenoprofen and acetaminophen. J.A.M.A., *237:*976, 1977.
132. Schmid, F.R., and Culic, D.D.: Anti-inflammatory drugs and gastrointestinal bleeding: a comparison of aspirin and ibuprofen. J. Clin. Pharmacol., *16:*418, 1976.
133. Arsenault, A., et al.: Effect of naproxen on gastrointestinal microbleeding following acetylsalicylate medication. J. Clin. Pharmacol., *15:*340, 1975.
134. Halvorsen, L., Dotevall, G., and Sevelius, H.: Comparative effects of aspirin and naproxen on gastric mucosa. Scand. J. Rheumatol., Suppl. 2:43, 1973.
135. Roth, S.H., and Boost, G.: An open trial of naproxen in rheumatoid arthritis patients with significant esophageal, gastric and duodenal lesions. J. Clin. Pharmacol., *15:*378, 1975.
136. Cuthbert, M.F.: Adverse reactions to non-steroidal antirheumatic drugs. Curr. Med. Res. Opin., *2:*600, 1974.
137. Brooks, C.D., Schlagel, C.A., Sekhar, N.C., and Sobota, J.J.: Tolerance and pharmacology of ibuprofen. Curr. Ther. Res., *15:*180, 1973.
138. Nadell, J., Burno, J., Varady, J., and Segre, E.J.: Effect of naproxen and of aspirin on bleeding time and platelet aggregation. J. Clin. Pharmacol., *14:*176, 1974.
139. McIntyre, B.A., Philp, R.B., and Inwood, M.J.: Effect of ibuprofen on platelet function in normal subjects and hemophiliac patients. Clin. Pharmacol. Ther., *24:*616, 1978.
140. Rhymer, A.R., and Gengos, D.C.: Indomethacin. Clin. Rheum. Dis., *5:*541, 1979.
141. Hvidberg, E., Lausen, H.H., and Jansen, J.A.: Indomethacin: plasma concentrations and protein binding in man. Eur. J. Clin. Pharmacol., *4:*119, 1972.
142. Shen, T.-Y., and Winter, C.A.: Chemical and biological studies on indomethacin, sulindac, and their analogs. Adv. Drug Res., *12:*89, 1977.
143. Brogden, R.N., et al.: Sulindac: a review of its pharmacological properties and therapeutic efficacy in rheumatic diseases. Drugs, *16:*97, 1978.
144. Duggan, D.E., et al.: The disposition of sulindac. Clin. Pharmacol. Ther., *21:*326, 1977.
145. Selley, M.L., et al.: Pharmacokinetic studies of tolmetin, a new anti-inflammatory agent (abstract). Clin. Pharmacol. Ther., *17:*599, 1975.
146. Cressman, W.A., Wortham, G.E., and Plostnieks, J.: Pharmacokinetics of tolmetin, a new anti-inflammatory agent (abstract). Clin. Pharmacol. Ther., *15:*203, 1974.
147. O'Brien, W.M.: Indomethacin: a survey of clinical trials. Clin. Pharmacol. Ther., *9:*94, 1968.
148. Bross, H., Tausch, G., and Eberl, R.: Long term treatment of rheumatoid arthritis with indomethacin. *In* Huskisson, E.C., and Velog, G.P. (Editors): Inflammatory Arthropathies. Amsterdam, Excerpta Medica, 1976, p. 178.
149. Smyth, C.J., Velayos, E.E., and Amososo, C.: A method for measuring swelling of hands and feet. Part II. Influence of new anti-inflammatory drug, indomethacin, in acute gout. Acta Rheum. Scand., *9:*306, 1963.
150. Hart, F.J., and Boardman, P.L.: Indomethacin: a new nonsteroid anti-inflammatory agent. Br. Med. J., *2:*965, 1963.

151. Emmerson, B.T.: Regimen of indomethacin therapy in acute gouty arthritis. Br. Med. J., 2:272, 1967.
152. Boardman, P.L., and Hart, F.D.: Indomethacin in the treatment of acute gout. Practitioner, 194:560, 1965.
153. Smyth, C.J., and Percy, J.S.: Comparison of indomethacin and phenylbutazone in acute gout. Ann. Rheum. Dis., 32:351, 1973.
154. Pinals, R.S., and Frank, S.: Relative efficacy of indomethacin and acetylsalicylic acid in rheumatoid arthritis. N. Engl. J. Med., 276:512, 1967.
155. Haslock, I., Omar, A.S., and Wright, V.: A comparison of microencapsulated aspirin and indomethacin in the treatment of rheumatoid arthritis. Br. J. Clin. Pract., 29:311, 1975.
156. Kogstad, O.: A double-blind crossover study of naproxen and indomethacin in patients with rheumatoid arthritis. Scand. J. Rheumatol., Suppl. 2:159, 1973.
157. Percy, J.S., Stephenson, P., and Thompson, M.: Indomethacin in the treatment of rheumatic diseases. Ann. Rheum. Dis., 23:226, 1964.
158. Hart, F.D., and Boardman, P.L.: Indomethacin and phenylbutazone: a comparison. Br. Med. J., 2:1281, 1965.
159. Wright, V., Walker, W.C., and McGuire, R.J.: Indomethacin in the treatment of rheumatoid arthritis: a controlled trial comparing indomethacin, phenylbutazone and placebo. Ann. Rheum. Dis., 28:157, 1969.
160. Hahn, K.-J.: A comparison of phenylbutazone and indomethacin in the treatment of rheumatoid arthritis. Arzneimittelforsch., 23:851, 1973.
161. Smyth, C.J., and Percy, J.S.: Comparison of indomethacin and phenylbutazone in acute gout. Ann. Rheum. Dis., 32:351, 1973.
162. Calin, A., and Britton, M.: Sulindac in ankylosing spondylitis. Double-blind evaluation of sulindac and indomethacin. J.A.M.A., 242:1885, 1979.
163. Huskisson, E.C., et al.: Evening indomethacin in the treatment of rheumatoid arthritis. Ann. Rheum. Dis., 29:393, 1970.
164. Hobkirk, D., Rhodes, M., and Haslock, I.: Night medication in rheumatoid arthritis. Part ii. Combined therapy with indomethacin and diazepam. Rheumatol. Rehabil., 16:125, 1977.
165. Berkowitz, S.S., et al.: Tolmetin versus placebo for the treatment of rheumatoid arthritis: a sequential double-blind clinical trial. Curr. Ther. Res., 16:442, 1974.
166. Brooks, P.M., et al.: Clinical evaluation of tolmetin. Curr. Med. Res. Opin., 2:323, 1974.
167. Brown, J.H., Hull, J., and Biundo, J.J.: Results of a one year trial of tolmetin in patients with rheumatoid arthritis. J. Clin. Pharmacol., 15:455, 1975.
168. Cordrey, L.J.: Tolmetin in sodium, a new antiarthritis drug: double-blind and long term studies. J. Am. Geriatr. Soc., 24:440, 1976.
169. Bain, L.S., et al.: Tolmetin: an evaluation of a new preparation in the treatment of rheumatoid arthritis. Br. J. Clin. Pract., 29:208, 1975.
170. Huskisson, E.C., et al.: Tolectin for rheumatoid arthritis. Rheumatol. Rehabil., 13:132, 1974.
171. Muller, F.O., Gosling, J.A., and Erdmann, G.H.: A comparison of tolmetin with aspirin in the treatment of osteoarthritis of the knee. S. Afr. Med. J., 51:794, 1977.
172. Maibach, E.: European experiences with tolmetin in the treatment of rheumatic diseases. Curr. Ther. Res., 19:350, 1976.
173. McMillen, J.I.: Tolmetin sodium vs. ibuprofen in rheumatoid arthritis patients previously untreated with either drug: a double-blind crossover study. Curr. Ther. Res., 22:266, 1977.
174. Cardoe, N., and Steele, C.E.: A double blind crossover comparison of tolmetin sodium and phenylbutazone in the treatment of rheumatoid arthritis. Curr. Med. Res. Opin., 4:688, 1977.
175. Huskisson, E.C., and Scott, J.: Sulindac: trials of a new anti-inflammatory drug. Ann. Rheum. Dis., 37:89, 1978.
176. Reynolds, P.M.G., Rhymes, A.R., MacLeod, M.M., and Buchanan, W.W.: Comparison of sulindac and aspirin in rheumatoid arthritis. Curr. Med. Res. Opin., 4:485, 1977.
177. Chahade, W.H., and Jose, S.H.: Clinical evaluation of the efficacy and tolerance of sulindac in patients with osteoarthritis of the hip and/or knee during 144 weeks: comparative study with aspirin during the first 96 weeks. Eur. J. Rheum. Inflam., 1:41, 1978.
178. Dieppe, P.A., et al.: Sulindac in osteoarthrosis of the hip. Rheumatol. Rehabil., 15:112, 1976.
179. Brackertz, B., and Busson, M.: Comparative study of sulindac (Clinoril) and ibuprofen (Brufen) in osteoarthritis. Br. J. Clin. Pract., 32:77, 1978.
180. Broll, H., et al.: Preliminary results with the new nonsteroidal anti-inflammatory agent sulindac compared to phenylbutazone in the treatment of ankylosing spondylitis. In Huskisson, E.C., and Franchimont, P. (Editors): Clinoril in the Treatment of Rheumatic Disorders. New York, Raven Press, 1976, p. 123.
181. Gadomski, M., Singer-Bakker, H., and Braun, H.D.: Sulindac: a double blind clinical study of a new anti-inflammatory agent in the treatment of ankylosing spondylitis compared with phenylbutazone. In Huskisson, E.C., and Franchimont, P. (Editors): Clinoril in the Treatment of Rheumatic Disorders. New York, Raven Press, 1976, p. 133.
182. Diamond, H.S., and Bankhurst, A.D.: Double-blind comparison of sulindac and phenylbutazone in acute gouty arthritis. A special report. West Point, Pennsylvania, Merck, Sharp and Dohme, 1979, p. 75.
183. Sharma, B.K., and Haslock, I.: Night medication in rheumatoid arthritis. III. The use of sulindac. Curr. Med. Res. Opin., 5:472, 1978.
184. Boardman, P.L., and Hart, F.D.: Side effects of indomethacin. Ann. Rheum. Dis., 26:127, 1967.
185. Beirne, J.A., et al.: Gastrointestinal blood loss caused by tolmetin, aspirin and indomethacin. Clin. Pharmacol. Ther., 16:821, 1974.
186. Bianchi-Porro, G., et al.: Sulindac and gastric mucosa. Lancet, 1:1152, 1977.
187. Cohen, A.: Intestinal blood loss after a new anti-inflammatory drug, sulindac. Clin. Pharmacol. Ther., 20:238, 1976.
188. Green, D., Ts-ao, C., and Ross, E.C.: Sulindac. Lancet, 1:804, 1977.
189. Orme, M.L.E.: Phenylbutazone: plasma concentrations and effectiveness in patients with rheumatoid arthritis. J. Int. Med. Res., 5(Suppl. 2):40, 1977.
190. Orme, M., et al.: Plasma concentration of phenylbutazone and its therapeutic effects—studies in patients with rheumatoid arthritis. Br. J. Clin. Pharmacol., 3:185, 1976.
191. Brooks, P.M., et al.: Phenylbutazone: a clinicophar-

macological study in rheumatoid arthritis. Br. J. Clin. Pharmacol., 2:437, 1975.
192. Dick, W.C., Brooks, P.M., and Buchanan, W.W.: Phenylbutazone dose response in patients with rheumatoid arthritis. J. Int. Med. Res., 5(Suppl. 2):48, 1977.
193. Pavelka, K., et al.: Double-blind comparison of ibuprofen and phenylbutazone in a short term treatment of rheumatoid arthritis. Arzneimittelforsch., 23:842, 1973.
194. Scharff, E.U.: A double blind comparison of phenylbutazone and aspirin in osteoarthritis. Curr. Ther. Res., 16:1264, 1974.
195. Rotstein, J.: Phenylbutazone and aspirin in osteoarthritis: a controlled study. Curr. Ther. Res., 17:444, 1975.
196. Committee on the Review of Medicines: Recommendations on phenylbutazone, oxyphenbutazone, feprazone, allopurinol, colchicine, probenecid, and sulfinpyrazone. Br. Med. J., 1:1466, 1978.
197. Sperling, I.L.: Adverse reactions with long-term use of phenylbutazone and oxyphenbutazone. Lancet, 2:535, 1969.
198. Ward, J.R., et al.: Sodium meclofenamate (Meclomen) dose determining studies. Curr. Ther. Res., 23:S60, 1978.
199. Multz, V.C., Brobyn, R.D., and Caldwell, J.R.: Sodium meclofenamate (Meclomen) vs. aspirin for rheumatoid arthritis. Curr. Ther. Res., 23:S72, 1978.
200. Wolf, R.: European studies of sodium meclofenamate (Meclomen) in the treatment of rheumatoid arthritis. Curr. Ther. Res., 23:S113, 1978.
201. Eberl, R.: European studies of sodium meclofenamate (Meclomen) in long-term treatment. Curr. Ther. Res., 23:S131, 1978.
202. Schleyer, I.: European studies of sodium meclofenamate (Meclomen) in the treatment of osteoarthritis. Curr. Ther. Res., 23:S121, 1978.
203. Eberl, R.: European studies of sodium meclofenamate (Meclomen) for the treatment of ankylosing spondylitis. Curr. Ther. Res., 23:S126, 1978.
204. Gowant, J.D.C., Miniter, M., and Mills, D.M.: Early studies of sodium meclofenamate (Meclomen) for gout. Curr. Ther. Res., 23:S138, 1978.
205. Preston, S.N.: Safety of sodium meclofenamate (Meclomen). Curr. Ther. Res., 23:S107, 1978.
206. Smith, T.C.: Clinical pharmacology studies of sodium meclofenamate (Meclomen). Curr. Ther. Res., 23:S42, 1978.
207. Forestier, J.: Rheumatoid arthritis and its treatment by gold salts. J. Lab. Clin. Med., 20:827, 1935.
208. Freyberg, R.H., Block, W.D., and Wells, G.S.: Gold therapy for rheumatoid arthritis. Clinics, 1:537, 1942.
209. Freyberg, R.H.: Gold salts in the treatment of chronic arthritis: metabolic and clinical studies. Proc. Staff Meet. Mayo Clin., 17:534, 1942.
210. Adams, C.H., and Cecil, R.L.: Gold therapy in early rheumatoid arthritis. Ann. Intern. Med., 33:163, 1950.
211. Empire Rheumatism Council: Gold therapy in rheumatoid arthritis; report of a multi-center controlled trial. Ann. Rheum. Dis., 19:95, 1960.
212. American Rheumatism Council: A controlled trial of gold salt therapy in rheumatoid arthritis. Arthritis Rheum., 16:353, 1973.
213. Sigler, J.W., et al.: Gold salts in the treatment of rheumatoid arthritis. Ann. Intern. Med., 80:21, 1974.
214. Rothermich, N.O., et al.: Chrysotherapy; a prospective study. Arthritis Rheum., 19:1321, 1976.
215. Furst, D.E., et al.: A double-blind trial of high versus conventional dosages of gold salts for rheumatoid arthritis. Arthritis Rheum., 20:1473, 1977.
216. Luukkainen, R., Osomaki, H., and Kajander, A.: Gold treatment of an early stage of rheumatoid arthritis. Rheum. Rehab., Suppl. 94, 1978.
217. Kean, W.F., and Anastassiades, T.P.: Long term chrysotherapy. Incidence of toxicity and efficacy during sequential time periods. Arthritis Rheum., 22:495, 1975.
218. Srinivasan, R., Miller, B.L., and Paulus, H.E.: Long-term chrysotherapy in rheumatoid arthritis. Arthritis Rheum., 22:105, 1979.
219. Halla, J.T., Cassady, J., and Hardin, J.G.: Gold and penicillamine therapy in rheumatoid arthritis: a clinical comparison of effectiveness and toxicity. Arthritis Rheum., 23:686, 1980 (abstract).
220. Hill, D.F.: Gold therapy for rheumatoid arthritis. Med. Clin. N. Am., 52:733, 1968.
221. Bland, J.H.: Drug treatment of rheumatoid arthritis. Semin. Drug Treat., 1:93, 1971.
222. Myers, A.R.: Chrysotherapy in rheumatoid arthritis. Mod. Treat., 8:761, 1971.
223. Bluhm, G.B.: The treatment of rheumatoid arthritis with gold. Semin. Arthritis Rheum., 5:147, 1975.
224. Gottlieb, N.L.: Chrysotherapy. Bull. Rheum. Dis., 27:912, 1977.
225. Rothermich, N.O.: Chrysotherapy in rheumatoid arthritis. Clin. Rheum. Dis., 5:631, 1979.
226. Allegretti, J.E.: The role of chrysotherapy in active rheumatoid arthritis. Postgrad. Med., 28:623, 1960.
227. Gerber, R.C., et al.: Gold kinetics following aurothiomalate therapy. J. Lab. Clin. Med., 83:778, 1974.
228. Gottlieb, N.L., Smith, P.M., and Smith, E.M.: Pharmacodynamics of Au labeled aurothiomalate in blood; correlation with course of rheumatoid arthritis, gold toxicity, and gold excretion. Arthritis Rheum., 17:171, 1974.
229. Gold revalued (editorial). Lancet, 1:789, 1974.
230. Palmer, D.G., and Dunckley, J.V.: Gold levels in serum during treatment of rheumatoid arthritis with gold. Aust. N.Z. J. Med., 3:461, 1973.
231. Gottlieb, N.L., Smith, P.M., and Smith, E.M.: Tissue gold in a rheumatoid arthritic receiving chrysotherapy. Arthritis Rheum., 15:16, 1972.
232. Mascarhenes, B.R., Grand, J.L., and Freyberg, R.H.: Gold metabolism in patients with rheumatoid arthritis treated with gold compounds—reinvestigated. Arthritis Rheum., 15:391, 1972.
233. Gottlieb, N.L., Smith, P.M., and Smith, E.M.: Gold excretion correlated with clinical course during chrysotherapy in rheumatoid arthritis. Arthritis Rheum., 15:582, 1972.
234. Gold for rheumatoid arthritis (editorial). Br. Med. J., 1:471, 1971.
235. Lawrence, J.S.: Factors in gold dosage and toxicity in rheumatoid arthritis. Ann. Rheum. Dis., 12:129, 1953.
236. Lawrence, J.S.: Comparative toxicity of gold preparations in treatment of rheumatoid arthritis. Ann. Rheum. Dis., 35:171, 1976.
237. Gottlieb, N.L., and Major, J.C.: Ocular chrysiasis correlated with gold concentrations in the crystalline lens during chrysotherapy. Arthritis Rheum., 21:704, 1978.
238. Huskisson, E.C.: Penicillamine and the rheu-

matologist: a review. Pharmacotherapeutics, *1*:24, 1976.
239. Lyle, W.H.: Penicillamine. Clin. Rheum. Dis., *5*:569, 1979.
240. Huskisson, E.C., et al.: Trial comparing D-penicillamine and gold in rheumatoid arthritis. Ann. Rheum. Dis., *33*:532, 1974.
241. Baum, J.: The use of penicillamine in the treatment of rheumatoid arthritis and scleroderma. Scand. J. Rheum., Suppl. 28:65, 1979.
242. Multicenter Trial Group: Controlled trial of D-penicillamine in severe rheumatoid arthritis. Lancet, *1*:275, 1973.
243. Day, A.T., et al.: Penicillamine in rheumatoid disease; a long term study. Br. Med. J., *1*:180, 1974.
244. Zuckner, J., et al.: D-penicillamine in rheumatoid arthritis. Arthritis Rheum., *13*:131, 1970.
245. Golding, J.R., Wilson, J.V., and Day, A.T.: Observations on the treatment of rheumatoid disease with penicillamine. Postgrad. Med. J., *46*:599, 1970.
246. Huskisson, E.C., and Hart, D.F.: Penicillamine in the treatment of rheumatoid arthritis. Ann. Rheum. Dis., *31*:402, 1972.
247. Hill, H.L.H.: Selection of patients with rheumatoid arthritis to be treated with penicillamine and their management. Curr. Med. Res. Opin., *2*:573, 1974.
248. Jaffe, I.A.: The effect of penicillamine on the laboratory parameters in rheumatoid arthritis. Arthritis Rheum., *8*:1064, 1965.
249. Jaffe, A.I.: The treatment of rheumatoid arthritis and necrotizing vasculitis with penicillamine. Arthritis Rheum., *13*:436, 1970.
250. Jaffe, I.A.: D-penicillamine. Bull. Rheum. Dis., *28*:948, 1977–1978.
251. Webley, M., and Coomers, E.W.: An assessment of penicillamine therapy in rheumatoid arthritis and the influence of previous gold therapy. J. Rheumatol., *6*:20, 1979.
252. Bunch, T.W., and O'Duffy, J.D.: Disease-modifying drugs for progressive rheumatoid arthritis. Mayo Clin. Proc., *55*:161, 1980.
253. Evens, R.P.: Therapeutics of antirheumatic agents. Am. J. Hosp. Pharm. *37*:346, 1980.
254. Stein, H.B., et al.: Adverse effects of D-penicillamine in rheumatoid arthritis. Ann. Intern. Med., *92*:24, 1980.
255. Kean, W.F., et al.: The toxicity pattern of D-penicillamine therapy. Arthritis Rheum., *23*:158, 1980.
256. Jaffe, I.A., et al.: Nephropathy induced by penicillamine. Ann. Intern. Med., *69*:549, 1968.
257. Bucknall, R.C., et al.: Myasthenia gravis associated with penicillamine treatment for rheumatoid arthritis. Br. Med. J., *1*:600, 1975.
258. Sternlieb, I., Bennett, B., and Scheinberg, I.H.: D-penicillamine induced Goodpasture's syndrome in Wilson's disease. Ann. Intern. Med., *82*:673, 1975.
259. Jaffe, I.A., and Smith, R.W.: Rheumatoid vasculitis—report of a second case treated with penicillamine. Arthritis Rheum., *11*:585, 1968.
260. Zvaifler, N.J.: Antimalarials in the treatment of rheumatoid arthritis. Mod. Treat., *8*:769, 1971.
261. Popert, A.J.: Chloroquine: a review. Rheumatol. Rehabil., *15*:235, 1976.
262. Swosh, I.L., et al.: Azathioprine in early rheumatoid arthritis. Comparison with gold and chloroquine. Arthritis Rheum., *20*:685, 1977.
263. Wollheim, F.A., Hanson, A., and Laurell, C.-B.: Chloroquine treatment in rheumatoid arthritis. Scand. J. Rheum., *7*:171, 1978.
264. Mackenzie, A.H.: An appraisal of chloroquine. Arthritis Rheum., *13*:280, 1970.
265. Marks, J.S., and Power, B.J.: Is chloroquine obsolete in treatment of rheumatoid disease? Lancet, *1*:371, 1979.
266. Brinkley, J.R., Jr.: Long-term course of chloroquine retinopathy after cessation of medication. Am. J. Ophthalmol., *88*:1, 1979.
267. Gifford, R.H.: Corticosteroid therapy in rheumatoid arthritis. Med. Clin. N. Am., *57*:1179, 1973.
268. Burry, H.C.: Use and abuse of corticosteroids in rheumatic diseases. Drugs, *19*:447, 1980.
269. Myles, A.B., Schiller, L.F.G., Glass, D., and Daly, J.R.: Single daily dose corticosteroid treatment. Ann. Rheum. Dis., *35*:73, 1976.
270. Klinefelter, H.F., Winkenwerdes, W.L., and Bledsoe, T.: Single daily dose prednisone therapy. J.A.M.A., *241*:2721, 1979.
271. Murthy, M.H.V., Rhymer, A.R., and Wright, V.: Indomethacin or prednisolone at night in rheumatoid arthritis? Rheumatol. Rehab., *17*:8, 1978.
272. David, D.S., Grieco, M.H., and Cushman, P.: Adrenal glucocorticoids after twenty years; a review of their clinically relevant consequences. J. Chronic Dis., *22*:637, 1970.
273. Thompson, E.B., and Lippman, M.E.: Mechanism of action of glucocorticoids. Metabolism, *23*:159, 1974.
274. McCarty, D.J.: Intrasynovial therapy with adrenocorticosteroid esters. Wiscon. Med. J., *77*:S75, 1978.
275. Balch, H.W., et al.: Repeated corticosteroid injections into knee joints. Rheumatol. Rehab., *16*:137, 1977.
276. Urowitz, M.B.: Immunosuppressive therapy in rheumatoid arthritis. J. Rheumatol., *1*:364, 1974.
277. Andreis, M.: Immunosuppression in the treatment of rheumatoid arthritis. Adv. Clin. Pharmacol., *6*:81, 1974.
278. DeSeze, S., and Kahn, M.F.: Immunosuppressive drugs in rheumatoid arthritis: clinical results. Adv. Clin. Pharmacol., *6*:89, 1974.
279. Davis, J.D., Muss, H.B., and Turner, R.A.: Cytotoxic agents in the treatment of rheumatoid arthritis. S. Med. J., *71*:58, 1978.
280. Williams, J.H., et al.: Comparison of high and low dose cyclophosphamide therapy in rheumatoid arthritis. Arthritis Rheum., *23*:521, 1980.
281. Currey, H.L.F.: Immunosuppressive drugs in rheumatoid arthritis—toxicity. Adv. Clin. Pharmacol., *6*:98, 1974.
282. Fox, I.H.: Hypouricaemic agents in the treatment of gout. Clin. Rheum. Dis., *3*:145, 1977.
283. Diamond, H.S., and Paolino, J.S.: Evidence for a postsecretory reabsorptive site for uric acid in man. J. Clin. Invest., *52*:1491, 1973.
284. Fanell, F.M.: Uricosuric agents. Arthritis Rheum., *18* (Suppl.):853, 1975.
285. Gaines, L.M., and Shulman, L.E.: The failure of uricosuric drugs to reduce attack rate in primary nontophaceous gout. Presentation before American Rheumatism Association, Interim Session, Tucson, Arizona, 1969.
286. Kadar, D., et al.: Comparative drug elimination capacity in man—glutethimide, amobarbitol, antipyrine and sulfinpyrazone. Clin. Pharm. Ther., *14*:552, 1973.
287. Dieterle, W., et al.: Biotransformation and pharmacokinetics of sulfinpyrazone (Anturan) in man. Eur. J. Clin. Pharmacol., *9*:135, 1975.

288. Miller, R.R., and Greenblatt, D.J.: Drug Effects in Hospitalized Patients. New York, John Wiley & Sons, Inc., 1976, p. 168.
289. Wallace, S.L.: Colchicine. Semin. Arthritis Rheum., 3:369, 1974.
290. Wallace, S.L.: Colchicine and new anti-inflammatory drugs for the treatment of acute gout. Arthritis Rheum., 18 (Suppl.):847, 1975.
291. Paulus, H.E., et al.: Prophylactic colchicine therapy of intercritical gout. Arthritis Rheum., 17:609, 1974.
292. Wallace, S.L., Omokoku, B., and Ertel, N.H.: Colchicine plasma levels. Implications as to pharmacology and mechanism of action. Am. J. Med., 48:443, 1970.
293. Ellwood, M.G., and Robb, G.H.: Self poisoning with colchicine. Postgrad. Med. J., 47:129, 1971.
294. Heaney, D., Derghazarian, C.B., Pince, G.F., and Al, M.A.: Case report. Massive colchicine overdose; report on the toxicity. Am. J. Med. Sci., 271:233, 1976.
295. Hitchings, G.H.: Pharmacology of allopurinol. Arthritis Rheum., 18 (Suppl.): 863, 1975.
296. Loebl, W.Y., and Scott, J.T.: Withdrawal of allopurinol in patients with gout. Ann. Rheum. Dis., 33:304, 1974.
297. Rodnan, G.P., Robin, J.A., Tolchin, J.F., and Elias, G.B.: Allopurinol and gouty arthritis. Efficacy of a single daily dose. J.A.M.A., 231:1143, 1975.
298. Kersley, G.D.: Long-term use of allopurinol in the treatment of gout. Ann. Rheum. Dis., 29:89, 1970.
299. Serre, H., Simon, L., and Claustre, J.: Uric acid inhibitors in the therapy of gout. Sem. Hop. Paris, 50:3295, 1970.
300. Kantor, G.L.: Toxic epidermal necrolysis, azotemia and death after allopurinol therapy. J.A.M.A., 212:473, 1970.
301. Bird, H.A., and Dixon, A.S.: Failure of D-penicillamine to affect peripheral joint involvement in ankylosing spondylitis or HLA B27-associated arthropathy (letter). Ann. Rheum. Dis., 36:289, 1977.
302. Jaffe, I.A.: Penicillamine in seronegative polyarthritis (letter). Ann. Rheum. Dis., 36:593, 1977.
303. Golding, D.N.: D-penicillamine in ankylosing spondylitis and polymyositis. Postgrad. Med. J., 50 (Suppl. 2):62, 1974.
304. Golding, D.N.: D-penicillamine in spondylitis and sacro-iliitis. Scand. J. Rheum., 4 (Suppl. 8), abstract 12, 1975.

CHAPTER 9

ANEMIAS

James W. Linman

Anemia may be defined as a decrease in the hemoglobin per unit volume of blood below the level established as normal with respect to age, sex, and geographic locale. Although this definition is not necessarily synonymous with a decrease in the total body hemoglobin, the ratio of body to venous hematocrit values is sufficiently stable to permit clinical usage of the foregoing definition. Although the peripheral erythroid values differ between children and adults, there exists no compelling support for the widely held belief that hemoglobin levels decrease with advancing age. The mean hemoglobin and hematocrit levels in men 62 to 80 years old are 14.8 gm. per 100 ml. and 44.8 per cent, respectively. In women of similar ages the mean hemoglobin level is 13.5 gm. per 100 ml. and the mean hematocrit value is 41 per cent. Recognition of anemia in the elderly is based on the same criteria for any adult population, and a decrease in the erythroid values demands appropriate clinical evaluation to determine its cause.

Anemia is a manifestation of some underlying disorder and is not a disease of advancing age. Because the causes of anemia are many, a simple and workable etiologic classification is needed (Table 9–1). Although all anemias result from production failing to keep pace with need, they can be divided into two groups based on loss or impaired production; however, it is not unusual for an anemia to reflect both mechanisms.

Despite the technologic advances of recent years and the availability of a large number of diagnostic procedures, the evaluation of anemic patients remains a basically simple task that begins with a history and physical examination and relies heavily on hematologic morphology. In most instances these maneuvers alone point clearly to the type of documentation needed to confirm the diagnosis. It is inappropriate to approach either the diagnosis or the treatment of anemia in a "shotgun" fashion (e.g., routine use of a battery of tests or a therapeutic trial with a number of hematinic drugs; the former unnecessarily inflates the cost of health care, and

TABLE 9–1. Etiologic Classification of Anemia*

I. Blood loss	
A. Hemorrhage	
B. Hemolysis	
II. Impaired erythropoiesis	
A. Deficiencies	Vitamin B_{12}, folates, and iron
B. Destruction	Hypoplastic anemia
C. Diversion of growth potential	Nonlymphocytic leukemias
D. Displacement	Lymphocytic leukemia and metastatic carcinoma
E. Defective	Hereditary hemoglobinopathies
F. "Depression" (etiology unclear)	Anemia of chronic infection and liver disease

*From Linman, J.W.: Hematology. New York, Macmillan Publishing Co., Inc., 1975. (Copyright © 1975 by James W. Linman. Reprinted by permission of Macmillan Publishing Co., Inc.)

the latter is more apt than not to be harmful). The workup and treatment of an anemic patient depends on specific cause, and the success of the therapies to be discussed are, of course, predicated on accurate diagnoses.

BLOOD LOSS ANEMIAS

Blood loss anemias are due to removal of red cells from the circulation prior to the end of their normal life span. The decrease in red cell mass activates the humoral erythropoietic regulatory mechanism, which in turn increases erythropoiesis; the latter is reflected in the peripheral blood by polychromasia, reticulocytosis, and nucleated red cells and in the marrow by erythrocytic hyperplasia. There are only two mechanisms by which red cells can be lost; one is hemorrhage and the other is premature destruction (i.e., hemolysis). Because of the long survival time of normal red cells, a sudden decrease in the peripheral erythroid values always indicates acute blood loss whether by hemorrhage or hemolysis.

Acute Hemorrhagic Anemia

The clinical manifestations of acute hemorrhage depend on the amount of blood lost, the rapidity of bleeding, and the status of the patient before the hemorrhage. If an anemia develops gradually, an otherwise normal person can tolerate as much as a 50 per cent reduction in red cell mass without conspicuous untoward effects. On the other hand, the sudden loss of 40 to 50 per cent of the blood volume is followed by shock and, unless treated promptly, by death.

The immediate effect of acute hemorrhage is an equivalent decrease in both red cell mass and plasma volume. Anemia (i.e., a decrease in the hemoglobin level per unit volume of blood) does not become evident until extravascular fluid begins to enter the intravascular compartment to correct the hypovolemic state (Fig. 9–1). Hence, the early manifestations of acute hemorrhage reflect hypovolemia rather than a decrease in the oxygen carrying capacity of the blood. Cardiac, pulmonary, and vascular adjustments are brought into play, and if these mechanisms are unable to maintain the oxygen supply to vital organs, as is often the case in the elderly, shock ensues.

Plasma refill begins immediately after

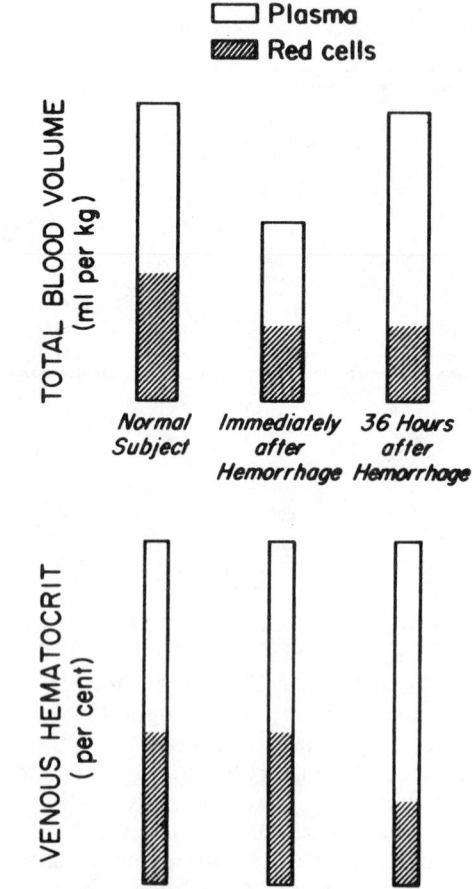

Figure 9–1. Effects of acute hemorrhage on the plasma volume, red cell mass, and venous hematocrit. (From Linman, J.W.: Hematology. New York, Macmillan Publishing Co., Inc., 1975. Copyright © by James W. Linman. Reprinted by permission of Macmillan Publishing Co., Inc.)

acute hemorrhage, and a normal total blood volume is ordinarily restored within 20 to 60 hours after a single episode of bleeding. The speed with which fluids enter the intravascular compartment is largely contingent on the rate at which protein from pre-existent pools is added to the circulation. Consequent to expansion of the plasma volume, the reduced red cell mass is diluted, and over a period of one to three days the peripheral erythroid values fall and a normochromic normocytic anemia develops. The latter evokes increased erythropoietin elaboration, which in turn increases marrow erythropoietic activity. If all requirements for erythropoiesis are met, if no other disorder exists that impairs erythropoiesis, and if hemorrhage does not recur, the peripheral erythroid values will be normal in three to six weeks.

The diagnosis of acute hemorrhagic anemia rarely presents a problem, for bleeding is ordinarily evident. The initial treatment consists of measures to stop the bleeding and to maintain an adequate blood volume. For the latter purpose, whole blood is the treatment of choice, although other volume expanders may be needed until whole blood is available. Once bleeding has ceased and the symptoms of shock or acute anemic hypoxia have abated, further transfusions are not needed. As noted, plasma expansion occurs promptly after an acute bleeding episode consequent to a shift of fluid from the extravascular to the intravascular compartment. If bleeding has stopped, continued transfusions are quite apt to bring about circulatory overload with disastrous results, especially in patients with an impaired cardiac reserve. Because older persons are more liable to have underlying cardiovascular disease, the treatment of acute hemorrhagic anemia in the elderly poses special problems less apparent in a younger population.

During the recovery phase in acute hemorrhagic anemia, treatment with iron is advisable in order to replenish the body iron stores. Ferrous sulfate in doses of 0.3 gm. three times daily after meals is preferred. Iron therapy should be continued for at least two to three months or longer if bleeding recurs or if hypochromia, which indicates prior blood loss, is present.

Hemolytic Anemias

Normally erythrocytes survive in the circulation for about 120 days, during which time they are subjected to severe mechanical buffeting and metabolic stresses and must expend considerable energy in order to maintain their functional and physical integrity. Although red cells cannot undergo mitosis, they are very much alive and carry on numerous metabolic processes, some of which are necessary for their survival. A variety of intrinsic and extrinsic defects, which may be inborn or acquired, can shorten the red cell life span and interfere with the normal erythroid steady state. A compensatory increase in erythropoiesis follows by way of the humoral erythropoietic regulatory mechanism in a manner like that already described for acute hemorrhage. Because a normal marrow can increase erythrocyte production six to eight times, red cell survival times must be shortened to 15 to 20 days (one-eighth to one-sixth of normal) before anemia results.

The causes of hemolysis are many and varied, but the hematologic findings are similar regardless of the nature of the underlying disease or red cell defect (i.e., manifestations of accelerated erythropoiesis [increased polychromasia, reticulocytosis, circulating nucleated red cells, and marrow erythrocytic hyperplasia] and of increased erythrocyte destruction [hyperbilirubinemia due to indirect reacting or unconjugated bilirubin, increased fecal and urine urobilinogen levels, decreased plasma haptoglobin, and shortened red cell survival times]). A clinical classification of the hemolytic disorders is shown in Table 9–2.

As a rule, a hemolytic anemia can be recognized with relative ease, but because of the similarities in the clinical manifestations of hemolysis, differential diagnosis (i.e., a precise etiologic diagnosis) may be difficult. However, knowledge of the cause of hemolysis is essen-

TABLE 9–2. Classification of the Hemolytic Disorders*

I. Hereditary
  A. Hereditary spherocytosis
  B. Hereditary elliptocytosis
  C. Hereditary hemoglobinopathies
  D. Hereditary glycolytic enzyme deficiencies
    1. Pentose phosphate pathway
      a. Glucose-6-phosphate dehydrogenase
        (1) "Primaquine sensitive" anemias
        (2) Favism
      b. Others
    2. Embden-Meyerhof pathway
      a. Pyruvate kinase
      b. Others
  E. Erythropoietic porphyria

II. Acquired
  A. Isoimmune
    1. Hemolytic transfusion reactions
    2. Erythroblastosis fetalis
  B. Autoimmune
    1. Primary (idiopathic)
    2. Secondary (lymphoma, chronic lymphocytic leukemia, collagen diseases)
  C. Drug induced immunohemolytic anemia
  D. Chemical and physical factors
  E. Mechanical factors (fragmented red cell hemolytic syndromes)
  F. Infections
  G. Splenomegaly ("big spleen" syndromes)
  H. Vitamin B_{12} or folate deficiency
  I. Paroxysmal nocturnal hemoglobinuria

*From Linman, J.W.: Hematology. New York, Macmillan Publishing Co., Inc., 1975. (Copyright © by James W. Linman. Reprinted by permission of Macmillan Publishing Co., Inc.)

tial, for such information may determine the type of treatment that is indicated. Erythrocyte morphology plays an important role in this process. Of these morphologic aberrations, spherocytes are most important, and their presence usually points to hereditary spherocytosis or an autoimmune hemolytic anemia. Schistocytes reflect red cell fragmentation, hypochromia suggests a thalassemia syndrome or paroxysmal nocturnal hemoglobinuria, oval macrocytes with hypersegmented neutrophils indicate vitamin B_{12} or folate deficiency, and so forth. It should be noted that all such deformed red cells have impaired pliability and decreased life spans. Normal red cells are easily deformable, biconcave discs that can successfully navigate the small openings in the microvasculature (e.g., the interendothelial slits in the walls of the splenic sinusoids). On the other hand, a spheroidal cell or an erythrocyte fragment is rigid and incapable of surviving in the circulation.

The diagnosis of a hemolytic anemia is ordinarily evident on the basis of the peripheral blood cell counts (including a reticulocyte count) and study of a stained blood smear. Such information, especially if strengthened by splenomegaly or jaundice due to indirect reacting bilirubin, usually precludes the need for other diagnostic procedures (e.g., ^{51}Cr labeled red cell survival times and plasma haptoglobin levels). However, other data are needed to establish the cause of the hemolytic process.

The direct Coombs or antiglobulin test is most useful, for a positive test result is the most consistent finding in patients with acquired isoimmune and autoimmune hemolytic disorders, both primary (or idiopathic) and secondary, and in drug induced immunohemolytic anemias. A search for a similar problem in family members is essential in the workup of patients suspected of having a hereditary disorder (e.g., hereditary spherocytosis and thalassemia). Specialized procedures (e.g., measurement of red cell glycolytic enzyme levels) are indicated only when simpler, routine studies suggest a process such as glucose-6-phosphate dehydrogenase deficiency.

Treatment of the hemolytic anemias is dependent on the nature of the underlying cause(s). There are no forms of treatment or support that are generally applicable. Even such therapeutic measures as transfusions may be at least relatively contraindicated if the cause of the decreased red cell survival time is an antibody injurious to all erythrocytes regardless of their antigenic properties (i.e., an autoimmune hemolytic anemia). It should also be noted that certain drugs commonly used to treat anemia (e.g., iron, folic acid, and vitamin B_{12}) are indicated only if the hemolytic process is complicated by a deficiency of iron, folates, or vitamin B_{12}. In fact, patients with a chronic hemolytic anemia assimilate greater than normal quantities of iron, and if treated inappropriately with inorganic iron, their body iron stores may increase to the point of organ dysfunction. Specific therapy for certain of the hemolytic syndromes is considered in the following sections.

Hereditary Spherocytosis

Although the course of hereditary spherocytosis varies greatly, it is generally one of relative benignity as attested to by the frequency of the diagnosis in the elderly. Because severe disease will be recognized in childhood or early adult life and requires treatment at that time, recognition of hereditary spherocytosis in an older person alters therapeutic principles, for the disease will be mild. There is no drug therapy for hereditary spherocytosis, and the treatment is splenectomy.

Even though the primary defect is within the red cell (presumably an abnormal protein in the erythrocyte membrane), the spleen is requisite for a clinically significant shortening of the life span of these defective erythrocytes. Splenectomy does not affect the intrinsic defect, and spherocytes persist after splenectomy. However, following removal of the spleen, the life span of the red cells is only slightly decreased; the marrow compensates for this minor change, and the anemia and other changes of hemolysis disappear. Splenectomy is completely effective, and overt hemolysis ceases in virtually all patients. In fact persistent hemolysis after splenectomy points to another diagnosis or an accessory spleen that may have been missed at the time of surgery. For this reason, failure to recommend splenectomy in a person with an uncompensated hemolytic anemia due to hereditary spherocytosis or some complication thereof, (e.g., cholelithiasis) cannot be condoned unless the patient has some other disease that greatly increases the operative risk or could logically be expected to cause his death before he encounters serious trouble consequent to the hemolytic disorder. Elderly patients are more likely to meet the latter requirements and are, as already noted, also more apt to have mild disease. Therefore, the recommendation to remove the spleen in older patients must be individualized and requires the judgment of an experienced clinician.

Despite the knowledge that some persons with hereditary spherocytosis reach an advanced age without serious untoward effects, the advantages to be gained by removing the spleen outweigh in most patients the possible risks of surgery. There is evidence that young children and persons with altered immune mechanisms (e.g., an individual being treated with a cytotoxic drug) may be more susceptible to certain infections after splenectomy, and this fact must also be considered in determining the risk versus benefit ratio. It is the consensus of most hematologists that the diagnosis of hereditary spherocytosis in a person without another disease or contraindication to surgery is, regardless of age, an indication for elective splenectomy.

Rare patients with hereditary spherocytosis develop hypoplastic crises, presumably owing to superimposed viral infections. These self-limited episodes are characterized by reticulocytopenia and a dramatic fall in the peripheral erythroid values, and such patients ordinarily require red cell transfusions to maintain acceptable circulating hemoglobin levels; otherwise there is little need for blood transfusions. Some patients with this hemolytic disorder develop superimposed folate deficiency; they should be treated with folic acid.

Hereditary Hemoglobinopathies

The hemoglobinopathies, both qualitative (e.g., sickle cell disease) and quantitative (e.g., the thalassemia syndromes), reflect abnormal or impaired globin chain synthesis as well as hemolysis. The most serious forms (i.e., homozygous disease) are not seen in the elderly because survival is shortened. Heterozygous forms are seen in older persons. Specific therapy is not available, and if treatment is needed, these patients can be offered only general supportive measures.

Hereditary Glycolytic Enzyme Deficiencies

The chemical, functional, and physical integrity of an erythrocyte is dependent on glycolysis, which in turn is contingent on a number of enzymes and coenzymes. Interference with glucose metabolism shortens the life span of red cells; genetically determined enzyme deficiencies occur and are manifested clinically by a hemolytic anemia. Deficiencies of enzymes participating in the Embden-Meyerhof glycolytic pathway (e.g., pyruvate kinase) are uncommon and usually produce severe disease; thus, they are ordinarily recognized early in life and rarely pose therapeutic problems in the elderly. On the other hand, abnormalities of the pentose phosphate pathway (e.g., deficiencies of glucose-6-phosphate dehydrogenase) are more common, are more apt to produce episodic, less severe hemolysis, and do not impair longevity; therefore, these types of hemolytic anemia are seen in all age groups and are clinically significant problems in the elderly.

The diagnosis of hereditary glucose-6-phosphate dehydrogenase deficiency is based on the demonstration of reduced red cell glucose-6-phosphate dehydrogenase activity or one of the consequences of a reduction in this enzyme; it must be considered in all patients with episodic, nonspherocytic, hemolytic anemia. Clinically significant hemolysis is contingent on exposure to a redox compound; some of the more common offenders include antimalarial drugs (e.g., primaquine), sulfonamides, nitrofurans, analgesics or antipyretics (e.g., aspirin and phenacetin), sulfones, chloramphenicol, water soluble vitamin K analogues, quinidine, naphthalene (moth balls), trinitrotoluene, and certain plants (e.g., fava beans). Treatment consists of recognition of the responsible agent and discontinuance of exposure thereto. Transfusions may, on occasion, be lifesaving (e.g., some patients with favism), but they are otherwise rarely needed. There is no role for corticosteroids or splenectomy in the management of these patients.

Idiopathic (Primary) Autoimmune Hemolytic Anemias

Therapeutic options in the treatment of idiopathic autoimmune hemolytic anemias include corticosteroids, splenectomy, immunosuppressive drugs, and blood transfusions.

Corticosteroids. In general the diagnosis is an indication for treatment with a corticosteroid; the usual starting dosage in an adult is 15 to 20 mg. of prednisone orally every six hours (or an equivalent amount of a comparable compound); in addition, acutely anemic, severely ill patients should receive hydrocortisone intravenously during the first 24 to 48 hours. Most patients with warm-reactive antibodies respond to these large doses of corticosteroids, and the anemia is corrected or at least significantly decreased in 80 to 90 per cent of the patients treated with 60 mg. or more of prednisone daily. The deleterious side effects of such corticosteroid therapy must be anticipated and the patients provided with appropriate support; such adverse reactions (e.g., fluid retention, electrolyte disturbances, hyperglycemia, increased susceptibility to infection, peptic ulceration, emotional disturbances, osteoporosis, and other assorted musculoskeletal, gastrointestinal, endocrine, ophthalmic, neurologic, and dermatologic disorders) constitute special problems in older patients, who may have pre-existing diseases such as diabetes mellitus and organic heart disease.

The corticosteroids also have a significant potential for interacting with other drugs the elderly patient may be consuming. In the diabetic patient corticosteroids may increase requirements for insulin or orally administered hypoglycemic drugs. The metabolic clearance of corticosteroids may be enhanced by phenytoin, phenobarbital, and ephedrine, thus resulting in decreased blood levels and lessened physiologic activity. Upward adjustment in the dose of the corticosteroid may be necessitated in such circumstances. The prothrombin time should be checked frequently in patients receiving corticosteroids and coumarin anticoagulants, for there have been reports of corticosteroids inhibiting the response to coumarin anticoagulants (e.g., warfarin, dicumarol, and phenprocoumon). Finally, when corticosteroids are administered concomitantly with potassium depleting diuretics (e.g., thiazides and loop diuretics), patients should be observed closely for the development of hypokalemia.

An adequate trial of corticosteroids appears to be about 21 to 28 days; if hemolysis has not lessened by this time, it is unlikely that more prolonged therapy will be effective, and other therapeutic options should be considered (i.e., splenectomy or immunosuppressive drugs). At this juncture a trial of massive corticosteroid therapy (e.g., 200 to 400 mg. of prednisone daily for five to seven days) may be justified in certain patients; however, the results leave much to be desired, and such treatment may introduce unacceptable risks, especially in elderly persons.

In patients in whom the anemia is corrected or in whom at least acceptable peripheral erythroid values are achieved, the corticosteroid dosages should be gradually tapered, the goal being discontinuance. Some patients may remain in remission even after steroid therapy is stopped; these patients require no further treatment but should be followed closely. More often hemolysis recurs, and retreatment is needed. In patients who exhibit only a partial response to full doses of corticosteroids, it is unlikely that such improvement will persist if prednisone is stopped. Under these circumstances the prednisone dosage should be reduced to the smallest amount that will maintain a satisfactory circulating hemoglobin level. It then becomes necessary to weigh carefully the undesirable side effects of long term corticosteroid therapy against the risks of other forms of treatment (i.e., splenectomy and immunosuppressive therapy).

Patients with idiopathic autoimmune hemolytic anemia due to cold reactive agglutinins respond much less well to corticosteroids than do patients with antibodies that are most reactive at 37° C. Although some of these patients deserve a trial of corticosteroids and a few improve, avoidance of exposure to cold is often more effective.

Splenectomy. Removal of the spleen is a much less effective therapeutic maneuver in the acquired autoimmune hemolytic anemias than in hereditary spherocytosis. In about half the patients hemolysis ceases or lessens; the remaining patients are not benefited significantly. Even so, splenectomy remains a viable option in those who fail to respond to corticosteroids or who cannot be maintained on continuous, long term therapy; in the absence of clear-cut contraindications to surgery consequent to age or the presence of other disease(s), removal of the spleen is preferred over the only other form of treatment available (i.e., immunosuppressive drugs).

Splenectomy offers two theoretical advantages in the acquired autoimmune hemolytic anemias—removal of an organ that sequesters and destroys antibody-damaged red cells and removal of a large collection of antibody-producing cells. An autoimmune hemolytic anemia due to cold reactive agglutinins rarely responds to splenectomy.

Immunosuppressive Drugs. Because the autoimmune hemolytic anemias reflect the presence of antibodies that damage red cells and decrease their life spans, it is reasonable to presume that control of such a process might be achieved with cytotoxic drugs, which decrease proliferation of cells that synthesize antibodies. Several such drugs have been shown to be variably effective and should be considered in patients who are unresponsive to corticosteroids or splenectomy or in individuals in whom these types of treatment cannot be used. The widest experience exists with azathioprine (Imuran), cyclophosphamide (Cytoxan), and chlorambucil (Leukeran); the daily dosages for average sized adults are 50 to 100 mg. of azathioprine, 50 to 100 mg. of cyclophosphamide, and 6 to 8 mg. of chlorambucil. Treatment must be continued for weeks to months. Toxicity is an ever present threat, and dosages must be monitored closely to prevent serious marrow depression. An additional hazard is the oncogenic potential of such cytotoxic drugs as the alkylating drugs.

Blood Transfusions. In the management of the acquired autoimmune hemolytic anemias, red cell transfusions are only palliative, usually ineffective, and not without risk; consequently, they should be avoided insofar as possible. Because most erythrocyte antibodies affect all red cells irrespective of their antigenic properties, donor cells survive no longer in patients with autoimmune hemolytic anemias than do their own cells. In fact the larger number of older, less resistant donor cells often survive less well than do the younger, more resistant cells of the patients. For this reason a transfusion is often followed by increased hemolytic activity with little or no increase in oxygen carrying capacity. Nonetheless, transfusions may be essential in certain critically ill patients, in patients being prepared for surgery, and so forth. Insofar as possible, corticosteroids should be started prior to giving a transfusion. It should also be noted that serious problems are often encountered in typing and cross matching, and they frequently cause much anxiety and concern. Unless massive hemolysis has taken place over a very short period of time, these patients are not hypovolemic. Therefore, if transfusions are deemed necessary, only packed red cells should be used; otherwise circulatory overload may ensue.

Other Therapy. If a patient with an autoimmune hemolytic anemia develops folate deficiency, treatment with folic acid is indicated. There is no indication for any other type of treatment. As already noted, iron therapy is contraindicated, for in the absence of some other disease associated with bleeding, long term iron therapy may cause tissue hemosiderosis and dysfunction of such organs as the liver, pancreas, and heart.

Secondary Autoimmune Hemolytic Anemias

The disorders associated with secondary autoimmune hemolytic anemias include hematologic neoplasms (e.g., lymphoma, chronic lymphocytic leukemia, and plasmacytic myeloma), connective tissue disorders (e.g., systemic lupus erythematosus), infections (e.g., infectious mononucleosis and mycoplasmal pneumonia), miscellaneous tumors (e.g., ovarian neoplasms), and other disorders (e.g., ulcerative colitis). The clinical and laboratory manifestations in these patients differ from those of primary (idiopathic) autoimmune hemolytic anemia only insofar as the underlying disease contributes to the clinical pictures of the secondary forms.

The principles underlying the treatment of the secondary autoimmune hemolytic anemias are those already described for the idiopathic form. There are, however, certain differences:

1. Treatment of the underlying disease is of primary importance and may be followed by a lessening of hemolytic activity (e.g., decreased hemolysis after chemotherapy for lymphoma.)

2. Treatment of the underlying disease may aggravate the anemia (e.g., erythropoietic suppression following chemotherapy for lymphoma).

3. Corticosteroids are less effective in the secondary autoimmune hemolytic anemias (e.g., normal peripheral erythroid values are rarely restored because of the limitations imposed by the underlying disease).

4. There is a greater tendency to avoid splenectomy and deny the patient any benefit of splenic removal because of the prognosis of the basic disease and the fact that many of these patients are poorer surgical risks than those with idiopathic autoimmune hemolytic anemia.

5. Blood transfusions play a more important role in the treatment of the secondary (autoimmune) hemolytic anemias.

Drug Induced Immunohemolytic Anemias

Although a large number of drugs have been implicated in the pathogenesis of immunohemolytic anemias, the incidence of these disorders is low. There are four mechanisms by which drugs can cause hemolysis; they are best designated by the drug that serves as the prototype for each:

Stibophen Type. Hemolysis secondary to stibophen (Fuadin) appears to reflect destruction of erythrocytes as "innocent bystanders." A drug-plasma factor complex functions as the antigen that evokes the elaboration of an IgM immunoglobulin; the antibody joins with additional drug and attaches to the red cell membrane, activates complement, and brings about cell injury and a decreased life span. The direct Coombs test result is positive with anticomplement specificity. The hemolytic episode is one of acute intravascular lysis. Treatment consists of stopping the drug and providing support as needed (e.g., red cell transfusions).

Penicillin Type. In this type of drug induced hemolytic disorder, the drug (i.e., penicillin) acts as a hapten and binds tightly to the red cell membrane; the latter complex evokes antibody production, which upon subsequent or continued exposure to the drug reacts with drug-coated red cells and brings about their destruction. The direct Coombs test result is positive with anti-IgG reagents. Large doses of penicillin over a long period of time are needed to bring about hemolysis. Usually the only treatment that is needed is to stop the drug. Although relatively few recipients of penicillin manifest hemolysis, the widespread use of this antibiotic makes it the most common cause of drug related immunohemolytic anemias.

Methyldopa Type. Alpha-methyldopa (Aldomet) is the cause of a positive direct Coombs test result (anti-IgG specificity) in about one-third of the persons who have taken this drug for periods of three to six months or longer. Despite the relatively high frequency of positive Coombs test results in recipients of methyldopa, only a few (about 1 to 2 per cent) manifest an overt hemolytic anemia. The mechanism is not completely understood, and the drug appears to impart some nonspecific stimulus to antibody elaboration; the latter may reflect a greater than normal propensity for the recipient to form autoantibodies. In patients who develop this phenomenon secondary to Aldomet therapy, an alternative drug should be found. Because the antibody remains for a long time after the drug is discontinued, hemolysis subsides slowly after the drug is stopped; in some cases corticosteroids may be helpful.

Cephalothin Type. Positive direct Coombs test results (anti-IgG specificity) occur in the majority of patients treated with large doses of cephalothin (Keflin) and in smaller numbers of persons given other cephalosporins. Because Coombs positivity occurs rapidly and is not dependent on prior exposure, it seems unlikely that it reflects an immune mechanism. Because most patients do not display hemolysis, the major clinical significance is the diagnostic confusion caused by the positive antiglobulin test result. The full meaning of this reaction is not yet clear, and it seems probable that other drugs will be implicated in similar responses.

Hemolytic Anemias Caused by Chemical, Physical, and Mechanical Factors

Red cell life spans can be decreased by a variety of chemicals (e.g., phenylhydrazine and arsenic hydride), physical agents (e.g., heat and breathing 100 per cent oxygen), and mechanical factors (e.g., prosthetic heart valves and fibrin strands consequent to disseminated intravascular coagulation). Treatment consists of removing the responsible agent or factor. It should be noted that the fragmented red cell hemolytic syndromes (e.g., hemolysis due to a prosthetic heart valve) are characterized by intravascular hemolysis. Consequently, iron is lost in the urine, body iron stores are reduced, and an iron deficiency anemia may ensue. Because most patients with valvular prostheses lose significant amounts of iron in the urine, it is reasonable to give all such patients iron, as described in the section dealing with iron deficiency anemia. These patients are also in jeopardy of the development of folate deficiency because of the increased requirements needed to maintain increased erythropoietic activity. Routine folic acid supplementation cannot be recommended; however, physicians must be constantly alert to this complication of a cardiac hemolytic anemia, for it is easily treated.

Hemolytic Anemias Caused by Infections

Certain infections (e.g., malaria) are consistently associated with hemolysis, for the micro-organisms invade the red cells and bring about their destruction. Other infectious processes impair erythrocyte viability by producing hemolytic substances (e.g., *Clostridium welchii*) or by evoking the formation of proteins that function as red cell antibodies (e.g., the cold agglutinins associated with mycoplasmal pneumonia). The treatment of these hemolytic anemias is the treatment needed to eradicate the responsible micro-organisms (e.g., antimalarial drugs).

Hemolytic Anemias Caused by Splenomegaly

The "big spleen syndromes" are characterized by splenic enlargement and expansion of the stasis compartment of the spleen. As a result, the time spent by red cells in the hostile environment of the spleen is increased, with resultant injury to the cell and a decrease in its life span. Such hypersplenism can result in an overt hemolytic anemia. Examples of disorders that may be accompanied by this type of hemolytic anemia include portal hypertension with chronic congestive splenomegaly, agnogenic myeloid metaplasia, Gaucher's disease, and kala-azar. The treatment is aimed at reducing splenic size or by eliminating the responsible organ (i.e., splenectomy). However, it should be noted that in many of these situations hemolysis may not be the predominant pathophysiologic manifestation and that splenectomy may not be without risk (e.g., removal of the major site of hematopoiesis in a patient with agnogenic myeloid metaplasia with myelofibrosis and increasing the susceptibility of serious infection, most notably pneumococcal septicemia).

Paroxysmal Nocturnal Hemoglobinuria

This rare acquired hemolytic disorder of unknown cause is characterized by red cells with an increased susceptibility to lysis by complement, hemoglobinuria occurring during sleep superimposed on a chronic hemolytic anemia, leukopenia, thrombocytopenia, recurrent infections, and venous thrombosis. Because the hemolysis is intravascular, iron is lost in the urine, and iron deficiency usually ensues. The disorder occurs most often in the third to fourth decade of life, but it may begin at any age. It should be noted that demonstration of complement sensitive erythrocytes by the acid-serum or sugar-water tests is not pathognomonic of paroxysmal nocturnal hemoglobinuria and may occur in other disorders such as the preleukemic syndrome. Thus, findings suggestive of paroxysmal nocturnal hemoglobinuria in an elderly patient demands exclusion of a myeloproliferative disorder, which would be statistically more likely in older persons. There is no effective treatment for the disorder other than support directed at specific pathophysiologic manifestations (e.g., transfusions with washed red cells if the anemia is severe and treatment with inorganic iron if iron deficiency is present).

IRON DEFICIENCY ANEMIA

Iron is an integral part of the hemoglobin molecule (0.347 per cent). In order to maintain the erythroid steady state, enough hemoglobin must be synthesized each day to replace that lost consequent to normal red cell attrition. If body iron stores are unable to meet this need, the amount of hemoglobin produced by each developing red cell is decreased; the total marrow output of hemoglobin falls, and a hypochromic microcytic anemia ensues. Iron deficiency is one of the most frequently encountered problems in clinical medicine. Because most of the body's iron is contained in hemoglobin and because this metal is tenaciously conserved, iron deficiency generally reflects chronic blood loss.

There is approximately 4 gm. of iron in a normal sized adult (Table 9–3). Because about two-thirds of this iron is incorporated in the hemoglobin molecule, requirements are largely determined by the amount of hemoglobin needed to replace that lost as a result of normal red cell catabolism. For this purpose 20 to 25 mg. of elemental iron is required daily; however, an equivalent amount is made available by the destruction of red cells that have reached the end of their finite life span, and this iron can be reutilized for the synthesis of new hemoglobin. Consequently, exogenous iron requirements reflect the amount lost from

TABLE 9–3. Average Distribution of Iron in a Normal Sized Adult*

	Percentage	Milligrams
Hemoglobin	65.0	2600
Storage iron (ferritin and hemosiderin)	29.0	1160
Myoglobin	3.5	140
Iron in transit (iron-transferrin complex)	0.1	4
Labile iron pool	2.2	88
Enzyme iron	0.2	8
Total	100.0	4000

*From Linman, J.W.: Hematology. New York, Macmillan Publishing Co., Inc., 1975. (Copyright © 1975 by James W. Linman. Reprinted by permission of Macmillan Publishing Co., Inc.)

the body. The retentive capacity of the body for iron is great, and there is no normal excretory mechanism.

Small amounts of iron are lost in the urine, feces, and sweat and in shed cells, hair, and nails. In order to maintain a positive iron balance, adult males and nonmenstruating females must acquire 0.5 to 1.0 mg. of new iron each day. Since a "normal" diet in the United States contains 10 to 20 mg. of elemental iron, it would seem that the task of maintaining body iron stores would be an easy one. However, a normal person can absorb only 10 per cent or less of dietary iron, and even in the face of depleted body stores, only 30 per cent or so of food iron can be extracted from the diet. Consequently, there is available from normal dietary sources barely enough iron to counteract the daily obligatory loss. This fact, coupled with knowledge that 1.0 ml. of blood contains approximately 0.5 mg. of elemental iron, emphasizes the ease with which increased loss (e.g., chronic bleeding), can cause an iron deficiency anemia.

In the face of negative iron balance, stores are affected first and gradually give up their iron to supply the body's needs; thus, the storage compartment must be exhausted (or nearly exhausted) before altered physiology occurs. Because most of the body's iron is contained in hemoglobin, it is not surprising that the pathophysiologic manifestations of iron deficiency are basically hematologic. When there is less iron available than is needed to maintain a normal hemoglobin level, anemia is inevitable. Iron deficiency curtails the quantity of hemoglobin synthesized and does not significantly affect other aspects of erythropoiesis. When the level of circulating hemoglobin falls, the humoral erythropoietic regulatory mechanism (i.e., erythropoietin) is responsible for marrow erythrocytic hyperplasia. Since the nucleated red cells are unable to synthesize normal amounts of hemoglobin, the more mature nucleated red cells exhibit impaired hemoglobinization. The decreased concentration of hemoglobin in the red cells is manifested morphologically by hypochromia. Hemoglobin synthesis fails to keep pace with cellular proliferation, yielding microcytes in addition to hypochromia. Consequently, the hemoglobin and hematocrit levels are disproportionately lower than the red cell count, and the hematologic manifestation of iron deficiency is a hypochromic microcytic anemia.

The symptoms and physical findings of iron deficiency anemia are basically those attributable to a decrease in the oxygen carrying capacity of the blood in addition to those of the primary disease responsible for the depleted iron stores. Tissue iron deficiency may be reflected in some patients by additional abnormalities (e.g., tongue changes and koilonychia), but such findings are rare and are associated with profound deficiency states.

Iron deficiency may result from inadequate intake, increased requirements (e.g., infants, adolescents, and pregnant women), or excessive loss. Because of the size of the storage compartment and the efficiency with which iron is reused, most iron deficiency anemias reflect increased loss. Since there are no effective excretory mechanisms and most of the body iron is contained in hemoglobin, increased loss is, for all practical purposes, contingent on bleeding. Therefore, the diagnosis of an iron deficiency anemia indicates blood loss until disproved, although multiple factors in some cases may act conjointly (e.g., dietary inadequacy in a chronically bleeding person). Aging does not increase normal physiologic iron requirements; thus this mechanism does not contribute to iron deficiency in the elderly. The latter persons do, of course, have a greater frequency of diseases that may cause blood loss, and iron deficiency anemias are common geriatric problems.

Steps in the evaluation of the hypochromic anemias are depicted in Figure 9–2. Although the diagnosis of an iron deficiency anemia is predicated on the demonstration of depleted iron stores, recognition is facilitated because hypochromia and microcytosis are the easily demonstrable morphologic features of an iron deficiency anemia and most (over 90 per cent) hypochromic anemias are the result of iron deficiency. Therefore, the simplest, easiest, and least expensive diagnostic procedure is the examination of a stained peripheral blood smear. In the face of an obvious cause for iron deficiency (e.g., chronic gastrointestinal bleeding), the morphologic diagnosis of a hypochromic microcytic anemia may be considered synonymous with an etiologic diagnosis of iron deficiency anemia.

In most patients other hematologic studies are not needed unless the patient fails to respond to adequate replacement therapy; in these instances or in patients without obvious causes for iron deficiency, body iron stores must be assessed by measuring the serum ferritin level, determining serum iron and iron

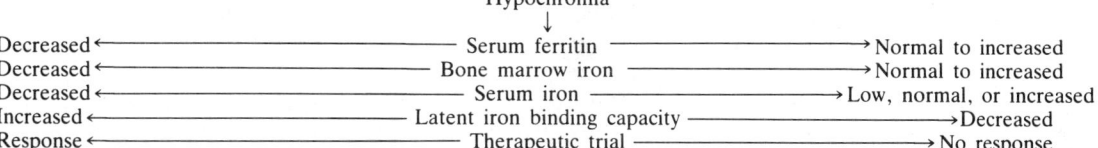

Figure 9-2. Steps in the diagnosis of a hypochromic anemia. (From Linman, J.W.: Differential diagnosis of the hypochromic anemias. Postgrad. Med., *49*:88–94, 1971. By permission.)

binding capacity, or quantifying bone marrow iron using special stains. Each of these tests yields comparable data, and there is ordinarily no reason to perform more than one. However, each test has its shortcomings; serum ferritin levels are preferred because of accuracy, simplicity, and reproducibility. If body iron stores are not decreased, some other cause for a hypochromic anemia must be sought, such as the thalassemia syndromes, the sideroblastic anemias, or the anemia of chronic disease.

An iron deficiency anemia is always a secondary manifestation of some other disorder. The importance of finding the cause cannot be overemphasized, for all such anemias respond to iron replacement therapy, and restoration of normal peripheral erythroid values may obscure the nature of the primary disease until remedial therapy is precluded (e.g., a bleeding colonic carcinoma). Consequently, the workup of a patient with an iron deficiency anemia is never complete until the pathogenesis of the iron deficiency is identified.

The treatment of iron deficiency anemia consists of supplying the missing substance (i.e., iron). The response is prompt, dramatic, predictable, and fully effective. In fact, the response is such that it may actually be used as diagnostic confirmation. For example, if the hemoglobin deficit due to iron deficiency is at least 5 gm. per dl. of blood and the patient is not actively bleeding, the hemoglobin content of the blood should increase 2 gm. per dl. or more during the first three weeks of therapy. A hypochromic microcytic anemia is the only anemia that responds to iron and the only anemia for which iron is indicated. With the possible exception of acute hemorrhagic anemia, all other anemias are associated with normal or increased iron stores, and long term therapy given inappropriately could result in tissue hemosiderosis and organ dysfunction.

The drug of choice is an inorganic bivalent salt given by mouth. In adults ferrous sulfate, 0.3 gm. three times daily after meals, is the standard with which all other iron preparations should be compared; it is completely effective, ordinarily well tolerated, and least expensive, with one of the widest margins of safety of any potent medicinal. The hydrated salt (20 per cent elemental iron) is available in 300 mg. tablets; three such tablets provide 180 mg. of iron, which is the optimal daily dosage. An iron deficient person treated according to this schedule assimilates 20 to 60 mg. of elemental iron a day. Larger amounts of iron offer no advantage; the rate of response is determined by the capacity of the marrow, and the foregoing dose provides more than enough to support maximal erythropoietic activity.

Because absorption of iron is less efficient about four hours after a single large dose, ferrous sulfate should be given in divided doses (i.e., one tablet three times daily). Ferrous sulfate tablets are coated to prevent oxidation; however, there is no place for the use of enteric coated or prolonged released preparations, because most of the iron would not be available for absorption until it had passed by the optimal absorptive sites (i.e., the duodenum and proximal jejunum). Liquid preparations are available for use in certain patients in whom tablets may not dissolve before they have gone beyond the upper small intestine (e.g., patients with a gastroenterostomy).

Despite the many advantages of ferrous sulfate, there exists a plethora of proprietary iron compounds, each with a dubious claim to greater effectiveness or better toleration. Since ferrous sulfate is completely effective, the former claim lacks meaning. As to poor patient tolerance, the belief that ferrous sulfate frequently produces unacceptable gastrointestinal side effects appears to be largely unfounded. Only 5 to 10 per cent of persons receiving ferrous sulfate in divided doses after meals manifest such effects (e.g., anorexia, nausea, and constipation or diarrhea), and it is noteworthy that in most such patients, similar complaints persist even though iron is given in some other form. Should another preparation be needed, the best one to select is a simple one (e.g., ferrous gluconate [11.6 per cent elemental iron] or ferrous fumarate [33 per cent elemental iron]). Any increase in absorption that might follow the addition of such substances as ascorbic acid and succinic acid is inconsequential and does not warrant the increased cost of such supplementation.

As with other di- and trivalent cations, orally administered iron products interact with concurrently administered oral doses of tetracyclines to decrease the absorption of the antibiotic. Antacids administered concomitantly with iron compounds result in decreased absorption of iron. Both these interactions can be minimized or prevented by separating ingestion of each by at least two hours.

The response to iron replacement is prompt and orderly. The reticulocyte count begins to increase two to four days after treatment is begun; the height of the reticulocyte response varies inversely with the level of the pretreatment erythroid values and may reach values as high as 20 per cent in severely anemic patients. As the reticulocytosis subsides, the hemoglobin level increases at a rate of about 0.2 gm. per dl. of blood per day, and normal erythroid values are restored within four to eight weeks. If the cause of the negative iron balance cannot be corrected, treatment with inorganic iron should be continued indefinitely. Even if the cause can be eliminated (e.g., surgical removal of a bleeding lesion), treatment should be continued for six to 12 months because all data indicate that the storage compartment is repleted slowly.

Most patients can and should be treated with oral doses of iron. Effective parenteral preparations are available (e.g., iron-dextran [Imferon]). However, there exist very real objections to their use. These objections include adverse reactions such as discoloration of skin, pain at the injection site, and anaphylactoid reactions; even death has been attributable in a few instances to parenteral iron administration. Epinephrine should be immediately available in the event of an acute hypersensitivity reaction. Other adverse effects from parenteral administration of iron-dextran include dyspnea, urticaria, arthralgia, myalgia, febrile episodes, sterile abscesses at the intramuscular injection site, hypotensive episodes, paresthesias, headache, and rash. In addition, parenterally administered iron may be recoverable from storage sites with difficulty.

Patient or physician convenience is not a valid reason to give iron by injection. Appropriate indications include a lack of response to orally administered pharmacologic doses in persons with unequivocal iron deficiency, a need for rapid repletion of iron stores, and clear-cut gastrointestinal intolerance. Psychogenic intolerance to oral doses of iron is very rarely, if ever, an indication to give iron parenterally; even patients with gastrointestinal disease (e.g., peptic ulcer) generally tolerate oral doses of iron, but a few may be better treated with parenteral doses. Formulas are available to determine the dosage of iron-dextran; initial dosages should be small and gradually increased as tolerated.

One formula frequently utilized to determine the dosage of iron-dextran necessary to restore hemoglobin and body stores of iron is the following:

$$0.3 \times \text{body weight (lb.)} \times \left(100 - \frac{\text{patient's hemoglobin in gm. per 100 ml} \times 100}{14.8}\right) = \text{mg. iron}$$

MEGALOBLASTIC ANEMIAS

A megaloblastic anemia is the hematologic manifestation of impaired proliferation of blood cell precursors; when fully developed, such anemias are characterized by normochromia, oval macrocytes, leukopenia with large hypersegmented neutrophils, thrombocytopenia with giant platelets, and distinctive bone marrow morphology. The mitotic defect, which reflects impaired DNA synthesis, also affects other proliferating cellular systems (e.g., the gastrointestinal mucosa). Over 95 per cent of the megaloblastic anemias are caused by a deficiency of vitamin B_{12} or folates. The metabolic functions of these coenzymes are related, but they do differ (e.g., vitamin B_{12} is needed to maintain nerve tissue integrity, a role not shared by folates). However, the hematologic pictures caused by deficiencies of vitamin B_{12} and folates are identical, and the precise etiology of a megaloblastic anemia cannot be established on the basis of hematologic criteria alone.

Vitamin B_{12}

Cyanocobalamin was isolated from liver in 1948. Vitamin B_{12} is synthesized only by certain bacteria and other micro-organisms, and all other living things depend on these sources for their supply of this essential substance. The primary natural producers of vitamin B_{12} are rumen bacteria; such vitamin B_{12} is absorbed by the host and stored in liver, muscle, and other tissues. Thus, man's major sources of vitamin B_{12} are foodstuffs of animal origin (e.g., meat, fish, milk, cheese, and eggs); vegetables and other plant products are not sources of vitamin B_{12}. The average diet in the United States provides about 5 to 30 μg. of vitamin B_{12} per day; about 1 to 5 μg. are absorbed. Normal body stores are about 2 to 5 mg., and daily attrition is about 0.1 to 0.2 per cent of body stores, or about 1 to 5 μg. in a normal adult. Daily attrition decreases as body stores are depleted, and clinical manifestations of vitamin B_{12} deficiency do not occur until body stores are reduced to 5 to 10 per cent of normal. Therefore, daily assimilation from dietary sources of 1 μg. or less will maintain a positive balance. The average diet is quite adequate to meet all needs, provided the absorptive mechanism is intact.

Absorption of dietary vitamin B_{12} is complex; it takes place in the distal ileum and requires the presence of a glycoprotein, intrinsic factor, which is elaborated independently of acid or pepsin by the parietal cells in the fundus of the stomach. During the first phase of absorption, a molecule of intrinsic factor binds tightly to two molecules of vitamin B_{12}. The second step involves the adherence of the intrinsic factor–vitamin B_{12} complex to the mucosal cells of the distal ileum. The manner by which vitamin B_{12} traverses the ileal mucosa is poorly understood. Massive or suprapharmacologic amounts of vitamin B_{12} (e.g., 500 to 1000 μg.) are absorbed by simple diffusion in the upper small intestine. Intrinsic factor does not participate in this absorptive mechanism, which is inefficient and not physiologically operative; however, it does possess pharmacologic significance.

After vitamin B_{12}, unattached to intrinsic factor, enters the circulation, it is bound to one of a group of proteins termed transcobalamins and transported to storage sites, mainly the liver, where it has a biologic half-life of about one year. Serum vitamin B_{12} levels can be quantified by microbiologic techniques or by radioimmunoassay; the latter is preferred, and normal values are about 200 to 800 ng. per 1. There is some evidence that serum vitamin B_{12} levels are below the usual lower limits of normal in a significant proportion of elderly persons, even though such individuals are not anemic and vitamin B_{12} absorption appears to be normal.

Folates

Folic acid (pteroylglutamic acid) is a synthetic substance made up of a pteridine grouping linked by p-aminobenzoic acid to a single glutamic acid residue. The term is also used by some to designate a group of naturally occurring conjugated polyglutamates; all substances with folic acid-like activity most appropriately are termed "folates." Folic acid was isolated from spinach in 1941 and synthesized in 1945. Natural folates contain one to 10 additional glutamic acid residues attached to the single glutamic acid of the folic acid molecule.

Folates, which are widely distributed in nature, are most abundant in fresh green vegetables, liver, kidney, yeast, beans, nuts, grains, and certain fresh fruits, and these foodstuffs are man's source of folates. Although normal, well balanced diets contain abundant folates (e.g., the daily diet in the United States contains 800 to 1000 μg.), the amount assimilated varies greatly, for cooking and processing procedures may inactivate more than 90 per cent of dietary folates. It should also be noted that persons not consuming "average" or "normal" diets are more apt to avoid foods containing folates than those that are good sources of vitamin B_{12}.

The normal adult folate stores are approximately 6000 to 8000 μg., with the largest amounts in the liver. Daily attrition (the folate contents of bile and urine are relatively high) is about 50 to 100 μg. Because of the variability in usable dietary folates, the daily diet should contain at least 400 μg. in order to prevent negative folate balance. Physiologic amounts of folic acid are absorbed in the upper jejunum, and pharmacologic doses are absorbed along the entire small intestine. About 80 per cent of a physiologic quantity of folic acid is absorbed. Dietary polyglutamates are not absorbed so completely or efficiently (e.g., only 50 per cent of orally administered heptaglutamates are absorbed). Although certain aspects of folate absorption remain unclear (i.e., an energy dependent mechanism versus passive diffusion), a substance such as intrinsic factor is not involved.

Following absorption, folates disappear rapidly from the blood. In contrast to the inability of plasma to retain folates, most other tissues and body fluids display a great avidity for binding folates. Nonetheless, serum folate levels are measurable, and such determinations are of diagnostic significance. Both microbiologic and isotope dilution assays are available; normal values are about 6 to 20 μg. per l. of serum. Less than normal values have been noted in a small number of nonanemic elderly persons; however, similar findings have been described in young persons, and the significance of these observations is conjectural.

Following absorption, monoglutamates are reduced first to dihydrofolate and then to tetrahydrofolate (both steps are catalyzed by the same enzyme, dihydrofolate reductase). Tetrahydrofolate is methylated in the liver to N^5-methyltetrahydrofolate; most of the folate in the body is in this form, and the other folate coenzymes are derived therefrom. Tetrahydrofolate acts as an acceptor-donor of one-carbon units in a variety of reactions involving movement of such units from one site or compound to another. The metabolic systems in mammalian cells known to require folate coenzymes include pyrimidine, purine, and methionine synthesis and histidine catabolism. The major manifestations of folate deficiency are attributable to the essential role of N^5-,N^{10}-methylenetetrahydrofolate in thymidylate biosynthesis, thereby affecting DNA anabolism and cellular proliferation.

Pathophysiology

The major clinical manifestations of vitamin B_{12} deficiency are due to imperfect mitosis and neurologic disease. In all probability the former is due to defective DNA synthesis involving the joint role of vitamin B_{12} and the folate coenzymes in methionine biosynthesis. This hypothesis, which has been designated the "methyltetrahydrofolate trap," is based on the presumption that vitamin B_{12} deficiency would reduce the availability of tetrahydrofolates and especially N^5-, N^{10}-methylenetetrahydrofolate by restricting the conversion of N_5-methyltetrahydrofolate to tetrahydrofolate. According to this scheme, vitamin B_{12} deficiency would then impair folate coenzyme-dependent reactions such as thymidylate synthesis and would produce the same effect on cellular proliferation as does folate deficiency. The identical hematologic pictures of vitamin B_{12} and folate deficiency attest to the correctness of this hypothesis.

Vitamin B_{12} deficiency affects all dividing cells, but abnormalities are most prominent in those cell systems with the fastest rates of growth (e.g., the marrow and the gastrointestinal mucosa). Hematologic aberrations dominate and are characterized by pancytopenia and the symptoms and physical findings attributable thereto together with a hypercellular marrow displaying megaloblastic abnormalities. The products of a megaloblastic marrow are also abnormal, and a megaloblastic anemia is first suspected on the basis of findings in the stained peripheral blood smear. Changes in other proliferating cellular systems also contribute to the clinical picture of vitamin B_{12} deficiency (e.g., the smooth or sore, uncoated tongue and gastrointestinal symptoms).

The precise pathogenesis of the neurologic manifestations of vitamin B_{12} deficiency are unknown, but they most likely reflect defective propionate metabolism. This feature of vitamin B_{12} deficiency has often been termed "subacute combined degeneration of the cord," but "vitamin B_{12} neuropathy" is more appropriate, for the brain and peripheral nerves are also involved. Both the posterior or dorsal columns of the cord (ascending fibers) and the lateral columns or pyramidal tracts (descending fibers) are involved; defects of the former are responsible for such symptoms and findings as weakness, numbness and tingling of the feet and hands, decreased vibratory sense, impaired position sense, and hyporeflexia. Lesions affecting the lateral columns cause hyperreflexia, positive Babinski signs, and muscle spasticity; impaired superficial sensation and hyperesthesias may be due to peripheral nerve changes. Consequently, the clinical picture of vitamin B_{12} neuropathy is mixed and quite variable.

Cerebral involvement is much less common than spinal cord or peripheral nerve lesions. Psychiatric symptoms have been attributed to vitamin B_{12} deficiency (especially in elderly populations) and have been given the euphonious designation of "megaloblastic madness." However, such occurrences are rare and appear to be features mainly of marked, long standing deficiencies, for the psychiatric status has not been shown to be affected by vitamin B_{12} in patients without a megaloblastic anemia or evidence of vitamin B_{12} neuropathy.

The major clinical manifestations of folate deficiency are due to defective pyrimidine synthesis and altered cellular proliferation; they are identical to those already described for vitamin B_{12} deficiency. However, there is a major difference, for folates have not been shown to be required to maintain the functional integrity of nerve tissue. Despite scattered reports of neuropathy and psychiatric symptoms attributable to folate deficiency, proof of such causal relationships has not been provided, and such manifestations most likely reflect the inadequacies of other vitamins that commonly accompany folate deficiency.

Diagnosis

The causes of the megaloblastic macrocytic anemias are listed in Table 9–4; over 95 per cent are due to vitamin B_{12} or folate deficiency. Classification of the megaloblastic anemias in the past has been confusing, because it was once thought that a response to replacement with either vitamin B_{12} or folic acid established that substance as the cause of the anemia. This assumption is no longer tenable, for pharmacologic amounts of either substance are capable of evoking a hematologic response in a person who is deficient in the other.

Although a megaloblastic anemia is often suggested by the complaints or physical findings (e.g., the symptoms of anemia and the smooth uncoated tongue), the diagnosis is based on the characteristic findings in the peripheral blood and the demonstration of a megaloblastic marrow. Because the hematologic findings in vitamin B_{12} and folate deficiency are indistinguishable, it now becomes necessary to identify the exact cause of the megaloblastic anemia. There may exist important clinical clues such as evidence of neuropathy, which points strongly to vitamin B_{12} deficiency, and dietary inadequacies, which suggest folate deficiency.

Because of the nature of foods containing the largest quantities of vitamin B_{12}, the small daily requirements, and the generous body stores, nutritional vitamin B_{12} deficiency is almost nonexistent; on the other hand, folate deficiency consequent to nutritional inadequacies is achievable within a few weeks and is quite common. However, a precise distinction between vitamin B_{12} and folate deficiency can

TABLE 9–4. Causes of Megaloblastic Macrocytic Anemia*

I. Deficiency of vitamin B_{12} or folates	
A. Decreased intake	
1. Nutritional deficiency	Folates
	Vitamin B_{12}
B. Impaired absorption	
1. Pernicious anemia	Vitamin B_{12}
2. Gastrectomy	Vitamin B_{12}
3. Severe gastric disease	Vitamin B_{12}
4. Small bowel resection	Vitamin B_{12}
5. Intestinal blind loops, diverticula, or strictures	Vitamin B_{12}
6. *Diphyllobothrium latum* infestation	Vitamin B_{12}
7. Malabsorption syndromes (e.g., sprue, drugs)	Folates
	Vitamin B_{12}
C. Increased requirements	Folates
1. Pregnancy	
2. Hemolytic anemias	
3. Malignant tumors	
4. Hyperthyroidism	
5. Skin diseases	
II. Impaired utilization	Folates
A. Folic acid antagonists	
B. Anticonvulsant drugs	
C. Liver disease	
D. Ascorbic acid deficiency (?)	
III. Miscellaneous causes	
A. Cytotoxic therapy (e.g., alkylating drugs, ionizing radiation, antipurines, antipyrimidines)	
B. Congenital orotic aciduria	
C. Formiminotransferase deficiency	
D. Nonlymphocytic leukemia and the preleukemic syndrome ("megaloblastoid" marrow)	

*From Linman, J.W.: Hematology. New York, Macmillan Publishing Co., Inc., 1975. (Copy © 1975 by James W. Linman. Reprinted by permission of Macmillan Publishing Co., Inc.)

be made only by measuring serum levels or by determining responses to replacement with physiologic doses.

In view of the current widespread availability of accurate serum vitamin B_{12} and folate measurements, these tests are mandatory in the workup of all patients with a megaloblastic anemia. In addition to their vital role in differentiating between vitamin B_{12} and folate deficiency, serum vitamin B_{12} and folate levels have assumed additional importance as a means for separating the treatable megaloblastic anemias from the refractory anemia that characterizes the preleukemic syndrome (or hemopoietic dysplasia). It has become clear over the past few years that the morphologic features of the latter panmyelopathy resemble closely the peripheral blood and marrow findings of vitamin B_{12} and folate deficiency; it has also become increasingly evident that the preleukemic syndrome is a relatively common cause of anemia in the elderly.

After the etiology of a megaloblastic anemia has been established (i.e., vitamin B_{12} or folate deficiency), it then becomes necessary to determine the cause of the deficiency. Knowledge of the disorders associated with these deficiency states (Table 9–4) is ordinarily adequate to indicate what other clinical or laboratory data may be needed (e.g., assessment of vitamin B_{12} absorption with a Schilling test, a gastric analysis, and tests for a malabsorption syndrome). The commonest cause of vitamin B_{12} deficiency is pernicious anemia, and most folate deficiency anemias reflect, at least in part, nutritional inadequacies.

Treatment

The treatment of a megaloblastic anemia due to vitamin B_{12} or folate deficiency is simple and straightforward (i.e., replacement therapy with the deficient substance). However, in the absence of unequivocal evidence of the exact cause, the following facts assume vital importance.

Only patients with vitamin B_{12} deficiency manifest hematologic responses to physiologic amounts of vitamin B_{12} (i.e., 1 μg. or less per day), and only patients with folate deficiency respond to physiologic amounts of folic acid (i.e., 100 μg. or less per day). On the other hand, patients with vitamin B_{12} deficiency exhibit hematologic responses to pharmacologic dosages of folic acid (i.e., 1000 or more μg. per day), and patients with folate deficiency respond to the doses of vitamin B_{12} used to treat vitamin B_{12} deficiency (i.e., injections of 100 to 1000 μg.).

The explanation for these phenomena appears to involve the biochemical reaction in which the folate and cobamide coenzymes act jointly (i.e., methionine synthesis). Large amounts of the coenzyme that is present in normal quantities apparently divert the limited quantities of the deficient coenzyme into the metabolic activity in which both coenzymes participate. In the case of vitamin B_{12} deficiency, pharmacologic doses of folic acid correct the block in cellular division, and hematologic normalcy is restored; however, the resultant hematologic response is costly, for other metabolic functions requiring vitamin B_{12} suffer (e.g., propionate catabolism), and neurologic damage may progress (sometimes with great speed) despite hematologic improvement. Such occurrences are unacceptable, for the neurologic manifestations of vitamin B_{12} deficiency may not be completely reversible. If pharmacologic doses of folic acid are continued, hematologic relapse will eventually recur once the limited supplies of vitamin B_{12} are exhausted. Large doses of vitamin B_{12} will evoke at least partial hematologic responses in folate deficient patients; however, no significant adverse effects comparable to the progressive neuropathy in vitamin B_{12} deficient persons given large doses of folic acid has been noted. If replacement therapy cannot be delayed until the type of deficiency is known with certainty, patients with a megaloblastic anemia should be treated temporarily with both vitamin B_{12} and folic acid.

Vitamin B_{12} Deficiency. All instances of vitamin B_{12} deficiency reflect absorptive problems with the exception of nutritional inadequacies (see Table 9–4). Consequently, oral doses of vitamin B_{12} are effective only in the treatment of a megaloblastic anemia secondary to nutritional deficiency of vitamin B_{12}; all other deficient states require parenteral therapy. Nutritional vitamin B_{12} deficiency is a rare happening, and even in such cases, parenteral therapy is preferable in order to more rapidly and completely replenish vitamin B_{12} stores.

Vitamin B_{12} deficient patients respond to very small amounts of vitamin B_{12} (e.g., 1 μg. a day or less). Because vitamin B_{12} is nontoxic, inexpensive, and readily available, it is wise to overtreat in order to replenish body stores and prevent progressive or recurrent neurologic damage. When pharmacologic doses of vitamin B_{12} are administered parenterally, a relatively large proportion is excreted in the urine. Despite this loss, supraphysiologic doses are justified because the body gain is significantly greater.

The following regimen is appropriate: 100 μg. intramuscularly daily during the first week, 100 μg. twice weekly until hematologic values have returned to normal, and 100 μg. monthly thereafter. Depending on the cause of the vitamin B_{12} deficiency, replacement therapy may be required for the lifetime of the patient (e.g., pernicious anemia and following total gastrectomy); less often, treatment of the primary lesion may effect a permanent cure, and replacement therapy can be stopped (e.g., a small intestinal diverticulum or blind loop that can be surgically removed).

Equivalent amounts of cyanocobalamin and hydroxycobalamin evoke comparable clinical responses. Although larger amounts of hydroxycobalamin appear to be retained and higher serum vitamin B_{12} levels have been attributed to this cobalamin, it is not clear that the patient gains by such minor differences. Therefore, one vitamin B_{12} preparation cannot be recommended at the exclusion of the other.

The response to replacement therapy is prompt and most gratifying. Within a few hours after treatment is begun, the serum vitamin B_{12} level rises, the serum iron level falls, and reversion to a normoblastic morphology in the marrow begins. Mitotable megaloblastic precursors may undergo mitosis, yielding two normal cells of comparable maturity, but cells that have already matured to a postmitotable stage retain their megaloblastic features. Within two to five days, marrow morphology reverts to normal.

Reticulocytes begin to appear in the peripheral blood within 24 to 48 hours, and the maximal response, which varies inversely with the level of the pretreatment erythroid values, is reached in seven to 10 days. The reticulocyte response subsides during the second and third weeks, and the erythroid values increase rapidly. Barring some other hematologic abnormality, blood cell counts become normal in four to six weeks.

Rapid clinical improvement accompanies the hematologic response. Symptoms subside, and all physical and laboratory abnormalities disappear with the exception of the atrophic gastritis and achlorhydria in patients with pernicious anemia; the latter findings are permanent, as is the defect in intrinsic factor elaboration and vitamin B_{12} absorption (e.g., the Schilling test result is always abnormal in a patient with pernicious anemia irrespective of the presence or absence of anemia or other hematologic abnormalities).

It should also be noted that the manifestations of vitamin B_{12} neuropathy may fail to resolve completely. Patients who do not respond in this manner require study to identify an incorrect diagnosis or some other abnormality that is preventing a complete response.

Vitamin B_{12} is relatively nontoxic. However, hypokalemia has occurred in some patients following the institution of replacement therapy (presumably consequent to a shift of potassium intracellularly), and sudden death has been attributed to this phenomenon. Although death may have been due to other causes, physicians should be aware of possible problems, and potassium levels should be monitored before and during the early phases of treatment. Other adverse effects possibly attributable to vitamin B_{12} injections include pruritus, transitory exanthema, and anaphylaxis.

There is no justification for the use of any other vitamin B_{12} preparation (e.g., hydroxycobalamin) or route of administration other than the intramuscular route. Many oral treatment programs have been evaluated (e.g., vitamin B_{12}–intrinsic factor combinations), but none can be recommended because of less than optimal control, the development of refractoriness with relapse, and the likelihood that asymptomatic patients may neglect to take oral doses of medications. Liver extract should no longer be used (it was effective because of the vitamin B_{12} contained therein), and there is no good support for the contention that a cobamide coenzyme (e.g., methylcobalamin) is superior to cyanocobalamin or hydroxycobalamin.

No other treatment is indicated unless some complication exists (e.g., iron should be given only if there is associated iron deficiency). Because of the prompt response to replacement therapy, red cell transfusions are rarely needed and should be avoided for all but a few exceptional cases (e.g., profound anemia in the face of heart failure or myocardial ischemia). Although folic acid is innocuous when given together with vitamin B_{12}, there is no reason to give it unless there is a combined deficiency of both vitamin B_{12} and folates. Depending on the cause of the vitamin B_{12} deficiency, treatment of the basic disease is, of course, needed (e.g., *Diphyllobothrium latum* infestation).

Folate Deficiency. Although parenteral forms of folic acid are available, there are few indications for their use. Folate deficient persons respond to very small oral dosages of folic acid (e.g., 0.1 mg. per day). Larger amounts are virtually nontoxic, and oral dosages of 1.0 mg. per day, which are more than ample even in patients with malabsorption syndromes, are ordinarily used. Although dosages of 5.0 mg. per day or more have been used, there is little, if any, justification for their use.

The response to treatment is identical to that described for vitamin B_{12} deficiency. The duration of therapy is contingent on the etiology. Thus, treatment for two to four weeks is adequate for nutritional deficiency provided the dietary inadequacy is corrected, whereas treatment for several months may be needed in patients with celiac sprue. When folate deficiency is secondary to the administration of a drug (e.g., cycloserine, phenytoin, glutethimide, isoniazid, nitrofurantoin, orally administered contraceptives, phenobarbital, primidone, triamterine and trimethoprim), treatment with the drug can be continued as long as oral doses of folic acid are also given.

Other Megaloblastic or Megaloblastoid Anemias. Normochromic macrocytic anemias not due to vitamin B_{12} or folate deficiency do not respond to treatment with vitamin B_{12} or folic acid (see Table 9–4). Anemia is rarely the major clinical problem, and treatment should be directed to the primary disease (e.g., nonlymphocytic leukemia). It should be noted that a folate coenzyme (N^5-formyltetrahydrofolate; folinic acid or the citrovorum factor) is effective in counteracting toxicity attributable to a folate antagonist such as methotrexate.

APLASTIC ANEMIA

An aplastic (or hypoplastic) anemia is the clinical syndrome resulting from bone marrow failure; it may be idiopathic, congenital, or secondary to a variety of marrow toxins such as drugs, chemicals, ionizing radiation, certain infectious agents, and immune mechanisms. It is characterized by quantitatively inadequate (but qualitatively normal) marrow activity with too few mature cells in the peripheral blood and marrow hypocellularity without atypical precursor cells, maturation defects, or evidence of space occupying lesions. It should be noted that this definition demands anatomic hypoplasia and sets the disorder apart from peripheral blood cytopenias due to functional failure (e.g., the megaloblastic anemias). Ordinarily all marrow elements are affected with a resultant pancytopenia. Although much less common, erythrocytic aplasia occurs singly, and rare instances of isolated granulocytic and megakaryocytic hypoplasia have been observed. The discussion to follow is restricted to the acquired aplastic anemias, for the congenital forms do not produce problems compatible with survival to old age (i.e., the patient experiences either a remission or premature death).

About half the patients with an acquired aplastic anemia deny contact with any injurious substance, and no reason for the marrow failure can be found; these cases must be classified as primary or idiopathic. Such cases are ordinarily attributed to an unknown injury(ies) to the hematopoietic stem cell, but a defect(s) in the microenvironment has also been suggested as a possible pathogenic mechanism. Recent observations in a few patients indicate that aplasia may sometimes reflect cellular or humoral immune mechanisms directed against the marrow stem cell or its progeny.

In the remaining patients it is possible to incriminate some chemical or physical agent or some other disorder such as a viral infection. Marrow toxins can be divided into two groups. The first includes those agents that consistently produce marrow hypoplasia in man, provided the exposure is adequate (i.e., dose dependent mitotic poisons); examples of such toxins include ionizing radiation, alkylating drugs (e.g., cyclophosphamide and chlorambucil), antimetabolites (e.g., methotrexate and azathioprine), and a number of miscellaneous compounds (e.g., benzene). The degree of marrow hypoplasia varies directly with the dose, and the more severe the hypoplasia, the greater the chance that the marrow failure will be irreversible.

The second group of agents that has been implicated in the pathogenesis of acquired aplastic anemia is heterogeneous and large. Only rare individuals develop marrow aplasia on exposure, and these idiosyncratic reactions show no consistent relationship between dose or length of exposure and the development of aplastic anemia. The manner in which marrow hypoplasia is produced is unknown, and studies have been seriously limited by the lack of a suitable animal model. Drugs and chemicals that have been associated with marrow aplasia include antimicrobials (e.g., chloramphenicol), antimalarials (e.g., quinacrine), antihistaminics, antithyroid drugs, anticonvulsants, tranquilizers, insecticides, heavy metals (e.g., gold), industrial solvents, analgesics, orally administered hypoglycemic drugs, and diuretics. In most instances only a few cases have been reported in which there exists strong support for a causal relationship. Exposure to several rather than one drug is the rule not the exception, and proof of a cause and effect relationship (i.e., recovery with recurrent marrow aplasia on re-exposure) is precluded by the high mortality rate of aplastic anemia and the lack of effective therapy. One drug, chloramphenicol, deserves special consideration, for it has been implicated more often than any other drug in the causation of aplastic anemia (it has been estimated that 1 in 20,000 to 30,000 persons given chloramphenicol will develop aplastic anemia).

The infectious process that has been associated most often with aplastic anemia is viral hepatitis. Although such cases are rare, it is difficult to deny a causal relationship. The mechanism responsible for marrow failure is unclear, but it most likely reflects direct injury to the marrow stem cell by the hepatitis virus.

The clinical manifestations of aplastic anemia are directly attributable to marrow failure and the resultant pancytopenia. Thus, the symptoms and physical findings are those of anemia (e.g., weakness, exertional tachycardia, and pallor), neutropenia (e.g., superimposed infections), and thrombocytopenia (e.g., epistaxis and dermal hemorrhage). Such findings as splenomegaly and adenopathy suggest some explanation for pancytopenia other than anatomic marrow aplasia. Peripheral blood findings include a normochromic normocytic anemia without significant anisocytosis, poikilocytosis or nucleated red cells, leukopenia without immature cells, thrombocytopenia, and reticulocytopenia. The demonstration of a hypocellular marrow with increased fat confirms the diagnosis. Marrow cells display normal morphology without discernible abnormalities in maturation; there is ordinarily a relative increase in lymphocytes and plasma cells, and mast cells are sometimes increased in number.

Treatment

The management of patients with aplastic anemia is a most difficult task, and the outlook is bleak, for the mortality rate in adults is about 75 per cent. Although data for different age groups are not available, it is reasonable to presume that older patients fare less well than younger ones; certainly the prognosis in children is much better than in adults.

Recent studies have shown clearly that the treatment of choice for severe aplastic anemia is a bone marrow transplant from a compatible donor. Many problems remain to be solved (e.g., graft versus host reactions), and older patients present special problems (e.g., unavailability of suitable donors and the presence of associated disorders that may make the rigorous side effects of marrow transplantation less tolerable). Nonetheless, all patients with severe marrow aplasia and an HLA matched sibling should be considered for bone marrow transplantation and referred to an appropriate center. Transplantation should take place early before the patient has been sensitized by transfusions, thereby increasing the likelihood of graft rejection.

For patients who are not candidates for a marrow transplant, the primary goal of treatment is to support the patient, hoping for a spontaneous remission; a remission may occur within a short time or may not be evident for months or even years. Such support includes removing the patient from exposure to any possible causative agent, red cell transfusions as needed to maintain a satisfactory circulating hemoglobin level, and appropriate antibiotics for intercurrent infections. The indications for platelet or granulocyte transfusions are not straightforward because of the chronicity of the disorder and the fact that consequent to antibody formation, the effectiveness of such transfusions varies inversely with the number of transfusions the patient has received. Each case must be considered separately, and thrombocytopenia or neutropenia alone (i.e., low counts without significant bleeding or superimposed infections) is not an adequate reason to administer platelets or granulocytes.

No form of treatment (with the exception of marrow transplantation) will reverse marrow aplasia or impart a primary stimulus to hematopoiesis. However, the list of substances or techniques with which success has been claimed is lengthy and includes, among others, corticosteroids, androgens, cytotoxic drugs, plasmapheresis, yellow bone marrow, splenectomy, phytohemagglutinin, cobalt, spleen extracts, iron, and vitamin B_{12}. Only the first four deserve further discussion, for there is no reasonable evidence that the others are effective; instead, patients in whom success has been claimed appear to reflect spontaneous remissions or misdiagnoses. As noted, iron and vitamin B_{12} affect erythropoiesis only in deficient subjects, and they play no role in other situations. In fact, iron stores in patients with aplastic anemia are apt to be increased consequent to increased assimilation of dietary iron, transfusions, or prior inappropriate therapy; under these circumstances treatment with iron is contraindicated.

Corticosteroids. The corticosteroids appear to be effective in some children with aplastic anemia (both congenital and acquired forms) and in some adults with acquired erythrocytic aplasia. However, the evidence that they work in adults with acquired aplastic anemia is scant, and in most patients the adverse effects of the corticosteroids outweigh any discernible gain. Despite the lack of response in most, a few patients do appear to improve, and a trial is indicated in most cases. This trial should be limited (i.e., two to four weeks) and carried out with adequate dosages (in an average size adult, 60 to 80 mg. per day of prednisone or its equivalent). If the patient does not respond, the dosage should be tapered rapidly and the corticosteroids discontinued. If a response ensues, the dosage should be decreased to the smallest amount capable of maintaining adequate marrow activity (it is to be hoped that the hormone can be discontinued). If a responsive patient is shown to be steroid dependent, it will become necessary to decide whether the benefit warrants the risks of the side effects of long term corticosteroid therapy; such a decision requires advice from an experienced clinician. As noted, the undesirable effects of corticosteroids are magnified in older patients.

Androgens. Androgens affect erythropoiesis, and they have been used widely in the treatment of a variety of anemias. Unfortunately their popularity as erythropoietic stimulants far exceeds any benefits attributable to them. The mechanisms by which androgens stimulate erythropoiesis are unclear; some data support an effect on erythropoietin elaboration, and other observations indicate that the marrow stem cells may also be stimulated. In regard to the former, it is noteworthy that plasma and urine erythropoietin titers are increased in patients with aplastic anemia; it is unlikely that any additional increase consequent to androgen therapy would benefit the patient.

Androgens have been recommended in the past in aplastic anemia. However, reports claiming responses have been outnumbered by others that have failed to support a beneficial effect. Aplastic anemia is rare, and most studies have involved small numbers of patients; the tendency for the disease to undergo spontaneous remission has also contributed to difficulties in resolving this issue. More importantly, a recent multi-institutional study involving an adequate number of patients failed to demonstrate any value of androgens in the treatment of aplastic anemia, and they can no longer be recommended for all patients. In selected cases a trial may be justified; oxymetholone (3 to 5 mg. per kg. orally per day) and nandrolone decanoate (3 to 5 mg. per kg. intramuscularly per week) are the preferred forms, and treatment should be continued for three to four months. In deciding to use androgens, their unwanted effects must be weighed carefully against the anticipated benefit.

The androgens have great potential for producing adverse endocrinologic effects. In the mature male these include inhibition of testicular function, testicular atrophy, oligospermia, gynecomastia, epididymitis, and bladder irritability. Mature females may experience hirsutism, male pattern baldness, deepening of the voice, and enlargement of the clitoris. Other adverse effects common to both sexes may include acne, decreased libido, insomnia, chills, hypercalcemia (particularly in immobile patients and in patients with metastatic breast cancer), nausea, vomiting, and diarrhea.

Androgenic-anabolic steroids may interact with anticoagulants to produce an exaggerated anticoagulant effect. These steroids are contraindicated in patients with known or suspected prostatic carcinoma, in elderly patients in whom overstimulation is to be avoided, in hypercalcemia, and in the presence of significant cardiac, hepatic, or renal impairment.

Immunosuppression. A few patients undergoing immunosuppressive therapy prior to receiving a marrow transplant have been observed to develop remissions. On the basis of the assumption that marrow aplasia in such patients reflected an immune mechanism, trials with cytotoxic drugs (e.g., cyclophosphamide [Cytoxan]) and antithymocyte globulin have been carried out in a few patients. Plasmapheresis, a procedure that has been effective in a variety of immune mediated disorders, has also been reported to be effective. Further investigations along these lines are indicated and may provide information bearing on both the pathogenesis and treatment of aplastic anemia.

ACQUIRED ERYTHROCYTIC APLASIA (PURE RED CELL ANEMIA)

A normochromic normocytic anemia with normal leukocyte and platelet counts and erythrocytic aplasia in the marrow with active, orderly granulopoiesis and abundant megakaryocytes are the findings in this rare type of anemia. Thymomas are present in about half these patients, and thymectomy may be curative. Drugs (e.g., chloramphenicol and phenytoin [Dilantin]) appear to be responsible in a few cases, and occasionally erythrocytic aplasia may be a manifestation of the preleukemic syndrome. However, most such cases must be classified as idiopathic. There exists significant support that many of these cases reflect the presence of antibodies directed against nucleated red cells, and responses have followed treatment with corticosteroids or cytotoxic (i.e., immunosuppressive) drugs such as azathioprine (Imuran) and cyclophosphamide (Cytoxan).

OTHER ANEMIAS DUE TO IMPAIRED ERYTHROPOIESIS

Anemias consequent to defective erythropoiesis caused by other primary diseases are secondary manifestations (see Table 9–1). The treatment is that of the primary disease, and there exists no therapy for the anemia other than appropriate support (i.e., red cell transfusions). Drug therapy is not available, and the usual hematinic drugs (e.g., iron and vitamin B_{12}) are indicated only if a deficiency exists as a complicating factor.

The anemias of chronic disease deserve special comment, for they constitute a clinical problem of considerable magnitude, especially in the elderly. These anemias are secondary to renal insufficiency, chronic infections, liver disease, occult neoplasms, rheumatoid arthritis, and certain endocrinopathies (e.g., hypothyroidism). They are characterized by a normochromic normocytic anemia (mild hypochromia is sometimes present) without other hematologic abnormalities. Although the serum iron level may be decreased, iron stores are normal or increased (e.g., the serum iron binding capacity is decreased, serum ferritin levels are normal or increased, and there is abundant stainable iron in the marrow). Multiple factors appear to act together to cause the anemia; such mechanisms include abnormalities in the reutilization of iron derived from the catabolism of effete red cells, decreased erythropoietin production, and a decrease in red cell life span.

The diagnosis of these secondary anemias is contingent on nonhematologic data (e.g., evidence of renal dysfunction), and treatment is that of the primary disease (e.g., antibiotics for a chronic urinary tract infection). Anemia is rarely a limiting factor in the management of these patients, and they should not be subjected to the expense, discomfort, and possible harm that may accompany the administration of such "routine" antianemic drugs as vitamin B_{12} and iron. A number of other drugs have been recommended from time to time; none has been effective. Androgens are widely used, and in selected cases a trial may be warranted (e.g., oxymetholone, 3 to 5 mg. per kg. orally per day); however, the unwanted side effects of androgens usually dominate such treatment programs without significant change in the circulating hemoglobin level. If preparations of erythropoietin that can be given to man become available (none now exists), the secondary anemias are those that might be expected to respond. Among the other drugs with which success has been claimed is cobalt. In experimental situations the cobaltous ion does stimulate erythropoiesis, apparently by interfering with cellular oxygen utilization, producing histotoxic hypoxia and thereby stimulating erythropoietin formation. Because clinical responses attributable to cobalt have been inconstant, infrequent, and at best inconsequential, the potential toxicity of this metal precludes its use.

REFERENCES

1. Camitta, B.M., Storb, R., and Thomas, E.D.: Aplastic anemia: pathogenesis, diagnosis, treatment and prognosis. N. Engl. J. Med., 306:645–652, 712–718, 1982.
2. Fairbanks, V.F., Fahey, J.L., and Beutler, E.: Clinical Disorders of Iron Metbolism. Ed. 2. New York, Grune & Stratton, Inc., 1971.
3. Goodman, L.S., and Gilman, A. (Editors): The Pharmacological Basis of Therapeutics. Ed. 6. New York, Macmillan Publishing Co., Inc., 1980.
4. Harris, J.W., and Kellermeyer, R.W.: The Red Cell: Production, Metabolism, Destruction: Normal and Abnormal. Cambridge, Harvard University Press, 1970.
5. Linman, J.W.: Hematology. Physiologic, Pathophysiologic, and Clinical Principles. New York, Macmillan Publishing Co., Inc., 1975.
6. Williams, W.J., Beutler, E., Erslev, A.J., and Rundles, R.W. (Editors): Hematology. Ed. 2. New York, McGraw-Hill, Inc., 1977.
7. Wintrobe, M.M., et al.: Clinical Hematology. Ed. 8. Philadelphia, Lea & Febiger, 1981.

CHAPTER 10

ENDOCRINE DISORDERS

Irma H. Ullrich

OSTEOPOROSIS

Osteoporosis is a problem of great magnitude among the elderly and accounts for large expenditures in direct medical costs as well as indirect loss of productivity. It has been estimated that osteoporosis accounts for 70 per cent of the one million fractures that occur annually, at a cost of over $1 billion.[1]

Although osteoporosis occurs in a worldwide distribution, there are many regional differences. Some of these differences may reflect variations in racial constitution and length of average life span in the area. Six per cent of the world's population is over 65 and may be affected; this number increases to 10 per cent in North America and 14 per cent in Western Europe.[2] A lower rate has been noted in areas of high calcium intake, and vegetarians appear to be affected less frequently than omnivores.[2] Other dietary constituents may also be of importance, a high protein intake being associated with an increase in incidence.

Elderly women are most often affected by both asymptomatic and symptomatic osteoporosis. The early stages of osteoporosis are asymptomatic but may be detected by loss of height or radiologic changes of the spine. The patient may later experience spinal deformity, a chronic "backache," or more acute pain due to a fracture. The bones most often fractured are the vertebral bodies, femoral head and neck, and the distal radius.

Clinical Presentation

A compression fracture of the spine in an osteoporotic person usually follows minimal trauma, such as coughing or lifting a light object. The lower thoracic or upper lumbar vertebrae are the vertebral bodies involved most often, although any area of the spine may be affected.[3] Compression fractures usually wedge anteriorly and are stable fractures without nerve root compromise. The acute fracture is associated with severe pain in the immediate and surrounding area due to paravertebral muscle spasm, as well as pain that radiates to the abdominal or chest region. The pain usually responds to analgesics and bed rest but requires four to six weeks for complete resolution. Multiple fractures of the spine, either symptomatic or subclinical, eventually result in spinal deformity—the so-called "dowager's hump." The marked kyphosis may result in a protuberant abdomen and ribs that nearly rest on the pelvic brim. This deformity may cause the patient significant mental anguish as well as difficulty in finding attractive clothing to fit an altered frame.

Of more medical significance are fractures of the hip. Nearly 200,000 Americans sustain hip fractures annually. Over 75 per cent of these fractures are due to associated osteoporosis. Although these are well treated surgically with nails or prostheses, as many as one-sixth of all patients die of complications. Femurs may fracture with minimal trauma, or the trauma may occur during a fall from a standing height. It has been suggested that osteoporotic patients may fall more frequently than those not affected, and this may account for some of the increase in fractures seen in these patients.

In addition to vertebral and hip fractures, the forearm is another common site of fracture in postmenopausal women. The incidence of these fractures is much higher in elderly women than in men of similar ages. In younger individuals these rates are comparable between the sexes.

Not all compression vertebral or hip fractures are due to idiopathic osteoporosis. Other disorders that may present in a similar manner include multiple myeloma, lymphoma, leukemia, metastatic carcinoma, Paget's disease, and osteomalacia. Other less common disorders in which osteoporosis may be a complication include hyperthyroidism, Cushing's syndrome (iatrogenic or endogenous), and the adult form of osteogenesis imperfecta tarda. Primary hyperparathyroidism also reaches a peak incidence in middle aged persons, is more common in women, and may present with generalized osteoporosis; thus this should be included in the differential diagnosis as well. Obviously these disorders require considerably different diagnostic as well as therapeutic maneuvers. The low prevalence of some of the disorders means that a high index of suspicion is required to make a diagnosis.

Diagnosis

Because a decrease in bone mass appears to be a normal component of aging, it may be difficult to determine at which stage it becomes pathologic. A compression fracture of the spine or hip or a forearm fracture can be visualized easily by plain x-ray techniques and is presumptive evidence of pathologic bone changes. However, making a diagnosis prior to such a morbid event is obviously more desirable. A diffuse decrease in bone density (osteopenia) may be noted on plain radiologic films, but this decrease is apparent only when 30 per cent or more of the bone mass is lost and therefore is of little value in detecting early changes or in following regression or progression of the disorder. A more sensitive technique that would correlate with the "fracture threshold" would be advantageous.

The fracture threshold is that level of bone mass below which the bone no longer serves an adequate structural function. This stage of osteoporosis is advanced yet may be asymptomatic. The fracture threshold correlates with a bone mass more that 2 standard deviations below the mean in young women. By age 65, half of all women and all those over age 85 have a bone mineral density in the vertebrae below the threshold for fracture.[4]

Hip and vertebral fractures occur in bone that is predominantly trabecular, yet access to these areas for measurement of bone is difficult. The radius is more readily accessible. Although the midshaft contains primarily cortical bone, at a more distal location 25 per cent or more is trabecular bone. These two features, accessibility and trabecular bone content, have led to attempts to correlate bone mineral content of the distal radius with that in trabecular bone as measured by biopsy. Photon absorptiometry using ^{125}I or ^{241}Am as a measure of the mineral content of the radius correlates well with various measurements of iliac biopsy specimens.[5] These measurements are reproducible and may be repeated with little patient morbidity.

Other qualitative findings on plain films include a greater prominence of vertical than horizontal trabeculae, a relative prominence of the end plates compared to the central parts of the vertebral bodies, and expansion of the intervertebral disks to form "codfish" vertebrae. In the long bones there is widening of the marrow cavity and narrowing of the cortical portion, which results in a decrease in the cortex to marrow ratio (normally this is 1:1).

The value of computed tomography in determining bone mineral content has not yet been established, but this promises to be a useful modality. Evaluation of total bone mass using in vivo neutron activation analysis is useful as a research tool but requires sophisticated instrumentation. Occasionally the clinical presentation and radiographic findings are not typical and bone biopsy is required. In order to differentiate among the bone disorders, undecalcified sections must be studied by a person familiar with such specimens.

Etiology

Studies of bone turnover and metabolism are difficult because of regional differences in types of bone (trabecular versus cortical) as well as differences between sexes and ages of the subjects. Bone tissue is 50 to 55 per cent mineral and 30 to 35 per cent organic material (primarily collagen); the remaining 10 to 15 per cent is water. Changes in any of these compartments may be important. In order to study changes in bone metabolism, both bone accretion and resorption must be evaluated, because they are coupled in bone remodeling; minor changes in the rate of one or the other over many years may result in profound skeletal alterations.

Bone reaches a maximal mass at maturity in both sexes. Men lose an insignificant amount of bone until age 60 or more, with a gradual decline thereafter. In women there are differences in the decreases in bone in the axial and appendicular skeleton. There is little loss from the appendicular skeleton until after age 50. A gradual loss occurs from age 50 to 65, with a deceleration of the rate of loss thereafter. Bone loss from the axial skeleton occurs in young adulthood, with more rapid loss in the three to five years after menopause, followed by a return to a more gradual rate of loss. The loss of vertebral bone is nearly 50 per cent in women from age 20 to 80. Women also lose relatively more trabecular than cortical bone.[4]

Two causes of idiopathic osteoporosis have been proposed. One suggests that the loss of bone is a normal concomitant of aging. Those who reach maturity with a small bone mass are therefore at risk for the development of symptoms when the bone mass is below the fracture threshold. This model gains support from cross sectional studies of bone mineral content and would explain why small, thin women are at greater risk than large, obese women, or men, all of whom have a greater bone mass at maturity. The second theory proposes that the development of osteoporosis involves a pathologically increased rate of bone loss.

Other factors that have been implicated include deficient dietary intake or absorption of calcium. According to a National Health Survey, postmenopausal women typically consume less than 500 mg. of calcium daily. This may reflect a general decrease in food intake, perhaps in part due to a decrease in the acuity of the senses of taste and smell in the elderly. An increase in lactose intolerance that is not clinically recognized has been demonstrated in osteoporotic persons.[6] This may contribute to a decrease in the consumption of dairy products, which are the primary source of calcium in the diet. A normal diet that does not contain dairy products contains about 300 mg. of calcium per day. Furthermore, the consumption of processed foods that are high in phosphates, such as flour and macaroni, rice, and potatoes, may impair calcium absorption further as well as increase bone resorption. Postmenopausal women also have a decreased rate of intestinal calcium absorption, which is reversible with estrogens, suggesting at least a permissive role for these hormones.[7,8]

Groups who consume a diet high in meat (e.g., Eskimos) tend to have a lower bone mineral content than age matched white subjects. This mechanism has been postulated to involve buffering by bone of a systemic acidosis caused by ingested protein, especially the sulfur containing amino acids. The resulting mobilization of bone calcium is accompanied by an increase in urinary calcium excretion. This, however, is modified by the high phosphorus content of meat, which tends to decrease urinary calcium excretion. Fecal calcium, however, may be increased, with a net increase in calcium loss. Another mechanism postulated to be involved in the difference in the incidence of osteoporosis in vegetarians (18 per cent) compared with omnivores (35 per cent) is the intestinal "recycling" of estrogens in the vegetarians, which would make omnivores relatively more estrogen deficient.[2]

The influence of the calcium regulating hormones—parathyroid hormone, vitamin D, and calcitonin—is clearly also of interest. Measurement of parathyroid hormone with several different assays that measure the amino and carboxy terminal ends and intact parathyroid hormone have all shown an increase in serum levels with increasing age in both normal and osteoporotic women.[9] The higher level among elderly normal women is postulated to reflect the decrease in intestinal calcium absorption that occurs with age. The lesser increase noted with age in the osteoporotic women was thought to be a normal response due to an increased release of calcium from bone.

Furthermore, the production of 1,25-dihydroxy-vitamin D during parathyroid hormone infusion is decreased in osteoporotic subjects as compared with normals despite a similar level at baseline. This decreased reserve may contribute to the impaired intestinal calcium absorption in the elderly, which may be even more impaired in osteoporotic subjects. Other investigators have found 1,25-dihydroxy-vitamin D levels to be lower than normal, although 25-hydroxy vitamin levels were normal.[7] Estrogen therapy normalizes both the level of 1,25-dihydroxy-vitamin D and intestinal calcium absorption.[1]

Serum calcitonin levels decrease with age. Furthermore, the infusion of calcium produces less of a rise in the serum calcitonin level in older women aged 50 to 70 compared with that in a group 20 to 39 years of age.[11] Whether these alterations in calcitonin secretion are important in the etiology of osteoporosis or are secondary to it is not clear.

Because of the rapid loss of bone that occurs after menopause, serum levels of estrogenic hormones have been studied. The serum level of androstenedione, which is the principal source of estrogens in postmenopausal women, is lower in osteoporotic and corticosteroid treated women than in normal women.[12] Androstenedione levels decrease with advancing age. This suggests that osteoporotic subjects are relatively more estrogen deficient than normal controls. The increased frequency of osteoporosis in thin, as compared with obese, women may be related to decreased conversion of androstenedione to estrone in fat tissue. Early menopause or castration contributes markedly to an earlier onset of osteoporosis.

Postmenopausal women who smoke have more bone loss than nonsmokers. Osteoporotic fractures are also more common in thin smokers than in thin nonsmokers. The mechanism by which this occurs is not clear, but systemic acidosis due to smoking and hypoxemia may contribute.

Inactivity is a well recognized cause of either localized (as occurs in an immobilized limb) or generalized osteoporosis (as in the subject who requires prolonged bed rest). Decreased exercise may contribute to postmenopausal osteoporosis.

It is likely that multiple factors influence the development of osteoporosis in an individual patient.

Therapy

In such a disorder in which the basic etiology is so poorly understood, it has been difficult to devise effective therapy. The problems involved with establishing a diagnosis apply to therapy as well. It is difficult to measure small changes expected to occur over several months of therapy. Many of the therapies that have been evaluated do not result in new bone formation; rather, they prevent the age related decrease in bone mass. These must therefore be given prophylactically in order to achieve benefit. A legitimate concern about such preventive therapy is that it is presently impossible to predict which individuals will be disabled by osteoporosis. Preventive therapy should be without significant side effects, or at least the benefits should outweigh the risks. Thus far, none of the therapies except for supplemental calcium intake and exercise approaches these goals.

Estrogens

Albright was the first to suggest that a decrease in the production of gonadal hormones was important in the development of osteoporosis.[13] Since that time many studies have been conducted that show a maintenance of bone mass as well as a decrease in the incidence of fractures with estrogen administration. In retrospective survey studies, the risk of forearm and hip fractures was 50 to 60 per cent lower in women who had taken 0.625 or 1.25 mg. of conjugated estrogens daily for at least six years than in nonusers or those who had taken estrogens for a shorter time.[14]

Another similar epidemiologic study showed that menopausal estrogen use protected against hip fracture, especially in oophorectomized women who took them for longer than five years.[15]

A prospective study compared a group of postmenopausal women treated for two years with 0.625 mg. of conjugated estrogen and 5 mg. of methyltestosterone for 21 days of each month, with an untreated control group.[16] The control group lost bone at a rate of 1.18 per cent annually; the estrogen treated group showed no bone loss. Both calcium accretion and resorption decreased with hormonal therapy, and although the external calcium balance was improved, it was still negative.

A 10 year follow-up of estrogen treated postmenopausal women compared them with a similar group of control subjects.[17] Those treated with estrogens less than three years after the last menstrual period gained bone mass as measured by photon absorptiometry. Those treated more than three years after the last menstrual period maintained the original bone mass compared with both placebo groups, which lost mass.

A five year study using mestranol compared to placebo showed an increase in bone as measured by photon absorption if hormones were started before six years after menopause.[18] Bone loss in the oophorectomized group was most rapid in the initial three years after surgery.

Estrogen therapy does seem to be of benefit in decreasing bone loss and perhaps increasing bone accretion if given soon after menopause. It, however, is not without complications, the most significant of which are estrogen dependent tumors of the breast or uterus, atherosclerotic cardiovascular disease, deep vein thrombosis, and pulmonary emboli. Infrequently liver tumors may also be associated with estrogen therapy. Hyperlipidemia, diabetes, hypertension, migraine headaches or seizure disorders may be worsened. Pancreatitis may develop. Among factors that predispose a woman to endometrial carcinoma are nulliparity, obesity, diabetes mellitus, and liver disease. Present evidence suggests that the risk of endometrial carcinoma is increased with estrogen therapy but is still low. The intermittent administration of a progestogen, which results in edometrial sloughing, is protective and may be used in combination with estrogens.[19] A useful regimen is to give 0.625 mg. of conjugated estrogens for three of four consecutive weeks. A progestogen, such as 10 mg. of Provera, may be given on days 17 to 21.

Calcium

Supplemental calcium either as food or as oral or intravenous medication has been used to treat osteoporosis. The postmenopausal calcium balance has been estimated to be negative, with a daily loss of 43 mg. The daily requirement of calcium in postmenopausal women is 1.27 to 1.73 gm. per day.[8] The administration of 1 gm. of supplemental calcium daily for two years in postmenopausal women resulted in a decrease in bone remodeling when compared with controls.[16] Changes in the amount of bone surface were noted on biopsy specimens obtained after three to four months of 2 to 2.5 gm. per day of supplemental calcium.[20] The addition of 50,000 units of vitamin D twice weekly resulted in hypercalcemia but similar bone improvement. An increase in the intestinal absorption of calcium has been achieved in osteoporotic patients treated with 1,25-dihydroxyvitamin D.[7] Similar results were noted with the addition of cheese containing 360 mg. of calcium and supplemental calcium (350 mg.) in osteoporotic elderly women who were consuming a diet containing less than 500 mg. of calcium daily.[21]

Alternating intravenous infusions of calcium and phosphorus in osteoporotic subjects resulted in an increased thickness of cortical bone in iliac crest biopsy specimens obtained one year after the beginning of therapy.[22] This finding also was associated with a decrease in the fracture rate and symptomatic improvement. However, this method is clearly not as convenient as oral calcium supplementation.

A useful method of giving additional calcium is as a combination of foods and calcium supplements to provide a total of 1 to 2 gm. of elemental calcium daily. Eight ounces of milk contains 240 mg. and five slices of American cheese 600 mg. of calcium. For each 650 mg. tablet, calcium carbonate yields 260 mg. of calcium; calcium lactate, 84.5 mg.; calcium gluconate, 58.5 mg.; and OsCal, 250 mg. of calcium and 125 units of vitamin D_2. Side effects of calcium therapy potentially include nephrolithiasis due to increased urinary calcium excretion, but this has not proved to be a significant problem.

Exercise

Exercise among the elderly may improve cardiovascular fitness as well as promote a sense of well-being. Whether such exercise stimulates new bone formation is questionable. Athletes, especially those who engage in weight lifting, have an increased bone density when compared to controls. Even within control groups in one study there was a higher bone density in those who exercised compared to those who did not. An exercise program lasting one hour, three times each week for one year was associated with a positive calcium balance in a small group of postmenopausal women.[23] Such vigorous exercise may not be possible in an elderly person who is otherwise disabled, but even walking should be encouraged. Osteoarthritis may be exacerbated, but otherwise exercise in moderation is without serious side effects.

Fluoride

Therapy with fluoride in combination with calcium or estrogen resulted in a marked decrease in the incidence of fractures in a group of postmenopausal osteoporotic women who were treated for four years.[24] This was given as sodium fluoride, approximately 55 mg. daily. However, 40 per cent of those treated with fluoride had no increase in bone mass and no decrease in the fracture rate. About 20 per cent of the patients had adverse reactions to fluoride that caused them to discontinue therapy. Although this therapy has promise for promoting the formation of new bone, it requires further study.

Other Forms of Therapy

Therapy with thiazide diuretics was thought to be of possible benefit in treating osteoporosis because of its known effect in decreasing urinary calcium excretion. Its effect in maintaining bone mineral content is short-lived, however, and probably of little clinical value.[25]

Androgen therapy with 5 mg. daily of methandrostenolone for three or four weeks has been reported to be beneficial.[26] Although this study reported no significant side effects, there remains concern about the development of hepatoma and peliosis hepatis with such therapy.

Therapy with porcine calcitonin in a dose of 1 MRC unit per kg. twice daily for three months has been reported to result in a decrease in symptoms and a positive calcium balance.[27] In this study, however, calcitonin was combined with 1 gm. of supplemental calcium daily. Because there was no control group treated with calcium alone, it is difficult to ascribe the effects to calcitonin. The result remains to be tested in a double blind study with quantitative bone evaluation.

DIABETES MELLITUS

Diabetes mellitus occurs in approximately 3 per cent of the population in the United States. Although in many persons it may not be associated with any apparent increase in morbidity or mortality, in others it contributes to multiple hospitalizations and early death.

Diabetes has been called a "disease of civilization" because it is found far more frequently among groups living in an "advanced" society.[28] Movement from a rural to a primarily urban population and the technological changes involved in such advancement have resulted in the development of many labor saving devices, with a resultant decrease in personal energy expenditures. This decreased expenditure, accompanied by an increase in the availability of high calorie foodstuffs, is contributory to, if not entirely responsible for, the initiation and maintenance of obesity that is so common among middle aged and elderly persons and that predisposes them to the development of diabetes. The influence of obesity must be considered in any evaluation of the pathogenesis and therapy of diabetes, because it, as well as the high caloric intake required to maintain the obese state, is very much involved in the impaired glucose or insulin tolerance noted with both states.

Although it has been recognized for many years that there are different types of diabetes, the classification has been recently revised to allow better communication among and between investigators and clinicians.[29] The two types seen most frequently are type I, which includes those who are insulin dependent, and type II, or noninsulin dependent diabetes.

Diagnosis

The criteria for the diagnosis of diabetes are as follows:[30]

1. Unequivocal elevation of the plasma glucose level ($\geq$ 200 mg. per dl.) and classic symptoms of diabetes, including polydipsia, polyuria, polyphagia, and weight loss.

2. A fasting plasma glucose level $\geq$ 140 mg. per dl. on two occasions.

3. A fasting plasma glucose level < 140 mg. per dl. and a two hour plasma glucose level $\geq$ 200 mg. per dl. with one intervening value (one-half, one, or one and one-half hours) $\geq$ 200 mg. per dl. following a 75 gm. oral glucose tolerance test.

These revised criteria take into account numerous observations that glucose tolerance becomes impaired with age. Subjects over age 60 commonly have a higher blood glucose level after an oral glucose challenge than younger subjects. Generally the fasting glucose level remains normal with increasing age, and it is only the postprandial value that is increased. Insulin levels may also increase with age.

Type I Diabetes

Of all patients with diabetes mellitus, approximately 10 per cent have type I diabetes.

They are characterized by the propensity to develop ketoacidosis unless they receive exogenous insulin. The usual patient who develops this disorder is a child or young adult, although elderly individuals may also present with this type of diabetes. The progression through the early symptoms of weight loss despite polyphagia, polydipsia, and polyuria, to decreased mental alertness is ordinarily brief and encompasses only several weeks. Although other family members may have the disorder, the inheritance is not nearly as strong as in type II diabetes.

Etiology

The pathophysiology of type I disease is believed to involve a deficiency in insulin synthesis or secretion. Autopsy studies of persons with a recent onset of diabetes have shown an inflammatory involvement of the pancreatic islets, especially the beta cells.[31] This cellular response against the individual's own tissues has been variously suggested to involve autoimmune phenomena or an appropriate response to a viral or other infection of the islets. Several well documented cases of diabetes have been attributed to specific infectious agents, such as mumps or Coxsackie B virus.[32]

An animal model utilizing mice and encephalomyocarditis virus has been useful in studying the disorder.[33] In this case, infection with the organism results in a transient insulitis. As this resolves, the plasma insulin level decreases and the glucose level increases. Depending upon the dose of the infecting organism, as well as other factors, the animals may have diabetes, which ranges from a form that is ketosis-prone to only mild hyperglycemia. Alterations of viral characteristics by multiple in vitro passages and then infecting sensitive mice, which subsequently develop diabetes, has lent further support to the postulate that type I diabetes is due to an islet infection in a susceptible host.[34]

It is apparent that some aspect of individual susceptibility must also be involved because of the infrequency with which diabetes occurs despite a presumed high general viral attack rate. The reason proposed is that a particular gene composition predisposes the individual. This would also account for the increased occurrence of diabetes in certain families because of similar gene make-up.

The second theory involves consideration of autoimmune mechanisms. For no apparent reason, antibodies may be developed toward the beta cells of the islets that destroy these cells, resulting in insulin deficiency and diabetes. Antibodies to islet cell surfaces as well as to cytoplasm have been noted in the serum of the majority of patients with type I diabetes if they are evaluated shortly after the onset of clinical symptoms; the frequency with which these antibodies are detectable decreases with a longer duration of diabetes. They are, however, also found more often in asymptomatic relatives of type I subjects than in a comparable control group. This suggests that their presence is not sufficient for the development of diabetes.

Antibodies to other endocrine glands are found more frequently among diabetics and their families than in a nondiabetic control group. These may be associated with clinical disease, such as Addison's disease or Hashimoto's thyroiditis, or may be asymptomatic. The association of other diseases thought to be of an autoimmune nature is presumptive evidence that such a pathogenesis also may be involved in the development of type I diabetes.

Although the major problem in type I diabetes appears to be insufficient insulin secretion, recent work has also implicated peripheral insulin resistance in playing a role in the hyperglycemia.[35] At similar levels of plasma insulin, diabetics were noted to have evidence of decreased glucose metabolism compared to individuals without diabetes.

Regardless of etiology, the sine qua non for making the diagnosis of type I diabetes is the dependence on insulin to sustain life; without insulin the patient develops ketoacidosis.

Complications

Patients with type I disease are prone to develop complications after many years of disease. These complications are due to small vessel (microvascular) involvement, which results in the clinical findings of retinopathy, neuropathy, and nephropathy. Atherosclerotic complications are also more common in type I diabetes than in nondiabetic subjects (because they are responsible for most of the morbidity and mortality of type II diabetes they are discussed in that section). The retinopathy is evidenced on ophthalmoscopic examination as new vessel formation around the disk. Macular edema may be apparent only with fluorescein angiography but clinically is associated with a marked decrease in vision. Hemorrhage into the vitreous from the fragile new vessels similarly may result in loss of all useful vision. Retinal detachment and cataracts also occur with increased frequency and are additional causes of impaired vision in type I diabetes.

Theories of etiology of the ophthalmic complications are multiple. Retinal ischemia with elaboration of a local hormonal factor that stimulates vessel proliferation has been proposed. A decrease in the ischemia with infarction of selected areas of the retina with photocoagulation may be responsible for the improvement in the retinopathy with this therapeutic modality. The earlier onset of cataracts in diabetics compared to nondiabetics has been postulated to be due to sorbitol accumulation; the amount of this glucose metabolite within the lens is dependent upon the plasma glucose concentration. Sorbitol is only slowly metabolized and serves as an osmotic particle causing water uptake and swelling of the lens. Inhibition of aldose reductase, the enzyme required for sorbitol formation, inhibits cataract formation in experimental animals and lends support to this theory.

Complications of diabetes mellitus involving the nervous system may involve cranial nerves and peripheral or autonomic nerves. Any cranial nerve may be affected, but those most commonly affected are the third and the sixth nerves, with production of ptosis and diplopia. The involvement is usually acute in onset and is associated with periorbital pain, thereby assisting in the differentiation from increased intracranial pressure. It resolves after several months in most patients.

The more frequent peripheral neuropathy is gradual in onset and is usually most prominent in the feet and legs. It may be only mildly annoying, with paresthesias and numbness, or disabling, with such severe pain and burning that the patient is unable to walk. Although the sensory component is most prominent, motor nerves may also be affected, with resultant muscular weakness or only changes in nerve conduction. These abnormalities appear to correlate with the duration of diabetes, but many patients with type II diabetes have decreased peripheral sensation and absent Achilles reflexes at the time of diagnosis. The etiology of this neuropathy is poorly understood; vascular insufficiency, Schwann cell abnormalities, and biochemical abnormalities such as myoinositol deficiency or sorbitol accumulation have been postulated by various authors to be responsible.

Autonomic neuropathy may cause functional abnormalities in both type I and type II diabetes. Postural hypotension may not be accompanied by a normal reflex tachycardia; episodes of otherwise inexplicable diarrhea or impaired gastric emptying may occur; and symptoms of impotence or neurogenic bladder may be clinical manifestations of autonomic neuropathy. The pathogenesis of these common complications is poorly understood and they are even more poorly treated.

An unusual form of diabetic neuropathy is polyradiculopathy. In this disorder multiple nerve roots are involved, pain and dysesthesia being the most frequent symptoms. Isolated root involvement may present as localized pain in a thoracic or lumbar distribution similar to that which precedes herpes zoster. Alternatively it may be difficult to distinguish from intra-abdominal disease, but electromyography may be helpful in this differentiation.

Nephropathy may be present at the time of diagnosis, with proteinuria noted on urinalysis. Usually, however, the asymptomatic progression to renal insufficiency occurs only after 15 or more years of the diabetic state.

Therapy

Present scientific opinion tends to support the view that careful control of the blood sugar concentration may prevent the development of complications. The transplantation of pancreatic islets to animals with early renal disease has resulted both in normalization of the blood glucose level and reversal of some of the renal changes.[36] Evidence is less convincing that a similar improvement may occur in human diabetic renal disease if the glucose level is well controlled.[37]

The ocular abnormalities may also be less rapidly progressive with improved glucose control, but this has not been conclusively proven. Of demonstrated value for the treatment of retinopathy is photocoagulation. This has been shown in a controlled study to be associated with retention of more useful vision in eyes that were treated.[38] Other types of therapy for diabetic eye disease include cataract removal; less commonly used modalities such as vitrectomy may result in the restoration of useful vision in properly selected patients.

The multitude of therapies used for

diabetic neuropathy is evidence that none of them is curative. Vitamins, especially of the B complex group, trace minerals such as chromium, or other compounds such as myo-inositol have all been used with mixed results. Phenytoin and amitriptyline-fluphenazine in combination have been reported to relieve the pain that is a prominent component of some peripheral neuropathy. The improvement of diabetic control has also been reported to improve motor nerve conduction velocity.

Until recent years, the achievement of a normal blood sugar level was both difficult to measure as well as to attain. With the advent of home monitoring of blood glucose levels and multiple subcutaneous injections or continuous infusion of insulin, these goals have become realistic. Follow-up of such well controlled patients over the next several years should permit an answer to the question whether "tight" diabetic control prevents or improves diabetic complications. In the meantime most available evidence appears to support the postulate that poor control has little to recommend it, whereas good control may decrease the likelihood of occurrence of detrimental long term effects.

Diet. The therapy of hyperglycemia in type I diabetes involves alterations in diet, both in types of food and in patterns of consumption and exercise and, of course, administration of insulin.

Before the availability of insulin, the prime and essentially the only therapy used to sustain life was dietary manipulation. Because it was recognized that carbohydrate required insulin for its utilization, this was eliminated entirely from the diet and replaced with fat and protein. If the patient retained some ability to secrete insulin, he might show some improvement in the blood sugar regulation with such a regimen. As he did so, small amounts of carbohydrate were gradually added to the diet until glycosuria reappeared. The final diet, however, still contained large amounts of fat.

The isolation and purification of insulin on a large scale in 1922 made it available for use in many patients with type I diabetes. Although it was initially hailed as a life saving drug (as it indeed was), it soon became apparent that the longer diabetics survived, the more susceptible they were to the development of both small and large vessel complications. In nondiabetics it was recognized that plasma lipids, cholesterol and triglycerides, were of major importance in the pathogenesis of cardiovascular and peripheral vascular disease. Dietary fats, as well as intake of cholesterol, appear to be prime determinants of the plasma cholesterol level. Triglyceride levels are influenced by carbohydrate, sucrose, and alcohol ingestion. These observations in nondiabetics led to a reconsideration of the recommended diet for diabetics because of their propensity for developing atherosclerotic vascular disease. A historical review of the mortality rate from vascular disease, however, has shown it to have increased despite a more liberal allowance of carbohydrate at the expense of fat.

Recommendations by the American Diabetes Association have decreased the dietary allotment of fat from 40 per cent of the calories to 12 to 20 per cent (polyunsaturated fats should supply up to 10 per cent of the total kilocalories).[39,40] The calories deleted from fat are to be replaced with carbohydrate, primarily high fiber, complex carbohydrates; refined sugars should be restricted. The replacement of fats with carbohydrate has been noted to result in a decrease in cholesterol levels. The increased carbohydrate also appears to cause an improvement in glucose tolerance.

Food consumed during the day is divided into three meals and two or three snacks. The intent of this division is to avoid the large increases in plasma glucose that accompany ingestion of a large bolus of food in a diabetic subject. Complex carbohydrates are believed to be absorbed more gradually along the gastrointestinal tract than are simple sugars, once again aiming at elimination of rapid swings in blood sugar levels. The total caloric intake is designed to maintain a normal body weight.

Use of an exchange list has facilitated the ability of the patient to make the required changes in his diet. The exchange list is based on the division of foods into groups—bread, fruit, vegetables, milk, fat, and meat (low, medium, and high fat meat groups). Within each group specific amounts of the foods listed have a similar number of calories and the same proportions of carbohydrate, fat, and protein, and thus they may be exchanged for each other. A particular diet for a patient may be devised by taking foods from each group to arrive at specific total numbers of calories, carbohydrate, fat, and protein. Further modifications of the list enable ready calculation of fiber, cholesterol, and saturated and unsaturated fats as well. Although some patients may be able to plan their own diet using the lists, in most circumstances the process is more efficient if the patient receives detailed instructions from a dietitian or similarly trained person.

The major objection to the diet is that it eliminates the spontaneity of eating, which must now be done at a prescribed time in a specific amount. In most patients, however, the diet soon becomes familiar and easy to follow. Eating in restaurants or fast food establishments may be "worked into" the diet. No special or "dietetic" foods need be purchased because the diet utilizes "normal" foods that are readily available.

Because most types of hypertension are exacerbated or may be caused by a high sodium intake, it has been recommended that diabetics decrease their salt consumption. The addition of hypertension to diabetes causes more rapid progression of diabetic retinopathy and atherosclerotic vascular disease. Diabetics should be cautioned against the use of salt substitutes, which primarily contain potassium, unless they are prescribed. This is especially true if the patient has renal failure or hyporeninemic hypoaldosteronism, in which circumstances he will be susceptible to hyperkalemia.

Exercise. The role of exercise in improving the health or preventing complications in type I diabetes has recently been explored. Vigorous exercise may result in a decrease in blood pressure and lipid levels; it also improves the utilization of carbohydrate if sufficient insulin is available. These changes as well as alterations in clotting parameters have suggested that exercise may be useful in decreasing atherosclerotic vascular disease. Such exercise, however, may be contraindicated if there is active retinal bleeding or diffuse neovascularization. Failure to modify the insulin or dietary regimen may result in hypoglycemia.

Insulin Therapy. Insulin is required to prevent the development of ketoacidosis in type I diabetes. Several types of insulin are available for general use, and special insulins may be obtained for individual patients from pharmaceutical companies or other investigators (Table 10–1). The insulins commonly used are mixtures of insulin from beef and pork sources, but pure pork insulin is commercially available (at increased cost). The purification of insulin is much greater now than in preceding years; it is called single component insulin and is at least 99 per cent pure. This improved insulin is predicted to cause less lipoatrophy at injection sites and may be used to treat existing atrophy by injection into the site. IgG insulin antibody formation will probably not be affected because insulin is still a foreign protein.

Different formulations of insulin, by complexing it with protamine (as NPH) or varying the crystalline structure (lente insulins), have led to the development of insulins with different peaks and durations of action. Use of a combination of different insulins is necessary in many diabetics.

The insulins may be divided into two groups, one group containing ultralente, lente, and semilente and the other, PZI, NPH, and regular or crystalline insulin. The duration and peak action of the lente insulins are determined by the amount of zinc complexed to the insulin. Ultralente insulin has a peak action at 18 to 24 hours and a duration of action of 36 hours or more. It has received increased attention and use in achieving a continuous low "basal" level of circulating insulin. Because of its delayed and prolonged action, it cannot be used to achieve control of the blood sugar level without accompanying hypoglycemia between meals. Lente insulin is intermediate in action, peaks at six to 12 hours, and lasts for 24 to 28 hours. The short acting semilente insulin peaks in two to four hours and is active for 12 to 16 hours.

Regular or crystalline insulin is rapid acting, with a peak in two to four hours and a duration of action of five to seven hours. Neutral protamine Hagedorn (NPH) insulin is named after its discoverer. Its intermediate duration of action (24 to 28 hours) is the result of formation of a precipitate with the protein protamine at a pH of 7.2 (formed with a phosphate buffer). The peak activity is six to 12 hours. In protamine zinc insulin (PZI) there is an excess of protamine, which makes it more insoluble and prolongs its duration of action to 36 hours or more; peak activity occurs 14 to 24 hours after administration.

The studies that determined these peak and duration activities were performed in well controlled hospitalized diabetic patients with monitoring of the glucose lowering response of a single injection of insulin.

Sometimes, for no apparent reason, regular insulin has a duration of action comparable to that of NPH or lente insulin, or, conversely, the effect of intermediate insulin is only tran-

TABLE 10-1. Selected Characteristics of Insulin Formulations*

		Onset (hrs.)	Peak (hrs.)	Duration (hrs.)	pH
Rapid Acting	Insulin injection (regular)	½ to 1	2 to 5	6 to 8	7.0 to 7.8[1]
	Prompt insulin zinc suspension (semilente)	½ to 1½	5 to 10	12 to 16	7.2 to 7.5
Intermediate Acting	Isophane insulin suspension (NPH)	1 to 1½	8 to 12	24	7.1 to 7.4
	Insulin zinc suspension (lente)	1 to 2½	7 to 15	24	7.2 to 7.5
Long Acting	Protamine zinc insulin suspension (PZI)	4 to 8	14 to 20	36	7.1 to 7.4
	Extended insulin zinc suspension (ultralente)	4 to 8	10 to 30	>36	7.2 to 7.5

*Reprinted with permission from Facts and Comparisons, Inc., 1982.
[1] Neutral regular insulin. Although USP XX still recognizes acid regular insulin (ARI, pH 2.5–3.5), all regular insulins are now prepared at neutral pH.

sient. Clinical observation is of paramount importance in detecting a deviation from the expected duration of action, appropriate modification of the dosage interval being made if necessary.

Within the past several years there has been a change in both the type of insulin used in treatment and the frequency with which it is given. A few patients may have nearly normal blood sugar levels with a single morning injection of an intermediate insulin, but such a circumstance is unfortunately unusual. Most patients require at least two daily injections of mixtures of short and intermediate acting insulins for optimal control. A combination of NPH or lente insulin and regular or semilente insulin is most commonly used. Two-thirds of the total dosage may be given prior to breakfast, with the remainder given approximately 30 minutes before the evening meal. Further subdivision of each dose into two-thirds intermediate and one-third short acting insulin is a useful starting regimen. If, for example the total dosage is 45 units, 30 units would be given in the morning and 15 units in the evening. Of the 30 units, 20 could be given as NPH and 10 as regular insulin; the evening 15 units would be divided into 10 units of NPH insulin and 5 units of regular insulin. This should be used only as a rough guide, with modifications made as required by blood glucose determinations.

Another method makes use of ultralente insulin to achieve a low but constant level of insulin throughout the day to simulate basal pancreatic insulin secretion. The increase in the blood sugar level that occurs with meals is covered with three or more injections of a short acting insulin, such as regular or semilente insulin. The ultralente form is given in an amount sufficient to normalize the fasting blood glucose level; the short acting insulin dose is varied throughout the day, depending on the response and the size of the meal. This pattern of giving insulin allows more flexibility in the time and amount of meal ingestion than twice a day insulin regimens.

A still more frequently used insulin injection method is that achieved by continuous subcutaneous infusion with an indwelling catheter. A low rate of insulin administration is used throughout the day, with an additional bolus administered for each meal. This method allows the patient to avoid multiple injections, but requires that he carry a small gadget with him. Although some patients object to the public awareness of illness that such a device gives, in many circumstances, especially for men, it is easily possible to conceal it beneath clothing. Further, as the machinery becomes miniaturized, this becomes less of a problem. Obviously potential problems may arise with mechanical dysfunction of the pump or accidental dislodgment of the needle. If this occurs, the patient will be susceptible to the development of severe hyperglycemia and ketoacidosis. Some concern has been expressed because of the occurrence of several unexplained deaths in patients using the insulin pump.[41] It is postulated that some of these may have been due to nocturnal hypoglycemia.

Careful comparison of the regimens with multiple injections and the pump has shown that similar blood sugar levels may be obtained with either method.[42] Both require careful patient input and compliance, with the use of home glucose monitoring to determine the appropriate dose of insulin.

It has been documented that many other factors, in addition to the kind of insulin, modify its effect. Insulin antibodies are demonstrable in virtually all patients who have received insulin for several months. Although there may be a genetic predisposition to develop these antibodies, in most circumstances the level does not inactivate large amounts of the administered insulin and they are of little clinical importance. Occasionally such antibodies may cause marked insulin resistance, the requirement for insulin reaching several hundreds, or thousands, of units daily.

Local enzymes may inactivate insulin at the injection site. This development should be suspected if insulin is effective if given by the intravenous route but not when given subcutaneously. The use of trasylol to inactivate local insulinases, giving the insulin by continuous intravenous infusion (with a Hickman catheter), or giving the insulin intramuscularly are treatment alternatives in such a circumstance.

The absorption of insulin (and its effect) may be increased if the insulin has been injected into an exercised extremity instead of into the abdominal wall. Avoiding injection into an area to be exercised should ameliorate hypoglycemia due to this effect.

Renal insufficiency also tends to increase the duration of action of insulin because of elimination of a site of excretion. The effect of insulin in these patients, however, is affected by numerous other factors, such as the counterregulatory hormones and dialysis; thus the duration of action is not always predictable.

Another side effect of insulin is a local or systemic allergic response. Such may be treated by a change to pure pork insulin or desensitization if necessary. Local fat atrophy usually responds to injection of pork insulin into the atrophic area.

Recombinant DNA technology was used to synthesize human insulin in 1979. The A and B chains are synthesized by *Escherichia coli* fermentation with subsequent conversion to sulfate linked insulin. The amino acid sequence corresponds to that of human insulin, and in vitro and in vivo studies of normal and diabetic human subjects have been made. These indicate that this insulin is apparently similar in metabolism as well as hypoglycemic effect to pork insulin.[43] The major advantage of biosynthetic human insulin (BHI) will be to ensure an adequate supply of insulin to patients, with less concern for the vagaries of foreign governments in obtaining the raw materials (beef and pork pancreas). Prolonged use of BHI may also be associated with less antibody formation because it is not a foreign protein. Unforeseen side effects may become apparent with increased use.

If insulin resistance due to insulin antibodies is encountered, either BHI, pure pork, salmon, or sulfated insulin may be tried. There is less cross reactivity with insulin antibodies with these kinds of insulins than with beef insulin, which is also most antigenic. Insulin allergy or lipodystrophy at the injection site may also be treated with purified BHI when it becomes available.

Glucose Monitoring. The determination of the plasma glucose level by the diabetic patient has greatly facilitated the management of diabetes. The patient may obtain blood by a fingerstick and measure the glucose level by using either a visually interpreted strip that changes color depending on the level of glucose or a device that gives a digital readout of the glucose level. Both methods are much more useful than urine glucose measurements, which generally correlate poorly with the blood sugar level. This is especially true in diabetics who have diabetic or other renal disease in which the threshold of glucose reabsorption is higher than normal.

Although the attainment of a normal blood sugar level is desirable in young diabetics, with the hope being to avoid the development or progression of complications, in older persons this goal may not be an appropriate one. The complications of type I diabetes are dependent in large part on the duration of the diabetes. In an elderly person who has other diseases, the expected life span may not be such as to warrant the possible complications of extremely rigid glucose control. In such a subject perhaps the more appropriate goal would be to achieve control that is not associated with frequent hypoglycemic episodes while maintaining glucose levels that are not extremely elevated.

Type II Diabetes

Most (90 per cent) elderly diabetics have type II diabetes; that is, they are not dependent on insulin to prevent ketoacidosis. These patients frequently are unaware of their glucose intolerance and are commonly noted to be diabetic during evaluation for another medical problem. Frequently the other disorders involve atherosclerotic disease, with symptoms of angina, transient ischemic attacks, or claudication. Because the diabetes itself may not be associated with symptoms, in many cases it is difficult to estimate its duration.

Etiology

The etiology of type II diabetes does not involve deficient secretion of insulin; in fact, in many obese subjects with diabetes the circulating insulin level is above that seen in normal thin subjects. The abnormalities in this type of diabetes are integrally related to obesity because 60 to 90 per cent of those affected are obese.

In order for insulin to exert its biologic effect, it must first interact with a receptor on the cell surface. Following this, various intracellular events are stimulated that promote carbohydrate metabolism. Abnormalities at the insulin receptor as well as postreceptor defects have been reported in cells of type II diabetes. The decreased number of receptors described has been believed by some to be secondary to the increased caloric intake (and subsequent hyperinsulinemia) required to maintain the obese state. The number of receptors increases with fasting (which causes a decrease in insulin levels). Receptor affinity may be altered in unusual states in which an antibody to the receptor itself has been produced.

In most patients with type II diabetes the abnormality in insulin action lies in the postreceptor area. Despite pharmacologic doses of insulin, the rate of glucose metabolism is not normalized. Some investigators have recently suggested, however, that these abnormalities may be at least partially reversed with control of the blood sugar concentration.

In addition, the rate of plasma insulin removal may decrease with age. If true, part of the decline may be due to decreased renal function, which is known to occur with increasing age. It may also be due to a change in the relative degree of obesity or the degree of physical fitness and activity of elderly subjects.

As previously noted, the new criteria for the diagnosis of diabetes take into account the deterioration of glucose tolerance that occurs with age. Whether this is acceptance of what "is" the state of elderly persons rather than what is truly "normal" is controversial. The production of glycosylated hemoglobin increases with age, suggesting that the hyperglycemia is significant. The changes that occur in many, but certainly not all, elderly persons may reflect an increase in the amount of body fat at the expense of muscle, which is most likely due to inactivity. Physical conditioning and exercise promote glucose utilization.

Abnormalities in trace minerals such as chromium have also been linked to glucose intolerance. Chromium is believed to complex with amino acids to form "glucose tolerance factor," which along with insulin stimulates glucose utilization. Controlled studies in which brewer's yeast as a source of chromium or chromium itself was given have demonstrated improvement in both glucose and lipid levels.[44,45] The unavailability of plasma chromium levels, however, has made it difficult to predict whether or in how many diabetics the abnormalities in carbohydrate metabolism are due to chromium deficiency. Such a deficiency state remains hypothetical.

Dietary habits may change with age owing to economic conditions or personal situations. In some circumstances caloric intake may be inadequate to maintain body weight. Caloric absorption may be decreased by gastrointestinal disorders or edema due to congestive heart failure, but in otherwise normal elderly subjects, the absorption of nutrients does not change with age. Decreased intake may result in "starvation diabetes," although whether carbohydrate tolerance decreases with low carbohydrate intake is also controversial.

Complications

As previously noted, many subjects who are found to have type II diabetes are asymptomatic with respect to the hyperglycemia. However, they may have proteinuria and background retinopathy and the Achilles reflexes may be absent at the time of diagnosis. This obviously suggests that they already have developed some of the complications of diabetes.

The most common cause of death in diabetic patients is atherosclerotic disease. It accounts for three-fourths of deaths among those with diabetes, compared to only one-third of nondiabetic persons. This death rate has apparently increased over the past 50 years; this may be a true increase or may represent only the use of a different set of criteria for the diagnosis of diabetes.[46] The progression of the vascular disease may be entirely silent until the occurrence of a devastating event, such as a stroke or myocardial infarction. It may be at this time that diabetes is first discovered on routine screening studies. Clinically the glucose intolerance may be very mild and perhaps only apparent by documentation of elevated insulin levels, which will be evidence of insulin resistance.

Pathologically atherosclerosis associated with diabetes cannot be distinguished from that which occurs in nondiabetic patients. This of course does not mean that they are caused by the same mechanism or that they will respond to therapy in a similar manner.

Many abnormalities noted in type II diabetes have been implicated in the progression and acceleration of atherosclerotic vascular disease. These may be grouped into local vascular factors and systemic or circulating factors.

Local injury to the endothelial surface has been extensively used to induce atherosclerosis in animals. It has been postulated that similar mechanical injury occurs along the vessel daily. The initial response to experimental injury appears to be platelet aggregation at the site. After several days there is a migration of smooth muscle cells from the media, which proliferate to cover the defect. Eventually new endothelial cells reconstitute the intimal surface, but this may require several months for completion. Hypertension may promote atherosclerosis by causing an increased rate of damage due to turbulent blood flow. Endothelial damage due to hypoxemia has been postulated to occur because of alterations in 2,3-DPG or an increase in the production of glycosylated hemoglobin. Abnormal metabolism, with sorbitol formation, has also been advanced as an etiologic factor. The endothelial cells normally produce prostacyclin, which inhibits atherosclerotic plaque formation; decreased production of this substance, for whatever reason, may accelerate lesion development. Increased amounts of low density lipoprotein may potentiate vascular injury.

Among circulating factors, platelets and a normal clotting system are required for atherosclerosis to occur. Platelets have been found to function abnormally in diabetic patients. Release of a platelet-derived growth factor has been postulated to stimulate the migration and proliferation of smooth muscle cells into the intimal area. Lipoprotein levels may be increased in diabetics, or alternatively lipoproteins may be metabolized in an abnormal fashion with an increase in atherogenic potential. High density lipoprotein, which is protective against atherosclerosis, is decreased and abnormal in diabetic subjects. Lastly, the elevated insulin level itself, seen in most patients with type II diabetes and insulin resistance, has been implicated. Insulin stimulates smooth muscle cell proliferation; local fatty acid synthesis is increased with insulin, and fatty acids could be used to esterify cholesterol from the circulation and result in plaque formation.

A positive correlation has been found between an elevated insulin response to glucose and increased serum triglyceride levels. Other studies have found a positive relationship between fasting or postprandial insulin levels and the incidence of myocardial infarction.

Although there is experimental evidence of abnormalities in all the areas mentioned, the contribution of each of them to the final result of atherosclerosis is unknown. The effect of other risk factors, such as smoking and hypertension, is additive to the increase in atherosclerosis resulting from diabetes. The clinical concomitants of these pathologic abnormalities are cerebrovascular insufficiency with transient ischemic attacks or strokes, myocardial infarction, angina or heart failure, or peripheral vascular insufficiency with claudication or gangrene.

Another complication of type II diabetes is hyperosmolar hyperglycemic nonketotic coma. This occurs almost exclusively in noninsulin dependent patients who acquire another (usually acute) illness. Glucose levels are usually over 500 mg. per dl. and may be 1500 mg. per dl. or more. This increase is associated with extensive diuresis, which results in severe dehydration and prerenal azotemia. Despite the severe hyperglycemia, however, ketoacidosis does not develop. This has been variously attributed to the prevention of lipolysis by low levels of insulin, failure of secretion of counterregulatory hormones, or secretion of other substances that inhibit fat mobilization.

Subjects with hyperosmolar hyperglycemic nonketotic coma are usually very ill; the mortality rate in some series is 50 per cent. This high mortality rate may be due, at least in part, to the age of the persons involved as well as the seriousness of associated illnesses, such as myocardial infarction or stroke.

Therapy

Because the major clinical manifestations of type II diabetes are the result of atherosclerotic disease rather than hyperglycemia, therapy should be directed toward preventing the vascular disease. Owing to an inadequate understanding of the pathogenesis, however, exact determination of an appropriate form of therapy is difficult. Modification of lipid and insulin abnormalities is thought to be a useful beginning attack.

Diet. Because obesity is so common among patients with type II diabetes, the principal approach to therapy is weight reduction. Attainment of an ideal body weight may normalize both carbohydrate and lipid abnormalities so that no other therapy is indicated. The exchange diet system is useful in this group of patients; the caloric allotment is decreased to promote the desired weight loss, but the modifications mentioned previously are retained. It is especially important that the amount of fat be restricted, because of both its high caloric density and its propensity for causing hypercholesterolemia. The restriction of simple sugars and alcohol may decrease triglyceride levels. In type II diabetics not taking oral doses of hypoglycemic drugs or insulin, less emphasis is placed on the timing and frequency of meals. Although various types of diets have been popularized for weight loss, many of them depend on packaged, prepared foods or strange, monotonous regimens (e.g., the grapefruit diet) and are thus not suitable for lifelong use. The initial weight loss may be greater with these diets than with an exchange diet, but the gradual weight loss achieved with a more moderate regimen will allow the patient time to change his dietary habits. Many patients with mild diabetes also deteriorate and require additional therapy, in which case it would seem desirable to start on an American Dietetics Association exchange diet program initially.

High carbohydrate, high fiber diets have been found to both improve glucose metabolism and decrease the hyperlipidemia commonly seen in type II diabetes. These effects may be mediated by improved insulin binding, although it has also been speculated that the changes noted in insulin receptor numbers may be secondary to changes in insulin levels. The addition of an exercise program to the dietary regimen may enhance lipid and glycemic improvement.

If, as is the circumstance far too often, the patient is unable to achieve or maintain an ideal body weight and still is morbidly obese (more than 100 pounds above the ideal weight), further therapeutic options may be entertained. Surgical procedures in which the stomach is bypassed or decreased in size have largely replaced intestinal bypass operations because of a lower incidence of complications with the former. Because the weight loss is dependent primarily on a decrease in the consumption of calories, patients must be properly selected in order to achieve weight loss with any of the gastric procedures. Although age alone is not a contraindication to surgery, additional medical or psychiatric complications may make the patient an unacceptable surgical candidate. Hospitalization and more extreme caloric restriction or a total fast are other options for such patients.

If the patient has only mild or moderate obesity, is unable to lose weight, or is of normal weight but remains severely hyperglycemic, a decision must be made whether and how to treat the hyperglycemia. If the patient is very old and has no severe complications and the hyperglycemia is asymptomatic, the decision might be made to do nothing more than to observe him periodically. If, on the other hand, the hyperglycemia is associated with polyuria and polydipsia with or without other complications, he should probably be treated. Two options for therapy are available—oral doses of hypoglycemic drugs and insulin. Neither of these, however, should replace the continued emphasis on dietary changes.

Orally Administered Hypoglycemic Drugs. Sulfonylurea drugs and biguanides are separate classes of drugs that are active in lowering the blood glucose level (Table 10–2).[47] The biguanides have been withdrawn from the American market because of their association with lactic acidosis, and they will not be discussed further.[48]

The mechanism of action of the sulfonylureas appears to involve both pancreatic and extrapancreatic effects. Initial therapy results in a decrease in the fasting glucose level associated with an increase in the circulating insulin level. After several weeks to months, however, the insulin level returns to pretreatment values despite continued improvement in the fasting glucose level. An extrapancreatic effect has been demonstrated in in vitro studies of liver, muscle, and adipose tissue. An increase in the number of insulin receptors has

TABLE 10–2. Selected Characteristics of the Oral Hypoglycemic Drugs*

	Equivalent doses (mg.)	Doses/day	Serum t½ (hrs.)	Duration (hrs.)	Metabolism
Tolbutamide	500	2–3	4–5	6–12	Oxidized in liver to inactive metabolites
Acetohexamide	250	1–2	6–8 (parent drug plus metabolite)	12–24	Reduced in liver to potent active metabolite
Tolazamide	100	1–2	7	10–16	Several mildly active metabolites
Chlorpropamide	100	1	35	Up to 60	80% metabolized in liver; activity of metabolites unknown

*Reprinted with permission from Facts and Comparisons, Inc., 1982.

been reported by some investigators, but not all. Nevertheless sulfonylurea drugs have an effect on enhancing in vivo insulin action. They are, however, without effect in insulin dependent, type I diabetics, suggesting that their major effect may be a pancreatic one.[49] An alternative explanation may be that the effect of the drugs differs in the two types of diabetes. Although fasting glucose levels improve, the postprandial glucose level usually remains elevated.

Tolbutamide (Orinase) is a short-acting compound with a three to eight hour duration of action. It is metabolized in the liver to inactive compounds, which are then excreted by the kidneys. The 500 mg. tablets are given in a total dosage of 1000 to 3000 mg. per day.

Acetohexamide (Dymelor) and tolazamide (Tolinase) are intermediate in duration of action, with a biologic effect evident 12 to 24 hours after ingestion. This longer effect is the result of the hepatic metabolism of the parent compound into substances with hypoglycemic activity. About three-fourths of acetohexamide is metabolized by the liver to form hydroxyhexamide, which is a potent hypoglycemic compound. The activity is terminated by renal excretion. Administration of 500 to 1500 mg. daily in two doses is usually necessary with acetohexamide; it is available in 250 and 500 mg. tablets. Tolazamide likewise is given once or twice daily, 100 to 1000 mg. per day. Once a day dosage may be sufficient if 500 mg. or less is required. It is available in 100, 250, and 500 mg. scored tablets. It is metabolized in the liver to at least six products, some of which also have hypoglycemic effects.

The remaining drug, chlorpropamide (Diabinese), has a very long duration of action (24 to 36 hours). It is available in 100 and 250 mg. tablets and the daily dosage, given once daily, is 100 to 500 mg. It is poorly metabolized and significantly protein bound, thereby accounting for its prolonged activity. Renal excretion is primarily responsible for termination of the drug's effect. Because of the importance of renal excretion in intermediate (acetohexamide and tolazamide) and long acting (chlorpropamide) compounds, their use is contraindicated in the presence of renal insufficiency.

Two "second generation" hypoglycemic drugs have been used in Europe and are undergoing clinical trials in the United States. They are glibenclamide and glipizide. Their potency is 20 to 100 times that of the older drugs; they are metabolized differently and may have desirable properties such as being natriuretic. Side effects are similar to those with first generation compounds.

Drug induced side effects include skin rashes, nausea, and other gastrointestinal disturbances. Of more concern, however, are serious hypoglycemia, hyponatremia, and perhaps an increase in cardiovascular mortality. Although hypoglycemia is really a manifestation of drug toxicity rather than a side effect, it may be severe and unexpected. Possible explanations include physician, pharmacist, or patient errors in dosage, development of renal insufficiency, or the concomitant ingestion of alcohol. Other drugs such as sulfas, salicylates, phenylbutazone, coumarin, and monoamine oxidase inhibitors may potentiate the effect of sulfonylurea drugs, perhaps by causing a decrease in metabolism or excretion or diminished protein binding. Extreme caution should be used in choosing other drugs for treating patients who already are taking hypoglycemic drugs. If severe hypoglycemia does occur, the patient should be hospitalized. The duration of therapy with an intravenous glucose infusion should be at least 24 to 48 hours to prevent recurrence of hypoglycemia. Oral administration of the hypoglycemic drug and other offending medication should be discontinued.

Hyponatremia severe enough to cause seizures has been noted only with chlorpropamide. It requires the presence of antidiuretic hormone in the hypothalamic pituitary area as well as excessive water ingestion. This syndrome of inappropriate antidiuretic hormone secretion appears to be due to both increased release of the hormone and potentiation of its effect at the renal level. Chlorpropamide has been used to treat patients with partial diabetes insipidus, thereby capitalizing on this side effect.

The concern that the sulfonylureas may cause an increase in cardiovascular mortality was raised following a controlled study by the University Group Diabetes Program.[50] This multicentered study randomly assigned type II patients to one of several groups: placebo, tolbutamide, insulin standard (a fixed dose of insulin was given regardless of the blood sugar level), and insulin variable (the dose of insulin was adjusted according to the blood glucose). A phenformin group was added later. After several years the investigators noted an excess mortality from cardiovascular causes in the groups taking tolbutamide or phenformin when compared with the other groups, and because of this the study was terminated prior to its planned conclusion. Although there has continued to be active controversy regarding this study, the Food and Drug Administration has recommended the use of orally administered hypoglycemic drugs only when diet alone is inadequate and insulin therapy is either unacceptable or impractical; a package insert stating this is also required by the Food and Drug Administration and the patient should be informed of these recommendations.

An interesting side effect, facial flushing after alcohol ingestion, has been noted in some patients treated with chlorpropamide. This finding has been used to categorize patients with the objective of identifying those more susceptible to retinopathy or peripheral vascular disease. It was found that in some subjects with a positive chlorpropamide-alcohol flush, the flush was blocked with an opiate antagonist or indomethacin; these observations suggest that prostaglandins or opiates may also be involved in some of the complications of type II diabetes.

Insulin Therapy. If the patient with type II diabetes remains severely hyperglycemic despite dietary therapy, and perhaps a trial of orally administered drugs, the use of insulin is the next logical step. Careful evaluation of the patient's or a family member's ability to understand the use of this potentially hazardous drug is necessary first. If after such consideration it is determined that the potential complications (and likelihood) of severe hypoglycemia are greater than the possible benefits derived from improvement in blood glucose control, no therapy may be given. If this is the case, however, periodic measurement of the blood sugar level will need to be done in order to detect early development of hyperglycemic hyperosmolar nonketotic coma.

Usually sufficient community assistance in the form of visiting nurses or home health aides is availabale to ensure proper patient supervision. The insulin may be drawn up into syringes to give the patient several days' or a week's supply if he has difficulty in measuring or seeing the marks on the syringe. Age alone is certainly not a contraindication to the use of insulin, and despite initial apprehension, most elderly patients cope with daily insulin injections with ease. Compliance, in fact, seems better in many elderly than in young diabetics. Many thin or normal weight elderly subjects with type II diabetes may be adequately treated with a single daily dose of intermediate acting insulin. A trial of the most simple regimen should be undertaken before multiple doses are used. If it is noted that a mixture of intermediate and short acting insulin is best, this can be mixed in the same syringe in order to eliminate the need for two injections. This injection should be administered within 15 minutes after it is mixed, however. Obese subjects who are not compliant with dietary recommendations may require large amounts of insulin before any change occurs in the blood glucose level.

If the patient with type II diabetes who has been well controlled on diet or orally administered drugs requires surgery or develops a serious concomitant illness, additional or alternative therapy must be considered. If the surgical procedure is minor and of brief duration, no changes need be made. Complicated or prolonged surgery requiring general or regional anesthesia usually requires a switch to insulin therapy in patients with moderately severe diabetes. Admission to the hospital several days in advance of surgery is recommended for an orderly change to insulin. If the surgery is of an emergency nature, continuous intravenous infusion of 1 to 2 units of insulin hourly may be used; alternate methods are intravenous or subcutaneous injections. In either circumstance, frequent blood glucose levels should be obtained during the procedure. A portable glucose measuring device or visually interpreted strips are ideal for rapid and convenient determination of blood glucose levels during surgery. Postoperatively the same regimen may be continued until the patient is stable, at which time the method previously used may be restarted.

As noted previously, the complication of hyperglycemic hyperosmolar nonketotic coma may be treated with an insulin regimen comparable to that just discussed. In addition, because these patients are usually very dehydrated, they require large amounts of replacement intravenous fluids. Simultaneous therapy of the precipitating event (e.g., infection, myocardial infarction) is also of utmost importance.

The use of a completely implantable continuous infusion system has recently been used in type II diabetes, and although only a small number of patients were reported, there were few complications.[51] This delivery system holds promise for future long term therapy.

Cholesterol and triglyceride levels should be measured after optimal glucose control has been achieved in order to evaluate whether additional therapy is needed. A moderate amount of exercise should be encouraged, to control lipid levels, to increase carbohydrate tolerance, and perhaps to control body weight and composition.

THYROID DISORDERS

Alterations in thyroid function are responsible for a significant amount of morbidity and mortality among the elderly. Investigations suggest that although some changes in either structure or function of the thyroid gland may be a normal concomitant of aging, others represent pathologic changes. In order to better understand and appreciate abnormal function, a brief review of normal metabolism in the aging thyroid follows. Excellent reviews of the subject have been published.[52-54]

The weight of the thyroid, as determined by autopsy studies, is less in elderly subjects than in young persons. Microscopically this is seen as smaller follicles containing less colloid. There is also an increase in the amount of fibrous tissue.

Controversy continues with respect to the extent of change in thyroid function with aging. Some of the difficulties have arisen because although elderly subjects have been studied, they frequently were obtained from among hospitalized patients and therefore had associated illnesses. It has recently been recognized that acute and chronic diseases alter thyroid function tests without the presence of legitimate thyroidal disease, producing the "euthyroid sick." Furthermore, some investigators have described differing effects in men and women related to aging.

The uptake of ^{131}I has been shown to decrease with age. This has been attributed to a decrease in renal iodine clearance, resulting in increased plasma iodine levels rather than altered thyroid function per se. Alternatively the decrease in urinary iodine excretion may reflect a decrease in iodine intake. Although not all investigators have found a decrease in absolute iodine uptake, this suggests that not as much thyroid hormone is synthesized in the old as in the young.

Plasma levels of thyroxine have been found to be either normal or lower in the elderly (unless they are hospitalized and presumably have other illness) but there is a 50 per cent decrease in the metabolic clearance rate of thyroxine from age 20 to 80. Therefore, the presumed decrease in hormonal synthesis may be compensatory for a prolonged plasma half-life. Altered turnover rates might be due to decreased levels of free thyroxine, but measurement of free thyroxine as a free thyroxine index or by dialysis has shown either no change with age or an increase in men 70 to 90 years of age. Although thyroid binding globulin may be increased in the elderly, the total amount of bound thyroxine remains unchanged because of a decrease in binding to thyroid binding prealbumin.[55] An alternative mechanism for decreased thyroxine degradation is a decrease in the distribution space or perhaps a decrease in the number of degradation sites that occurs with age.

Thyroxine (T_4) undergoes deiodination peripherally to form triiodothyronine (T_3). T_3

has been considered by many to be responsible for most, if not all, of the metabolic effects of thyroid hormones. Plasma levels of total T_3 show a progressive decrease in men 60 to 89 years of age—but in women only after age 80—compared with healthy men and women aged 20 to 59 years. Unbound T_3, estimated by a free triiodothyronine index or measured by dialysis, shows a similar age related decline, which differs in men and women. Yet despite these decreases, there is little to suggest that healthy elderly people are hypothyroid.

One of the tests believed to be the most sensitive available for the detection of primary hypothyroidism is the thyrotropin releasing hormone (TRH) test. In this test the thyroid stimulating hormone response to an intravenous bolus of thyrotropin releasing hormone is measured. A response that is greater than normal is suggestive of primary hypothyroidism or decreased thyroid reserve. Although the thyroid stimulating hormone response is not related to age in women, in men there is a decrease with age. Basal thyroid stimulating hormone levels did not differ in groups of middle aged and elderly subjects, but it was measurable in all old people; it was undetectable in 40 per cent of the middle aged subjects.

Overall evidence, although incomplete, appears to suggest that normal elderly persons have normal thyroid function. The progressive decline in basal oxygen consumption with age may reflect a decrease in cell mass and body water rather than a decrease in metabolism due to otherwise subclinical hypothyroidism.

Hypothyroidism

Because the symptoms of hypothyroidism in the elderly may be very mild or attributed to other diseases or "old age," it is difficult to ascertain its prevalence. Of over 3400 patients seen in a geriatric unit, 1.7 per cent were found to have hypothyroidism.[56] The diagnosis of hypothyroidism was made in 2.9 per cent of 2000 patients on a geriatric inpatient service.[57] The Whickham survey reported a prevalence of 1.4 per cent among women and 0.1 per cent in men, but over 10 per cent of postmenopausal women (not men) had evidence of mild hypothyroidism detected as an increase in the basal thyroid stimulating hormone level.[58] Nearly 6 per cent of elderly persons seen at a senior citizens center were found to have elevated thyroid stimulating hormone levels, over 80 per cent of these being women.

Etiology

The etiologies of hypothyroidism in the elderly are similar to those seen in younger subjects and include iatrogenic causes such as surgical or radioactive iodine therapy for hyperthyroidism or carcinoma, antithyroid drugs, iodine induced hypothyroidism, and iodine deficiency. A frequent cause of spontaneous hypothyroidism is chronic thyroiditis (Hashimoto's thyroiditis). Evidence of this disorder may be obtained by biopsy of thyroid tissue or measurement of thyroid autoantibody levels (antimicrosomal or antithyroglobulin antibodies). Rarely hypothyroidism is the result of pituitary insufficiency.

Clinical Presentation

The symptoms of hypothyroidism may be so mild and so gradual in onset that they are easily overlooked. One of the common presentations is a nonspecific decrease in mobility and general health. Other central nervous system presentations include cerebellar ataxia and lethargy. Coma with hypothermia may be precipitated in individuals with long standing hypothyroidism who acquire another illness (usually infection). Deafness may be due to hypothyroidism and may be reversible with replacement therapy.

Myalgias, arthralgias, and generalized stiffness are easily ascribed, by both patient and physician, to aging or may suggest polymyalgia rheumatica. Cold intolerance may be difficult to evaluate in those who are saving money by turning down the thermostat. Peripheral numbness may be due to nerve entrapment in the carpal tunnel or peripheral neuropathy.

Dry skin and peripheral edema without cardiac failure may be prominent features. Scalp hair may become coarse and thin generally or may be lost in patches as alopecia areata. Vitiligo suggests the presence of autoimmune thyroid disease.

Among the cardiac changes, sinus bradycardia is common, but other bradyarrhythmias may occur and cause drop attacks. An increase in blood pressure may occur. Exposure to cold may precipitate peripheral vasospasm, although claudication may be independent of temperature. Physical examination frequently suggests cardiomegaly. This may be due to a combination of chamber dilation and pericardial effusion. Despite the large size of the effusion, it rarely is associated with cardiac tamponade. The patient may experience unexplained dyspnea, but may also have findings resulting from congestive heart failure with pleural effusion.

Constipation is such a common complaint generally among the elderly that hypothyroidism may not be suspected as its etiology. Ascites suggests intraabdominal malignant disease or cirrhosis. Although the appetite may increase or decrease, there may be little change in the body weight.

Hoarseness due to vocal cord edema may prompt referral to an ENT clinic. Sometimes elderly hypothyroid individuals may actually be hyperkinetic and agitated instead of lethargic. Because such a high index of suspicion is required to detect most cases, it may be appropriate to screen elderly subjects for hypothyroidism. The prevalence of thyroid failure appears to be especially high in elderly women with type I insulin dependent diabetes mellitus.

The diagnosis is suspected by the clinical symptoms. Physical findings such as bradycardia, thinning of the lateral eyebrows, myxedematous thickened skin, and a slow relaxation of deep tendon reflexes increase suspicion further. Unlike younger patients with hypothyroidism who usually have goiters, in the elderly the thyroid gland may not be palpable. Because these findings are not entirely reliable and are frequently absent, the diagnosis must be confirmed by appropriate laboratory studies. An elevated basal serum thyroid stimulating hormone level in association with decreased levels of thyroxine and triiodothyronine and a measure of protein binding (such as the T_3 resin uptake) is virtually diagnostic of primary hypothyroidism. In milder cases it may be helpful to do a thyrotropin releasing hormone test. An increased response may suggest decreased thyroidal reserve and, at the very least, identify the patient as being at risk for future development of hypothyroidism. Whether such an individual with decreased reserve but no other evidence of hypothyroidism should receive prompt treatment is controversial. In the elderly patient who is ill with another disease, the diagnosis of hypothyroidism may not be as straightforward.

Therapy

Two aspects of therapy for hypothyroidism will be considered—first, the effect of treatment on associated diseases and, second, the choice of the type of therapy.

Patients with hypothyroidism frequently have secondary hyperlipidemias; cholesterol level elevation is the most common, but hypertriglyceridemia or elevation of the levels of both lipids is also not unusual. These abnormalities predispose elderly hypothyroid patients to accelerated atherosclerosis, which may result in symptomatic or asymptomatic cardiovascular disease. Thyroid hormone has profound effects on the heart; it increases the heart rate and myocardial contractility. The increase in cardiac output that occurs after the administration of thyroid hormone in a patient with coronary artery disease may result in the precipitation or exacerbation of angina. It has been recommended that increases in the thyroid hormone dosage be more gradual in patients known to have cardiovascular disease. Infrequently angina may improve with the administration of increasing amounts of thyroid hormone, but usually angina is worsened. The addition of propranolol and nitrates to the therapeutic regimen may permit an increase in the thyroid hormone dosage. In many patients, despite combination therapy, it is not possible to control both angina and hypothyroidism satisfactorily. Furthermore, propranolol may worsen bradycardia, and the vasodilatory effects of nitroglycerin may be exaggerated in hypothyroid patients, with the production of syncope.

Evaluation and possible therapy of coronary artery disease in the presence of hypothyroidism have been considered hazardous. The sedatives, tranquilizers, and analgesics used during coronary angiography may have a prolonged duration of action and a heightened effect in hypothyroidism. Furthermore untreated myxedematous patients are prone to develop intraoperative cardiovascular collapse, postoperative respiratory depression, ileus, and inappropriate antidiuretic hormone secretion with hyponatremia. Yet the absence of better alternatives to angiography and surgery has prompted several investigators to evaluate this form of therapy in hypothyroid patients. Of four patients who had vascular grafts, none had intraoperative or perioperative complications.[59] It may, in fact, be more dangerous to delay surgery until adequate levels of thyroid hormone are achieved. Four of seven patients sustained their first myocardial infarction while receiving therapy with thyroid hormone.[60] Furthermore, there was no difference in operative morbidity or mortality in those who underwent coronary artery surgery before thyroxine therapy compared with those who were operated on after several months of therapy.

Another complication that may occur with hypothyroidism is myxedema coma. This is an endocrine emergency, because during coma the patient is susceptible to the development of aspiration pneumonia as well as malnutrition and potential abnormalities in fluid and electrolyte balance. Attention should be directed toward possible precipitating factors of the coma, such as pneumonia. Passive rewarming with blankets in a warm room is recommended for hypothermia, which, if severe enough, may predispose the patient to cardiac arrhythmias. Active rewarming with heating pads may cause hypotension because of the intravascular volume depletion. Alternatively, intravenous fluids or blood may be warmed prior to administration. Thyroxine therapy, using a large intravenous dose (420 to 750 μg.) initially followed by 100 to 200 μg. daily, was found to be associated with no complications.[61] Electrocardiograms and creatine phosphokinase measurements showed no evidence of cardiac ischemia or infarction during therapy. There was a more rapid response in the serum T_4 and thyroid stimulating hormone levels and basal metabolic rate in the group receiving larger amounts of thyroxine than in those receiving the smaller amount.

The cortisol response to stress, as measured by insulin hypoglycemia, is less than normal in hypothyroidism. It is therefore recommended that the patient receive corticosteroid supplements (100 mg. of hydrocortisone or the equivalent) for at least several days until he is alert. Obviously other disorders such as infection and electrolyte abnormalities should be treated simultaneously.

There are numerous preparations of thyroid hormone available for the treatment of hypothyroidism. Thyroid extract from bovine and porcine glands continues to be available today. The content of thyroxine varies according to the species, the season, and the availability of iodine in the animal's diet. The amount of iodine in each batch is regulated by law, but the amount of thyroxine or triiodothyronine or their ratio is not. For these reasons, desiccated thyroid has largely been replaced as the therapy of choice.

Synthetic preparations of thyroxine and triiodothyronine have avoided many of the concerns just noted. When it was noted that both T_4 and T_3 are found in the circulation, it was thought important to include both hormones in replacement preparations. Combinations in which the ratio of $T_4:T_3$ varied from 4:1 to 9:1 were developed. More recently, however, it was discovered that most (80 per cent) of circulating T_3 is derived from peripheral deiodination of T_4 rather than from thyroidal secretion. Athyreotic individuals maintained only on thyroxine had normal serum levels of both T_4 and T_3. Combination tablets may not only be unnecessary but also undesirable. Following ingestion of T_3, rapid absorption results in an unphysiologic peak in the serum and a gradual decline as it is metabolized and redistributed. These peaks and their potential for producing myocardial toxicity are avoided by the administration of only thyroxine.

Triiodothyronine is useful in determining thyroidal autonomy—as in the T_3 suppression test. It may also be required in patients who have a rare enzyme defect in which they are unable to deiodinate T_4 to form T_3. Other than these indications, because of its short half-life and greater cost, T_3 should not be used for long term replacement therapy.

L-Thyroxine is absorbed better in the fasting state (79 versus 68 per cent in the nonfasting state). Absorption is decreased in patients with malabsorption syndromes or in those taking cholestyramine. Triiodothyronine is more completely absorbed.

Several studies have addressed the question of how much thyroid hormone, as L-thyroxine, is sufficient yet not excessive to produce a euthyroid status. Cotton et al. treated 21 patients with increments of 0.025 mg. of L-thyroxine at three week intervals.[62] They found that serum T_4 and thyroid stimulating hormone levels were normalized with total dosages between 0.15 and 0.2 mg. daily. Stock et al. did a similar study in 44 patients and found that the dose of L-thyroxine that suppressed the serum thyroid stimulating hormone level to normal was weight related.[63] At a dosage of 2.25 μg. per kg., serum T_3 levels were slightly less than in age matched controls while T_4 levels were slightly higher. The age of those studied was 50 ± 13 years, and the group did not include large numbers of elderly people. A recent study by Rosenbaum of 23 subjects with a mean age of 75.7 years compared the replacement dose required with that in a younger group with a mean age of 48 years.[64] The older subjects required significantly less L-thyroxine to achieve the same levels of T_4 and thyroid stimulating hormone than the younger group (1.86 µg. per kg. versus 2.06 µg per kg.). This decrease in replacement dose may reflect the decrease in turnover that occurs with age.

A method that may be used to treat hypothyroidism in the elderly once the diagnosis has been firmly established is as follows:

If the patient is otherwise stable, one begins with oral dosages of 0.025 or 0.050 mg. of L-thyroxine daily. Increments of 0.025 mg. may be added at three to four week intervals. Adequacy of therapy should be judged by clinical evaluation as well as periodic measurement of serum thyroid stimulating hormone and T_4 levels. The final dosage will be approximately 1.85 to 2.25 µg. per kg. body weight.

If the patient develops or experiences an exacerbation of angina, the dosage should be decreased to the previous level. Consideration might be appropriately made at that time about the possibility of coronary artery bypass surgery.

In the patient with myxedema coma, an intravenous dose of L-thyroxine, 400 to 700 µg. should be given as an initial dose, with 100 to 200 µg. daily continued intravenously until the patient is able to continue a similar dosage orally. Corticosteroid therapy should also be given, as discussed earlier.

Hyperthyroidism

Because of the lack of "classic" findings, the diagnosis of hyperthyroidism may not be suspected among the elderly, despite the fact that the elderly may account for 9 to 17 per cent of all recognized cases. The prevalence of hyperthyroidism is about one-fifth or less that of hypothyroidism—4 per 1000—although in the Whickham survey, approximately equal numbers had hyperthyroidism as had hypothyroidism.[58] The Whickham survey was a population study and was not limited to elderly subjects.

Etiology

Hyperthyroidism in the elderly is usually due to diffuse goiter (Graves' disease) or toxic nodular goiter. Classic or painless subacute thyroiditis should also be considered. Iatrogenic or factitious hyperthyroidism, a single nodule, ectopic elaboration of thyroid stimulating hormone, and functioning thyroid carcinoma are less common causes of the clinical syndrome. About two-thirds of the patients have a nodular goiter with most of the remaining patients having a diffuse goiter.[65]

Clinical Presentation

The clinical presentation may not suggest hyperthyroidism at all. Rather than being hyperkinetic, as occurs among young hyperthyroid patients, the elderly subject may be listless and lethargic, a syndrome defined as apathetic hyperthyroidism. In some patients cardiovascular symptoms may predominate, whereas others have gastrointestinal or emotional symptoms. These differences in presentation appear to be due less to the etiology of the hyperthyroidism than to the age of the patient when he develops the disease. This may be due in part to associated diseases. Over half the elderly patients over 60 who have hyperthyroidism also have hypertension.

Although cardiac complaints may be the presenting or primary symptoms in both old and young patients, the type of symptom differs markedly between them. In one study all 48 hyperthyroid patients 20 to 29 years of age had palpitations, whereas only 60 per cent of those 50 to 78 years of age experienced this symptom.[66] Despite this, 22 per cent of a group over age 60 had congestive heart failure compared with only 2 per cent in a younger group. Atrial fibrillation occurs in 13 to 39 per cent of elderly hyperthyroid subjects. Yet tachycardia is frequently absent in elderly patients; the heart rate is less than 100 per minute in 42 per cent and less than 80 in 11 per cent. Evaluation of elderly patients who present with atrial fibrillation and few or no signs of hyperthyroidism should include thyroid function tests. Ten of 75 patients presenting in this way were found to be hyperthyroid, with reversion to sinus rhythm after therapy for hyperthyroidism occurring in three subjects.[67]

Symptoms of nervousness, tremor, heat intolerance, lack of energy, diarrhea, and muscle weakness were all noted more frequently among young than in old patients, although they are common in both groups.

Gastrointestinal symptoms may predominate in the elderly.[68] Although increased appetite is nearly the rule in young hyperthyroid subjects, anorexia is often present in those over age 60. Weight loss in the elderly may be impressive: it is present in approximately 75 per cent and is over 10 kg. in about 50 per cent. Although increased numbers of bowel movements occurred in 24 per cent, an equal number of patients had constipation. The combination of anorexia, weight loss, and constipation, which is suggestive of carcinoma, was present in 15 per cent.

The tremor that occurs in many elderly hyperthyroid subjects may be ascribed to "old age." Emotional disorders may be a presenting and single finding, "thyroid melancholia" with depression and paranoia responding to antithyroid therapy.

In some cases of hyperthyroidism the presenting features may be bizarre and include acute abdomen, osteoporosis, severe myopathy, confusion, or seizures. Optic neuritis may occur with Graves' disease, and thrombocytopenia may be a presenting feature with the presence of petechiae and ecchymoses.

Although a goiter is present in nearly all patients age 20 to 29 with hyperthyroidism, the thyroid is not palpable in over one-third of elderly subjects.[66] Elderly patients with subacute thyroiditis present in a similar manner with weight loss, depression, and palpitations.

In summary, the clinical presentation of the elderly patient with hyperthyroidism may be so atypical that it requires an astute clinician to suspect it.

Confirming the diagnosis may be difficult and requires laboratory testing. In one study clinical improvement and normalization of tests were evaluated after therapy.[69] Serum triiodothyronine values were normal in 34 per cent, and radioactive iodine uptake was normal in 41 per cent of elderly hyperthyroid patients. The serum thyroxine level and the free thyroxine index were the most consistently abnormal test results. Another study found that free T_4 levels were not different in young and elderly subjects.[70] This suggests that measurement of the serum thyroxine level as well as an estimate of protein binding, such as T_3 resin uptake, would be most appropriate to confirm the diagnosis. In some cases it may be necessary to do a thyrotropin releasing hormone test. If the thyroid is functioning autonomously, there will be no increase in the serum thyroid stimulating hormone level after the bolus of thyrotropin releasing hormone. Measurement of radioactive iodine uptake will assist in differentiating subacute thyroiditis with very low uptake from Graves' disease, which is characterized by a normal or increased iodine uptake. Patients with subacute thyroiditis also have an elevated erythrocyte sedimentation rate. Thyroid biopsy may clarify the diagnosis further but is rarely necessary. The presence of more unusual forms of hyperthyroidism requires specific testing.

Therapy

Therapeutic options in hyperthyroidism include radioactive iodine or surgical ablation, antithyroid drugs, or symptomatic therapy. Combinations of these are also frequently used. Therapy must be individualized, considering not only the type of thyroid disease but also the general condition of the patient. Graves' hyperthyroidism with diffuse thyroid involvement is best treated with radioactive iodine. The dose deemed appropriate varies among clinicians, depending on whether the aim is to maintain a euthyroid state or to render the patient hypothyroid. The amount of iodine to be given is calculated by measuring the 24 hour radioactive iodine uptake, estimating the weight of the gland by palpation, and then giving the desired amount (μCi per gram of tissue). This amount ranges from 50 to 100 μCi per gram to considerably more if hypothyroidism is desired. Radioactive iodine therapy has very few side effects and is well tolerated. A rare complication is thyroid storm, which may occur within one to two weeks after therapy and is due to release of stored thyroid hormone from the gland. A mild transient exacerbation of hyperthyroidism may occur at this time instead of the severe form. In order to prevent possible cardiovascular complications at this time, some physicians pretreat patients with antithyroid drugs for several months to deplete the glandular stores of hormones. In any case the patient should be evaluated following radioiodine treatment at four to six week intervals in the expectation that the effect of therapy will become apparent in four weeks and be complete by approximately three months. If necessary, retreatment may be given at this time.

In patients with toxic nodular goiter, opinion is divided as to whether surgery or radioactive iodine ablation is the treatment of choice. Proponents of surgery argue that because uptake of iodine within the gland is irregular, multiple or very large doses of radioactive iodine are often required to achieve cure. Concern is expressed that this may make the patient more susceptible to disorders due to radiation exposure (e.g., blood dyscrasias and thyroid carcinoma). Although this is a possibility, it does not appear to be a major concern—perhaps because elderly subjects have a shorter life span in which to develop delayed effects. Radioiodine would be the apparent treatment of choice in the elderly patient who is medically unfit or unwilling to undergo surgery.

Surgical removal of the thyroid has been used for many years to treat hyperthyroidism. The mortality due to thyroid surgery is 5 to 10 per cent above age 60 and increases to 20 per cent over age 70. Others have found that the mortality from thyroid surgery for hyperthyroidism in a group of patients over age 60 was only 2.5 per cent without pretreatment with propylthiouracil, and it was decreased to 0.8 per cent after propylthiouracil therapy. Hypothyroidism is a significant complication of subtotal thyroidectomy; of 100 patients followed after surgery for Graves' disease, 75 were hypothyroid within five months.[71] Because the therapy for hypothyroidism is relatively simple, this may not be viewed as a significant problem. Surgery is the therapy of choice if a goiter is causing obstruction—dysphagia or tracheal compression—or if there is concern about possible malignant disease.

Antithyroid drugs such as propylthiouracil and methimazole (Tapazole) are useful in achieving a euthyroid state prior to surgery or radioactive iodine in order to avoid exacerbation of cardiac symptoms. Both drugs inhibit incorporation of iodine and block coupling of monoiodothyronine and diiodothyronine. Propylthiouracil, but not methimazole, inhibits peripheral T_4 deiodination with a resultant decrease in circulating T_3 levels. Although the plasma half-life of propylthiouracil is two hours, and six to 13 hours for methimazole, both drugs appear to be concentrated within the thyroid and to have a much longer biologic half-life. The side effects of both drugs are usually minor and include skin rash, stiff joints, paresthesias, headache, nausea, and hair loss. Rarely fever, hepatitis, and nephritis may occur. The life threatening side effect of both drugs is agranulocytosis, which is seen in 0.44 per cent of the patients taking propylthiouracil and in 0.12 per cent of those taking methimazole. This appears to be an idiosyncratic reaction and cannot be predicted by periodic measurement of white blood cell counts. The dose of propylthiouracil is 75 to 100 mg. orally every eight hours, with up to 900 mg. used daily for thyroid storm. Methimazole is given in doses of 5 to 10 mg. every eight to 12 hours. It has been suggested that a single dose of methimazole may be as effective.

This regimen will achieve a euthyroid state in most patients within two to three months. If not, compliance may not be adequate, the dose interval should be decreased, or the dose should be increased.

Although antithyroid drug therapy may be given to induce a remission in younger subjects, this is probably not practical in most older subjects with Graves' disease because of a low remission rate. These drugs are ordinarily used in pretreatment for either surgical or radioiodine thyroid ablation.

Iodine is another antithyroid drug. The primary physiologic effect of iodine is to inhibit the release of thyroid hormone from thyroglobulin. It has therefore been used primarily to attain a rapid decrease in symptoms, such as in thyroid storm. The other major use is to decrease the vascularity of the thyroid gland prior to surgery. This aspect of increased vascularity may be less important than initially suspected, because surgery has been performed for hyperthyroidism using only propranolol as preoperative preparation with no operative or postoperative complications. Iodine is given as a saturated solution of potassium iodide, 5 to 10 drops in a glass of water once daily. This dose of iodine is probably excessive. It should be given after antithyroid drugs, because otherwise the gland will be overloaded with iodine, which may be subsequently used for new hormone synthesis.

Propranolol (Inderal), a nonselective beta blocking drug, has been useful in treating the tachycardia, stare, tremor, and anxiety of hyperthyroid patients. It has been used either alone, with iodine, or with antithyroid drugs in preparing patients for surgery.[72] The metabolism of propranolol is altered with hyperthyroidism, aging, and smoking. There is a positive correlation between plasma propranolol levels and age in both hyperthyroid and euthyroid patients; thus the dose may need to be modified, depending on these factors as well. Generally beta blocking drugs should be avoided in patients with asthma or in diabetics who are taking either insulin or orally administered hypoglycemic drugs. Caution should also be exercised in its use in elderly hyperthyroid patients with congestive heart failure. Propranolol has largely replaced reserpine, guanethidine, or alpha methyldopa in treating the sympathetic manifestations of hyperthyroidism. Additionally, it blocks the peripheral conversion of T_4 to T_3 and may be useful as a single drug in the treatment of mild hyperthyroidism. It is the therapy of choice for the transient hyperthyroidism of subacute thyroiditis. The dose must be modified according to patient response. An initial dosage of 20 mg. every six or eight hours may be increased as needed.

Other drugs such as lithium carbonate have not become popular because of the narrow therapeutic window. This drug is concentrated within the thyroid gland, interferes with the action of thyroid stimulating hormone on the gland, impairs thyroid hormone synthesis, and interferes with hormone release.

OBESITY

Unlike the majority of the world's population who must consider whether they and their family will have enough to eat, and among whom starvation still occurs, Americans suffer from the opposite form of malnutrition—obesity. Obesity contributes to an increased morbidity and mortality from various diseases as well as being costly in terms of personal happiness. Although the effect of obesity on health may decrease with age, the elderly are certainly not immune from its deleterious effects.

In this section possible etiologies of obesity, its complications, and various approaches to therapy are considered.

Definition

Although looking casually at an individual will give the observer the impression that the subject is fat or obese, the use of such terms in this context is imprecise and of little scientific value. Furthermore, weight measurement is also insufficient. The professional weight lifter may be overweight by most commonly used criteria, yet most would agree that he is not overfat; rather the increase in weight is due to increased muscle mass. Another example is the sedentary elderly person who weighs the same amount that he did at age 20 when he played rugby. Although his weight has remained constant, muscle has been replaced by fat, and he is probably at least overfat if not frankly obese.

The social definitions of desirable body weight are directed toward what is personally, sexually, or by other criteria a weight or build thought to be most attractive. This obviously depends on the age and social position as well as ethnic inheritance of the individual. For example, in Western countries, with increasing socioeconomic affluence, body weight decreases; in developing countries, however, weight may increase with improvement in social status. Among agricultural or lower socioeconomic communities in developed countries, body weight is relatively greater. These observations suggest that social or economic and cultural influences are very important determinants of body weight. Such considerations may be of great importance to the individual, but obesity is usually defined in terms that consider an increase in medical complications. There is further difficulty with this, however, because use of the same criteria to define obesity in different countries has illustrated that the risks are not the same.

In order to obtain information about large numbers of people and to determine the incidence of obesity as well as its complications, it is desirable to use the simplest measurements possible. Two that are easily obtained are height and weight. The relationship of these variables to obesity has been evaluated by several investigators. Researchers have determined the amount of body fat by several methods, among them weighing the subject submerged in water and comparing this weight with that obtained conventionally. Body fat and lean muscle mass can be then quantitated by considering their different densities. Since about half the total body fat is subcutaneous, the measurement of skin fold thickness may be useful in estimating the content of body fat. Measurements are complicated by the recent observation that fat distributed in the lower body segment may have a less deleterious effect than upper body fatness. Newer methodologies using computed tomographic scanning, sonography, or nuclear magnetic resonance may improve measurement in the future, but these by their nature are not useful for epidemiologic studies.

As noted, obesity is poorly defined. Keys et al. found the best correlation between body fat and the weight/height—the so-called body mass index (BMI).[73] Others have used $\sqrt[3]{W/H}$ (ponderal index) or the log of the skinfold thickness as correlating best with body density.[74] In using the body mass index, with weight measured in kilograms and height in meters, a value above 24.2 for women and 25.0 in men is defined as indicating overweight, and a value above 29.2 in both men and women is defined as indicating obesity.[75]

Much of the confusion regarding ideal weight stems from the method by which such values were derived. Early data are taken primarily from insurance company information in which the death rate among those insured was found to have a positive correlation with body weight. Recent observations have disputed these conclusions and have noted little or no increased risk among those in the mildly overweight category. It appears that those who were insured were not representative of the population at large and that the curve relating risk of death related to weight actually is U shaped; that is, there is increased mortality at both ends—both fat and thin—but not a direct linear relationship as the insurance company had found. Part of this U shape may be due to the inclusion of smokers in the lower weight group. Those who smoke are known to be more susceptible to many diseases, yet they are thinner than the average of the population. The nadir of death rates from all causes appears to occur at weights 12 to 19 per cent over "ideal" body weight.

These findings, like a redefinition of diabetes, have effectively "cured" many elderly persons of obesity. Even so, a significant number of elderly subjects are left in the obese category. The frequency of obesity is less among the elderly than in the middle aged—perhaps because those affected do not attain old age. This also may be the reason that the contribution of obesity to disease decreases with age. Among a group of 100 subjects examined from senior centers in Oregon with a mean age of 74 years, half were 20 per cent or more over the ideal weight.[76] A long term prospective study was conducted by enrollment of 750,000 persons by volunteers for the American Cancer Society.[77] Those over age 30 were questioned and followed by repeat questionnaires or death certificates. Of the men over age 60, 6 to 9 per cent were 120 per cent or more over the ideal body weight. Ten to 14 per cent of the women over age 60 were obese. This study found a tendency for less obesity with an increased level of education; women with more years of schooling tended to be underweight.

Etiology

Obesity reflects the storage of excess calories as fat. In a simplistic consideration then, obesity may be concluded to reflect an imbalance between energy intake and energy expenditure. An increase in energy intake or a decreased expenditure would, in this model, result in a similar positive energy balance.

In nonobese persons, energy intake matches output quite closely over a long period of time. The regulation is not quite perfect because there is a gradual increase in weight with age. Furthermore, in normal subjects there is a marked day to day variation in calorie consumption, which involves changes in appetite regulation. Appetite is perceived as a desire to obtain and consume food. It may be directed toward a specific food or a general hunger. Appetite and satiety may not be opposite terms, although in most circumstances they are used in this manner. Satiety may actually be perceived as a desire to avoid food or eating. Food consumption involves not only the appetite; eating may be further divided into eating rate as well as duration of eating. These aspects may involve different regulatory mechanisms.

The involvement of the central nervous system in the control of eating has been known since the discovery of the "satiety center" in the ventromedial hypothalamus and the "feeding center" in the lateral hypothalamus. Electrical stimulation of these areas results in starvation owing to lack of intake or hyperphagia and obesity, respectively. Since these initial observations, however, it has been noted that things are not so simple with only a dual control system. There is an additional contribution into each of these areas from much of the central nervous system. Both serotonergic and adrenergic systems are involved; increased serotonin levels promote decreased food intake primarily by decreasing the duration of eating. Increased catecholamine stimulation decreases food intake in animals by impairment in the initiation of eating behavior. These differing effects may be noted with the use of various anorectic drugs to be considered later.

The stimuli that influence the sensations of hunger or satiety may arise from either the cerebral cortex or the periphery. Those from the cerebral cortex may involve visual or other sensory receptors (smell or taste). Various other central nervous system stimuli such as pain, stress, or anxiety may also stimulate eating by an unknown mechanism.

Interesting observations considering the possible existence of peripheral hormone-like substances have come from parabiotic animal studies. Parabiotic animals have been connected surgically so that the peritoneal surface is in contact, but both animals can eat in a normal fashion. If one animal is fed through a gastrostomy to the point of obesity, the other becomes thin through decreased intake of readily available food.[78] Several substances have been nominated as being responsible for this effect—among them insulin, cholecystokinin, and other small peptides. Release of such a substance would be stimulated by food intake with the net result of impaired intake—a negative feedback loop. This may account for the decrease in the rate of eating that occurs during a meal. The infusion of insulin into the cerebral ventricles decreases food intake, and this has been postulated to be the active agent. In theory, the increased insulin that occurs after a mixed meal would diffuse into the central nervous system and inhibit eating. Although this may occur to some extent, central nervous system insulin levels appear to vary independently of serum levels. Genetically obese mice have high basal serum insulin levels, yet their brain insulin concentration is similar to that of their thin counterparts.

Another theory of weight and appetite regulation involves a signal of some kind that mediates the status of fat stores. Persons who are either starved or force-fed to an abnormal weight will, when allowed to eat ad libitum, gain or lose weight to their original starting weight. Among possible signals, glycerol has been implicated. The mobilization of fat results in an increase in circulating glycerol and free fatty acids, making the level of circulating glycerol a possible measure of the status of the total body fat. In fact, infusion of glycerol in rats results in a decreased food intake beyond that expected due to its caloric content. Similar results have been obtained in humans: a group given glycerol ate less than a placebo treated control group.[79]

Cholecystokinin (a gastrointestinal hormone) has been postulated to be involved as a hormone that regulates appetite. The intravenous infusion of a C-terminal octapeptide of cholecystokinin resulted in a decrease in food intake in men of normal weight.[80]

Endorphins in the central nervous system have also been implicated in appetite control. Studies in which genetically obese animals were treated with naloxone, an opiate antagonist, suggested a role for these drugs. The animals treated with the antagonist lost weight as compared with the control group of animals.[81] One possible explanation for these findings is that in obese, and perhaps nonobese individuals, eating results in a release of endorphins, which in turn reinforces eating behavior. The block at the receptor level impairs reinforcement and reduces the behavior.

We have postulated that the fiber content of food and the amount of insulin it stimulates may be of importance in the generation and maintenance of obesity.[82] A useful animal model of obesity simulates the circumstances in free-living humans. The animals, given free access to a variety of foods that have a high caloric density, gain weight by overeating by 30 to 50 per cent compared with their littermates who eat standard chow. One postulate might be that high calorie foods stimulate insulin secretion more than chow. The rapid peak and fall of the glucose level promotes relative reactive hypoglycemia, which once again stimulates hunger and food intake, resulting in obesity. The increased insulin levels also promote storage of excess calories as fat. If the diet is changed to one high in fiber, there is less insulin response—perhaps because fiber causes a slowing of absorption or a translocation to more distal intestinal sites. More distal absorption might decrease insulin secretion because of less gastric inhibitory polypeptide release; this intestinal substance, thought to be a local hormone that stimulates insulin release, is most concentrated in the upper small intestine. Much of the carbohydrate of high fiber foods may be metabolized in the colon to free fatty acids, which may be absorbed without stimulating insulin release.

High fiber foods, because of their lower caloric density, may also require more energy in chewing and intestinal transit than low fiber foods. The effect of their bulk may increase the sensation of satiety if the distention of the stomach is important. That this may play a role has been suggested by the results of gastric plication procedures. Substitution of the "usual" American diet (high in fat and sugar but low in fiber) with one that is high in carbohydrate and fiber may reverse these effects. Some support for this theory comes from epidemiologic studies in which societies that consume high fiber diets have a low occurrence of "Western" diseases, such as obesity and diabetes.

A third theory of metabolic regulation involves thermogenesis. Both animals and humans, if overfed, gain less weight than would be expected from the caloric content of the food. This excess energy is lost in heat production. It has been postulated that obese subjects are able to utilize energy more efficiently than thin people, and therefore any excessive energy consumed would be stored as fat rather than burned and lost as heat.

It has been considered that one of the effects of heat production is to maintain a normal body temperature despite changes in ambient temperature. Marked changes in metabolic rate are associated with changes in body temperature that occur in hibernating animals. In such animals, and perhaps man, much of the change in heat production is due to changes in activity of brown adipose tissue. It has been suggested that this system is responsible for the ability of some persons to eat excessively without a change in weight; the increased energy intake is burned as heat. If an individual has inherited a "thrifty trait" that enables him to conserve energy by regulating heat production, in times of plenty this would make him liable to develop obesity.

Metabolic processes are required to maintain the integrity of an organism; these include protein synthesis and the energy required by the Na^+K^+-ATPase pump, which maintains the gradient across cell membranes by extruding sodium from the interior of cells. Abnormalities of this pump have been noted in red cells of obese subjects; a decreased number of pump units was correlated with the degree of obesity as well as increased intracellular sodium.[83] This pump accounts for 20 to 50 per cent of the total cellular thermogenesis and if significantly impaired could account for the increased energy available for storage. Another group found, however, that there was a negative correlation between enzyme activity and the body mass index in liver tissue from control and obese subjects. These studies indicate that enzyme activity may differ among various body tissues, and findings in one tissue may not apply to the organism as a whole. Several of these thermogenic mechanisms are regulated by thyroid hormone or catecholamines. During overfeeding there is an increase in T_3 production, while reverse T_3 increases during starvation. Catecholamines also increase with overfeeding. Although obese subjects may not produce increased amounts of T_3 and catecholamines with overnutrition, as do nonobese, there is as yet little objective evidence to support this speculation.

Following ingestion of a meal, there is an increase in heat production called diet induced thermogenesis. Examination of this phenomenon in obese and normal men after sucrose and glucose ingestion showed no difference between the groups.[84] Furthermore, although sucrose appears to cause a larger amount of weight increase than a comparable amount of glucose, this was not accounted for by differences between glucose and sucrose in diet induced thermogenesis in either normal or obese subjects.

The second half of the equation of energy balance involves energy expenditure. Do fat people expend less energy than thin ones? Although it may seem by casual observation that obese people are less physically active, this actually may not be so. Because more energy is expended in moving the extra weight of fat for the same amount of activity (e.g., walking a mile), the obese person uses more calories. Furthermore, his resting metabolic rate is higher than that in a thin person. Measurements of the resting metabolic rate in moderately and very obese young people have found it to be increased compared with a normal weight control group. This is perhaps indicative that although obese persons have excess fat, they also have increased muscle mass (perhaps required to carry the additional weight). Despite the lack of evidence that obese persons expend less energy than normal, abnormalities in thyroid hormone metabolism have been frequently implicated to explain the increase in weight.

Short term (three weeks) overfeeding causes an increase in the serum T_3 level and a decrease in the reverse T_3. There is an increase in the production and clearance of T_3 but no change in T_4 levels. These changes are independent of whether carbohydrate, protein, or fat is used as the source of excess calories. Long term maintenance of weight in overfed subjects has shown that the T_3 level is higher in those fed carbohydrate than in those fed high fat diets. Conversely, starvation in both obese and thin subjects results in a decrease in T_3 while the reverse T_3 increases. This effect can be nullified by small amounts of dietary carbohydrate (50 gm.).

It is apparent from these studies that the state of the obese person—gaining or losing weight—as well as the particular diet being consumed, is of great importance in evaluating the status of thyroid function. In the nondieting obese, serum levels of T_4, T_3, and reverse T_3 are not different from those in normal subjects; free T_4 and free T_3 levels likewise are similar, and the normal thyroid stimulating hormone response to thyrotropin releasing hormone indicates that the hypothalamic-pituitary axis is normal.

Obese subjects require large amounts of calories in order to maintain their weight. If they are forced to consume less calories, weight is lost. Despite this, when the same patients are followed as outpatients, they may no longer lose weight despite their claims to be following the diet. One of the problems may be errors in estimating either portion size or caloric content. This was demonstrated in a group of 30 obese dieters: 64 per cent underestimated the quantities of food they consumed and 53 per cent underestimated the caloric content. Those who erred in quantity measurement tended to drop out of the program.[85]

It may be that the weight control mechanism is not as carefully regulated as initially thought. Small errors might be greatly magnified by foods that are calorically dense. Lack of such foods among less industrialized countries may account for the lack of obesity. A change in dietary habits in the population at large, and in obese subjects in particular, to a high carbohydrate, high fiber, low fat diet may be beneficial.

Complications

Although there is little effect of overweight on mortality except at both extremes, some studies have found a deleterious effect. The risk of obesity may be related to the associated factors of hyperlipidemia, glucose intolerance, or frank diabetes or hypertension, which are so common among obese subjects. Because these complications are frequently readily reversible with weight loss, it would seem ill advised not to implicate obesity as being related in some manner.

Obesity, especially if very severe, also causes social problems. In much of the United States obesity is socially undesirable, and the obese may be subjected to personal ridicule and embarrassment. This is not true in all societies; in some African countries potential brides are confined and force-fed to obesity in order to improve their social and financial value. Obesity similarly may be less of a stigma in some segments of American society, especially if it is very common.

Socioeconomically obesity may constitute a liability for advancement. Weight differences in favor of thin people have been shown both in salary levels as well as social position. Despite a vocal effort for "equal rights" by groups representing obese persons, they may be selected against—either initially and openly or subconsciously because of other unattractive traits, such as lack of self-confidence, which is a common accompaniment of obesity.

Concern has been expressed that obese persons may receive less thorough medical evaluation because of technical-mechanical difficulties (e.g., abdominal examination may be very difficult and x-ray examination frequently requires multiple exposures for an adequate examination). Only in computed tomographic evaluation may increased fat mass be beneficial because of increased density differences.

In addition to the social problems of marked obesity, significant medical problems are also more common; among these, coronary artery disease accounts for most of the increase in mortality due to obesity. Although much of this influence, as noted earlier, appears to be of most importance in middle life, the risk continues into older age categories. Among a group of white male employees of the Chicago Peoples Gas Company who were followed for 14 years, those who were 50 to 59 years of age at entry into the study showed an increase in total mortality related to both relative weight and body mass index.[86] In the American Cancer Society's study, among those over 60 years of age there was a 1.2 to 2 times higher mortality rate due to coronary artery disease in those over 120 per cent of the ideal body weight.[77] This rate was increased further in those who smoked.

Keys has found that for the middle 80 per cent of the weight distribution there is little increase in risk, and in middle aged Swedish women the death rate actually correlated negatively with obesity except with marked obesity.[87] Although the death rate for Pima Indians is higher than in the general population, the lowest mortality for this group was at 167 to 190 per cent of the ideal body weight for women and 145 to 176 per cent for men![88] Another study found a relationship between weight and myocardial infarction only among those aged 30 to 39, and angina only in the group aged 40 to 49. These relationships were not noted in older age groups.[89]

The risks of morbid obesity (variously defined as twice the ideal body weight or at least 100 pounds overweight) continue to be important with aging. Those aged 55 to 64 had a 150 per cent excess overall mortality during a seven and one-half year follow-up; this was due primarily to cardiovascular disease.[90] A possible mechanism for this increased risk may relate to circulatory changes. There is a linear increase in blood volume with increases in body weight. Cardiac output increases as do systolic and diastolic blood pressures. Because of pulmonary abnormalities resulting in hypoxemia, the red cell mass increases. The resultant increase in blood viscosity as well as the increase in myocardial work load (due to perfusion of the adipose "organ") may ultimately impair coronary artery flow rates. Coexisting hypertension and hyperlipidemia may increase coronary atherosclerosis, thereby further impairing myocardial perfusion.

Hypertension is related to obesity. This is true in epidemiologic studies, and improvement in hypertension generally occurs with a relatively small (10 kg.) weight loss. The frequency of strokes among those over age 60 is somewhat increased in obese subjects.

Obese subjects may have numerous respiratory problems. As previously noted, oxygen consumption and carbon dioxide production are higher in obese subjects than in normal subjects. The carbon dioxide is excreted in the lungs by increasing ventilation. Increased fat over the thoracic area increases the mechanical work of breathing as a result of less pulmonary compliance; this can be simulated in a thin person by strapping the thorax. Some investigations have noted that the muscles of respiration are either inefficient or dysfunctional. The pattern of breathing that consumes the least energy in an obese subject is a rapid and shallow one.

Obesity is associated with alterations in lung volume; the total lung capacity, functional residual capacity, and vital capacity are all reduced. Hypoxemia results from increased perfusion to dependent portions of the lung, which are not ventilated. These abnormalities are worsened when the supine position is assumed. Another syndrome called the obesity induced hypoventilation or pickwickian syndrome is complicated by a decreased sensitivity to carbon dioxide. This results in somnolence, severe hypoxemia, pulmonary hypertension, and ultimately cardiac failure. This syndrome may not be entirely related to obesity, although the clinical definition includes it. The response to carbon dioxide may be improved by progesterone therapy, suggesting that a central nervous system abnormality may be involved. The pulmonary abnormalities in simple obesity as well as in the pickwickian syndrome make these patients poor anesthesia risks. This risk may be increased further by limited cardiac reserve owing to factors previously mentioned.

Lipid abnormalities are common in obese subjects. Triglyceride synthesis is increased as a result of increased consumption of carbohydrates. Triglyceride levels correlate with various measures of body fat. Although not all investigators consider triglycerides to be an independent risk factor for coronary artery disease, their level correlates inversely with the high density cholesterol level, which is a protective factor. The abnormalities in triglyceride levels may occur more frequently during weight gain than if a steady weight is maintained. Lipid abnormalities may be more common if the upper body segment and abdomen are obese than when the lower body segment is the area primarily involved. This has been reported only among middle aged subjects; thus, whether this is also true among elderly obese cannot be stated.

Some of these abnormalities in lipid metabolism that correlate with obesity actually may be related more to physical fitness than to age. Matching of younger and older subjects for similar maximal aerobic capacity has shown no difference between them.

Diabetes mellitus is two to four times as common among persons over age 60 if they are obese than if they are of normal weight. It accounts for at least twice the mortality rate noted in normals, although its contribution to mortality decreases with age. Morbidly obese subjects had much higher (five to seven times) mortality rates than those less obese. There are alterations in insulin binding in obesity. Diminished red cell and monocyte receptor binding has been reported in association with increased circulating insulin levels. The decrease in numbers of receptors can be reversed in monocytes by brief periods of fasting. No change in receptor numbers on red cells has been noted, however, suggesting there may be a differential effect. Receptor abnormalities may not be primary, and intracellular glucose disposal rates have continued to be decreased despite either pharmacologic doses of insulin or normalization of the glucose tolerance by insulin administration for several days. Fat cells, on the other hand, may have an increased rate of glucose metabolism. The mechanism of the postreceptor abnormalities remains to be clarified but may be reversed with weight loss in some obese subjects. This suggests that they may be secondary to either the obesity itself or the high caloric intake required to maintain it.

Various abnormalities of other endocrine organ functions have been described. In many cases the alterations in serum hormone levels are due to altered turnover rates or protein binding of the hormones, or the state of weight stability or caloric intake, and may not necessarily reflect underlying hormone activity. The thyroidal system has already been described.

The results of plasma cortisol and urinary free cortisol determinations, the cortisol response to insulin and ACTH, the overnight dexamethasone suppression test, and the metyrapone test are usually normal in obese subjects. There is, however, an increased rate of cortisol turnover and a slight increase in ACTH secretion; the result of this is an increase in urinary 17-hydroxycorticosteroids. (This may be corrected by expressing the result in grams of creatinine excreted in the 24 hour urine collection.) 17-Ketosteroid excretion also may be slightly increased in obese persons. Overall, however, the hypothalamic-pituitary-adrenal axis is believed to be normal in simple obesity.

In massive obesity there is an inverse relationship between the serum testosterone level and body weight. In less severely obese men, testicular size and sexual function are normal. There may be a decrease in testosterone-estrogen binding globulin, which results in an increase in the percentage of free testosterone. Luteinizing hormone and follicle stimulating hormone levels are usually normal in the basal state and increase normally after luteinizing hormone–releasing hormone and clomiphene stimulation. Human chorionic gonadotropin results in the expected rise in the plasma testosterone level. The pituitary gonadotropin and testosterone levels may be abnormal in massive obesity—perhaps because of elevated estradiol and estrone levels resulting from increased metabolism of androgens to estrogens in adipose tissue.

Obese women also may have increased estrogen levels. This persistent estrogenic stimulation may be reflected in the increased frequency of uterine carcinoma known to occur.

Growth hormone levels are abnormally low in obese patients following the usual stimulation tests such as insulin or arginine. These responses are normalized following weight loss. They appear to be due only to excessive fat accumulation because they are normal in weight lifters. The administration of growth hormone results in the expected calorigenic and lipolytic effect. Somatomedin levels are normal.

Prolactin regulation appears to be normal; this is also true of the parathyroid gland and renin-angiotensin systems.

Obese subjects have an increased frequency of gallbladder disease, especially gallstones. Surgical morbidity and mortality of cholecystectomy may be significantly higher in the obese because of cardiac and pulmonary abnormalities noted earlier.

It might be hoped that there would be some advantage of obesity because of its ubiquitous nature; it has in fact been called a "thrifty trait." In times of famine an excess of stored calories would enable the obese subject to survive longer than the thin one. This may also be true in some forms of carcinoma, but the increase in frequency of diseases would seem to more than counteract this beneficial effect. Bronchogenic carcinoma occurs more commonly among thin subjects, but this may be related to smaller body weight noted among heavy smokers.

Osteoporosis is most common in thin elderly women; obesity may be protective against osteoporosis because of higher estrogen levels (there is increased estrogen formation in adipose tissue) or because of the mechanical effect of increased muscle tension on the bone required to support excessive weight. There is, however, an increased disability among the obese because of more osteoarthritis in the weight bearing joints, especially the knee and hip.

In sum, although in another society or at another time an increase in body fat may be beneficial, for most people in the United States it is more or less harmful.

Therapy

The therapy of obesity is generally unsatisfactory. An obvious illustration of this fact is the billions of dollars spent annually in diet clubs on formula diets with little in the way of permanent success being achieved. To be "on a diet" is almost the "American way," and interviews have found that it is a rare individual who has not been or is not presently on a diet of some sort. An interview with an obese subject will show the reason for his discouragement: although he has been on multiple diets with perhaps some weight loss, he remains obese. Although obesity is a frustrating disorder, which is resistant to treatment, attempts should continue because of its known deleterious effects on health and longevity.

The various types of therapy to be considered include dietary manipulation (including total or semistarvation), behavior modification (either medically or nonmedically supervised), anorectic medication, exercise therapy, surgical procedures, and new drugs used to inhibit starch absorption or to simulate the taste of fat without its caloric content.

Diet. Total fasting has been used therapeutically to achieve weight loss. The hunger noted on the first several days of such a regimen dissipates and starvation is usually well tolerated. Initially the large amounts of weight lost are accounted for in fluid shifts and volume and electrolyte loss. The rate of weight loss declines, but continues as long as the fast is maintained (3 to 4 kg. per week). The aim of any weight loss therapy is to cause loss of excess adipose tissue while retaining muscle mass. The problem with a fast is that much of the weight lost is actually from the lean body mass. Furthermore, the fluid shifts may be associated with electrolyte abnormalities (hypokalemia and hypomagnesemia especially) and cardiac arrhythmias. Severe hyperuricemia, liver function abnormalities and fatty infiltration, and postural hypotension also may occur. These may be complications not only during the fast but also when the patient is refed. Because of potential complications, such a regimen is best carried out by hospitalization of the patient. This greatly increases the cost and makes it unrealistic except in very unusual circumstances. Such a circumstance may be present in a morbidly obese person who is in urgent need of surgery or in the patient with severe pulmonary compromise who is unable to follow a weight loss regimen on his own. Patients require not only mineral supplements but vitamin replacement as well. Trace mineral deficiencies may also occur during a very prolonged fast.

Because of the problems noted with total starvation, various modifications have been devised. All are characterized by being deficient in calories—some contain primarily protein, others primarily carbohydrate. During fasting it was noted that the amount of protein lost was about 3 to 5 grams of nitrogen daily after the first three to four weeks. Diets devised to prevent this loss were called protein sparing modified fasts. Comparison of this diet with one in which the source of calories was carbohydrate instead of protein but equal in calories showed no difference between the diets with respect to protein loss.[91] In both circumstances it decreased markedly during the first month; by that time both groups of patients were essentially in zero protein balance. A difference between the diets was the much larger loss of sodium and water (with symptomatic postural hypotension) in the group consuming the protein diet.

Various liquid formula diets have also been used: all are calorically deficient. Concern was raised about liquid protein diets when a number of deaths occurred in persons who had lost large amounts of weight while consuming only this diet. The etiology of the deaths was thought to be related to myocardial damage and arrhythmias—perhaps as a result of deficient mineral supplementation with the incomplete protein, which was obtained from a hydrolysate of beef hides. Liquid formula diets such as the Cambridge diet are based on casein as the protein source, contain supplemental vitamins and minerals, and are said to be well tolerated. Patients for whom such diets of 300 to 400 calories daily are prescribed require careful medical supervision. The age of the patient should present no special contraindication for use of such a diet, but because of the frequent presence of underlying heart disease in elderly patients, extreme caution should be exercised.

For the majority of patients who are morbidly obese, less rigorous diets are more realistic. The aim of a dietary regimen is twofold. The first is to achieve the desired weight loss without serious complications. This is relatively easy compared to the second goal—that of maintenance of new weight. In order to achieve both goals, modification of not only the caloric intake but also the abnormal eating behavior found in many obese subjects is of importance.

Behavior Modification. Promoting a change of habits that have been present for 50 or more years in the elderly obese may be extremely difficult and may in part account for the low rate of "cure." Investigators have compared weight loss during therapy and follow-up in groups treated with similar diets but with one group receiving care by a physician and the other by a therapist who also gave instructions to describe and modify behavior.[92] They found that although the initial weight losses were nearly equal, the group receiving behavior therapy gained less weight during the follow-up period. The initial success of this therapy encouraged its adoption by many commercial and self-help weight loss groups. Detailed information is frequently not available from such groups, and results are generally not as spectacular as advertised. The attrition rate may be 70 per cent by 12 weeks. Overall it is estimated that less than 20 per cent achieve their goal weight, with few maintaining the weight loss.[93] One study found that only 48 of 367 persons had lost a mean of 6.2 kg.; 76 were above their initial weight in three years.[94] Persons who elect to participate in such groups or present for medical advice may represent a more refractory group of subjects than those who simply follow a self-prescribed diet. It has been estimated, by interviewing techniques, that at least 60 per cent of a group who weighed at least 15 per cent above their ideal weight had been able to lose at least 10 per cent and maintained that loss for an average of 11 years.[95] Although self-reporting techniques are generally unreliable, this study is somewhat more encouraging than the 5 per cent or less permanent cure rate reported by medical reviewers.[96]

Drugs Affecting Appetite. The use of pharmacologic therapy to promote weight loss is based upon the observations previously noted that serotonin and norepinephrine are important regulators of appetite. Structural modification of these compounds to retain their anorectic effects but eliminate side effects has resulted in the marketing of two groups of drugs. Fenfluramine (Pondimin) is the prototype of the first group, which increases serotonin transmission at nerve endings in the central nervous system by blocking its uptake at nerve endings. In animal studies fenfluramine reduces meal duration and stress related eating. It selectively decreases carbohydrate consumption while protein intake increases. In rats tolerance develops, which is associated with a decrease in serotonin receptor sites. Use of the drug in humans has shown that it produces a greater weight loss than placebo, but once it is discontinued, weight gain occurs. It may, in fact, result in more weight gain if used in association with behavior modification therapy than if behavior therapy is used alone. Withdrawal of the drug may also be associated with the occurrence of significant depression. Alterations in metabolism or activity of other medications, such as orally administered hypoglycemic or anxiety relieving drugs, indicate a need for caution in their use. On the other hand, its hypoglycemic effect may make fenfluramine the drug of choice in obese diabetic subjects.

Fenfluramine is available in a 20 mg. tablet and a 60 mg. sustained release capsule. The recommended initial dosage is 20 mg., three times daily with a gradual increase to a maximum of 120 mg. It is approved for short term (weeks) use only. Additional side effects include sedation, nausea, vomiting, diarrhea, and an altered taste sensation. The drug should be used with caution in the presence of hypertension or central nervous system disorders. It is contraindicated in patients with a history of drug abuse.

The second class of drugs includes those that appear to mediate their effect via the adrenergic system in the brain. The drugs included in this group are phentermine, phenylpropanolamine, diethylpropion, phendimetrazine, and mazindol. In animal studies these drugs have an effect on delaying the beginning of food intake but have no effect on stress related eating. The side effects of this class of drugs are related to their amphetamine-like activity and include nervousness, irritability, palpitations, and dry mouth.

Diethylpropion (Tenuate or Tepanil) is effective in producing an initial weight loss. The rate of weight loss decreases with time and by the third month of therapy does not differ from that achieved with placebo. Side effects are primarily of a stimulant nature—nervousness, irritability, palpitations, and dry mouth. These are usually well tolerated by the patients. Of more interest in the elderly are possible cardiac sympathetic side effects. Although these have not been noted to occur, caution should still be exercised in the use of the drug. It is marketed as 25 mg. tablets to be taken one hour before meals or as a sustained release capsule of 75 mg. taken once daily. The development of tolerance, or at least diminished effect, may limit use of the drug to several months.

Phentermine (Adipex, Fastin, and Ionamin) is another drug in this class. It is similar in both efficacy and side effects to diethylpropion. Its effect on weight loss is decreased with the duration of administration. It is available in 15 and 30 mg. tablets to be taken once daily.

Mazindol (Sanorex) is the third drug to be considered. Although in chemical structure it bears little resemblance to amphetamine, it has similar central nervous system effects in animal studies. Effects reported on improved carbohydrate metabolism, perhaps due to decreased glucose absorption, have suggested that it might be useful in the obese subject who is also diabetic. These effects have been inconsistently reported, however, and have been attributed to weight loss alone. The weight loss achieved is similar to that with the preceding drugs. Adverse effects include central nervous system changes such as irritability and nervousness as well as drowsiness, lethargy, and insomnia. Cardiac arrhythmias may be potentiated in those with known cardiac disease, and the drug probably should not be used in such patients. It may also worsen hypertension or interfere with hypertensive medications directed toward the sympathetic nervous system (e.g., guanethidine). It is available in 1 mg. tablets to be taken three times daily or 2 mg. tablets to be taken one hour before lunch.

Clortermine hydrochloride (Voranil) has anorectic properties.

Phenylpropanolamine is another anorectic drug marketed under the trade name Appedrine, Cenadex, Dexatrim, and Prolamine. It is available in timed release capsules taken once daily or tablets of 37.5 mg. taken two or three times a day.

Phendimetrazine is available in 25 to 35 mg. tablets taken two to four times daily or as a 75 mg. capsule taken once a day. It is marketed as Bontril, Melfiat, Plegine, or Preludin. The adverse effects of the last three compounds, clortermine, phenylpropanolamine, and phendimetrazine, are due to their amphetamine-like qualities. Their effect on weight loss decreases with time, and they are contraindicated in patients with a history of drug abuse.

Another drug with a different mechanism of action is sodium carboxymethylcellulose. This is to be taken with water and is said to produce satiety by a bulk effect of this non-metabolizable carbohydrate. Its effectiveness is unproved, and it may cause an increase in sodium and water overload in susceptible patients.

One of the effects of caloric restriction on thyroid hormone metabolism is to decrease circulating levels of triiodothyronine (T_3). This observation, in addition to a progressive decrease in weight loss, has suggested that therapy with thyroid hormone might be of value in treating obesity.

In a study in which 20 patients consumed an 800 calorie diet, half were give 40 μg. of T_3 while the remainder received placebo.[97] Although, as expected, T_3 levels were higher in the treated group, there was no difference in weight loss. Of note, however, was the observation that half the control group but none of the treated group dropped out of the study. If reproduced, these findings may indicate a place for low dose, short term thyroid hormone therapy. Other studies have found no additive effect of thyroid hormone therapy except when given in amounts that produce symptoms of hyperthyroidism. Its use is contraindicated in patients known to have cardiac disease because of the potential for producing tachyarrhythmias.

Exercise. The addition of an exercise program to caloric restriction may increase weight loss. The caloric expenditures may not account for all the effects noted. Exercise improves insulin effectiveness, changes body composition (increases muscle mass at the expense of adipose tissue), as well as perhaps improving mental attitude. It may also prevent the increase in reverse T_3 seen with caloric restriction alone. The effect on cardiovascular fitness is well known. Attainment of these effects may be limited by orthopedic or cardiac problems in the obese elderly subject, but a walking or nonweight bearing exercise such as bicycle exercise or swimming still may be useful. It has been noted that obese women who exercised regularly for two months failed to increase their ad libitum food intake and gradually lost weight.[98] The major difficulty with this therapy, as with many of the others, is the high drop-out rate.

Surgery. Several surgical procedures have been devised in order to increase weight loss, especially in morbidly obese subjects. These include jaw wiring, intestinal bypass procedures, and gastric operations designed to decrease the reservoir function of the stomach.

Jaw wiring limits the ability of the patient to eat solid foods. It nevertheless depends on patient cooperation because ingestion of high calorie liquids is still possible and may prevent weight loss. Dental side effects and possible aspiration of vomitus may limit its use. It is obviously not suitable for long term therapy.

The exclusion of segments of the small bowel limits the area available for nutrient absorption. Bile salt and osmotic diarrhea may further contribute to malabsorption. Despite these findings, most of the weight loss that occurs in surgical patients is actually due to a decrease in calorie consumption. This may be conditioned by the occurrence of diarrhea after ingestion of food. Although the various procedures are efficacious in producing weight loss, the high rate of complications has resulted in a gradual decrease in their use. Most of the complications are related to fluid, electrolyte, mineral and vitamin abnormalities, but liver failure, arthritis, and infectious complications also occur. This method has largely been superseded by gastric surgery.

A variety of gastric bypass and plication procedures have been devised. Their common feature is a small gastric reservoir, which empties slowly. This procedure, like jaw wiring, depends on patient cooperation because the pouch may be stretched by consuming meals that are larger than prescribed, or the patient may circumvent the barricade by ingesting liquids that are calorically dense. Elderly subjects have an increased surgical risk, and this procedure, like others, should be carefully considered in this age group. It is, however, associated with few of the problems mentioned previously with intestinal bypass procedures.

Inhibitors of Absorption. A substance that would result in a sensation of satiety but not be calorically active would result in weight loss. The inhibition of hydrolysis of starch and sucrose occurs when a glucosidase inhibitor is fed with a meal.[99] It is unclear whether the carbohydrate is absorbed more distally in the colon or whether it produces true malabsorption. This legitimate compound is to be differentiated from the "starch blocker," which is without significant effect.

Another compound that holds potential promise is a substance with the gustatory qualities of fat but without its caloric content.[100] Use of such a food additive may decrease caloric consumption without changes in dietary habits. It remains experimental.

Although obesity continues to be a significant medical problem into old age, therapies are less than optimum. An understanding, sympathetic approach by the physician is of great importance in assisting the patient in dealing with this difficult disorder and its complications.

REFERENCES

1. Seeman, B., and Riggs, B.L.: Dietary prevention of bone loss in the elderly. Geriatrics, 36:71–73, 75, 79, 1981.
2. Munro, H.N.: Nutrition and ageing. Br. Med. Bull., 37:83–88, 1981.
3. Gilmore, R.L.: Recognizing problems of the aging spine. Geriatrics, 35:83–84, 89–92, 1980.
4. Riggs, B.L., Wahner, H.W., Dunn, W.L., Mazess, R.B., Offord, K.P., and Melton, L.J., 3rd: Differential changes in bone mineral density of the appendicular and axial skeleton with aging; relationship to spinal osteoporosis. J. Clin. Invest., 67:328–335, 1981.
5. Manicourt, D.H., Orloff, S., Brauman, J., and Schoutens, A.: Bone mineral content of the radius: good correlations with physicochemical determinations in iliac crest trabecular bone of normal and osteoporotic subjects. Metabolism, 30:57–62, 1981.
6. Newcomer, A.D., Hodgson, S.F., McGill, D.B., and Thomas, P.J.: Lactase deficiency: prevalence in osteoporosis. Ann. Intern. Med., 89:218–220, 1978.
7. Gallagher, J.C., Riggs, B.L., Eisman, J., Hamstra, A., Arnaud, S.B., and DeLuca, H.F.: Intestinal calcium absorption and serum vitamin D metabolites in normal subjects and osteoporotic patients. Effects of age and dietary calcium. J. Clin. Invest., 64:729–736, 1979.
8. Heaney, R.P., Recker, R.R., and Saville, P.D.: Menopausal changes in calcium balance performance. J. Lab. Clin. Med., 92:953–963, 1978.
9. Gallagher, J.U., et al.: The effect of age on serum immunoreactive parathyroid hormone in normal and osteoporotic women. J. Lab. Clin. Med., 95:373–385, 1980.
10. Slovik, D.M., Adams, J.S., Neer, R.M., Holick, M.F., and Potts, J.T., Jr.: Deficient production of 1,25-dihydroxyvitamin D in elderly osteoporotic patients. N. Engl. J. Med., 305:372–374, 1981.
11. Shamonki, I.M., Frumar, A.M., Tataryn, I.V., Meldrum, D.R., Davidson, B.H., Parthemore, J.G., Judd, H.L., and Deftos, L.J.: Age-related changes of calcitonin secretion in females. J. Clin. Endocrinol. Metab., 50:437–439, 1980.
12. Crilly, R., et al.: Hormonal status in normal, osteoporotic and corticosteroid treated postmenopausal women. J. Roy. Soc. Med., 71:733–736, 1978.
13. Albright, F., Richardson, A.M., and Smith, P.H.: Postmenopausal osteoporosis: its clinical features, J.A.M.A., 116:2465–2474, 1941.
14. Weiss, N.S., Ure, C.L., Ballard, J.H., Williams, A.R., and Daling, J.R.: Decreased risk of fractures of the hip and lower forearm with postmenopausal use of estrogen. N. Engl. J. Med., 303:1195–1198, 1980.
15. Paganini-Hill, A., Ross, R.K., Gerkins, V.R., Henderson, B.E., Arthur, M., and Mack, T.M.: Menopausal estrogen therapy and hip fractures. Ann. Intern. Med., 95:28–31, 1981.
16. Recker, R.R., Saville, P.D., and Henney, R.P.: The effect of estrogens and calcium carbonate on bone loss in postmenopausal women. Ann. Intern. Med., 87:649–655, 1977.
17. Nachtigall, L.E., Nachtigall, R.H., Nachtigall, R.D., and Beckman, E.M.: Estrogen replacement therapy. I. A 10-year prospective study in the relationship to osteoporosis. Obstet. Gynecol., 53:277–281, 1979.
18. Lindsay, R., Aitken, J.M., Anderson, J.B., Hart, D.M., MacDonald, E.B., and Clarke, A.C.: Long-term prevention of postmenopausal osteoporosis by oestrogen. Lancet, 1:1038–1040, 1976.
19. Gambrell, R.D., Jr., and Greenblatt, R.B.: Hormone therapy for the menopause. Geriatrics, 36:53–61, 1981.

20. Riggs, B.L., Jowsey, J., Kelly, P.J., Hoffman, D.L., and Arnaud, C.D.: Effects of oral therapy with calcium and vitamin D in primary osteoporosis. J. Clin. Endocrinol. Metab., 42:1139–1144, 1976.
21. Lee, C.J., Lawler, G.S., and Johnson, G.H.: Effects of supplementation of the diets with calcium and calcium-rich foods on bone density of elderly females with osteoporosis. Am. J. Clin. Nutr., 34:819–823, 1981.
22. Popovtzer, M.M., Stjernholm, M., and Huffer, W.E.: Effects of alternating phosphorus and calcium infusions on osteoporosis. Am. J. Med., 61:478–484, 1976.
23. Aloia, J.F., Cohn, S.H., Ostuni, J.A., Cane, R., and Ellis, K.: Prevention of involutional bone loss by exercise. Ann. Intern. Med., 89:356–358, 1978.
24. Riggs, B.L., Seeman, E., Hodgson, S.F., Taves, D.R., and O'Fallon, W.M.: Effect of the fluoride/calcium regimen on vertebral fracture occurrence in postmenopausal osteoporosis. N. Engl. J. Med., 306:446–450, 1982.
25. Transbol, I., Christensen, M.S., Jensen, G.F., Christiansen, C., and McNir, P.: Thiazide for the postponement of postmenopausal bone loss. Metabolism, 31:383–386, 1982.
26. Chestnut, C.H., Nelp, W.B., Baylink, D.J., and Denney, J.D.: Effect of methandrostenolone on postmenopausal bone wasting as assessed by changes in total bone mineral mass. Metabolism, 26:267–277, 1977.
27. Cohn, S.H., Dombrowski, C.S., Hausen, W., Klopper, J., and Atkins, H.L.: Effect of porcine calcitonin on calcium metabolism in osteoporosis. J. Clin. Endocrinol. Metab., 33:719–728, 1971.
28. Trowell, H.: Hypertension, obesity, diabetes mellitus and coronary heart disease. In Trowell, H.C., and Burkett, D.P. (Editors): Western Diseases—Their Emergence and Prevention. Cambridge, Harvard University Press, 1981, pp. 3–33.
29. National Diabetes Data Group: Classification and diagnosis of diabetes mellitus and other categories of glucose intolerance. Diabetes, 28:1039–1057, 1979.
30. Shuman, C.R., and Spratt, I.L.: Office guide to diagnosis and classification of diabetes mellitus and other categories of glucose intolerance. Diabetes Care, 4:335, 1981.
31. Gepts, W., and Lecompte, P.M.: The pancreatic islets in diabetes. Am. J. Med., 70:105–115, 1981.
32. Yoon, J.W., Austin, M., Onodere, T., and Notkins, A.L.: Virus-induced diabetes mellitus. Isolation of a virus from the pancreas of a child with diabetic ketoacidosis. N. Engl. J. Med., 300:1173–1179, 1979.
33. Craighead, J.E.: Viral diabetes mellitus in man and experimental animals. Am. J. Med., 70:127–134, 1981.
34. Toniolo, A., Onodera, T., Jordan, G., Yoon, J., and Notkins, A.L.: Virus-induced diabetes mellitus: glucose abnormalities produced in mice by six members of the Coxsackie B virus group. Diabetes, 31:496–499, 1982.
35. DeFronzo, R.A., Hendler, R., and Simonson, D.: Insulin resistance is a prominent feature of insulin-dependent diabetes. Diabetes, 31:795–801, 1982.
36. Mauer, S.M., Steffes, M.W., Sutherland, D.E.R., Najarian, J.S., Michael, A.F., and Brown, D.M.: Studies of the rate of regression of the glomerular lesions in diabetic rats treated with pancreatic islet transplantation. Diabetes, 24:280–285, 1975.
37. Steno Study Group: Effect of 6 months of strict metabolic control on eye and kidney function in insulin-dependent diabetes with background retinopathy. Lancet, 1:121–124, 1982.
38. Liang, J.C., and Goldberg, M.F.: Treatment of diabetic retinopathy. Diabetes, 29:841–851, 1980.
39. Principles of nutrition and dietary recommendations for individuals with diabetes mellitus: 1979. Diabetes Care, 2:520–523, 1979.
40. American Heart Association: Diet and coronary heart disease statement, 1978.
41. Deaths among patients using continuous subcutaneous insulin infusion pumps. Morbidity & Mortality Weekly Report, No. 31, pp. 80–87, Centers for Disease Control, Feb. 26, 1982.
42. Rizza, R.A., Gerich, J.E., Haymond, M.W., Westland, R.E., Hall, L.D., Clemens, A.H., and Service, F.J.: Control of blood sugar in insulin-dependent diabetes: comparison of an artificial pancreas, continuous subcutaneous insulin infusion and intensified conventional insulin therapy. N. Engl. J. Med., 303:1313–1318, 1980.
43. Skyler, J.S., and Raptis, S. (Editors): Symposium on biosynthetic human insulin. Diabetes Care, 4:139–264, 1981.
44. Offenbacher, E.G., and Pi-Sunyer, F.X.: Beneficial effect of chromium-rich yeast on glucose tolerance and blood lipids in elderly subjects. Diabetes, 29:919–925, 1980.
45. Riales, R., and Albrink, M.J.: Effect of chromium chloride supplementation on glucose tolerance and serum lipids including high-density lipoprotein of adult men. Am. J. Clin. Nutr., 34:2670–2678, 1981.
46. Steiner, G.: Diabetes and atherosclerosis: an overview. Diabetes, 30 (Suppl. 2):1–7, 1981.
47. Prince, M.J., and Olefsky, J.M.: Direct in vitro effect of a sulfonylurea to increase human fibroblast insulin receptors. J. Clin. Invest., 66:608–611, 1980.
48. Vigneri, R., Pezzino, V., Wong, K.Y., and Goldfine, I.D.: Comparison of the in vitro effect of biguanides and sulfonylureas on insulin binding to its receptors in target cells. J. Clin. Endocrinol. Metab., 54:95–100, 1982.
49. Grunberger, G., Ryan, J., and Gorden, P.: Sulfonylureas do not affect insulin binding or glycemic control in insulin-dependent diabetes. Diabetes, 31:890–896, 1982.
50. The University Group Diabetes Program: Study of the effects of hypoglycemic agents on vascular complications in patients with adult-onset diabetes. Diabetes, 19 (Suppl. 2): 747–830, 1970.
51. Rupp, W.M., Barbosa, J.J., Blackshear, P.J., McCarthy, H.B., Rohde, T.D., Goldenberg, F.J., Rublein, T.G., Dorman, F.D., and Buchwald, H.: The use of an implantable insulin pump in the treatment of type II diabetes. N. Engl. J. Med., 307:265–270, 1982.
52. Havard, C.W.H.: The thyroid and ageing. Clin. Endocrinol. Metab., 10:163–178, 1981.
53. Sirota, D.K.: Thyroid function and dysfunction in the elderly: a brief review. Mt. Sinai J. Med., 47:126–131, 1980.
54. Ingbar, S.H.: Effect of ageing on thyroid economy in man. J. Am. Geriatr. Soc., 24:49–53, 1976.
55. Braverman, L.E., Dawber, N.A., and Ingbar, S.H.: Observations concerning the binding of thyroid hormone in sera of normal subjects of varying ages. J. Clin. Invest., 45:1273–1279, 1966.
56. Lloyd, W.H., and Goldberg, I.J.L.: Incidence of

hypothyroidism in the elderly. Br. Med. J., 2:1256–1259, 1961.
57. Bahemuka, N., and Hodkinson, H.M.: Screening for hypothyroidism in elderly inpatients. Br. Med. J., 2:601–603, 1975.
58. Tunbridge, W.M.G., Evered, D.C., Hall, R., Appleton, D., Brewis, M., Clark, I., Grimly, E.J., Young, E., Bird, T., and Smith, P.A.: The spectrum of thyroid disease in a community: the Whickham survey. Clin. Endocrinol., 7:481–493, 1977.
59. Paine, T.D., Rogers, W.J., Baxley, W.A., and Russell, R.O., Jr.: Coronary arterial surgery in patients with incapacitating angina pectoris and myxedema. Am. J. Cardiol., 40:226–231, 1977.
60. Hay, I.D., Duick, D.S., Vliestra, R.E., Maloney, J.D., and Pluth, M.D.: Thyroxine therapy in hypothyroid patients undergoing coronary revascularization: a retrospective analysis. Ann. Intern. Med., 95:456–457, 1981.
61. Ridgway, E.C., McCammon, J.A., Benotti, J., and Maloof, F.: Acute metabolic responses in myxedema to large doses of intravenous L-thyroxine. Ann. Intern. Med., 77:549–555, 1972.
62. Cotton, G.E., Gorman, C.A., and Mayberry, W.E.: Suppression of thyrotropin (h-TSH) in serums of patients with myxedema of varying etiology treated with thyroid hormones. N. Engl. J. Med., 285:529–533, 1971.
63. Stock, J.M., Surks, M.I., and Oppenheimer, J.H.: Replacement dosage of L-thyroxine in hypothyroidism: a re-evaluation. N. Engl. J. Med., 290:529–533, 1974.
64. Rosenbaum, R.L., and Barzel, U.S.: Levothyroxine replacement dose for primary hypothyroidism decreases with age. Ann. Intern. Med., 96:53–55, 1982.
65. Seed, L., and Lindsay, A.M.: Hyperthyroidism in the aged. A review of 120 cases over 60 years of age. Geriatrics, 4:136–145, 1949.
66. Kawabe, T., Komiya, I., Endo, T., Koizumi, Y., and Yomada, T.: Hyperthyroidism in the elderly. J. Am. Geriatr. Soc., 27:152–155, 1979.
67. Forfar, J.C., Miller, H.C., and Toft, A.D.: Occult thyrotoxicosis: a correctable cause of "idiopathic" atrial fibrillation. Am. J. Cardiol., 44:9–12, 1979.
68. David, P.J., and David, F.B.: Hyperthyroidism in patients over the age of 60; clinical features in 85 patients. Medicine, 53:161–181, 1974.
69. Caplan, R.H., Glasser, J.E., Davis, K., Foster, L., and Wickus, A.: Thyroid function tests in elderly hyperthyroid patients. J. Am. Geriatr. Soc., 26:116–120, 1978.
70. Croxson, M.S., Wilson, T.M., and Ballantyne, G.H.: TRH testing; T4-thyrotoxicosis and the aging thyroid gland. N. Engl. J. Med., 24:417–420, 1981.
71. Farnell, M.B., vanHeerden, J.A., McConahey, W.M., Carpenter, H.A., and Wolff, L.H., Jr.: Hypothyroidism after thyroidectomy for Graves' disease. Am. J. Surg., 142:535–538, 1981.
72. Feek, C.M., et al.: Combination of potassium iodide and propranolol in preparation of patients with Grave's disease for thyroid surgery. N. Engl. J. Med., 302:883–885, 1980.
73. Keys, A., Fidanza, F., Karvonen, M.J., Kimura, N., and Taylor, H.L.: Indices of relative weight and obesity. J. Chron. Dis., 25:329–343, 1972.
74. Durnin, J.V.G.A., and Womersley, J.: Body fat assessed from total body density and its estimation from skinfold thickness: measurements on 481 men and women aged from 16 to 72 years. Br. J. Nutr., 32:77–97, 1974.
75. Bray, G.A.: Obesity. In Current Concepts. Kalamazoo, The Upjohn Company, 1982.
76. Yearick, E.S., Wang, M.L., and Pisias, S.J.: Nutritional status of the elderly: dietary and biochemical findings. J. Gerontol., 35:663–671, 1980.
77. Lew, E.A., and Garfinkel, L.: Variations in mortality by weight among 750,000 men and women. J. Chr. Dis., 32:563–576, 1979.
78. Nishizawa, Y., and Bray, G.A.: Evidence of a circulating ergostatic factor: studies of parabiotic rats. Am. J. Physiol., 239:R344–351, 1980.
79. Björvell, H., and Rössner: Effects of oral glycerol on food intake in man. Am. J. Clin. Nutr., 36:262–265, 1983.
80. Kissileff, H.R., Pi-Sunyer, F.X., Thornton, J., and Smith, G.P.: C-terminal octapeptide of cholecystokinin decreases food intake in man. Am. J. Clin. Nutr., 34:154–160, 1981.
81. Mandenoff, A., Fumeron, F., Apfelbaum, M., and Margules, D.L.: Endogenous opiates and energy balance. Science, 215:1536–1537, 1982.
82. Ullrich, I.H., and Albrink, M.J.: The effect of dietary fiber and other factors on insulin response: role in obesity. In Mehlman, M.A., and Tobin, R.B. (Editors): Advances in Modern Human Nutrition. Park Forest South, Illinois, Pathotox Publishers, Inc., 1982, Vol. 2.
83. Bray, G.A., Kral, J.G., and Björntorp, P.: Hepatic sodium-potassium-dependent ATPase in obesity. N. Engl. J. Med., 304:1580–1582, 1981.
84. Sharief, N.N.: Differences in dietary-induced thermogenesis with various carbohydrates in normal and overweight men. Am. J. Clin. Nutr., 35:267–272, 1982.
85. Lansky, D.: Estimates of food quantity and calories: errors in self-report among obese patients. Am. J. Clin. Nutr., 35:727–732, 1982.
86. Dyer, A.R., Stamler, J., Berkson, D.M., and Lindberg, H.A.: Relationship of relative weight and body mass index to 14-year mortality in the Chicago Peoples Gas Company Study. J. Chronic Dis., 28:109–123, 1975.
87. Keys, A.: Overweight, obesity, coronary heart disease and mortality: WO Atwater Memorial Lecture. Nutr. Rev., 38:297–307, 1980.
88. Pettitt, D.J., Lesse, J.R., Knowler, W.E., and Bennett, P.H.: Mortality as a function of obesity and diabetes mellitus. Am. J. Epidemiol., 115:359–366, 1982.
89. Chapman, J.M., Coulson, A.H., Clark, V.A., and Boruh, E.R.: The differential effect of serum cholesterol blood pressure and weight on the incidence of myocardial infarction and angina pectoris. J. Chronic Dis., 23:631–647, 1971.
90. Drenick, E., Bale, G.S., Seltzer, F., and Johnson, D.G.: Excessive mortality and causes of death in morbidly obese men. J.A.M.A., 243:443–445, 1980.
91. DeHaven, J., Sherwin, R., Hendler, R., and Felig, P.: Nitrogen and sodium balance and sympathetic-nervous-system activity in obese subjects treated with a low-calorie protein or mixed diet. N. Engl. J. Med., 302:477–482, 1980.
92. Stunkard, A.J., Wilcoxon-Craighead, L., and O'Brien, R.: Controlled trial of behavior therapy, pharmacotherapy, and their combination in the treatment of obesity. Lancet, 2:1045, 1980.

93. Gotto, A.M., Jr., Foreyt, J.P., and Goodrick, G.K.: Evaluating commercial weight-loss clinics. Arch. Intern. Med., *142:*682–683, 1982.
94. Hylander, B., and Rössner, S.: Three year's follow-up of members of a Swedish commercial weight-reducing club. Acta Med. Scand., *210:*485–488, 1981.
95. Schachter, S.: Self-treatment of smoking and obesity. Can. J. Public Health *72:*401–406, 1981.
96. Stunkard, A.J., and McLaren-Hume, M.: The results of treatment for obesity. Arch. Intern. Med., *103:*79–85, 1959.
97. Moreira-Andrès, M.N., Del Canizo-Gomez, F.J., Black, E.G., and Hoffenberg, R.: Long-term evaluation of thyroidal response to partial calorie restriction in obesity. Clin. Endocrinol. (Oxf.), *15:*621–626, 1981.
98. Woo, R., Garrow, J.S., and Pi-Sunyer, F.X.: Effect of exercise on spontaneous caloric intake in obesity. Am. J. Clin. Nutr., *36:*470–477, 1982.
99. Caspary, W.F., and Kalisch, H.: Effect of alpha-glucosidehydrolase inhibition and intestinal absorption of sucrose, water and sodium in man. Gut, *20:*750–755, 1979.
100. Glueck, C.J., et al.: Sucrose polyester and covert caloric dilution. Am. J. Clin. Nur., *35:*1352–1359, 1982.

CHAPTER 11

RENAL DISEASE

Thomas J. Cali

Aging has a variety of effects on renal function. The elderly patient without intrinsic renal disease or secondary diseases affecting kidney function generally does not have symptoms or signs of impaired renal function. However, when the elderly patient's kidneys are stressed, possibly by concurrent illness, the response may not be as fast or of the same magnitude as when the patient was younger and renal reserve was intact. Likewise, with decreased glomerular filtration, the dose of a renally excreted drug may have to be reduced, since excretion would be decreased, prolonging the drug's half-life and potentially predisposing the patient to toxicity. (The effect of aging on renal function is reviewed in Chapter 2.)

Renal failure in geriatric patients is generally underappreciated, for various reasons. The diagnosis is often complicated by the presence of other systemic diseases producing similar symptomatology or by symptoms that are nonspecific. There is generally a lack of controlled studies, and very few trials of therapeutic modalities have been conducted in elderly patients with renal disease.

Some studies indicate an association between age and the development of chronic renal failure. Perlman in a study of a total community reported that 86.6 per cent of new patients with renal failure were over 45 years of age.[1]. Patients over 50 years of age represented 92 per cent of those with chronic renal failure reported by Branch et al.[2] Geriatric patients may develop renal failure secondary to causes that are relatively uncommon in younger age groups. Two examples of these situations, to be discussed in detail, are renal failure caused by renal calculi and the increased incidence of acute renal failure associated with the use of contrast media in older diabetic patients.

Institutionalized elderly patients may develop dehydration or hyponatremia more frequently than patients in acute care settings. This may reflect a decreased access to water and salt or a decreased level of self-care. Symptoms of hyponatremia in this population may be confined to the central nervous system and be manifested only as confusion. In a patient with other diseases causing confusion, worsening symptoms are easily attributed to pre-existing disease, thus lowering the index of suspicion for hyponatremia. Since the elderly frequently do not have "classic" symptoms, the index of suspicion for many renal diseases would be low.

The treatment of end stage renal disease generally involves hemodialysis, peritoneal dialysis, or renal transplantation. These forms of therapy historically have been withheld from elderly patients. Only recently have age requirements for dialytic therapy and transplantation been liberalized to include the older age groups. New studies in these areas should yield a better understanding of the management of renal diseases in older persons.

This chapter includes further description of the examples previously mentioned, as well as acute and chronic renal failure and the management of those disorders. Whenever possible, specific information relating to elderly patients is provided.

GENERAL PATIENT EVALUATION

Even in the presence of severe renal failure, the older patient is likely to have diseases that affect renal function and complicate or obscure signs and symptoms of kidney disease. Hematuria and dysuria are consistent indicators of urinary tract abnormalities. Anorexia, nausea, and anemia, although not indicative of direct urinary tract involvement, may be related to primary kidney disease. The elderly patient in a chronic care facility may not be able to communicate regarding specific symptoms, and testing may not occur frequently enough to discover or document signs of renal disease. The uremic patient may have neurologic signs, such as convulsions, coma, or asterixis as initial presenting signs of kidney disease. An understanding of such signs and symptoms may lead one to consider renal diseases in the absence of historical or laboratory data.

Laboratory testing may include assessment of the blood urea nitrogen and serum creatinine concentrations and the creatinine clearance. The blood urea nitrogen concentration may be slightly elevated as a result of increased protein intake or may be above normal catabolism in elderly patients. This elevation may occur in the absence of declining renal function.

The serum creatinine concentration, in the absence of primary renal disease, may still be within the normal range, although renal function and glomerular filtration have declined. Serum creatinine concentration does not rise because creatinine production has declined secondary to decreased muscle mass. Thus, at steady state, if creatinine production has declined in conjunction with a decrease in renal function, the creatinine serum concentration does not have to rise outside the normal range. This leads to the incorrect assumption that a "normal" serum creatinine means that renal function is normal.

Creatinine clearance should be assessed with a 24 hour collection of urine for creatinine, and the clearance should be calculated from serum and urinary creatinine concentrations. Care must be taken in elderly patients and in all patients with diminished renal function to collect precisely 24 hours of urine production, since the lower the clearance, the greater the percentage error encountered in faulty urine collection. Appropriate urine collection can be made by discarding the first urine sample and starting the collection at that time. All urine produced in 24 hours should be collected, the last sample being voided exactly 24 hours after the first sample and added to the collection. Accurate assessment of the creatinine clearance should be a better reflection of the magnitude of functional impairment than either the serum creatinine or blood urea nitrogen concentration.

Careful urinalysis may provide valuable information about ongoing renal processes. A clean catch urine specimen should be examined for cells, casts, bacteria, and other components that may indicate renal abnormalities. Proteinuria greater than 150 mg. per 100 ml. of urine is abnormal and may indicate a glomerular lesion or the nephrotic syndrome. Twenty-four hour quantification of the urine protein concentration may be necessary. Red blood cells may indicate urinary tract hemorrhage, glomerular lesions, or the presence of urinary tract stones. Red blood cell casts in the urine are consistent with glomerulonephritis. White blood cells and white blood cell casts indicate inflammation and may be consistent with pyelonephritis or interstitial nephritis. Oval fat bodies are also seen with the nephrotic syndrome. Renal tubular epithelial cells usually indicate some intrinsic renal disease, perhaps acute tubular necrosis. The urine should be evaluated to ensure proper collection. The presence of vaginal epithelial cells may indicate poor collection technique.

HYPONATREMIA

Elderly patients develop hyponatremia, often with some associated abnormality of water balance, as a result of various psychologic, disease, and drug factors. The hyponatremia may not be dramatic or if dramatic may appear to be well tolerated. Symptoms may be minimal, atypical, or absent. Although the actual incidence of this disorder is unknown, Kleinfeld and associates found that 22.5 per cent (36 patients) of 160 randomly selected elderly patients in a chronic care facility had hyponatremia that was documented to be chronic.[3] Patients with hyponatremia may be better understood with concurrent evaluation of water balance. The majority of patients have hyponatremia in conjunction with an increased total body water content, and this is usually associated with renal failure. The remaining patients have hyponatremia associated with dehydration or euhydration.

Unlike some other problems in the elderly, the etiology of the hyponatremia is usually identifiable. An initial assessment of hydration should be made. In the overhydrated hyponatremic patient, diseases causing water retention, such as congestive heart failure, hepatic cirrhosis, and increased antidiuretic hormone activity, should be sought. Whenever hyponatremic patients are dehydrated, consideration should be given to diseases or symptoms associated with the renal or extrarenal loss of extracellular fluid. Lastly, in the hyponatremic but appropriately hydrated patient, isotonic salt and water losses and causes of pseudohyponatremia should be evaluated.

Hyponatremia-Euhydration

The causes of hyponatremia with normal hydration include elevated serum glucose, protein, or lipid concentrations, isotonic loss of fluids and "resetting of the osmostat." Patients with a "reset osmostat" have hyponatremia but can dilute and concentrate urine appropriately only at a lower serum sodium concentration.[4] Three criteria are necessary to establish the diagnosis of "reset osmostat": normal excretion of a standard water load (20 ml. per kg.), maintenance of hyponatremia and sodium balance with salt loading, and the capacity to concentrate the urine at levels of serum tonicity above the reset osmostat. The latter is accomplished either by depriving the patient of water or by intravenous salt loading. Pre-existing renal or cardiovascular disorders may represent relative contraindications to tests necessary to establish one or more of these criteria.

Abnormalities of some components of blood may cause a decrease in the serum sodium concentration without decreasing tonicity—so-called pseudohyponatremia. Pseudohyponatremia is caused by elevated concentrations of osmotically active substances that cause the accumulation of vascular water and displace sodium from extracellular fluid. Correction of these abnormalities elevates the serum sodium concentration by reversing the dilutional effect on blood volume. Hyperglycemia is observed to be the primary cause of pseudohyponatremia in elderly patients. For every 100 mg. per deciliter of glucose, the serum sodium level changes by approximately 1.6 mEq. per liter.[5,6] Hyperlipidemia and hyperproteinemia result in hyponatremia, although the concentration of sodium per unit of water may be unchanged.[7] Lipids and proteins, by causing the accumulation of water and contributing to the plasma volume, reduce the quantity of water present per unit of volume. In the euhydrated patient the serum osmolality value may be helpful in evaluating the patient's hyponatremia. A normal or increased serum osmolality value suggests the presence of osmotically active substances other than sodium.

Hyponatremia-Dehydration

The causes of hyponatremia in the dehydrated elderly patient are often related to dietary restrictions complicating a disease or treatment process. A low salt diet would be unlikely to result in hyponatremia unless it were employed in conjunction with diuretic therapy or some acute process such as a recent urinary tract infection.

These acute changes lower the serum sodium level from a baseline that may already be low because of dietary restriction. Diuretics (thiazides, furosemide, bumetanide ethacrynic acid), in addition to contracting plasma volume, may result in hyponatremia by reducing the urinary diluting capacity. They may decrease glomerular filtration, decreasing solute delivery to the distal tubule, and inhibit chloride reabsorption in the ascending thick segment of the loop of Henle. Both these actions would result in impairment of renal dilutional capacity. Endocrine abnormalities, especially Addison's disease, produce hyponatremia by increasing renal losses of sodium and water. Vomiting or diarrhea may result in hyponatremia and dehydration. Often dehydration from these causes is assessed to be more severe than the hyponatremia. Although hyponatremia in the elderly is primarily chronic, occasionally it is acute. The acute causes are most frequently associated with dehydration through gastrointestinal losses of extracellular fluid.

Hyponatremia-Overhydration

Underlying chronic processes are usually involved in the production of hyponatremia in the overhydrated patient. Congestive heart failure, hepatic cirrhosis, and the nephrotic syndrome are likely etiologies. The hyponatremia in these disorders is complicated by a decrease in the effective plasma volume resulting in further water retention, possibly through increased distal tubular sodium reabsorption mediated by aldosterone.

The most frequent cause of hyponatremia in Kleinfeld's series was the syndrome of inappropriate antidiuretic hormone secretion, which caused hyponatremia in 15 of 36 patients. The following are the criteria necessary to establish the existence of inappropriate antidiuretic hormone secretion: hyponatremia with hypo-osmotic serum, urine that is not maximally dilute, a positive response of the serum sodium concentration with water deprivation, no other apparent causes of hyponatremia, and abnormal excretion of a standard water load. Once again, the elderly patient may not tolerate some tests necessary to establish the diagnosis.

Inappropriate antidiuretic hormone secretion may be caused by central nervous system disease, pituitary disease, tumors producing antidiuretic hormone, stress (such as stroke), and drugs.[8] Chlorpropamide and the other sulfonylureas, carbamazepine, acetaminophen, clofibrate, amitriptyline, thiothixene, and other drugs are frequently used in the elderly and have been implicated in the production of this syndrome.[9-18] The drug induced inappropriate antidiuretic hormone secretion syndrome is an underappreciated entity, even though it may be the most frequent cause of hyponatremia in the elderly. In hyponatremic, volume overloaded patients this syndrome should be considered and evaluated. If possible, the suspected drug should be discontinued and the patient re-evaluated.

Signs and symptoms of hyponatremia are difficult to assess because of complicating chronic diseases. Patients may exhibit gastrointestinal manifestations such as anorexia, nausea, and vomiting, central nervous system effects such as confusion, weakness, and lethargy, and neuromuscular signs such as muscle twitching and tremor. Geriatric patients may have symptoms of disorientation or apathy or no symptoms at all. Patients frequently show signs and symptoms of the underlying disease, possibly worsened by hyponatremia. Depending upon accompanying disorders of water balance, signs and symptoms of hyponatremia may be confused with those associated with dehydration or volume expansion and cardiovascular overload.

Treatment

The treatment of hyponatremia is designed according to the etiology, symptomatology, and severity of the disorder. Chronic hyponatremia that is asymptomatic may be treated conservatively by improving the underlying disease process. Whenever a reversible etiologic disorder is identified, it should be reversed if possible. Additional therapy is based upon the assessment of fluid balance. The overhydrated patient should have water restricted to an amount less than the sum of insensible losses and urine output. This should improve water balance and gradually restore the serum sodium concentration. Patients with the inappropriate antidiuretic hormone secretion syndrome who do not respond to water restriction may require therapy with demeclocycline or lithium carbonate.[19,20] Studies in elderly patients using these drugs have not been done. Dehydrated or euhydrated patients may respond to administration of these drugs or dietary liberalization of salt.

Concentrated sodium chloride solution may be indicated in the patient with central nervous system signs such as coma or seizure activity. An approximation of the sodium chloride dosage can be obtained by estimating the total body water (roughly 62 per cent of the body weight in the adult male and 53 per cent of the body weight in the adult female) and multiplying it by the desired increment in the serum sodium concentration. For example, a 60 kg. female with a serum sodium concentration of 115 mEq. per liter should receive an amount of sodium chloride equal to 32 liters times 5 mEq. (to raise the sodium level from 115 to 120 mEq. per liter), or about 160 mEq. Patients generally respond symptomatically when the serum sodium concentration is raised to 120 to 125 mEq. per liter. It is not necessary to completely correct the serum sodium concentration immediately. Although this is a general guideline for therapy, the therapeutic objective is reversal of life threatening symptomatology.

In emergency situations the approximated

dose of sodium chloride should be administered as a hypertonic solution. Dosing can take several hours, and symptoms should be monitored continually. After symptom reversal has lessened the patient's risk, less concentrated sodium chloride solutions can be used to further improve the patient's sodium balance gradually during the next few hours to several days. Elderly patients may not tolerate hypertonic sodium chloride solutions. Caution should be used to avoid the problems of fluid shifts and cardiovascular volume overload. Pseudohyponatremia rarely requires therapy other than attention to the underlying disorder.

RENAL CALCULI

The incidence of renal lithiasis increases with age. Approximately 14 per cent of all males have a symptomatic urinary tract stone by age 70.[21] After the first stone episode, the risk of recurrence is approximately 3 per cent per year for the next 15 years.[22] The majority of stones (about 90 per cent) in the elderly contain calcium, usually as the oxalate salt. Fewer than 10 per cent contain urate, and only a small number of stones will be found to contain cystine.[23]

Two general situations are known to predispose the patient to stone formation. The concentration of stone forming material in the urine may be increased as a result of various systemic diseases, dehydration, or idiopathic causes. Also continuing factors may be present that favor stone formation, such as urate crystal formation in aciduria.

Ettinger et al. have reported the presence of triamterene or its metabolites in renal calculi.[24] Triamterene appeared to form a nucleus for stone formation and was frequently deposited with calcium oxalate or uric acid. About one-third of 181 triamterene containing stones were composed of triamterene (or its metabolites) alone. The authors estimated the risk to be approximately one per 1500 users. Thus persons with a history of renal calculi may represent a relative contraindication to triamterene diuretic therapy, and in patients developing a stone while receiving triamterene, the drug should be discontinued. This complication should be considered when treating elderly patients with renal calculi.

When evaluating the geriatric patient with renal lithiasis, one must carefully search the history, the record of the physical examination, and laboratory as well as other test results for diseases predisposing the patient to metabolic abnormalities favoring stone formation. Questioning may reveal several historical patterns. Renal lithiasis beginning in childhood is suggestive of renal tubular acidosis, hyperoxaluria, or cystinuria. Idiopathic stone formation and hyperparathyroidism tend to begin in the second or third decade. A careful drug history may reveal the use of carbonic anhydrase inhibitors, vitamin D, or calcium containing preparations in conjunction with dairy products. The latter combination may possibly result in development of the milk-alkali syndrome.

The physician carrying out the physical examination should evaluate the patient for signs and symptoms of diseases predisposing to urinary tract obstruction or stone formation. These diseases include multiple myeloma, metastatic carcinoma, hyperparathyroidism, osteoporosis, renal tubular acidosis, and Paget's disease of bone. Although the presence of one of these diseases may be helpful in evaluating the patient with renal lithiasis, most elderly patients do not have physical evidence of systemic diseases associated with stone formation. The laboratory evaluation should include serum determinations, especially of calcium and uric acid concentrations. Urinalysis should be performed in a search for crystalluria. A 24 hour collection of urine for calcium, oxalate, uric acid, and cystine determinations should be done. Routine x-ray examination of the kidneys, ureters, and bladder should be performed. Obstruction and urinary tract infection complicating stone formation should be evaluated.

The pathophysiology of renal lithiasis depends upon the specific etiology. Since the majority of stones occurring in geriatric patients contain calcium, abnormalities of calcium metabolism should be investigated. In the hypercalciuric patient, appropriate disease etiologies should be evaluated. In the absence of demonstrable disease the patient may be determined to have idiopathic hypercalciuria. Albright first described idiopathic hypercalciuria as a syndrome characterized by renal lithiasis, increased urinary calcium excretion (more than 250 mg. per day on a diet without milk or dairy products), a normal serum calcium concentration, and a low serum phosphorus concentration.[25] Rose and Harrison found that a majority of patients with idiopathic renal lithiasis had hypercalciuria.[26] The 24 hour urinary excretion of calcium in a patient consuming a diet without dairy products should be less than 250 mg.

Urinary supersaturation with uric acid accounts for the majority of urate lithiasis.[27] Excessive urinary acidification increases the proportion of free uric acid. Patients with uric acid lithiasis may have an elevated serum uric acid concentration, a decreased urine pH, or an elevated 24 hour excretion of uric acid (more than 600 to 800 mg. of uric acid). Elderly patients with the onset of uric acid lithiasis should be evaluated for malignant disease, such as the myeloproliferative syndrome or leukemia. Uric acid lithiasis may be seen in elderly patients with chronic diarrhea.[28] Dehydration, causing decreased urinary volume, increases the urinary uric acid concentration. The potential for uric acid stone formation increases as metabolic base is lost in the stool, and the urinary pH declines. Diarrhea may also predispose the patient to the formulation of other types of renal stones, by similar general mechanisms.[29]

Renal stones may be formed in the patient with cystinuria, an inherited disorder more commonly seen in the young. Confirmation of cystinuria is made by the discovery of urinary crystals containing cystine and a subsequent 24 hour urinary collection for a cystine determination. Adults normally excrete less than 30 mg. of cystine per day. Cystine stones occur infrequently in geriatric patients.

The factors directly responsible for stone formation are numerous and complex. Patients may have supersaturated urinary concentrations of calcium, oxalate, phosphate, or uric acid. Stones require a nidus for initial precipitation. Cellular debris as well as other crystals (uric acid) may serve as a nidus for stone formation. Infection may predispose patients to stone formation by increasing urinary cellular debris or by altering the urinary pH and affecting ion solubility. Obstruction may be accompanied by urinary stasis, which favors crystal formation. Magnesium, citrate, and pyrophosphate are potential inhibitors of stone formation. Supplementation of these ions in patients who are deficient in one or more of them may increase urinary inhibitor activity, thus decreasing stone formation.

Regardless of the etiology, renal calculi may cause obstruction, hydronephrosis, and renal failure and predispose the patient to infection. All these complications have varying components of reversibility, depending upon factors such as the time of exposure to the insult, the severity of the resultant metabolic abnormalities, and structural damage. Infections may be extremely difficult to correct in patients with urinary tract stones. Organisms may live in the stones, causing relapsing urinary tract infections that remain refractory to therapy.

The clinical manifestations of renal lithiasis vary with the presenting complications. Urinary retention may accompany obstruction; pyuria, hematuria, and local symptoms may be seen with infection. Occasionally a patient presents with end stage renal failure due to calculus formation without pain or other symptoms. When a stone begins descending the urinary tract, the patient often experiences severe pain. This pain may be sharp and stabbing in nature in the flank region, possibly radiating through to the abdomen. Severe pain may occur in the abdomen as the stone moves through the ureter. The pain may involve the groin, testicles, labia, or urethra as the stone descends. A stone in the renal pelvis may be associated with intermittent severe flank pain or persistent dull flank pain. Hematuria, especially microscopic hematuria, is often present when the stone is moving.

The causative factors in the formation of urinary tract stones in the elderly patient often remain obscure. Attempts should be made to discover the common causes of stones in this age group. Documentation of continuous stone formation may take months or years. Stone analysis may be helpful in discovering the etiology and in further individualizing therapy.

After appropriate evaluation, patients are distributed within two general categories. In one group of patients stones are found to form as a complication of underlying systemic disease; the treatment of these patients should be directed toward improving or removing the primary disease. The other group is often labeled as having idiopathic renal lithiasis. This group may be subdivided according to clinical features affecting the therapeutic approach:

1. Patients with absorptive hypercalciuria. After the establishment of hypercalciuria, a two hour quantification of urinary calcium is carried out after a 16 hour fast. If the urinary calcium level is less than 10 mg. per hour, the patient has absorptive hypercalciuria. This test establishes a urinary calcium response to dietary calcium restriction.

2. Patients with nonabsorptive hypercalciuria. Testing as described in category 1 results in a one hour urinary concentration of calcium greater than 15 mg. These patients as well as patients excreting 10 to 15 mg. of calcium per hour generally do not respond to dietary calcium restriction.

3. Patients without hypercalciuria. Urinary calcium concentrations in these patients respond poorly, if at all, to dietary calcium restriction. Therapy in this group is likely to involve supplementation of inhibitor substances.

4. Patients with hyperuricosuria. High levels of urinary uric acid may decrease inhibitor activity or precipitate in the kidney, allowing calcium oxalate deposition by epitaxial growth. In patients with documented uric acid abnormalities there is an increased incidence of calcium stones. Dietary restriction of protein to reduce the urinary concentration of uric acid may prove beneficial, although further study of this method is necessary.[29,30]

Treatment

Treatment of patients with idiopathic renal lithiasis needs to be individualized. All patients may derive benefit from fluid supplementation sufficient to produce a urine volume of 2 to 2.5 liters per day, provided a specific contraindication to additional hydration does not exist. If supersaturated urinary solutions of substances are found, dietary management of these disorders should be attempted. Concentrations of urinary inhibitors should be assessed and supplemented when indicated. Careful attention to these aspects of therapy should maintain the majority of patients in a metabolically inactive state of stone formation. Yearly x-ray evaluation of the kidneys, ureters, and bladder and more frequent urinalysis are essential to document the absence of stone formation.

In patients with absorptive hypercalciuria the fluid intake should be increased, as previously discussed. Fluid supplementation should occur frequently, perhaps as often as every hour while the patient is awake, with additional supplementation at night. Dietary calcium should be restricted to less than 100 mg. per day. This can usually be accomplished by avoiding the intake of dairy products. Inhibitor supplementation may be necessary. Thorough patient follow-up is essential.

The treatment of patients with nonabsorptive hypercalciuria also involves fluid supplementation as already described and inhibitor supplementation if indicated. Dietary calcium restriction usually does not reduce the urinary calcium level and may result in a negative calcium balance. Hydrochlorothiazide in doses of 50 mg. given twice daily effectively decreases urine calcium concentrations by approximately one-third. Sodium restriction may augment the hypocalciuric effect of thiazide diuretics and should be attempted in patients who are not adequately responding to hydrochlorothiazide.

Patients without hypercalciuria do not have apparent abnormalities of the serum or urinary calcium level and generally do not respond to treatment with thiazide diuretics or dietary calcium restriction. Dietary calcium restriction may be detrimental in these patients, since it increases the urinary oxalate concentration. Dietary oxalate restriction should be considered if calcium is restricted. Fluid therapy as previously described is also essential for patients without hypercalciuria.

These patients may respond to inhibitor supplementation, particularly phosphorus. Ideally the patient should receive 2 gm. of elemental phosphorus per day. Several forms of phosphorus supplementation are available. Dibasic sodium and potassium phosphate with monobasic sodium and potassium phosphate is available as Neutra-Phos powder, solution, and capsules. Dibasic and monobasic potassium phosphate is available as Neutra-Phos K solution, powder, and capsules. The potassium preparation is intended for sodium restricted patients, although Neutra-Phos supplies only 7.125 mEq. of sodium per 250 mg. of phosphorus. Eight capsules daily would result in the administration of 57 mEq. of sodium and 2 gm. of phosphorus. Both capsule preparations provide 250 mg. of elemental phosphorus. Patients should receive two capsules four times daily. If diarrhea becomes prohibitive, the dosage can be slowly increased from 1 to 2 gm. of elemental phosphorus. Patients in whom active formation of calcium phosphate stones is occurring may benefit from acidification of the urine, especially if the urinary pH is alkaline.

Elemental magnesium supplementation, if necessary, can be supplied as magnesium oxide capsules. The usual dosage is 200 mg. given twice daily. This dosage provides about 14 mEq. of magnesium per day. Inhibitor supplementation should be monitored both in terms of decreased stone formation and with serum or urinary concentrations of the respective ion. The elderly patient should be assessed for the presence of relative contraindications to therapy, such as renal failure for magnesium and phosphorus administration or severe congestive heart failure for sodium administration.

Patients with an elevated 24 hour excretion of uric acid require fluid therapy as previously described as well as the reduction of dietary protein to decrease the major source of urinary uric acid. They are also potential candidates for dietary calcium restriction. If stone formation continues, allopurinol (Zyloprim) in dosages of 100 to 300 mg. per day may be added to decrease uric acid formation and subsequent excretion. If additional therapy is required, citrate supplementation and alkalinization of the urine can be achieved by using a commercial citrate solution. These solutions (Polycitra, Polycitra-K, and others) contain various quantities of citrate salts. One milliliter of solution contains 2 mEq. of citrate (equivalent to 2 mEq. of bicarbonate) with 2 milliequivalents of cation—sodium and potassium, or potassium alone. Urinary alkalinization should be accomplished slowly. Care should be taken not to increase the urine pH above 6.5, since this may predispose the patient to the formation of calcium stones. An initial dose of 10 to 15 ml. for adults should be mixed with water and taken four times daily. The urinary pH should be monitored with nitrazine paper.

There is a minimal amount of objective information characterizing geriatric patients with renal lithiasis. Treatment approaches have not been specifically designed for the aged patient. Care should be taken to characterize complications in the geriatric patient that may affect all forms of therapy, including presumably safe treatments such as oral fluid supplementation. Although the elderly patient may benefit from all forms of therapy discussed, the therapeutic objective may be realized with a less rigorous approach to treatment that may eliminate stone formation while avoiding adverse effects of therapy. Adequate time should be allowed for each therapeutic maneuver, and monitoring should be frequent.

ACUTE RENAL FAILURE

Available sources demonstrate few differences in the course of patients with acute renal failure when analyzed by age. Some differences in etiology are apparent, such as the increased risk of acute renal failure in elderly diabetic patients studied with contrast media. The pathophysiology, course, prognosis, mortality, and causes of mortality in patients with acute renal failure do not appear to vary with age. In all patients developing acute failure of renal function, the prerenal and postrenal causes should be evaluated. The prompt discovery and reversal of the cause may favorably affect both recovery of renal function and morbidity.

Prerenal failure of kidney function generally involves two mechanisms. Patients either have a decreased extracellular fluid volume with a decreased plasma volume, or an increased extracellular fluid volume with a decreased effective plasma volume. Extracellular fluid losses occur in renal disease, adrenal disease, and gastrointestinal disease, with diuretic therapy, and in burned patients. A decreased effective plasma volume is associated with hypotensive episodes, shock, cardiac failure, and hepatic failure. Patients may develop prerenal failure despite the presence of peripheral edema or other interstitial ("third space") fluid accumulation.

Since all patients with prerenal failure have real or perceived plasma volume deficits, the signs and symptoms reflect vascular volume contraction. Patients should be evaluated for hypotension. Orthostatic blood pressures should be obtained if possible, and symptoms such as dizziness and syncope should be assessed. Tachycardia may be present, as well as signs and symptoms of cellular water loss like poor skin turgor, dry mouth, thirst, and diminished axillary or groin sweating. The urine should be concentrated and contain only a small amount of sodium, less than 20 mEq. per liter.[31] The urine sediment should be normal. Prerenal failure should respond to vascular rehydration. When the patient is rehydrated, the urinary volume should increase and the serum creatinine and blood urea nitrogen concentrations should fall. If they do not return to normal, there is a likely component of intrinsic renal failure.

The ratio of the blood urea nitrogen level to the serum creatinine level may be helpful in evaluating the patient with prerenal failure. This ratio is often elevated (greater than 10 or 15 to 1). Caution should be used in evaluating the blood urea nitrogen level or the ratio, since the former may be increased by hemolysis of red blood cells, increased dietary protein intake, catabolism, gastrointestinal hemorrhage, total parenteral nutrition, or drugs such as tetracyclines and corticosteroids. Severe hepatic disease may decrease the blood urea nitrogen level because the liver is responsible for urea synthesis.

Postrenal failure of kidney function is associated with obstruction. Obstruction may be due to renal stone formation, urologic or gynecologic surgery, gastrointestinal or pelvic malignant disease, or retroperitoneal fibrosis. Postrenal failure should be considered in the oliguric or anuric patient. Rather than defining a lower limit of urinary volume as oliguria (usually 400 ml. of urine output over 24 hours), the urine output should be assessed in the context of water and osmotic homeostasis. Adults consuming an "average" diet require a minimum of about 400 ml. of urine output in 24 hours to excrete the soluble waste products from intake and metabolism. Geriatric patients may consume less soluble excretable waste, thus obligating less water as urinary volume. Acutely ill patients may have additional water losses through pathologic or insensible mechanisms, potentially diminishing the urinary volume. Functionally, oliguria is that amount of urine flow that is unable to maintain renal excretory function. It varies with the dietary intake of food and water.

Patients with anuria should be evaluated for obstruction to differentiate the lack of urine production from absence of urine excretion. Anuria may also occur in rapidly progressive glomerulonephritis, not associated with postrenal obstruction.

Patients may experience symptoms associated with urinary stones and hydronephrosis, such as abdominal pain with swollen tender kidneys, or they may be asymptomatic. The blood urea nitrogen to serum creatinine ratio may be elevated, and the urine sediment, except with urinary stones, may be normal. Treatment is directed at the primary cause of the obstruction.

Patients with acute renal failure require evaluation of possible etiologies. Prerenal and postrenal failure should be ruled out. Some patients thought to have acute renal failure may be discovered to have chronic renal failure. Owing to the prevalence of these situations and the variance in definitions of "acute renal failure," little objective information is available concerning elderly patients with acute renal failure.

The causes of acute renal failure can be found in Table 11-1. Glomerulonephritis in the elderly and the risk of contrast media induced acute renal failure are to be discussed subsequently. The diagnostic possibilities in acute renal failure in the elderly have been reviewed.[38] Drug usage is frequently identified as being temporally related to, as well as causing, acute renal failure. A thorough review of drug induced nephrotoxicity and its implications in elderly patients is not available. Antibiotic associated nephrotoxicity has been reviewed by Appel and Neu.[39]

The signs and symptoms of acute renal failure may be referable to the underlying cause or may be generalized. Often signs and symptoms may be more difficult to recognize or assess in the older patient. In contrast to prerenal azotemia, urinalysis in acute renal failure usually reveals a level higher than 20 mEq. of sodium per liter. Urine sediment containing cells, cellular debris, casts, and protein is common. Serum creatinine and blood urea nitrogen concentrations are elevated or are rising, and the ratio of the blood urea nitrogen to creatinine is usually 10 or 15 to 1. Differentiation of acute renal failure from prerenal failure by the urinary sodium concentration may be complicated by diuretic therapy, which increases urinary sodium excretion. Urine composition is often not useful in differentiating acute renal failure from postrenal failure, since the findings may be similar. Obstruction should be readily identified by history, physical examination, or evaluative procedures such as excretory urography, catheterization, or cystoscopy.

The urine volume may be diminished in acute renal failure, but often is not. Classically acute renal failure is associated with an initial oliguric phase, averaging 12 to 14 days in length, and a diuretic or high output phase.

TABLE 11-1. Causes of Acute Renal Failure*

Obstruction with hydronephrosis
Interstitial nephritis (including drug induced)
Tubular impairment induced by drugs
Acute glomerulonephritis
Papillary necrosis (as in analgesic nephropathy)
Acute pyelonephritis
Malignant hypertension
Contrast media induced tubular dysfunction
Renal artery obstruction (embolism)
Hepatorenal syndrome
Multiple myeloma
Poststreptococcal glomerulonephritis

*Adapted from references 32 to 37.

Treatment

Aside from acute uremic syndrome symptoms, the management of fluid and electrolyte balance is of utmost importance. Hyperkalemia is more common with oliguria, while hyponatremia may occur during the diuretic phase. The volume status must be continually monitored to avoid dehydration, with its risk of further renal insult, and to avoid overhydration and cardiovascular overload. Frequent qualification and quantification of urinary volume and constituents must be made, with subsequent and precise replacement. Occasionally this is necessary every four to six hours. Strict intake and output records must be maintained as well as daily weights and assessments of fluid and electrolyte balance. If the patient's environment precludes careful attention to any of these parameters, the patient should be transferred to a location where appropriate facilities are available. Patient transfer should also occur if the need for hemodialysis or peritoneal dialysis is anticipated and cannot be accomplished in the present location. The symptoms of the uremic syndrome are best treated by dialysis (see page 379). Maintenance and support of the patient, with or without dialysis, through the episode of acute renal failure may result in the reversal of the renal insult, with partial or complete return of renal function.

The mortality in acute renal failure is often related to the underlying disease process and is due primarily to infection. Care must be taken to avoid or to monitor factors increasing the patient's risk of infection. Vascular and urinary catheters are necessary, but should be used cautiously and changed according to predetermined guidelines. Patients in whom oral nutrition is inadequate should receive parenteral supplementation, especially with essential aminoacids, with appropriate care of any vascular access sites.[40] The mortality in acute renal failure is high, 55 to 60 per cent, and does not appear to be any different in the elderly.[41]

IATROGENIC RENAL FAILURE

One cause of acute renal failure seems to be increasing as a consequence of more aggressive medical evaluation in elderly patients. The use of tests employing contrast media is associated with a small but significant risk of acute renal failure in elderly patients, particularly elderly diabetic patients.[42] The risk appears to be directly related to the state of hydration and inversely related to renal function. Previously patients were dehydrated prior to intravenous pyelography in order to concentrate the contrast medium and improve the quality of the study. This practice should be avoided, if possible, in the elderly patient. Geriatric patients, for a variety of reasons, may be somewhat hydropenic at the outset. If possible, this should be corrected prior to the use of contrast media. Although the risk increases as glomerular filtration decreases, it is not known whether a threshold for risk exists. Likewise it is not possible to estimate risk according to the magnitude of renal function impairment. A serum creatinine concentration of 5 mg. per dl. has been proposed as an absolute contraindication to intravenous pyelography.[43] Consideration should be given to the information to be gained by intravenous pyelography in the elderly and its utility in making therapeutic decisions.

As indicated in Chapter 2, numerous drugs possess the potential for causing nephrotoxicity (e.g., aminoglycoside antibiotics, bacitracin, cephaloridine, neomycin, penicillamine, polymyxin B, and viomycin). These drugs should be administered with extreme caution in the elderly with reduced renal reserve, doses should be individualized in view of the physiologic parameters of the patient, and therapy should be monitored for early signs of renal toxicity.

GLOMERULONEPHRITIS INDUCED ACUTE RENAL FAILURE

Acute glomerulonephritis is a cause of acute renal failure in the elderly that may be more common than previously suspected. According to early reports, glomerulonephritis was a disease occurring in childhood through early adulthood.[44] No well controlled epidemiologic reports have analyzed the occurrence of this disease in the elderly. Most reported series deal specifically with referred patients or autopsy cases. In one series of 74 autopsies, 23 patients (average age 56 years) had acute glomerulonephritis, and 10 of these were over 60 years of age.[45] In spite of increasing numbers of elderly patients reported with glomerulonephritis, the index of suspicion remains low.

Arieff analyzed reports involving 70 patients.[46] Although most commonly the disease was idiopathic, patients also developed glomerulonephritis in association with streptococcal infections, Henoch-Schönlein purpura, Goodpasture's syndrome, Wegener's granulomatosis, and other diseases. Glomerulonephritis also has been associated with pneumococcal pneumonia, a disease frequently encountered in the elderly.[47] Samiy reported seven cases of glomerulonephritis in patients over 60 years of age.[48] Four of those patients had associated streptococcal infections or elevated antistreptolysin titers. One patient had evidence of poststreptococcal glomerulonephritis with a temporal relationship to a close relative who also had poststreptococcal glomerulonephritis, suggesting a potential risk of the spread of streptococcal infection in the elderly.

The diagnosis of classic glomerulonephritis involves finding red blood cells and red blood cell casts in the urine, proteinuria, hypertension, and signs of volume overload. The elderly patient with glomerulonephritis may manifest signs of renal infection, pulmonary edema, or congestive heart failure, and renal disease is often not suspected.

The institutionalized geriatric patient may not have frequent urinalyses, and therefore urinary signs such as red blood cells and casts as well as proteinuria may be missed. Although most patients exhibit urinary signs, glomerulonephritis has been reported in a patient without urinary findings.[49] Oliguria may actually be more common in elderly patients with glomerulonephritis.[50] Anuria may also be present but is uncommon. The variety of etiologies, presentations, and symptoms makes diagnosis difficult. Renal biopsy is necessary to confirm and classify the glomerulonephritis. Whether the complications of the biopsy procedure (namely, bleeding and infection) occur more frequently in older patients is unknown.

The prognosis in glomerulonephritis in the elderly is ambiguous, but generally is considered to be poor. The prognosis may vary with the etiology of glomerulonephritis. Jennings and Earle reported that all their patients over age 50 recovered from poststreptococcal glomerulonephritis, but all six of Boswell and Eknoyan's patients with glomerulonephritis not associated with streptococcal infections expired.[51,52] As with treatment, better epidemiologic evaluation should clarify the prognosis in glomerulonephritis in the elderly.

Treatment of Glomerulonephritis

The treatment of the manifestations of glomerulonephritis involves supportive therapy, diuretics, and dialysis and is monitored by signs and symptoms of renal impairment and serum and urine testing. The treatment of the glomerulonephritis has been attempted with corticosteroids and immunosuppressive drugs. The results in younger adult patients have been disappointing, and there have been no objective trials of the therapy of glomerulonephritis in geriatric patients. Systematic and objective evaluation of therapy should be obtained before definitive guidelines for therapy are established.

CHRONIC RENAL FAILURE

The transition from acute renal failure to chronic renal failure may be rapid but often is not. Potentially any cause of acute renal failure may result in chronic renal failure. The patient with chronic renal failure may have moderate impairment of function above the level at which dialysis and transplantation are considered, but may still be symptomatic or may have end stage renal disease. Patients with moderate renal failure may demonstrate signs and symptoms of the nephrotic syndrome resulting from various disorders.

The nephrotic syndrome is characterized by proteinuria greater than 3.5 gm. per 24 hours, hypoalbuminemia less than 3.0 gm. per 100 ml, hypercholesterolemia greater than 300 mg. per 100 ml., lipiduria, and edema.[53] The nephrotic syndrome was thought to be uncommon in elderly patients, but Fawcett reported that 25 per cent of newly diagnosed cases of the nephrotic syndrome occurred in patients over 60 years of age.[54] The diagnosis is often obscured in the elderly for various reasons, including the presence of cardiovascular disease, as evidenced by the report of an elderly patient thought to have congestive heart failure refractory to diuretics who actually had an unrecognized nephrotic syndrome.[55]

The nephrotic syndrome may be associated with primary renal disease or with other systemic diseases involving the kidney. The renal disease that most frequently results in the nephrotic syndrome in the elderly is probably glomerulonephritis. Other primary renal diseases causing the nephrotic syndrome such as lipoid nephrosis are usually seen in children and only rarely in adults. Malignant tumors, renal vein thrombosis or embolic phenomena, amyloidosis, and diabetes mellitus are frequent secondary causes of the nephrotic syndrome in the elderly. Any disease producing primary or secondary glomerular lesions may result in the nephrotic syndrome.

Proteinuria develops as a result of enhanced glomerular permeability, allowing filtration of large molecular weight substances, primarily albumin. The amount of proteinuria varies considerably and may be in excess of 10 to 15 gm. daily. Hypoalbuminemia develops when hepatic synthesis no longer can keep pace with metabolic demands and urinary losses. The level of proteinuria associated with hypoalbuminemia varies with the protein intake and anabolic capacity. Hyperlipidemia results from proteinuria and hypoalbuminemia and represents an attempt to restore plasma oncotic pressure by synthesis of larger molecular weight lipoproteins. Declining lipid concentrations in the absence of declining proteinuria may represent further changes in glomerular permeability and is considered to be a poor prognostic sign. Edema results from several inter-related factors. Decreased plasma oncotic pressure favors fluid transudation into interstitial spaces. This may result in further declines in glomerular filtration with a subsequent decline in filtered sodium load. Excessive salt and water reabsorption in the nephron, perhaps partially mediated by aldosterone, may also contribute to edema formation. Patients often have edema and slightly abnormal aldosterone plasma volumes.

The patient evaluation should be designed to discover both primary and secondary causes of the nephrotic syndrome and often involves renal biopsy. Assessment should include intravenous pyelography, estimation of the glomerular filtration rate by creatinine clearance, and quantification of urinary protein excretion. Complications exacerbating a decrease in renal function, such as urinary infection, hypertension, and congestive heart failure, should be identified and reversed if possible. The etiology of the nephrotic syndrome in geriatric patients is often idiopathic glomerulonephritis or irreversible secondary causes such as diabetes mellitus.

Treatment

The treatment of the underlying cause of the nephrotic syndrome involves corticosteroids, usually prednisone, 1 to 2 mg. per kg. per day, and has been disappointing except in lipoid nephrosis. It is not known whether elderly patients benefit from corticosteroid therapy, and there may be contraindications because of the potential side effects of treatment. In patients in whom the nephrotic syndrome results from secondary causes, improvement may be effected with treatment of the underlying disorder. Primary treatment of the nephrotic syndrome in elderly patients requires further evaluation but because of specific secondary causes is not promising.

Symptomatic improvement may be obtained through manipulation of sodium and water intake and the careful use of diuretics. Bed rest and salt and water restriction may decrease edema formation. Patients who do not respond to conservative measures may require diuretic therapy. Small doses of spironolactone (Aldactone) with or without a thiazide diuretic may be beneficial. In patients with severely reduced glomerular filtration rates, more potent loop diuretics or metolazone may be necessary for symptomatic control. Adverse effects should be monitored and avoided if possible. Elderly patients may be more sensitive to vascular fluid shifts associated with diuretics; thus therapy should be initiated gradually and assessed frequently.

Since the nephrotic syndrome eventually results in end stage renal failure, every attempt should be made to manage the patient conservatively and avoid further renal insult prior to the need for dialysis.

As renal function declines further, regardless of etiology, patients with end stage renal failure manifest signs and symptoms secondary to the failure of renal excretory function, declining renal endocrine function, and accumulation of nitrogenous waste products. Management of these disorders should occur prior to and with the use of hemodialysis or peritoneal dialysis.

The urine volume in end stage renal failure varies widely and has therapeutic implications in regard to fluid balance. Anuric or severely oliguric patients may require stringent fluid restriction. In other patients the urinary output may be 2 to 3 liters per day, although this is not "quality urine" since tubular processes have not been involved. These patients may have more liberal amounts of fluid. Generally the daily fluid intake should be an amount equal to the daily urinary output in addition to insensible losses (normally 0.25 to 0.5 ml. per kg. of body weight per hour).

Not all patients retain sodium; indeed some waste significant amounts of sodium.[56] Attempts should be made to assess sodium elimination and avoid a further decline in renal function associated with rigid sodium restriction. The sodium need varies and occasionally as much as 10 to 12 gm. of salt intake per day is required.

Hyperkalemia. The renal capacity to eliminate potassium is usually adequate except when the patient develops oliguria, at which time hyperkalemia may ensue. Assessment of exogenous potassium sources (e.g., banked blood, salt substitutes, or spironolactone or triamterene use) should be carried out.

The emergency treatment of hyperkalemia involves one or more of the following:

1. The intravenous administration of glucose, 25 to 100 gm., with approximately 1 unit of regular insulin per 5 gm. of glucose.

2. The intravenous administration of sodium bicarbonate, 44.6 mEq. given over approximately two to five minutes.

3. The intravenous administration of calcium gluconate, 4.8 mEq. given over approximately two to five minutes.

Each modality must be monitored for toxic effects and efficacy and may need to be repeated. Calcium is thought to inhibit the effect of potassium on the myocardium, thus preventing or reversing lethal rhythm disturbances. Glucose and insulin as well as sodium bicarbonate work by causing the movement of potassium from the extracellular fluid to the intracellular fluid, obviously only a temporary intervention. Dialysis against potassium free solutions removes potassium but requires much time. Potassium is removed from the body by the use of sodium polystyrene sulfonate (Kayexalate). The dosage depends upon the symptoms of hyperkalemia and the serum potassium level, and patients may require 20 to 50 gm. once or more daily, orally or rectally. Sorbitol is often given currently to prevent constipation and produce an osmotic diarrhea, which would also eliminate potassium as well as prevent sodium reabsorption. Two to 3 mEq. of sodium may be liberated for each gram of resin used, potentially causing significant sodium reabsorption.[57] Prolonged therapy may be necessary.

Hypokalemia. Hypokalemia in end stage renal failure is uncommon and usually results from gastrointestinal losses. Caution should be used when replacing potassium, since renal excretory capacity is limited.

Metabolic Acidosis. Metabolic acidosis associated with increased amounts of unmeasured anions is frequently present. Often the acidosis is chronic and stable. Acidosis may be responsible for some anorexia or nausea and may exacerbate hyperkalemia when it exists. When the arterial blood pH becomes too low, the patient becomes symptomatic, or the carbon dioxide content falls below 16 to 18 mM per liter, treatment is indicated. Depending upon the current calcium status (discussed later), alkaline salts of calcium may be used; otherwise sodium bicarbonate can be used, in most cases orally. The therapeutic objective is the restoration of chronic acidosis, pH 7.2 to 7.3, or a carbon dioxide content of 16 to 18 mM per liter—not the correction of the acidosis. Although sodium absorption with potential cardiovascular overload is a consideration, evidence suggests that sodium absorption from sodium bicarbonate is not as significant as sodium absorption from sodium chloride.[58] The dosage level should be individualized according to the patient's response and the results of arterial blood gas determinations.

Hypocalcemia. The primary abnormality of calcium balance in end stage renal failure is hypocalcemia. The pathophysiology of hypocalcemia is complex, involving altered renal excretion of phosphates, abnormal vitamin D function secondary to the lack of renal activation of vitamin D to 1, 25-dihydroxycholecalciferol, resorption of bone secondary to the stress of metabolic acidosis, alteration of the feedback mechanisms for parathyroid hormone secretion, and altered metabolism of parathyroid hormone.

Although a majority of patients have histologic evidence of bone disease, few have symptoms.[59] This may be because of a normal ionized calcium concentration with decreased protein bound calcium. Immediate correction of the calcium balance is indicated only if signs and symptoms of hypocalcemia or tetany are present. Any calcium salt can be used, although calcium gluconate may be preferred since it is an alkaline salt.

Attempts at prolonged restoration of the calcium balance must consider all the pathophysiologic factors. If phosphate levels are elevated, they must be reduced prior to calcium supplementation to prevent metastatic calcification. This can be accomplished with the use of phosphate binding drugs, such as aluminum hydroxide or aluminum carbonate. The dosage level is determined by the response of the serum phosphate concentration. Aluminum salts may complicate the course by causing constipation and may exacerbate neurologic sequelae of chronic renal failure in dialysed patients.[60] After normalization and maintenance of the serum phosphate concentration, supplementation of calcium (as an alkaline salt) with vitamin D is indicated. Again the dosage level is based upon the serum calcium concentration and manifestations or radiologic evidence of bone disease. If autonomous hyperparathyroidism is present, it must be surgically corrected to prevent hypercalcemia. Owing to the complex relationship of calcium, phosphate, vitamin D, bone disease, and parathyroid hormone, monitoring should be frequent, and improvement may be slow with numerous setbacks.

Anemia. Anemia is a frequent if not a constant feature of chronic renal failure. Pathophysiologic considerations include decreased erythropoietin synthesis, gastrointestinal blood loss, blood loss during dialysis, decreased red blood cell survival, inability to utilize stored iron, and dialysis of folic acid.

Geriatric patients should also be evaluated for vitamin B_{12} abnormalities, since they may be more common in this age group. Such a patient may require supplementation with iron and folic acid; a reasonable objective is a hemoglobin concentration of 7 to 8 gm. per 100 ml. or a hematocrit level of 20 to 25 per cent. If the patient is still severely symptomatic or is not responding to iron and folic acid, transfusions of packed red blood cells may be required.

Uremic Syndrome. The uremic syndrome involves many metabolic, gastrointestinal, cardiopulmonary, and neurologic abnormalities. Specific information addressing the issues of uremia in geriatrics is not available. It does not appear that the uremic syndrome differs considerably in elderly patients. Uremia appears to be severe and debilitating in all patients regardless of age. The uremic syndrome is not to be specifically discussed; suffice it to say that it is most amenable to dialytic therapy.

Patients with chronic renal failure have a multitude of problems often requiring multiple drug therapy. These patients are known to have altered drug pharmacokinetics, as are geriatric patients. The occurrence of chronic renal failure in a geriatric patient presents a particularly complicated problem of drug dosing. Patient pharmacokinetics should be individualized whenever possible. Bennett and coworkers published a useful guide to drug dosing in patients with all levels of renal impairment.[61]

HEMODIALYSIS AND PERITONEAL DIALYSIS

During early experience with hemodialysis and peritoneal dialysis, the elderly were often excluded from this therapy, frequently on the basis of age alone. Most dialysis programs had an upper age limit for eligibility; this limit was occasionally as low as 45 years. Initially dialysis programs were not prevalent enough to meet demand. There was a shortage of machines, money, and trained personnel. Dialysis committees often made decisions, based upon age, to favor the younger applicant. The implied advantage of youth was the increased rehabilitation potential and thus a better chance to resume a productive life. As the age criteria for dialysis and transplantation have been liberalized, the presumed disadvantages of age have become less apparent.

Although the older patient may be more likely to have pre-existing cardiovascular disease, recent evidence indicates that the accelerated development of vascular disease is a problem associated with dialysis populations in general.[62] Reports of dialysis in patients over 50 years of age have been encouraging. The results in terms of treatment and rehabilitation in older patients may be more favorable than those in the young. Whether survival by the use of dialysis is a function of age has been controversial, at least since Keleman's report of successful hemodialysis in a 77 year old man in 1959, and the controversy continues because of the lack of epidemiologic and statistical data concerning geriatric patients who have undergone hemodialysis.[63]

Dramatic improvement in the techniques for both hemodialysis and peritoneal dialysis has occurred recently. The procedures do not require as much time as previously—three to six hours three times a week for hemodialysis as opposed to 10 to 12 hours three times a week in the past. Thus the procedure, although rigorous, represents less total stress time than before. Although this may prove beneficial to the entire population of patients with chronic renal failure with various degrees of impaired organ function reserve, it has particular applicability to the elderly patient with age related declines in organ function.

Rather than undertake a complete discussion of dialysis technique, the pertinent areas of hemodialysis, peritoneal dialysis, and home dialysis as they relate to the elderly patient are to be reviewed. The majority of information available concerning dialysis involves the younger population. Although they do not deal specifically with the elderly, several reports make favorable reference to the dialytic care of the older patient.[64-66] An occasional report shows poor results of dialysis in the elderly.[67]

Ghantous et al. reported 60 patients aged 50 to 80 years selected for hemodialysis.[68] Circulatory access was established with a Scribner-Quinton shunt or by the creation of a subcutaneous arteriolar-venous fistula. Problems encountered secondary to shunt access were as expected—infection and clotting, as are also seen with younger patients. Several older patients had arteriolar-venous fistulas with no apparent symptomatic compromise in cardiovascular function.

The dialysate potassium dosage was usually 2.6 mEq. per liter but could be individualized. Patients received systemic heparinization unless a contraindication existed. Patients ate a normal diet with the exception of potassium restriction, and fluid intake was adjusted to allow a weight gain of no more than 1 to 1½ pounds per day. All patients were dialyzed for six hours three times weekly. Patients had a variety of renal disorders including glomerulonephritis, polycystic renal disease, pyelonephritis, nephrosclerosis, and gouty nephropathy.

Complications of hemodialysis involved several major organ systems, typical of the patient with end stage renal disease. Cardiovascular complications were diverse and common, although in several patients there was improvement in terms of cardiac symptoms. For example, improvement in pericarditis was noted with more frequent hemodialysis, improvement in congestive heart failure was seen with ultrafiltration and the resulting better fluid balance, and improvement in angina pectoris occurred when the hematocrit level was elevated to 25 to 30 per cent. About half the patients required transfusions to remain asymptomatic from angina or anemia. In the remaining patients a satisfactory hematocrit level was maintained. This incidence of transfusion was assumed to be higher in elderly symptomatic patients than in younger patients, but actual comparison was not made. Infection was common; 25 per cent of the patients had at least one shunt infection, increasing the morbidity and mortality in that group. Additional complications involved the gastrointestinal system, neurologic system, bone disease, and the psychologic outlook of the patient.

Thirteen patients also received 15 homotransplants. The overall mortality was 33 per cent (20 deaths in the original 60 patients). Cardiovascular and infectious complications accounted for the majority of deaths. Thirteen deaths occurred in the dialysis population, eight within the first year. Twenty-four patients were rehabilitated to gainful employment, 20 patients continued normal household duties, and 10 patients were retired and able to lead active lives; in 6 patients progressive worsening occurred and they died soon after beginning dialysis.

Although data were not available allowing a specific comparison of this population with a younger dialysis population, it was believed that the older group tolerated dialysis and was psychologically more stable than younger patients. Unfortunately the elderly were thought to tolerate cardiovascular and infectious complications less well. The study indicated that some patients may benefit from a trial of peritoneal dialysis initially, with a subsequent change to hemodialysis if the patient tolerates the procedure well.

Walker retrospectively compared 154 patients aged 50 or over at the start of hemodialysis with 420 patients under 50 years of age at the beginning of dialysis.[69] No significant difference in survival rates between young and old patients could be found during the first three years of hemodialysis. The aged had a one year survival rate of 92 per cent, a two year survival rate of 75 per cent, and a three year survival rate of 64 per cent. The younger population had one, two, and three year rates of 90, 77, and 75 per cent, respectively. The younger group had a significantly higher survival rate from the fourth year on. The five year survival rates for the aged and the young were 30 and 62 per cent, respectively. Cohen and associates reported similar findings.[70]

Cardiovascular disease was the leading cause of death. Of 154 aged patients undergoing hemodialysis, 82 were dialyzed at home; the remaining 72 patients were dialyzed in a medical center. The survival in patients over age 50 undergoing hemodialysis was 84 per cent at three years. This agrees with the reported 75 per cent three year survival of patients regardless of age.[71] Unfortunately the five year survival rate in patients over age 50 undergoing hemodialysis was 38 per cent. Although the mortality rate was higher at five years, the deaths were evenly distributed among the 50 to 65 year old group, suggesting that although the five year mortality increases after age 50, the mortality rate does not continue to rise solely as a function of age. The over-50 year old patients undergoing dialysis at home were thought to have adapted to dialysis better than any other age group. Increased maturity and social stability were cited as reasons for this group's excellent adjustment. When comparing these home hemodialysis survival rates to that in the general population undergoing hemodialysis, one must consider that certain factors in patient selection, namely, pre-existing medical problems, symptoms during dialysis, and patient preference, may favor survival in the patient undergoing dialysis at home.

Rehabilitation was satisfactory in the entire population. Patients who are self-employed, white collar workers, or professionals have a greater rehabilitation potential than blue collar workers. This observation does not change with age, even though it might be psychologically more acceptable for an aged person to receive supplemental disability funds. The need for transfusion was greater in the younger population—0.29 transfusions per patient month, as compared to 0.14 transfusions per patient month for those aged 50 or over. This is partially explained by the larger number of younger anephric patients (35 of 99 patients) than older anephric patients (4 of 38 patients). Regardless of age, patients receiving hemodialysis who have not had nephrectomies need few transfusions, especially after stabilization. The need for hospitalization was greater among the young (0.93 day hospitalized per patient month) as compared to the old (0.74 day hospitalized per patient month). This is partially explained by the higher incidence of operative procedures among the young. It is also believed that the young patient may spend more time hospitalized for problems related to noncompliance with the prescribed medical regimen than the aged, supposedly more mature and better adjusted patient.

Although the results of this investigation appear to be favorable, elderly patients may manifest symptoms of problems that require medical center hemodialysis even though they would otherwise be excellent candidates for treatment at home. Several situations can be anticipated and require special attention in the elderly:

1. Acute hypotension with or without loss of consciousness may occur more frequently. This may be more severe, more symptomatic, and more difficult to treat.

2. The elderly may be more sensitive to the effects of anemia, manifesting symptoms of congestive heart failure or angina pectoris. The lower the hematocrit level, the greater the risk of the complications.

3. The elderly may be more sensitive to fluid shifts (even with mild weight gain) and may develop acute pulmonary edema.

4. Neurologic complications, including transient cerebral ischemic attacks, may be more common or more severe in the elderly.

5. Dialyzers that require large priming volumes or that produce rapid ultrafiltration rates may be poorly tolerated by the aged.

It appears that home hemodialysis should be offered to patients regardless of age, provided they are suitable candidates. Kolodner et al. reviewed the variables involved in good home hemodialysis.[72] Several advantages of this program apply to the elderly, among them the flexibility of hemodialysis scheduling, the lack of need for travel, and the more constructive use of time while being dialyzed. The psychosocial adjustment of the patient and family should be assessed. Adjustment may proceed smoothly in some patients, whereas for others the responsibility and psychologic implications of home dialysis may be more than friends or relatives can cope with. The stress involved relates to issues of patient independence and dependence—on both a machine and technical personnel—and rehabilitation. The elderly may experience different psychosocial problems related to their life style at an older age, and thus would require different kinds of understanding and support.[73] Patients undergoing hemodialysis at home have a lower incidence of mortality and morbidity. The incidence of hepatitis in patients dialyzed at home is lower than that in medical center dialyzed patients. Although this issue has not been specifically studied in the elderly, it is assumed that age does not determine the incidence of hepatitis. Indeed the incidence of hepatitis associated antigen positivity in this population is better correlated with the number of years the patient has been receiving hemodialysis treatments. Every home hemodialysis program requires the use of stringent criteria for selection as well as continuing supportive services. There appears to be no reason for the elderly to be deprived of the advantages of such a program. The elderly may be better candidates for home hemodialysis than some younger patients in a less settled environment.

As with hemodialysis, peritoneal dialysis in the past was often reserved for the younger, medically less complicated patient. Problems of solution leakage and peritonitis were thought to be more significant in the elderly. The elderly patient also had cardiovascular disease, a relative contraindication to peritoneal dialysis, and was less able to adjust to fluid shifts. Because of the possibility of overhydration in patients with reduced cardiovascular reserve, the elderly were often excluded from peritoneal dialysis treatment. With the increased availability of commercial solutions and equipment, and a subsequent reduction in the types and severity of complications of peritoneal dialysis, the age contraindication of the elderly in regard to peritoneal dialysis became less restrictive.

Vertes et al. reported the results of 25 peritoneal dialysis episodes in 11 geriatric patients.[74] Conservative management of fluid and electrolyte balance was begun in all patients. When this management failed to maintain a therapeutic objective, peritoneal dialysis was begun. It was carried out in the usual manner with two exceptions. Each dialysis involved 25 exchanges in a 36 hour period, exposing the geriatric patient to fewer volume exchanges than standard therapy. Also, each time a course of peritoneal dialysis was begun, there was a repeat peritoneal puncture. Indwelling peritoneal catheters were not used. The indications for peritoneal dialysis were acute exacerbation of chronic renal failure, advanced chronic renal failure, and control of edema associated with chronic renal failure. All patients were aged 60 years or older, and all had clinically apparent cardiovascular disease.

Nine patients had congestive heart failure, nine had diabetes mellitus, and four had severe hypertension. In all 11 patients in this study, peritoneal dialysis successfully restored fluid and electrolyte balance and removed edema fluid. The blood urea nitrogen concentration declined in all patients; the average concentration at the start of therapy (161 mg. per dl.) declined to an average of 60 mg. per dl., even though fewer exchanges were completed in 36 hours. One 71 year old patient was maintained for approximately one year by periodic peritoneal dialysis treatments. The most common complication was pain (15 of 31 dialyses), usually associated with catheter placement and fluid removal. Mental confusion occurred during six of 31 sessions of peritoneal dialysis. There was one episode of hypotension. There was a notable absence of mechanical complications, e.g., leakage, inadequate drainage, and perforation. The catheter could not be inserted in one extremely obese patient. There were also no infectious complications reported.

With a larger study population, aged or not, more mechanical complications as well as infectious complications would be expected. It is not known whether these complications would occur more often in the elderly, but it is assumed that when they do occur, they are more serious.

Peritoneal dialysis has demonstrated efficacy and safety in the geriatric patient, often in spite of pre-existing cardiovascular disease. The time required to accomplish peritoneal dialysis is longer than for hemodialysis, but peritoneal dialysis does not incur the risks of heparinization and dramatic fluid shifts seen with hemodialysis. Regardless of their age, patients undergoing peritoneal dialysis need to be monitored for mechanical problems (solution leakage), infectious problems (peritonitis), and metabolic problems (fluid overload). Strict fluid intake and output monitoring is necessary and may be more essential in the geriatric patient undergoing peritoneal dialysis. Peritoneal dialysis is a useful treatment modality in patients initially or in those in whom there are contraindications to hemodialysis. It appears that selection criteria for peritoneal dialysis based upon presumed complications of the aging process are unwarranted.

CONCLUSION

The elderly patient with renal disease poses a variety of unique therapeutic problems. Elderly patients often have diseases that may predispose to complications of therapy. In the past, therapeutic intervention was largely withheld from this population. Observations of patients receiving dialysis have been favorable and indicate that instead of withholding hemodialysis and peritoneal dialysis, they should be used but with an understanding of the elderly patient's altered physiology and with better monitoring techniques. Progress is needed in dialysis, drug dosing, and the treatment of primary renal disease in the elderly patient. An increased awareness of the prevalence of renal disease, its complications, and its treatment in elderly patients should benefit this population by increasing the index of suspicion for renal disease and also by stimulating much needed research in this area.

REFERENCES

1. Perlman, L.V.: Primary and secondary renal failure in a total community (Tecumseh, Michigan): preponderance in the elderly and possible antecedent factors. J. Am. Geriatr. Soc., 22:25, 1974.
2. Branch, R.A., et al.: Incidence of uremia and requirements for maintenance hemodialysis. Br. Med. J., 1:249, 1971.
3. Kleinfeld, M., et al.: Hyponatremia as observed in a chronic disease facility. J. Am. Geriatr. Soc., 27:156, 1979.
4. DeFronzo, R.A., et al.: Normal diluting capacity in hyponatremic patients. Ann. Intern. Med., 84:538, 1976.
5. Crandall, E.D.: Serum sodium response to hyperglycemia. N. Engl. J. Med., 290:465, 1974.
6. Katz, M.A.: Hyperglycemia-induced hyponatremia—calculation of expected serum sodium depression. N. Engl. J. Med., 289:843, 1973.
7. Fuisz, R.E.: Hyponatremia. Medicine, 42:149, 1963.
8. Bay, W.H., and Ferris, T.F.: Hypernatremia and hyponatremia: disorders of tonicity. Geriatrics, 31:53, 1976.
9. Miller, M., and Moses, A.M.: Mechanism of chlorpropamide action in diabetes insipidus. J. Clin. Endocrinol. Metab., 30:488, 1970.
10. Rado, J.P., et al.: Clinical value and mode of action of chlorpropamide in diabetes insipidus. Am. J. Med. Sci., 260:359, 1970.
11. Czako, L., and Laszlo, F.A.: Antidiuretic effect of carbamazepine in diabetes insipidus. Int. J. Clin. Pharmacol., 11:58, 1975.
12. Nusynowitz, M.L., and Forsham, P.H.: The antidiuretic action of acetaminophen. Am. J. Med. Sci., 252:429, 1966.
13. Bonnici, F.: Antidiuretic effects of clofibrate and carbamazepine in diabetes insipidus: studies of free water clearance and response to a water load. Clin. Endocrinol., 2:265, 1973.
14. Moses, A.M., et al.: Clofibrate-induced antidiuresis. J. Clin. Invest., 52:535, 1973.
15. Luzecky, M.H., et al.: The syndrome of inappropriate secretion of antidiuretic hormone associated with amitriptyline administration. South. Med. J., 67:495, 1974.
16. Moses, A.M., and Miller, M.: Drug-induced dilutional hyponatremia. N. Engl. J. Med., 291:1234, 1974.
17. Ivy, H.K.: The syndrome of inappropriate secretion of antidiuretic hormone. Med. Clin. N. Am., 52:817, 1968.
18. Miller, M., et al.: Drug induced states of impaired water excretion. Kidney Int., 10:96, 1976.
19. Singer, I., and Rotenberg, D.: Demeclocycline-induced diabetes insipidus. Ann. Intern. Med., 79:679, 1973.
20. White, M.G., and Fetner, C.: Treatment of the syndrome of inappropriate secretion of antidiuretic hormone with lithium carbonate. N. Engl. J. Med., 292:390, 1975.
21. Van Den Berg, C.J.: Clinical evaluation of renal lithiasis. Geriatrics, 34:35, 1979.
22. Wilson, D.M.: Medical treatment of urolithiasis. Geriatrics, 34:65, 1979.
23. Rosen, H.: Renal disease in the elderly. Med. Clin. N. Am., 60:1105, 1976.
24. Ettinger, B., et al.: Triamterene nephrolithiasis. J.A.M.A., 244:2443, 1980.
25. Albright, F., et al.: Idiopathic hypercalciuria. Proc. R. Soc. Med., 46:1077, 1953.
26. Rose, G.A., and Harrison, A.R.: The incidence, investigation and treatment of idiopathic hypercalciuria. Br. J. Urol., 46:261, 1974.
27. Gutman, A.B., and Yu, T.F.: Uric acid nephrolithiasis. Am. J. Med., 45:756, 1968.
28. Reisner, G.S.: Uric acid lithiasis in the ileostomy patient. Br. J. Urol., 45:340, 1973.
29. Earnest, D.L.: Enteric hyperoxaluria. In Year Book of Medicine, Chicago, Year Book Medical Publishers, Inc., 1979, pp. 407–427.
30. Coe, F.L., and Kavalach, A.G.: Hypercalciuria and hyperuricosuria in patients with calcium nephrolithiasis. N. Engl. J. Med., 291:1344, 1974.
31. Harrington, J.T., and Cohen, J.J.: Measurement of urinary electrolytes—indications and limitations. N. Engl. J. Med., 293:1241, 1975.
32. Murray, T., and Goldberg, M.: Chronic Interstitial nephritis: etiologic factors. Ann. Intern. Med., 82:453, 1975.
33. Linton, A.L., et al.: Acute interstitial nephritis due to drugs. Ann Intern. Med., 93:735, 1980.
34. Lyons, H., et al.: Allergic interstitial nephritis causing reversible renal failure in four patients with idiopathic nephrotic syndrome. N. Engl. J. Med., 288:124, 1973.
35. Abel, J.A.: Analgesic nephropathy—a review of the literature, 1967–1970. Clin. Pharmacol. Ther., 12:583, 1971.
36. Wollam, G.L., and Gifford, R.W.: The kidney as a target organ in hypertension. Geriatrics, 31:71, 1976.
37. Veranasi, U.R., et al.: "Spontaneous" atheroembolic disease as a cause of renal failure in the elderly. J. Am. Geriatr. Soc., 27:407, 1979.
38. Luke, R.G.: Diagnostic possibilities in acute renal failure in the elderly. Geriatrics, 31:92, 1976.
39. Appel, G.B., and Neu, H.C.: The nephrotoxicity of antimicrobial agents. N. Engl. J. Med., 296:663 (part 1), 296:784 (part 2), 1977.
40. Abel, R.M., et al.: Improved survival from acute renal failure after treatment with intravenous essential L-amino acids and glucose. N. Engl. J. Med., 288:695, 1973.
41. Kumar, R., et al.: Acute renal failure in the elderly. Lancet, 1:90, 1973.
42. Weinraugh, L.A., et al.: Contrast media-induced acute renal failure. J.A.M.A., 239:2018, 1978.
43. Harkonen, S., and Kjellstrand, C.: Exacerbation of diabetic renal failure following intravenous pyelography. Abstracts, American Society of Nephrology. Annual Meeting, Washington, D.C., 1976.
44. Ellis, A., and Toronto, M.D.: Natural history of Bright's disease. Clinical, histological, and experimental observations. Lancet, 1:1, 1942.
45. Nesson, H.R., and Robbins, S.L.: Glomerulonephritis in older age groups. Arch. Intern. Med., 105:23, 1960.

46. Arieff, A.I., et al.: Acute glomerulonephritis in the elderly. Geriatrics, 26:74, 1971.
47. Seegal, D.: Acute glomerulonephritis following pneumococcal lobar pneumonia. Arch. Intern. Med., 56:912, 1935.
48. Samiy, A.H., et al.: Acute glomerulonephritis in elderly patients: report of seven cases over sixty years of age. Ann. Intern. Med., 54:603, 1961.
49. Goorno, W., et al.: Acute glomerulonephritis with absence of abnormal urinary findings. Ann. Intern. Med., 66:345, 1967.
50. Lee, H.A., et al.: Acute glomerulonephritis in middle-aged and elderly patients. Br. Med. J., 2:1361, 1966.
51. Jennings, R.B., and Earle, D.P.: Post-streptococcal glomerulonephritis: histopathologic and clinical studies of the acute, subsiding acute and early chronic latent phases. J. Clin. Invest., 40:1525, 1961.
52. Boswell, D.C., and Eknoyan, G.: Acute glomerulonephritis in the aged. Geriatrics, 23:73, 1968.
53. Schreiner, G.E. (Editor): Clinician: The Nephrotic Syndrome. San Juan, Puerto Rico, Searle and Co., 1972.
54. Fawcett, I.W.: Nephrotic syndrome in the elderly. Br. Med. J., 1:387, 1971.
55. Flynn, V.J., and Roland, A.S.: Nephrotic syndrome in a 92-year old woman. Geriatrics, 22:119, 1967.
56. Slatopolsky, E., et al.: Studies on the characteristics of the control system governing sodium excretion in uremic man. J. Clin. Invest., 47:521, 1968.
57. Berlyne, G.M., et al.: Dangers of resonium A in the treatment of hyperkalemia in renal failure. Lancet, 1:167, 1966.
58. Husted, F.C., et al.: $NaHCO_3$ and NaCl tolerance in chronic renal failure. J. Clin. Invest., 56:414, 1975.
59. Eastwood, J.B., et al.: Some biochemical, histological, radiological, and clinical features of renal osteodystrophy. Kidney Int., 4:128, 1973.
60. Alfrey, A.C.: The dialysis encephalopathy syndrome. Possible aluminum intoxication. N. Engl. J. Med., 294:184, 1976.
61. Bennett, W.M., et al.: Drug therapy in renal failure: dosing guidelines for adults. Ann. Intern. Med., 93:62 (part 1), 93:286 (part 2), 1980.
62. Lindner, A., et al.: Accelerated atherosclerosis in prolonged maintenance hemodialysis. N. Engl. J. Med., 290:697, 1974.
63. Keleman, W.A., and Kolff, W.J.: The use of the artificial kidney in the very young, the very old and the very sick. J.A.M.A., 171:530, 1959.
64. Retan, J.W., and Lewis, H.Y.: Repeated dialysis of indigent patients for chronic renal failure. Ann. Intern. Med., 64:284, 1966.
65. Thomas, G.E., et al.: Hemodialysis for chronic renal failure—clinical observations. Arch. Intern. Med., 120:153, 1967.
66. Schupak, E., et al.: Chronic hemodialysis in "unselected" patients. Ann. Intern. Med., 67:708, 1967.
67. Shaldon, S.: Haemodialysis in chronic renal failure. Postgrad. Med. J., 42:669, 1966.
68. Ghantous, W.N., et al.: Long-term hemodialysis in the elderly. Trans. Am. Soc. Artif. Intern. Organs, 17:125, 1971.
69. Walker, P.J.: Long term hemodialysis for patients over 50. Geriatrics, 31:55, 1976.
70. Cohen, S.L., et al.: The effect of age on the results of regular hemodialysis treatment. Proc. Eur. Dial. Transplant Assoc., 7:254, 1970.
71. Walker, P.J., et al.: Self dialysis 1974. Proc. Dial. Transplant Forum, 4:22, 1974.
72. Kolodner, L., et al.: Screening and supportive techniques for home dialysis in the treatment of renal failure. J. Am. Geriatr. Soc., 24:32, 1976.
73. Lowenhaupt, E.: Psychic reactions to long-term hemodialysis: evaluation in the elderly by means of the draw-a-person test. J. Am. Geriatr. Soc., 25:358, 1977.
74. Vertes, V., et al.: Peritoneal dialysis in the geriatric patient. J. Am. Geriatr. Soc., 15:1019, 1967.

CHAPTER 12

NEUROLOGIC DISORDERS

*Elliott L. Mancall
and Timothy R. Covington*

Elderly individuals may develop virtually any form of disease involving the central or peripheral nervous system, the neuromuscular junction, or muscle. It is clear, however, that many neurologic diseases common in youth and middle age, such as demyelinating diseases, muscular dystrophy, or myasthenia gravis, to name but a few, are infrequent beyond the fifth decade; disorders such as these will receive little or no attention herein. Many other neurologic diseases ranging, for example, from meningitis to peripheral neuropathy may occur at any age, and evidence no special attributes, either pathogenetically or therapeutically, in the elderly; these too merit scant attention here. On the other hand, a number of neurologic diseases in fact either are particularly common beyond the age of 60 or, alternately, pose special problems in management in the later decades of life. It is to these that attention is primarily directed in this chapter. In the absence of absolute chronologic benchmarks, the selection of disorders for consideration here is to at least some extent arbitrary, but in general corresponds to ordinary clinical experience.

It is a commmonplace observation that little drug therapy is available in the management of neurologic disease. Although it is true that much current therapeutic effort in disease of the nervous system remains mechanical (surgical) or restorative in emphasis, an increasing number of pharmacologic agents may be identified that function either as primary specific therapies or as vital supportive modalities. Admittedly, even today such treatment is all too often symptomatic rather than corrective, a distinction that will become increasingly clear as this chapter progresses. Nonetheless, knowledge of such drugs, the indications for their use, and the adverse effects that may be encountered is basic to a rational approach to the treatment of the patient with disease of the nervous system. The therapeutic nihilism long considered a characteristic of classic clinical neurology can no longer be appropriately applied to the practice of neurology today.

CEREBROVASCULAR DISEASE

Cerebral Thrombosis

Of the many forms of cerebrovascular disease, the occlusive varieties are most common later in life. Thrombosis involving either the intracranial or extracranial (vertebral, carotid) vasculature is of particular importance. Appearing especially on a background of hypertension, diabetes, or hyperlipidemia, the phenomenon of thrombosis is based on an evolutionary process of atherosclerotic degeneration involving especially large and medium size arteries, leading to progressive stenosis and, ultimately, thrombus formation with complete obliteration of the vessel lumen. Any part of the cerebral hemispheres, brain stem, or cerebellum may be affected by the infarction that results from complete occlusion. The extent and severity of the resulting clinical syndrome, i.e., the stroke, are determined by two factors, viz., the distribution of the involved vessel(s) and the availability of collateral circulatory channels, which may limit the extent of the infarction. Parenchymatous edema may accompany the process of infarction, thus intensifying the clinical deficit, and is responsible at times for significant intracranial hypertension. The problem of thrombo-occlusive disease is not a simple one; a number of related but distinct clinical aspects require individual attention. It must be emphasized at the outset, however, that the most effective form of management of this and of other major forms of cerebrovascular disease is unequivocally preventative, based effectively on the long term control of hypertension and, although perhaps to a lesser extent, of diabetes.

The Established Stroke

When a patient presents with a completed (i.e., established) stroke, the therapeutic options are limited. The integrity of the airway, blood pressure control, and supportive measures directed particularly to maintenance of an adequate cardiac output, fluid-electrolyte and metabolic status, pulmonary function, and cerebral edema take precedence.[1] In hypertensive individuals the use of antihypertensive medication must be carefully monitored to prevent systemic hypotension. There are no specific measures that may be undertaken to limit the extent of the infarction once established. Stellate ganglion block is of no benefit. Vasodilators for the most part have no significant effect vis-à-vis the intracranial vasculature and thus offer no benefit. Carbon dioxide is an efficient cerebral vasodilator, but its use is, at the least, potentially hazardous. The widespread cerebral vasodilation resulting from inhalation of this agent effectively shunts blood away from the area of compromise to other portions of the brain and thus has an effect precisely the opposite from that intended (this chain of events is sometimes referred to as an intracerebral "steal").[2] Thrombolytic drugs (e.g., streptokinase) similarly play no therapeutic role in the management of cerebral thrombo-occlusive disease; in fact, the risk of intracerebral bleeding consequent to their use is significant. Steroid preparations such as dexamethasone (Decadron) may effectively reduce cerebral edema in some patients, but their routine use is to be deplored. Such drugs are properly utilized only under circumstances in which increasing intracranial pressure as suggested by deepening stupor or papilledema is evident, or when computed tomography demonstrates major swelling surrounding the area of infarction. When used, dexamethasone is generally given in a dosage of 4 to 6 mg. every four to six hours, following an initial parenteral dose of 10 mg.

Despite vigorous supportive measures, even when initiated early in the patient's course, the completed stroke is unfortunately best looked upon as a fait accompli. Meaningful therapeutic measures are primarily restorative. In any given individual neither the degree nor the rate of recovery can be predicted with certainty. Early institution of physical therapy should be encouraged, generally as soon as the patient is clinically stable and able to cooperate. Speech therapy and occupational therapy are utilized as necessary. During the more chronic phases of management, many patients require substantial psychologic support, and psychiatric referral is often sought.

A special form of occlusive vascular disease centers about the appearance of multiple small (lacunar) infarcts scattered in the cerebral white matter and basal ganglia in hypertensive individuals. Patients with infarcts of this type often exhibit a progressive dementing disorder referred to as multi-infarct dementia. With the exception of control of hypertension and maintenance of adequate cardiac function, no effective therapeutic measures are available.

The Stroke in Evolution

At times it is possible to identify the disorder in the course of an actively evolving occlusion, particularly during the stuttering progression of thrombosis involving the basilar or carotid artery. The vigorous use of heparin has been advocated under these circumstances, but results remain unsettled. All too often the disorder progresses to a fully completed stroke regardless of the form of therapy utilized. The dosage of heparin should be adjusted to the individual patient on the basis of laboratory test values and the clinical response. Table 12–1 may be used as a guideline for achieving therapeutic anticoagulant effect.

Heparin acts at multiple sites in the nor-

TABLE 12–1. Guidelines for Achieving a Therapeutic Anticoagulant Effect from Heparin*

Method of Administration	Frequency	Recommended Dose[1]
Subcutaneous[2]	Initial dose	10,000–20,000 units[3]
	Every 8 hours	8,000–10,000 units
	or Every 12 hours	15,000–20,000 units
Intermittent IV	Initial dose	10,000 units[4]
	Every 4 to 6 hours	5,000–10,000 units[4]
IV infusion	Continuous	20,000–40,000 units/day in 1,000 ml. of isotonic sodium chloride solution[3]

*Reprinted with permission from Facts and Comparisons, Inc., 1982.
[1] Based on a 150 lb. (68 kg.) patient.
[2] Use a concentrated solution.
[3] Immediately preceded by intravenous loading dose of 5,000 units.
[4] Administer undiluted or in 50 to 100 ml. isotonic sodium chloride.

mal coagulation system to inactivate clotting factors IX, X, XI, XII, and thrombin, thus inhibiting the conversion of fibrinogen to fibrin. Heparin also prevents the formation of a stable fibrin clot by inhibiting the activation of factor XIII (fibrin stabilizing factor). Heparin is not fibrinolytic, will not lyse existing clots, but will prevent the extension of existing clots.

Heparin is not active orally. Intravenous bolus injections produce an immediate anticoagulant effect. The duration of action of heparin is dose dependent, the normal half-life being 60 to 90 minutes. The half-life may be prolonged to approximately 2.5 hours at doses of 400 units per kg.

Heparin is contraindicated in individuals who are hypersensitive to it, during uncontrolled bleeding episodes, and in patients in whom suitable blood coagulation tests (e.g., whole blood clotting time or partial thromboplastin time) cannot be performed at the required intervals. Heparin should not be administered intramuscularly owing to the danger of hematoma formation. It should be used with extreme caution in coexisting disease states in which there is increased danger of hemorrhage, such as subacute bacterial endocarditis, dissecting aneurysm, suspected intracranial hemorrhage, shock, severe hypertension, thrombocytopenia, peptic ulcer disease, ulcerative colitis, and severe hepatic, renal, or biliary disease. Heparin should be used with caution if the patient has been taking any drug that might interfere with platelet aggregation, including aspirin, dextran, phenylbutazone, indomethacin, ibuprofen (and numerous other nonsteroidal anti-inflammatory drugs), dipyridamole, and hydroxychloroquine.

Hypersensitivity reactions to heparin have been reported. Manifestations of these reactions include chills, fever, urticaria, rhinitis, lacrimation, asthma, and rarely an anaphylactic reaction. Hemorrhage is the chief complication. An overly prolonged clotting time or minor bleeding during therapy usually can be controlled by withdrawing the drug. If not, or if there is evidence of bleeding from an occult lesion, protamine sulfate may be administered by slow intravenous infusion. Each milligram of protamine sulfate neutralizes approximately 100 USP heparin units. Decreasing amounts of protamine sulfate are required as the elapsed time from the last heparin dose increases. No more than 50 mg. of protamine should be administered in any 10 minute period. Thirty minutes after a dose of heparin only approximately 0.5 mg. of protamine is required to neutralize each 100 units of heparin administered. Protamine sulfate is an anticoagulant itself and has a longer half-life than heparin; therefore, if protamine sulfate doses are excessive, it may cause bleeding.

The dosage of heparin should be adjusted according to coagulation test results determined just prior to each injection or infusion. The dosage is adequate when the whole blood clotting time is approximately two and one-half to three times the control value or when the partial thromboplastin time is one and one-half to two and one-half times the control value. When heparin is administered intermittently by the intravenous or subcutaneous route, coagulation tests should be performed before each dose early in treatment and daily thereafter.

Transient Ischemic Attacks

The patient with transient ischemic attacks, i.e., intermittent episodes of cerebrovascular insufficiency, poses a special therapeutic problem. A transient ischemic attack is defined as an episode of reversible neurologic deficit with clear-cut lateralizing and focal neurologic signs, lasting from a few minutes to 24 hours and disappearing without appreciable neurologic residual. Attacks occur at unpredictable intervals. The episodes are usually repetitive and tend to produce the same reversible neurologic symptoms. They are best looked upon as a fragmentary expression of what in some individuals will eventuate as a full-blown stroke. Ischemic attacks must be distinguished from focal epileptic seizures, on the one hand, and attacks of migraine, particularly hemiplegic migraine without headache, on the other. Since transient ischemic attacks represent the only meaningful warning signal in instances of cerebrovascular disease, their recognition provides, at least theoretically, an opportunity to undertake preventative measures in hopes of forestalling an ultimate stroke. Assessment of therapeutic efforts in the patient with transient ischemic attacks must be based on a knowledge of the natural history of the disorder. Studies suggest that no more than 30 per cent of all patients with transient ischemic attacks in fact develop full-blown strokes. Nonetheless, in view of the fact that the attack does provide a warning otherwise lacking in cerebrovascular disease, the temptation to intervene vigorously is great.

Carotid endarterectomy is widely utilized, although opinions differ substantially in terms of selection of patients. Such surgery is probably best reserved for the patient in good general physical health with little if any appreciable cardiac disease, with no significant fixed neurologic deficit, with an isolated, hemodynamically significant stenotic lesion occupying a single (and appropriate) carotid artery, and without appreciable intracranial vascular disease. Patients often fail to conform to these rigid parameters, however, and surgery is often undertaken under other and less well defined circumstances, perhaps most appropriately when an ulcerating plaque, a potential source of intravascular microembolization, is demonstrated angiographically. In patients with transient ischemic attacks who by virtue of extensive vascular disease within the neck or within the cranial vault are not acceptable candidates for endarterectomy, temporal artery–middle cerebral artery bypass utilizing microsurgical techniques may offer benefit.

In patients in whom no form of surgery can be undertaken, the use of anticoagulants (primarily Coumadin) for periods of up to one year promises a reduction in the frequency and severity of transient ischemic attacks. However, anticoagulants may not appreciably alter the statistical likelihood of stroke per se, and in fact considerable controversy has surrounded their use.[3] Long term anticoagulant therapy is usually achieved with a coumarin derivative such as warfarin.

The coumarin anticoagulants (dicumarol, warfarin, phenprocoumon) act by depressing hepatic synthesis of vitamin K dependent clotting factors (e.g., factors VII, IX, X, and II). It takes five to seven days for optimal depletion of clotting factors from the plasma and a full anticoagulant effect to be achieved.

Warfarin sodium (Coumadin) is generally considered to be the anticoagulant of choice. It has predictable bioavailability and a half-life of one and one-half to two days and is 97 to 98 per cent bound to plasma protein. The elderly are more sensitive than young adults to the orally administered anticoagulants. This could be the result in large part of a physiologic decrease in the concentration of plasma protein with advancing age that is independent of diet. The consequence may be an exaggerated response to the usual dose because more of the anticoagulant is circulating in its unbound active form. The physician must be particularly mindful of the possible need to adjust the dosage downward to achieve the desired pharmacologic response with no hemorrhagic sequela.

The orally administered anticoagulants are contraindicated in any situation involving a decrease in the concentration of plasma coagulation factors, reduced platelets, leukemia with pronounced bleeding, recent or contemplated surgery, aneurysm, severe uncontrolled hypertension, hepatic insufficiency, subacute bacterial endocarditis, or ulcerative lesions. The oral administration of anticoagulants in the following conditions, although not contraindicated, may be associated with increased risk: severe trauma, infectious disease with associated broad spectrum antibiotic therapy (which may suppress vitamin K producing bacteria), prolonged dietary insufficiency, moderate hypertension, severe diabetes, or after major surgery.

The orally administered anticoagulants interact with many other drugs. Indeed this class of drugs has greater potential for producing clinically significant drug interactions than any other class of drugs. Among the drugs that may enhance the anticoagulant effect of the orally administered anticoagulants by decreasing the availability of vitamin K are broad spectrum antibiotics, cholestyramine (Questran), and mineral oil. The drugs that enhance the effects of such anticoagulants by displacing them from plasma protein binding sites include phenylbutazone (Butazoladin), salicylates, sulfonamides, sulfonylureas, ethacrynic acid (Edecrin), mefenamic acid (Ponstel), nalidixic acid (NegGram), oxolinic acid, and diazoxide (Hyperstat). The drugs that potentiate these anticoagulants by inhibiting their metabolism by hepatic microsomal oxidative enzymes include allopurinol (Zyloprim), chloramphenicol (Chloromycetin), nortriptyline (Aventyl), disulfiram (Antabuse), metronidazole (Flagyl) alcohol, phenylbutazone, and clofibrate (Atromid-S). An increase in the bleeding tendency may occur if drugs such as salicylates, phenylbutazone, ibuprofen (Motrin), indomethacin (Indocin), oxyphenbutazone (Tandearil), sulfinpyrazone (Anturane), and dipyridamole (Persantine), which inhibit platelet aggregation when given alone, are administered concurrently with the orally administered anticoagulants. Thyroid drugs, anabolic steroids, quinidine, glucagon, and cimetidine (Tagamet) enhance anticoagulant effects by unknown mechanisms.

The drugs that decrease the anticoagulant effects of the orally administered anticoagulants by inducing hepatic microsomal enzymes that accelerate metabolism of such anticoagulants include the barbiturates, phenytoin (Dilantin), griseofulvin (Fulvicin), glutethimide (Doriden), carbamazepine (Tegretol), rifampin (Rifadin), and ethchlorvynol (Placidyl). Estrogens, orally administered contraceptives containing estrogens, and vitamin K promote coagulation.

All patients should be warned about the potential hazards of drug interactions. They should be instructed to avoid any drug, including nonprescription drugs, until they have consulted their physician or pharmacist. Additionally, they should be advised against any sudden change in diet or alcohol consumption.

The principal adverse effect of oral doses of anticoagulants is hemorrhage. Other adverse effects are infrequent and include nausea, vomiting, diarrhea, urticaria, abdominal cramps, fever, leukopenia, mouth ulcers, and agranulocytosis. Uncooperative, alcoholic, senile, and emotionally unstable patients are usually not suitable for therapy on an outpatient basis.

The dosage should be individualized and adjusted according to the one stage prothrombin time. The dosage should be adjusted to achieve and maintain a prothrombin time one and one-half to three times the control value, or prothrombin activity of 20 to 30 per cent of normal. If rapid anticoagulation is necessary, heparin should be used. Oral loading doses of anticoagulants are frequently associated with bleeding complications. Such anticoagulants should be started at anticipated maintenance dosage levels. Dosage adjustments can be made every three to five days on the basis of prothrombin time values. The usual maintenance dosage of warfarin sodium is 2 to 10 mg. daily (less in the elderly).

Antiplatelet drugs, including aspirin, dipyridamole, and sulfinpyrazone, may play a useful prophylactic role in the occurrence of transient ischemic attacks, although the ultimate effectiveness of these drugs has not been well established. Aspirin appears to be of significant benefit in males, but its value in females has not been clarified.[4]

In attempting to evaluate these various therapeutic modalities in patients with cerebrovascular insufficiency, mortality statistics are of little use, since patients with transient ischemic attacks generally die from underlying cardiac disease rather than cerebrovascular disease per se.

Even more problematic than the management of the elderly patients with transient ischemic attacks is the issue of the patient with an asymptomatic carotid bruit. The wisdom of invasive evaluation (angiography) in such patients remains questionable, and the role of vascular surgery is virtually impossible to determine. Patients with asymptomatic bruits are probably best managed by careful clinical observation, with neither pharmacologic nor surgical manipulation. Careful real-time ultrasonic carotid imaging may be very helpful in determining appropriate diagnostic and therapeutic efforts.

Cerebral Embolism

Embolic occlusion of the intracranial vessels is particularly prevalent in the early and middle decades of life, tending to be much less frequent than thrombo-occlusive disease in the elderly. The majority of cerebral emboli arise in the heart, in patients with chronic atrial fibrillation with a clot in the auricular appendage, subendocardial infarction with a mural thrombus, rheumatic valvular disease with or without active endocarditis, and cardiac myxoma. Cerebral emboli may appear in the course of cardiac surgery, especially during valve replacement. Additionally, leakage during circulatory bypass may account for some instances of air embolization. Embolic material may also originate in the pelvic or deep leg veins, such paradoxical embolization generally indicating a cardiac septal defect or shunt in the pulmonary circulation that permits embolic material to bypass the pulmonary circulatory bed. Other embolic events, such as air emboli with penetrating wounds of the carotid artery, are rarely encountered in the elderly. As in thrombotic disease, the nature and extent of the clinical stroke in instances of cerebral embolism are determined by the distribution of the vessel occluded as well as by the available collateral circulation; since embolic occlusion is an acute process, generally without pre-existing vascular stenosis, the collateral circulation has little opportunity to increase its effective functional capacity and may thus play only a limited role.

The management of the acute embolic stroke is essentially supportive. When cerebral edema is significant, the use of steroids is suggested, utilizing dexamethasone in dosages up to 24 mg. per day. Anticoagulants are of importance as a prophylactic measure to prevent further episodes of embolization. Heparin may be used initially, but in general warfarin sodium (Coumadin) is the drug of choice, particularly for prolonged use. Since the infarction with cerebral embolism is often hemorrhagic in quality, the early use of anticoagulants carries some risk of converting such a hemorrhagic infarct to a frank hemorrhage. For this reason it is often believed best to defer the use of anticoagulation for five to seven days following the acute embolic stroke; this is, however, an arbitrary decision and no firm deadline or treatment protocol is recognized.

Hypertensive Intracerebral Hemorrhage

Hypertensive intracerebral hemorrhage is a common occurrence in mid- and late life in the hypertensive individual. Such hemorrhages tend to occur in remarkably stereotyped fashion, particularly in the basal ganglia and thalamus and less commonly in the tegmentum of the pons and in the cerebellum. The cause of hypertensive hemorrhage is not known; it has been suggested that miliary (Charcot-Bouchard) aneurysms may play a significant role in the pathogenesis. Physical or emotional stress may precede the episode of bleeding. By virtue of the proximity of the sites of bleeding to the ventricles, extension of blood into the spinal fluid is common; signs of meningeal irritation may thus appear as part of the clinical presentation, along with increasingly severe headache, stupor, and coma. As demonstrated by the computed tomographic scan, smaller hemorrhagic foci are probably more common than has previously been suspected. With such small lesions, extension into the cerebrospinal fluid may not occur.

The management of the patient with hypertensive intracerebral hemorrhage is almost entirely supportive. Maintenance of the airway and of cardiovascular function is a paramount consideration. The use of steroids (dexamethasone in an average dosage of 24 mg. per day) is widely advocated but of uncertain benefit. Glycerol in a dosage of 1 mg. per kg. every six hours is sometimes used to reduce brain swelling. When herniation is impending, the short lived drugs, mannitol or urea, may be valuable. Despite vigorous therapy, the prognosis in patients of this sort is very poor; a large proportion of such patients die within seven days. Neurosurgical intervention for the most part has little to offer in this patient group; however, in the patient with cerebellar hemorrhage, the removal of the hematoma may be lifesaving.

Subarachnoid Hemorrhage

Blood in the subarachnoid space may be found under many circumstances and at any age, as, for example, in the patient with hypertensive bleeding or in the individual who has sustained head trauma. Primary subarachnoid hemorrhage due to rupture of an intracranial congenital ("berry") or mycotic aneurysm or of an arteriovenous malformation is relatively common in the third, fourth, and fifth decades but is unusual in the elderly. The management of the patient with subarachnoid hemorrhage is, at least initially, supportive. Dexamethasone or glycerol may play a role in reducing concomitant cerebral edema. Aminocaproic acid (Amicar) is widely used as an antifibrinolytic drug, although with uncertain benefit; it is given in an initial dose of 5 gm. orally or intravenously, followed by repeated doses of 1.0 to 1.25 gm. at hourly intervals up to a total of 30 gm. in 24 hours if necessary. A sustained aminocaproic acid plasma level of 0.13 mg. per ml. is apparently necessary for the inhibition of systemic hyperfibrinolysis.

Control of blood pressure with antihypertensive drugs may be necessary. Sedation with such drugs as diazepam or phenobarbital is often required.

Intense cerebral vasospasm may occur in the patient with a ruptured aneurysm. Vasodilators have been advocated, but their therapeutic role remains uncertain. The use of nitroprusside has been suggested in established instances of vasospasm, but the risk of systemic hypotension is great, and pressor drugs such as dopamine or Neo-Synephrine may be required. Close monitoring is vital in patients so treated. Volume expanders such as albumin may be used, either prophylactically at the time of intracranial clipping of an aneurysm, or therapeutically when one is dealing with already established vasospasm.

Temporal Arteritis

Among the many recognized forms of arteritis, temporal arteritis is of particular concern in the elderly. Occurring most often in females in the later decades of life, temporal arteritis presents with severe, often intractable, headache associated with palpable alterations of the temporal artery, including thickening, nodularity, tortuosity, and tenderness; leukocytosis and elevation of the sedimentation rate are typically found. Commonly part of a more widespread giant cell arteritis, temporal arteritis is frequently associated with occlusion of the ophthalmic or intracranial arteries. The risk of blindness or stroke is thus substantial in untreated individuals. The drug of choice is prednisone in dosages of 40 to 60 mg. per day for the first week, gradually tapering over the next few weeks to a maintenance level of 10 to 20 mg. per day, continued for periods of six, 12, or on occasion 24 months or longer. The dosage of steroid required is determined by the disappearance of headache and return of the sedimentation rate to normal. By following the sedimentation rate and trials of reduced dosage, the physician can determine when to terminate steroid therapy.

Hypertensive Encephalopathy

A rapidly rising systemic blood pressure, generally associated with renal failure, may precipitate a disorder characterized by intense headache, seizures, alterations of consciousness, and variable neurologic signs, usually associated with severe hypertensive retinopathy with papilledema. Prompt management of the blood pressure with specific antihypertensive therapy is critical. The adjunctive use of dexamethasone or mannitol (50 mg. in a 20 per cent solution intravenously, repeated every 12 hours as necessary) to reduce intracranial pressure may be necessary.

CRANIOCEREBRAL TRAUMA

The older individual is particularly susceptible to head injuries, whether incurred in spontaneous falls or in the course of personal assault. Acute or chronic subdural hematoma is especially common in the elderly. Epidural hematomas with skull fracture and tearing of the middle meningeal artery, traumatic subarachnoid hemorrhage, cerebral concussion, contusion, and laceration may occur as well, depending upon the nature and severity of the traumatic incident. With the acute head injury, rapid diagnostic evaluation is essential in order to identify immediately such life threatening processes as epidural or acute subdural hematomas. When neurosurgical intervention is not urgently required, the management is largely supportive. The use of dexamethasone, mannitol, or urea derivatives for the control of intracranial pressure is commonly necessary. Erosion of the gastric mucosa with hemorrhage (the Curling ulcer) may occur in such patients, perhaps potentiated by the concomitant use of steroids.

Following recovery from acute cranial injuries, patients commonly experience a variety of troublesome symptoms, including headache, impaired concentration, insomnia, defective memory, blurred vision, dizziness, and at times true vertigo. The treatment of this so-called post-traumatic or postconcussive syndrome is for the most part supportive. Vertigo may be relieved by the use of drugs such as meclizine (Bonine), 25 to 50 mg. daily; diphenhydramine (Benadryl), 50 mg. up to four times daily; or dimenhydrinate (Dramamine), 50 mg. four times daily. Promethazine (Phenergan), 25 mg. four times a day, may be effective. With most of these drugs, drowsiness is an unpleasant side effect, and anticholinergic effects occasionally appear. Mild analgesics may be required for the relief of headache. Antidepressants such as amitriptyline (Elavil) in doses of 25 to 50 mg. two to four times daily may alleviate some of the associated depressive symptoms. In general, such postconcussive symptoms gradually subside spontaneously over a period of weeks to months and no further therapeutic intervention is necessary.

NEOPLASMS

Virtually any form of intracranial tumor may be found in the elderly. Metastatic carcinoma is the most frequent intracerebral neoplasm, tumors of the glioma group tending to be relatively infrequent in this age group. Meningioma is not uncommon and may achieve a remarkable size with only minimal clinical manifestations. It is evident that the management of intracranial neoplasms is primarily neurosurgical or radiologic. The medical management is confined to the adjunctive use of drugs designed to control edema, such as dexamethasone or glycerol. The use of cancer chemotherapeutic drugs in general has been disappointing.

In patients with systemic (visceral) malignant disease, paraneoplastic neurologic syndromes may appear as so-called remote nonmetastatic effects. These include carcinomatous myopathy, the Lambert-Eaton syndrome, carcinomatous neuropathy, carcinomatous necrotizing myelopathy, motor system disease, and subacute cerebellar degeneration. Opportunistic infections and progressive multifocal leukoencephalopathy may also appear in immunosuppressed individuals, most commonly those with lymphomatous disease. There is no specific treatment for the majority of these disorders; it has been suggested, however, that progressive multifocal leukoencephalopathy may respond to the use of antiviral drugs such as cytarabine (Cytosar arabinoside) or ara-A (adenosine arabinoside).

MOVEMENT DISORDERS

Parkinson's Disease

Parkinson's disease (paralysis agitans) and the various related forms subsumed under the rubric of parkinsonism (e.g., postencephalitic parkinsonism, toxic or symptomatic parkinsonism, "arteriosclerotic parkinsonism") compose the most common movement disorder of the elderly. All types present typically with a combination of hyperkinesia (resting tremor) and hypokinesia (e.g., rigidity, akinesia, masked facies, shuffling gait, impaired dexterity, difficulty in initiating movements, faulty ocular convergence). Significant dementia occurs in 15 to 20 per cent of the patients with Parkinson's disease. Morphologic changes predominate in the substantia nigra but may involve other parts of the basal ganglia as well. A deficiency of dopamine in the striatum (caudate and putamen) has been well documented, reflecting neurotransmitter deficiency in the nigrostriatal dopaminergic fiber system. The therapy is based primarily on the restoration of dopamine; however, since dopamine and acetylcholine appear to compose a functional balance within the striatum, ancillary therapy utilizing anticholinergic drugs often proves valuable as well.

Levodopa. Replacement of dopamine may be accomplished by the use of levodopa (Larodopa). Dopamine itself cannot cross the blood-brain barrier; however, levodopa, which is the metabolic precursor of dopamine, does cross the blood-brain barrier and is converted into dopamine in the basal ganglia. Levodopa is indicated in the treatment of idiopathic Parkinson's disease, postencephalitic parkinsonism, symptomatic parkinsonism following injury to the central nervous system by carbon monoxide, and parkinsonism in elderly patients associated with cerebral arteriosclerosis. Some neurologists favor the use of levodopa early in the course of the disease. Others prefer to reserve the drug until symptoms are severe, utilizing other drugs in the initial phase of the illness.

Levodopa is well absorbed orally. It is extensively metabolized and excreted primarily in the urine. Its use is contraindicated in narrow angle glaucoma; it may be used in chronic wide angle glaucoma provided the intraocular pressure is monitored closely. Levodopa is also contraindicated in patients receiving monoamine oxidase inhibitor therapy.

Levodopa interacts with many drugs. Levodopa used concurrently with anticholinergic drugs may result in a mild degree of synergy. Gradual reduction in the anticholinergic dosage may be necessary. Episodes of postural hypotension have been reported when levodopa has been administered concurrently with certain antihypertensive drugs. The dosage of guanethidine (Ismelin) or diuretics may be reduced in patients receiving levodopa. Methyldopa (Aldomet) inhibits dopa decarboxylase mildly and may potentiate the effects of levodopa. Reserpine depletes brain dopamine and may interfere with the normal action of levodopa. Benzodiazepines may reduce the effectiveness of levodopa. Levodopa may interfere with the action of the orally administered hypoglycemic drugs, and diabetic patients taking levodopa therapy should be monitored closely. Monoamine oxidase inhibitors should be withdrawn at least 14 days prior to levodopa therapy to avoid significant increases in blood pressure. Low doses of the phenothiazines, butyrophenones and thioxanthenes may reduce the efficacy of levodopa. Phenytoin (Dilantin) decreases the effectiveness of levodopa. Pyridoxine hydrochloride (vitamin B_6) in daily oral dosages of 10 to 25 mg. rapidly reverses the therapeutic effects of levodopa. Levodopa may potentiate the pharmacologic effects of ephedrine, amphetamines, epinephrine, and isoproterenol, resulting in adverse cardiovascular effects.

Many adverse effects with levodopa have been documented. The more common effects are anorexia, nausea, vomiting, abdominal pain, choreiform and dystonic movements, dry mouth, dysphagia, ataxia, increased hand tremor, headache, orthostatic hypotension, dizziness, weakness, faintness, bruxism, mental confusion, insomnia, nightmares, delusions, hallucinations, anxiety, and euphoria. Less frequent adverse effects include cardiac irregularities, bradykinetic episodes (on-off phenomena), paranoia, dementia, depression, urinary retention, intestinal bleeding, hemolytic anemia, agranulocytosis, convulsions, diarrhea, constipation, flatulence, skin rash, diplopia, blurred vision, and edema.

Patients must be routinely counseled to take levodopa with food in order to avoid gastrointestinal upset and to avoid vitamins containing pyridoxine (vitamin B_6). They should observe caution while driving or performing other tasks requiring mental alertness and notify the physician if faintness, lightheadedness, or dizziness occurs. Levodopa may cause darkening of the urine or perspiration, but this is not cause for alarm. The medication may interfere with urine tests for sugar or ketones: levodopa yields false positive urine glucose test results using the copper reduction method (Clinitest tablets) and false negative urine glucose results with the glucose oxidase method (Tes-Tape, Clinistix). The physician should be notified immediately if the patient experiences uncontrolled movements of the face, eyelids, mouth, tongue, neck, arms, hands or legs; if mood or mental changes occur; if irregular heartbeats and palpitations are noted; if the patient has difficulty in urinating; or if severe or persistent nausea and vomiting occur.

The optimal daily dosage of levodopa alone must be titrated for each patient. The usual initial dosage is 0.5 to 1.0 gm. daily in two or more divided doses taken with food. The daily dosage may be increased in increments of not more than 0.75 gm. every three to seven days as tolerated. The dosage of levodopa should seldom exceed 8.0 gm. per day. A full therapeutic response may not be observed for weeks to months.

Levodopa-Carbidopa. Carbidopa may be used with levodopa to decrease the amount of levodopa required to control symptoms of parkinsonism. Carbidopa is a dopa decarboxylase inhibitor. It inhibits decarboxylation of peripheral levodopa and does not affect the metabolism of levodopa within the central nervous system. The net effect is that more levodopa is available for transport to the brain. Carbidopa therefore decreases the dosage of levodopa required by 75 to 80 per cent.

Carbidopa has no significant pharmacologic or pharmacodynamic effect when given alone. If carbidopa and levodopa are given together, levodopa should be discontinued at least eight hours before concurrent therapy is started. Additionally the dosage of levodopa should be decreased to 20 to 25 per cent of the previous dosage. The suggested starting dosage of carbidopa-levodopa (Sinemet) is one tablet containing 25 mg. of carbidopa and 250 mg. of levodopa three to four times daily. The dosage may be adjusted by adding or omitting one-half or one tablet a day.

Most patients respond to a 1:10 proportion of carbidopa to levodopa, provided the dose of carbidopa is adequate to saturate peripheral dopa decarboxylase, usually 70 to 100 mg. per day. If the patient has not received levodopa previously, a usual starting dosage of carbidopa-levodopa is 10 mg./100 mg. or 25 mg./100 mg. three times daily. The dosage may be increased by one tablet daily or every other day until a dosage of six tablets a day is reached. No more than eight tablets daily of carbidopa (25 mg.)-levodopa (250 mg.) should be utilized. At the present time the combination of carbidopa with levodopa (Sinemet) is most widely used in the management of parkinsonism.

Levodopa used alone or in combination with carbidopa generally produces a significant reduction in muscular rigidity, with improvement in dexterity and movement. Many patients achieve little if any relief of tremor. The efficacy of levodopa tends to wane with the passage of years, and gradual increases in the dosage are often required. Although it improves the patient's immediate clinical status, the protracted use of levodopa probably does not materially affect the progression of the disease itself. If a patient becomes refractory to levodopa, he may benefit substantially from a "drug holiday" in which all medication is stopped for several days or weeks and then reinstituted at a lower dosage level.

Anticholinergic Drugs. Anticholinergic drugs may be very helpful in the management of all forms of Parkinson's disease, although they are generally less effective than levodopa. All pharmacotherapy of Parkinson's disease is directed toward correcting an imbalance of neurotransmitter within the central nervous system, an imbalance comprising a relative dopamine deficiency and acetylcholine excess in the corpus striatum.

The elderly patient frequently develops an increased sensitivity to anticholinergic drugs, and strict monitoring for side effects should be undertaken. Downward dosage adjustments are often necessary. The elderly may tolerate antihistamines with central anticholinergic effects better than an anticholinergic per se in the management of parkinsonism. The use of anticholinergic drugs is frequently associated with the appearance of acute confusional states or psychotic behavior in the elderly.

Anticholinergic drugs are contraindicated if the patient is hypersensitive to these drugs or has known or suspected angle closure glaucoma; they should not be used in patients with pyloric or duodenal obstruction, stenosing peptic ulcer, prostatic hypertrophy, bladder neck obstruction, known tardive dyskinesia, or myasthenia gravis. Although not contraindicated for patients with hypertension, angina, cardiac arrhythmias, liver disease, and renal dysfunction, these drugs should be used with great caution in such individuals. Anticholinergic drugs may dilate the pupil and thus fix vision for distant objects at the expense of near vision. Patients should be cautioned about driving or operating machinery. Tasks requiring mental alertness may become more difficult owing to the drowsiness or dizziness associated with these drugs.

Anticholinergic drugs have the potential for interacting adversely with many other drugs. When anticholinergics are given with other drugs possessing significant anticholinergic activity (e.g., phenothiazines, tricyclic antidepressants), serious obstructive and adverse mental effects are much more likely to occur. By delaying gastric emptying, large doses of anticholinergic drugs may increase the gastric degradation of levodopa. Trihexphenidyl has been associated with decreased plasma chlorpromazine levels by as much as 40 per cent.

The more frequently occurring adverse effects of anticholinergic drugs alone include dry mouth, blurred vision secondary to mydriasis, dizziness, nausea, nervousness, loss of appetite, constipation, tachycardia, palpitations, headache, and decreased perspiration. Less frequently occurring adverse effects include skin rash, paralytic ileus, delusions, hallucinations, paranoia, mental confusion, agitation, urinary retention, giddiness, fever, mild but transient postural hypotension, depression, memory loss, and muscle cramping. Gastrointestinal side effects may be averted by taking the medication with food. The patient should be advised to avoid alcohol and other unprescribed central nervous system stimulants while receiving anticholinergic drugs. The physician should be notified if rapid or pounding heartbeat, confusion, eye pain, or rash occurs or if the side effects of dry mouth, difficult urination, or constipation become bothersome.

The anticholinergic drug most widely used in idiopathic Parkinson's disease is trihexphenidyl hydrochloride (Artane). As initial therapy, 1.0 mg. the first day is recommended. The dosage may be increased by 2.0 mg. increments every three to five days until a total of 6 to 10 mg. per day is reached; this is the dosage range at which most patients derive maximal benefit. Trihexphenidyl is tolerated best if taken three times daily at mealtime. If trihexphenidyl is taken with levodopa, the dosage of both drugs may have to be reduced. Trihexphenidyl in dosages of 3 to 6 mg. daily is usually adequate when taken with levodopa.

Other anticholinergic drugs that are often used include benztropine mesylate (Cogentin) whose usual dosage in idiopathic parkinsonism is 2.0 to 6.0 mg. daily, biperiden (Akineton) in a dosage of 2.0 mg. three or four times daily, ethopropazine hydrochloride (Parsidol) in a dosage of 100 to 400 mg. daily, orphenadrine hydrochloride (Disipal) in a dosage of 50 mg. three times daily, and chlorphenoxamine hydrochloride (Phenoxene) in a dosage of 50 to 100 mg. three to four times daily.

Benztropine mesylate should be started at a dosage of 0.5 to 1.0 mg. at bedtime. Some patients experience the greatest relief from benztropine by taking the entire dosage at bedtime. The long duration of action of this drug makes it particularly suitable for bedtime dosing if the dosage is not so high as to induce adverse effects.

Amantadine. Amantadine hydrochloride (Symmetrel) is sometimes useful as adjunctive therapy in the management of Parkinson's disease. This drug acts to facilitate dopamine release from presynaptic terminals. Amantadine is less effective than levodopa in the management of Parkinson's disease, and its clinical superiority to anticholinergics is not obvious. The concurrent use of amantadine and anticholinergic drugs may provide benefit beyond the marginal benefits obtained from each drug administered alone.

Amantadine is excreted unchanged in the urine to the level of approximately 90 per cent of the dose administered. The drug's elimination half-life is approximately 20 hours. A special precaution should be observed in the elderly because this drug has such a great tendency to accumulate in patients with impaired renal function. Marked dosage adjustments downward may be necessary. Patients with a history of seizure disorders should be observed closely for a possible increase in seizure activity, and those with congestive heart failure should be carefully monitored.

Adverse effects of a serious nature that occur relatively frequently with amantadine therapy include mental depression, congestive heart failure, orthostatic hypotension, psychosis, urinary retention, leukopenia, and neutropenia. Less frequent adverse effects include convulsions, confusion, hallucinations, anxiety, anorexia, nausea, constipation, ataxia, dizziness, peripheral edema, dry mouth, headache, insomnia, fatigue, skin rashes, slurred speech, and visual disturbances.

The usual dosage of amantadine in parkinsonism when used alone is 100 mg. twice daily. Some patients receive relief of symptoms at 100 mg. daily, and therapy should be initiated at this dosage level. Rarely a patient requires up to 400 mg. daily in divided doses. A fall-off in effectiveness after a few months is not uncommon. Effectiveness may be regained by increasing the dosage or discontinuing therapy for several weeks and then reinitiating the regimen.

When amantadine and levodopa are used concurrently, the patient may exhibit rapid therapeutic benefit. The dosage of amantadine should be held constant at 100 mg. once or twice daily while the daily dosage of levodopa is increased to achieve optimal benefit.

Bromocriptine. Bromocriptine mesylate (Parlodel), a dopamine receptor agonist, has been used in patients with severe parkinsonism who are refractory to levodopa. Approximately 30 per cent of a dose of bromocriptine is absorbed from the gastrointestinal tract; it is 90 to 96 per cent bound to serum albumin, is completely metabolized prior to excretion, and is excreted almost totally in the bile. It may be used alone or with levodopa. The combination may prove valuable in the patient currently taking optimal doses of levodopa who is developing tolerance to levodopa. Bromocriptine may allow a reduction in the maintenance dosage of levodopa, thus minimizing or preventing serious adverse effects associated with long term levodopa use (e.g., dyskinesias and the "on-off" phenomenon). Patients who are unresponsive to levodopa are poor candidates for therapy with bromocriptine alone.

Significantly more adverse effects occur with bromocriptine therapy than with either carbidopa-levodopa or levodopa therapy. The most common adverse effects induced by bromocriptine include hypotension, nausea, abnormal involuntary movements, hallucinations, confusion, "on-off" phenomena, dizziness, drowsiness, faintness, vomiting, asthenia, abdominal discomfort, visual disturbance, ataxia, insomnia, depression, shortness of breath, constipation, and vertigo. Less frequent adverse effects include anorexia, dry mouth, edema, epileptiform seizures, fatigue, headache, nasal stuffiness, nightmares, paresthesias, rash, urinary frequency, urinary retention, cold feet, muscle cramps, and exacerbation of Raynaud's syndrome.

The patient utilizing bromocriptine should be advised to take the drug with food. Since dizziness or fainting may occur following the first dose, the patient should be advised to take the first dose at home, preferably at bedtime, and to avoid sudden changes in posture. Use of this drug with any other drug known to lower blood pressure requires extreme care and careful monitoring. The drug should be used with caution in hepatic dysfunction, since the liver is the principle organ of metabolism and the major route of elimination. Impaired renal function should not significantly influence the elimination of bromocriptine.

Bromocriptine therapy should be started

at a dose of 1.25 mg. given twice daily with meals. Assessment every two weeks is required. If necessary, the dosage may be increased every 14 to 28 days by 2.5 mg. daily in divided doses with meals. The safety of bromocriptine at dosages exceeding 100 mg. daily has not been demonstrated. Many of the adverse effects are dose related, and the benefits of high dosage therapy generally do not outweigh the risks. The safety of bromocriptine beyond two years of continuous therapy has not been established. Bromocriptine is not recommended for routine clinical application in the treatment of Parkinson's disease at this time.

Miscellaneous Drugs. Other drugs may be of occasional value in patients with parkinsonism. The antihistamine diphenhydramine (Benadryl) may alleviate the tremor when used in conjunction with levodopa. Occasional patients seem to benefit from the use of propranolol in doses of 10 to 40 mg. four times daily.

Parkinsonian features may appear in other neurologic disorders, such as olivopontocerebellar atrophy or progressive supranuclear palsy (Steele-Richardson-Olszewski syndrome). Antiparkinsonian drugs may provide some relief, but patients tend to become increasingly incapacitated by virtue of the primary disease processes, which are, unfortunately, themselves not amenable to specific therapy.

Huntington's Disease

Sometimes looked upon as the biochemical opposite of Parkinson's disease, Huntington's disease presents clinically with a progressive movement disorder, generally chorea or choreoathetosis, associated with severe depression and progressive intellectual impairment. A rigid form resembling parkinsonism is recognized. Huntington's disease is inherited as a classic mendelian dominant trait with full penetrance. Pathologically changes are found particularly in the caudate nuclei and cerebral cortex. The disease is predominantly one of midlife; its onset in the very young or quite late in life has also been recorded. Dopamine levels in the striatum are normal, but there is a significant reduction in the gamma-aminobutyric acid level. A similar movement disorder involving especially elderly individuals, affecting the limbs, trunk, and particularly the orofacial musculature but with little if any mental change and without a positive family history, is senile chorea. The pathologic substrate of this disorder and its relationship to Huntington's disease are unclear. Also encountered late in life, albeit rarely, is the syndrome of posthemiplegic chorea, characterized by choreic movements of a paretic limb following recovery from hemiplegia, generally due to capsular infarction.

The treatment of the movement disorder of Huntington's disease is based on the use of dopamine antagonists, in particular, those that act at postsynaptic receptor sites. Effective in many patients, at least early in the course of the disease, are haloperidol (Haldol), 1 to 5 mg. four times daily, or fluphenazine (Prolixin) in a similar dosage. Reserpine, 0.5 mg. daily, gradually increased as necessary, may be beneficial, as is chlorpromazine in relatively small doses, although to a lesser extent. Propranolol (Inderal) generally proves ineffective. Management of the associated depression requires the use of appropriate antidepressants. There is, unfortunately, no medication that can alleviate the progressive dementia.

Drug Induced Movement Disorders

It has long been recognized that the long term use of phenothiazines may be associated with the appearance of the typical extrapyramidal syndrome of parkinsonism. The concomitant use of antiparkinsonian drugs, in particular anticholinergic drugs such as trihexphenidyl or benztropine, is often of substantial assistance in alleviating or preventing such parkinsonian features. The prolonged administration of phenothiazines or other antipsychotic dopamine antagonists may also be responsible, particularly in older females, for the appearance of tardive dyskinesia, characterized by a variety of abnormal movements involving the face, tongue, jaw, head, and neck. Management of this complication is unsatisfactory, and many patients so afflicted remain permanently disabled despite discontinuation of the precipitating drug and trial of medications such as choline, lecithin, reserpine, and deanol (the latter in doses of 100 mg. three times daily, gradually increasing to a maximum of 1.0 gm. daily). The efficacy of these drugs is uncertain and the results, disappointing. In some patients benefit is paradoxically derived from reinstitution of the same antipsychotic medication that appeared to induce the movements initially.

Following the initiation of antidopaminergic, antipsychotic, or antiemetic medication, a patient may suddenly develop severe dystonic movements; discontinuance of the offending drug and the prompt parenteral use of an anticholinergic such as benztropine or diphenhydramine may dramatically stop the movements.

Senile Tremor

Senile tremor is best looked upon as a form of so-called benign or essential tremor. This movement disorder, which may make an appearance at any age, consists of fairly rapid, predominantly distal tremors of varying amplitude, appearing primarily when the limbs are sustained against gravity and at times persisting through volitional movements. Tremor of the head may appear, and the voice may become tremulous. The tremor typically subsides following the ingestion of alcohol, the only movement disorder to do so. The disorder is at times familial, inherited as a dominant characteristic. It is ordinarily present for many years, gradually increasing in severity, often embarrassing, and at times of sufficient intensity to prove incapacitating. Therapeutically, tranquilizers such as diazepam (Valium) or chlordiazepoxide (Librium) have been used, but with little appreciable relief. Propranolol in dosages of 10 to 40 mg. four times daily is remarkably effective in many patients.

Hemiballismus

Among the many other involuntary movements that may appear in the course of disease of the basal ganglia, hemiballismus is especially noteworthy. This is a dramatic movement disorder characterized by flinging or circling movements of a limb, or limbs, as a consequence of a focal lesion, generally infarction or hemorrhage, within the subthalamic nucleus (corpus luysii). Haloperidol, reserpine, phenothiazines, and tetrabenazine have all been recommended, but with little significant benefit in the majority of patients. The movements generally subside spontaneously, within a period of days to weeks.

DEMENTIA

Dementia should be looked upon as a clinical manifestation, i.e., a symptom, rather than as a disease *sui generis*. Simply put, dementia may be defined as an impairment of intellectual (cognitive) functioning that is generally progressive and ordinarily is associated with impairment of memory and alterations of mood. It may develop at any age; Table 12–2 outlines many of the disorders associated with dementia. Those most commonly encountered in elderly patients include multi-infarct dementia, traumatic encephalopathies (most importantly subdural hematoma), anoxia, normal pressure hydrocephalus (either primary, i.e., idiopathic, or symptomatic, resulting from meningitis or subarachnoid hemorrhage, for example), Alzheimer's disease, and Parkinson's disease.

The effective management of the demented individual depends on precise definition of the underlying cause of the intellectual abnormality; the axiom that rational therapy is based on accurate diagnosis is nowhere better applied than in this group of patients. The necessity for prompt and thorough investigation of the demented patient is clear. When a disease such as myxedema or general paresis can be identified, specific drug therapy directed toward the primary disorder is, of course, utilized. In other patients specific therapy is mechanical rather than pharmacologic. Thus, the features of normal pressure hydrocephalus may be apparent, based on a clinical syndrome of rapidly advancing dementia associated with pyramidal tract signs in the legs, sphincter disorder, and gait apraxia (or ataxia), coupled with the observation on computed tomography of enlarged ventricles with little if any cerebral convolutional atrophy. In such patients shunting of spinal fluid from the ventricles to one of several extracranial sites may suitably be undertaken, although admittedly one cannot predict with certainty, even in typical instances, the degree of resulting clinical improvement. A shunt procedure, it should be emphasized, is not without complications and risks. Shunting may result in the development of acute subdural hemorrhage when the ventricular decompression is rapid. Later the shunt may become infected, with the subsequent development of ventriculitis or meningitis, or the catheter may become dislodged from the ventricle with subsequent shunt failure.

In many older individuals a specific cause of dementia cannot be identified, and when cerebral convolutional atrophy with increased size of ventricles (hydrocephalus ex vacuo) is observed with the computed tomographic scan, a diagnosis of Alzheimer's disease is most appropriate. A distinction between Alzheimer's disease, as a putative "presenile" de-

TABLE 12–2. Causes of Dementia

Cerebrovascular disease
    Multi-infarct dementia (lacunar state)
    Arteritis
    Subarachnoid hemorrhage leading to normal pressure hydrocephalus

Craniocerebral trauma
    Subdural hematoma
    Multiple contusion foci
    Delayed demyelination

Infections
    Purulent meningitis leading to normal pressure hydrocephalus
    Granulomatous meningitis
        Tuberculous meningitis
        Cryptococcal meningitis
    General paresis (tertiary lues)
    Viral encephalitis (arthropod-borne)
    Slow virus infections
        Kuru
        Jakob-Creutzfeldt disease
        Subacute sclerosing panencephalitis
        Progressive multifocal leukoencephalopathy
    Parasitic infections
        Toxoplasmosis
        Trypanosomiasis
        Trichinosis
        Malaria

Toxic and metabolic disorders
    Heavy metal intoxication
        Lead
        Mercury
        Thallium
    Drug intoxication
        Bromides
        Alcohol
    Anoxia
    Hypoglycemia
    Hepatolenticular degeneration (Wilson's disease)
    Kernicterus
    Uremia
        Dialysis dementia
    Neuronal storage diseases
        Sphingolipidoses
        Mucopolysaccharidoses
        Glycogenoses
    Leucodystrophies
        Metachromatic leucodystrophy
        Adrenoleucodystrophy
        Krabbe's disease
    Endocrine disorders
        Myxedema
        Addison's disease
        Cushing's disease
        Hypopituitarism
        Parathyroid disease
    Nutritional disorders
        Wernicke-Korsakoff syndrome
        Marchiafava-Bignami disease
        Pernicious anemia
        Pellagra

Demyelinating diseases
    Multiple sclerosis

Neoplasms
    Paraneoplastic dementia

Degenerative diseases
    Dementia as a primary characteristic
        Alzheimer's disease (including senile dementia)
        Pick's disease
        Normal pressure hydrocephalus (idiopathic)
        Progressive supranuclear palsy
        Huntington's disease
    Dementia as a secondary characteristic
        Paralysis agitans (parkinsonism)
        Friedreich's ataxia
        Olivopontocerebellar atrophy
        Amyotrophic lateral sclerosis
        Progressive myoclonus epilepsy

---

mentia, and "senile" dementia is without real value. The clinical and pathologic features are identical regardless of the age of onset, and a distinction on this basis alone appears spurious.

There is no specific medication of value in patients of this sort. Many drugs have been suggested, including vasodilating drugs, choline, lecithin, prostigmine, massive doses of vitamins, anticoagulants, dihydrogenated ergot alkaloids, and vasopressin; the benefits to be derived from such drugs is questionable at best. Since many patients with Alzheimer's disease are depressed, and since depression may contribute to the total clinical disability, the use of amitriptyline (Elavil) in a dose of 25 to 100 mg. at bedtime, or imipramine (Tofranil), 75 to 100 mg. or more at bedtime, often proves valuable. Haloperidol (Haldol), 1 to 2 mg. two or three times daily, may be helpful in the demented individual who is confused or agitated, and methylphenidate (Ritalin) in a dosage of up to 60 mg. daily or dextroamphetamine (Dexedrine) may be useful in the apathetic patient. Such measures are palliative only but may substantially assist in the day to day management of these patients. Clearly drugs such as these may be appropriately utilized not only in Alzheimer's disease, but also in other degenerative diseases such as paralysis agitans or spinocerebellar degeneration in which dementia may appear as an ancillary clinical phenomenon.

In elderly patients it is critical to exclude a simple depressive illness when assessing seeming intellectual deterioration, since depression may mimic dementia in a number of respects. It may be difficult to distinguish depression from dementia, since the psychomotor retardation typically encountered in the depressed individual seriously interferes with cognitive testing and may lead to a spurious impression of intellectual impairment when such in fact does not exist. A search for forced grasping or for perioral release phenomena, such as visual or tactile sucking or a positive snout reflex, may be helpful, since physical signs such as these often appear in the demented individual, but are lacking in the patient with a pure depression. Additionally, depressed individuals may exhibit some degree of insight into their level of performance, whereas patients with dementia typically lack such insight, generally being unaware of their cognitive defect. Early in the course of dementia, however, when memory problems are prominent, the patient is often aware of, and deeply concerned by, this deficit. When depression is present, vigorous therapy with antidepressive drugs, in particular, imipramine or amitriptyline, must be instituted.

EPILEPSY

As is the case with the demented individual, rational management of the elderly patient with seizures depends first and foremost on identification of the cause of the convulsive disorder. Seizures beginning in the later decades of life should never be accepted as "idiopathic" until a thorough search for focal brain disease has been undertaken. Tumors, whether primary or metastatic, must be rigorously excluded by appropriate testing. In the majority of elderly individuals developing seizures for the first time, cerebrovascular disease, in particular infarction, is the most common underlying cause. Other lesions not infrequently identified in the adult include meningocerebral scarring secondary to head injury and porencephalic cysts; on occasion seizures may appear in the course of a degenerative process such as Alzheimer's disease.

When no focal remediable lesion can be identified, management with anticonvulsant drugs must be initiated. Although a wide variety of anticonvulsants are presently available, relatively few are widely used. Those most effective in the treatment of seizures in the elderly, whether focal (focal motor, focal sensory, complex partial) or generalized, are to be described. As a general rule, it should be stressed that failure of anticonvulsant therapy in the elderly, as in all other patient groups, is most often attributable to a lack of compliance on the part of the patient. Other factors to be considered include inadequate dosage levels, the use of an inappropriate or ineffective anticonvulsant, and the presence of an evolving underlying cerebral lesion.

Phenytoin. Phenytoin (Dilantin) is widely used and is effective in a broad range of seizure disorders. It is easily administered by the oral route and remains the drug of choice in many patients. Phenytoin stabilizes the neurons of the brain against hyperexcitability, thereby preventing the spread of seizure activity.

Dosage titration is a very important factor in successful patient management. Therapeutic serum levels usually range between 10 and 20 mcg. per ml. Phenytoin is slowly absorbed from the small intestine. It is one drug whose bioavailability may vary widely from manufacturer to manufacturer. The prescriber is strongly encouraged to advise the patient that brand interchange, when cost is the only consideration, may have serious consequences.

Phenytoin is metabolized in the liver and excreted in the urine by tubular secretion. The half-life of phenytoin varies widely depending on dose, but the median half-life when the drug is administered in dosages of 300 to 600 mg. in three divided doses is 22 hours. Steady state serum levels are achieved seven to 10 days after the initiation of therapy at dosages of approximately 300 mg. per day. Phenytoin is 87 to 93 per cent bound to plasma protein.

Numerous precautions should be observed with the use of phenytoin. Because the liver is the chief site of biotransformation, elderly patients should be monitored closely for symptoms of toxicity. Blood tests at monthly intervals for the first several months of therapy should be conducted, for blood dyscrasias have been reported. The drug should be discontinued if any type of skin rash develops. Phenytoin may inhibit insulin release and therefore may complicate the management of diabetes. Abrupt withdrawal should be avoided because such an action may precipitate status epilepticus. Good oral hygiene can minimize gingival hyperplasia. Patients should be forewarned that the drug may impart a pink, red, or reddish brown color to the urine. Patients should be advised to exercise extreme caution while driving or performing tasks requiring mental alertness or dexterity because phenytoin may induce dizziness, drowsiness, and blurred vision.

Phenytoin may interact with many other drugs. Its effects may be increased by coumarin anticoagulants (e.g., Coumadin, Dicumarol), disulfiram (Antabuse), phenylbutazone (Butazolidin), isoniazid, chloramphenicol (Chloromycetin), cimetidine (Tagamet), sulfonamides, dexamethasone (Decadron), and large doses of salicylates. The effects of phenytoin may be decreased by carbamazepine (Tegretol), folic acid, chronic alcohol use, antacid therapy, oxacillin (Prostaphlin), vinblastine, cisplatin (Platinol), bleomycin (Blenoxane), and increased dietary calcium. Phenytoin may decrease the effects of dicumarol, disopyramide (Norpace), quinidine, digitoxin, furosemide (Lasix), and prednisolone. Concomitant infusions of dopamine and phenytoin may lead to hypotension and bradycardia. Phenytoin may increase the anticoagulant effects of warfarin. The concomitant administration of valproic acid (Depakene) and phenytoin may produce breakthrough seizures. Tricyclic antidepressants in large doses may precipitate seizures and require upward adjustments of phenytoin dosing.

The use of phenytoin is associated with a number of side effects, at times sufficiently severe to necessitate discontinuation of medication. An idiosyncratic morbilliform rash may occur early in therapy; exfoliative dermatitis is a rare complication. Features of lupus erythematosus may be manifest, and occasional patients develop thrombocytopenia, aplastic anemia, or agranulocytosis. Anemia may also appear as the result of a drug induced folic acid deficiency. Enlargement of lymph nodes, which mimics lymphomatous disease ("pseudolymphoma"), is well recognized, and features of hepatitis have been recorded. An adverse effect on thyroid function tests due to competition for the binding sites of thyroxin binding globulin has been described, and depressed adrenocortical activity has been noted.

Other well recognized adverse effects of phenytoin include gingival hypertrophy, hirsutism, nystagmus, cerebellar ataxia, and occasional hypocalcemia. Choreoathetosis may appear and polyneuropathy has been reported. Permanent cerebellar degeneration with loss of Purkinje cells has been claimed in individuals utilizing phenytoin over an extended period of time. Finally, many patients complain of lethargy or an ill defined loss of clarity of thought when taking phenytoin, even in the absence of other side effects.

The initial adult oral dosage is usually 300 mg. per day in three equally divided doses. Oral dosages up to 600 mg. daily may be required in rare circumstances. An oral loading dose of 1000 to 1200 mg. can achieve a therapeutic blood level within two to six hours after the dose has been taken.

The parenteral use of phenytoin is indicated if oral administration is not feasible. Intramuscular use must be avoided. Intramuscular absorption is very unreliable owing to precipitation of phenytoin in muscle tissue, and extensive necrosis may appear. Intravenous phenytoin therapy is indicated particularly in the management of status epilepticus; it, however, has been associated with hypotension, bradycardia, and sudden death. The rate of phenytoin infusion should not exceed 50 mg. per minute.

Phenobarbital. Phenobarbital is a widely utilized anticonvulsant either by itself or in combination with other anticonvulsants, particularly phenytoin. It is a long acting barbiturate whose peak central nervous system depressant effect is seen 10 to 12 hours after an oral dose. Phenobarbital is metabolized primarily by the liver and excreted in the urine; approximately 25 to 50 per cent of a dose of phenobarbital is excreted unchanged in the urine.

Phenobarbital should be administered with caution, if at all, to patients who are depressed or have suicidal tendencies or a history of drug abuse. The abrupt withdrawal of phenobarbital, even when administered in small doses, may precipitate status epilepticus. Elderly patients may react to phenobarbital in a paradoxical way with marked excitation or confusion. Because it is excreted partially unchanged in the urine, phenobarbital should be used with extreme caution in elderly patients with renal failure. This same caveat applies to persons with hepatic dysfunction who may not be able to metabolize the drug efficiently. Patients should be warned that barbiturates may significantly impair the performance of motor tasks.

Barbiturates have been reported to interact with numerous drugs. Because they induce hepatic microsomal enzymes, they may decrease the clinical response to orally administered anticoagulants, digitoxin, corticosteroids, and doxycycline. The absorption of griseofulvin appears to be impaired by phenobarbital. Valproic acid and monoamine oxidase inhibitors appear to potentiate the barbiturates. Additive depressant effects are likely if phenobarbital is taken with any other central nervous system depressant drug (e.g., sedatives, hypnotics, antihistamines, narcotics, tranquilizers, alcohol). The effects of phenobarbital on the metabolism of phenytoin are variable and unpredictable.

The usual oral adult dosage of phenobarbital as an anticonvulsant is 50 to 100 mg. given as a single night-time dose or in two or three divided doses. Dosages should be individualized, however. Reduced dosages in the elderly and in patients with impaired renal or hepatic function are generally indicated.

Primidone. Primidone (Mysoline) is useful in the treatment of generalized and focal (especially psychomotor) seizures. Primidone may be used alone or in combination with other anticonvulsants, usually phenytoin. Primidone and its two metabolites, phenobarbital and phenylethylmalonamide, possess anticonvulsant activity.

Primidone is well absorbed orally, reaches peak serum concentrations three to five hours after an oral dose, and is not significantly bound to plasma protein. Monitoring of primidone therapy should include determination of plasma concentrations of both primidone and phenobarbital. Phenylethylmalonamide is less active than primidone and phenobarbital as an anticonvulsant, and routine monitoring of plasma concentration is not essential. The therapeutic plasma concentrations of primidone and phenobarbital are 5 to 12 mcg. per ml. and 15 to 45 mcg. per ml., respectively.

All the contraindications, warnings, and precautions that apply to phenobarbital also apply to primidone therapy. The drug interactions that have been reported with the barbiturates also should be considered when using this drug.

Most side effects reported affect the central nervous system. These include ataxia, vertigo, nausea, anorexia, vomiting, diplopia, nystagmus, and drowsiness. The incidence of these adverse effects is not high at proper dosage levels, and the early side effects of ataxia and vertigo tend to disappear with continued therapy. A rare adverse effect is megaloblastic anemia, which responds readily to folic acid therapy.

The usual adult starting dose of primidone when there is no history of anticonvulsant drug therapy is 100 to 125 mg. at bedtime on days 1 through 3, then 100 to 125 mg. twice daily on days 4 through 6, increased to 100 to 125 mg. three times daily on days 7 through 9, and then leveled off at a maintenance dosage of approximately 250 mg. three to four times daily beginning on day 10. The dosage may be individualized but should not exceed 500 mg. four times daily. If the patient is already receiving another anticonvulsant, primidone should be started at a dose of 100 to 125 mg. at bedtime and gradually increased to maintenance levels over a 10 to 14 day period as the dosage of the other anticonvulsant is tapered. Because the metabolites of primidone are active and may accumulate if renal impairment exists, elderly patients should be dosed very carefully. Lower limits of the "normal" dosage range or doses below the usual may be all that is required for an optimal anticonvulsant response.

Carbamazepine. Carbamazepine (Tegretol) is useful in the management of both grand mal and focal seizures and has become the anticonvulsant of choice of many neurologists. Carbamazepine is absorbed slowly but almost completely when administered orally. Therapeutic levels in the plasma are between 4 and 12 mcg. per ml. The liver is the principal route of metabolism; the epoxide metabolite also has anticonvulsant activity.

There are several precautions to be observed if carbamazepine is prescribed. Patients with a history of bone marrow suppression should not receive carbamazepine. The drug should be discontinued at the earliest evidence of marrow supression. Carbamazepine has demonstrated some anticholinergic activity and should be used with caution in patients with increased intraocular pressure. Because the drug may cause drowsiness, dizziness, and blurred vision, patients should be cautioned about driving or performing tasks requiring alertness and sharp visual acuity. Baseline and periodic liver function and ophthalmologic testing should be undertaken. The patient should be encouraged to report to the physician the occurrence of unusual bleeding or bruising, jaundice, abdominal pain, pale stools, impotence, swelling of the hands or feet, fever, chills, sore throat, or mouth ulcers. When the drug is discontinued, the dosage should be tapered over several days.

Adverse hepatic, hematologic, and cardiac effects associated with carbamazepine therapy are the most serious. Cholestatic and hepatocellular jaundice has been reported. Adverse hematologic effects include aplastic anemia, leukopenia, agranulocytosis, eosinophilia, leukocytosis, and thrombocytopenia. Adverse cardiac effects include aggravation of pre-existing heart failure, aggravation of hypertension, hypotension, edema, and aggravation of coronary artery disease. The most frequently reported adverse effects include dizziness, drowsiness, unsteadiness, nausea, and vomiting and can often be managed readily by lowering the dosage without compromising the anticonvulsant activity of carbamazepine.

The dosage of carbamazepine should be adjusted to the needs of the individual patient. The usual initial dosage is 200 mg. twice daily. The dosage may be increased by daily increments of 200 mg. per day in divided doses until the best response is obtained. The usual maintenance dosage range is 800 to 1200 mg. daily in divided doses. Carbamazepine may be used alone or added to existing anticonvulsant therapy.

Valproic acid. Valproic acid (Depakene) is most effective in absence attacks; it is also useful in generalized, partial, and myoclonic seizures. Although the mechanism of action has not been precisely established, it appears to be related to increased brain levels of gamma-aminobutyric acid.

Valproic acid is rapidly absorbed from the gastrointestinal tract, peak serum levels occurring one to four hours after a single dose. The drug is approximately 90 per cent bound to plasma protein. The therapeutic serum concentration appears to be in the range of 50 to 100 mcg. per ml. The serum half-life is approximately eight to twelve hours, but may be increased substantially in cirrhosis, acute hepatitis, or other hepatic dysfunction. The drug, metabolized primarily by the liver, is excreted largely by the kidneys.

Numerous precautions should be observed while using valproic acid. Hepatic failure resulting in fatalities has been reported, usually during the first six months of treatment. Serious or fatal hepatotoxicity may be preceded by nonspecific symptoms, such as loss of seizure control, malaise, weakness, lethargy, anorexia, and vomiting. Hepatic disease, significant hepatic dysfunction, or hypersensitivity to valproic acid are thus absolute contraindications to its use. Liver function tests should be performed prior to therapy and at frequent intervals thereafter, especially during the first six months of therapy. Platelet counts and bleeding time determinations are also recommended before initiating therapy, at intervals during therapy and prior to surgery because of reports of valproic acid induced thrombocytopenia and platelet aggregation dysfunction. Any sign of a coagulation defect (e.g., bruising, hemorrhage) is an indication for lowering the dosage or discontinuing therapy. The incidence of dyspepsia upon initiation of therapy warrants the recommendation to take the drug with food. If the sedative effects persist, the patient should be cautioned about operating motor equipment.

Valproic acid interacts with several other drugs. It may potentiate the central nervous system depressant effects of alcohol and other depressant drugs. The serum levels of phenobarbital may be increased because valproic acid may impair nonrenal clearance of phenobarbital. Breakthrough seizures may occur if valproic acid and phenytoin are administered concurrently. Valproic acid may significantly potentiate the effects of drugs altering coagulation (e.g., aspirin, warfarin).

Other than the adverse central nervous system, hematologic, and hepatic effects mentioned earlier, the adverse effects from valproic acid are relatively rare and mild. The more common adverse gastrointestinal effects of nausea, vomiting, and indigestion typically occur at the initiation of therapy. These effects are usually transient and rarely require discontinuation of therapy.

The recommended initial dosage is 15 mg. per kg. per day, increased at one week intervals by 5 mg. per kg. per day until seizure control is optimized or side effects become intolerable. The maximal recommended dosage is 60 mg. per kg. per day. If the total dosage exceeds 250 mg. per day, it should be given in divided doses. The usual adult dosage is 250 mg. four times daily.

Ethosuximide. Ethosuximide (Zarontin) is considered quite effective in the treatment of absence seizures. Since the adverse effects are not as severe as those induced by valproic acid, the clinician may desire to initiate therapy for absence (petit mal) seizures with ethosuximide initially.

STATUS EPILEPTICUS

The treatment of status epilepticus requires special mention. Maintenance of airway patency is vital. Blood should be drawn for a glucose determination, and hypertonic glucose should be administered intravenously when the patient first appears in status epilepticus. Among anticonvulsant drugs, diazepam (Valium) is useful in arresting seizures for a short period of time; up to 10 mg. intravenously may be used for this purpose. Since the action of diazepam is short lived, it should always be used in combination with another longer acting anticonvulsant drug. The use of repeated intravenous doses of diazepam is to be avoided, since profound respiratory depression may develop.

Phenytoin is also effective in the management of status epilepticus. It is utilized intravenously, in a dosage of 15 mg. per kg. (approximately 1000 mg. in the adult) over a 20 minute period. The infusion rate should not exceed 50 mg. per minute. When it is administered in this manner, therapeutic blood levels are achieved within a few minutes. The drug should be given undiluted, since it has a tendency to precipitate out in intravenous solutions. The intravenous injection should be followed by an injection of sterile saline through the same catheter or needle to avoid local venous irritation secondary to the alkalinity of the drug. Under no circumstances should phenytoin be given intramuscularly in this emergency situation.

Phenobarbital utilized intravenously or intramuscularly may also be helpful in the management of status epilepticus. This drug may be given initially in a dose of 120 to 200 mg. intravenously, with a simultaneous equivalent dose intramuscularly. The intravenous medication should be repeated as necessary to control seizures. The patient receiving phenobarbital intravenously in large amounts must be monitored carefully to detect the development of respiratory depression.

Paraldehyde is only rarely used in the adult with status epilepticus, although it has a broader application in children. The use of general anesthesia is to be looked upon only as a last resort.

VERTIGO

Vertigo, defined as an illusory sense of movement of the self or of the environment—generally, although not invariably, rotatory—may appear in the course of a variety of disorders involving the inner ear, the vestibular portion of the eighth cranial nerve, the vestibular complex within the brain stem, and (although much less commonly) with disorders affecting the central vestibular connections, particularly the temporal lobe. Careful distinction must be drawn clinically between true vertigo and dizziness, the latter a nonspecific complaint lacking diagnostic precision, often used to describe feelings of giddiness or lightheadedness and generally of extracerebral origin.[5]

The specific treatment of vertigo depends upon appropriate isolation and identification of the underlying cause. Symptomatic relief may be obtained by the use of meclizine, 15 to 25 mg. two to four times daily; dimenhydrinate, 50 mg. four times daily; or promethazine, 25 mg. four times daily. Scopolamine, 0.6 mg. four times daily, is often helpful. Vasodilators such as nicotinic acid (100 mg. two or three times daily) or papaverine are claimed to be of occasional assistance, particularly in the elderly. Salt restriction and the judicious use of diuretics may prove of benefit in isolated cases. In incapacitating long standing vertigo, as in intractable instances of Meniere's disease, labyrinthotomy may be necessary for relief, but only when other therapeutic measures fail.

NEUROPATHY AND NEURALGIA

Turning briefly to disease of the peripheral nervous system, it need hardly be stated that specific therapy of the patient with polyneuropathy, or mononeuropathy, is dependent on precise identification and management of the underlying etiologic agent. Consideration of the numerous identifiable pathogenetic factors concerned with disease of the peripheral nervous system is beyond the scope of this presentation. Certain general principles of management, however, may be reviewed briefly. In some rapidly evolving neuropathies, such as the Landry-Guillain-Barré syndrome, or in the neuropathies of porphyria or diphtheria, respiratory failure may be life-threatening. Respiratory embarrassment must be recognized early and treated vigorously. Frequent monitoring of blood gas levels and of tidal volume and maximal breathing capacity are necessary and may provide early clues to impending failure. When continued surveillance indicates deterioration of pulmonary function, respiratory assistance must be instituted promptly. Particularly in patients with respiratory failure, the possibility of vasomotor collapse must always be borne in mind; a labile blood pressure as a manifestation of autonomic dysfunction is particularly common in the Landry-Guillain-Barré syndrome.

Pain is a prominent symptom in some patients with peripheral neuropathy, in particular those due to diabetes or nutritional depletion, with or without attendant alcoholism. Perversions of sensation (dysesthesias) may also appear. In addition to analgesics, phenytoin, 100 mg. three times daily, or carbamazepine, 200 mg. three to six times daily, may be of substantial benefit. A combination of fluphenazine, 1 mg. three times daily, and amitriptyline, 50 to 75 mg. at bedtime, has been found helpful in a number of such patients. Transcutaneous nerve stimulation is sometimes beneficial, especially in rapidly evolving pain syndromes. As a last resort, posterior root section (rhizotomy) may be necessary.

Some patients with polyneuropathy benefit from the use of vitamins on an empiric basis. Thiamin (vitamin B_1), 50 to 100 mg. two to three times daily, and cyanocobalamin (vitamin B_{12}), 1000 mg. parenterally once or twice weekly, appear useful from time to time, even in the absence of demonstrable nutritional depletion. In the management of most patients with neuropathy, proper nutrition with a high calorie, high protein, high carbohydrate diet is recommended.

Occasional patients with polyneuropathy complain of leg restlessness. Nocturnal discomfort in the legs necessitating repetitive movements of the limbs may seriously interfere with sleep in such individuals. Diazepam, up to 20 mg. or more orally per day, may be helpful.

In addition to the pain encountered in many instances of polyneuropathy, a more specific disorder characterized by chronic severe pain, often of a sharp lancinating (radicular) quality distributed along the course of an isolated dorsal spinal root or sensory cranial nerve, may be encountered. Such a chronic pain syndrome is referred to as neuralgia. It may develop following herpes zoster infection (shingles), but more often than not no precipitating factor can be identified. Among the more common forms of neuralgia encountered in clinical practice are trigeminal neuralgia, sphenopalatine neuralgia, glossopharyngeal neuralgia, occipital neuralgia, intercostal neuralgia, plexus neuralgia (especially brachial neuritis or neuralgic amyotrophy), and coccygeal neuralgia (coccydynia). Along with severe spontaneous pain, afflicted individuals often experience painful local dysesthesias as well. Carbamazepine, up to 1200 mg. daily in divided doses, or phenytoin, 300 to 600 mg. daily in divided doses, may be beneficial. In instances of intercostal neuralgia particularly, epidural block utilizing a combination of procaine and steroids may provide substantial symptomatic relief. Posterior rhizotomy may be necessary as a last resort.

Causalgia, a syndrome of severe pain associated with weakness, sensory impairment, and autonomic and trophic changes in the involved limb consequent to trauma to a peripheral nerve trunk, is treated in much the same way as neuralgia. Sympathetic block or sympathectomy may be especially helpful.

REFERENCES

1. McHenry, L.C.: New approaches to TIA's and strokes, Drug Ther., 67–73, 77–78, June 1980.
2. McHenry, L.C.: Cerebral Circulation and Stroke. St. Louis, Warren Green, 1978.
3. Ibid. p. 77.
4. Barnet, H.J.M.: A randomized trial of aspirin and sulfinpyrazone in threatened stroke: Canadian Cooperative Study. N. Eng. J. Med., *299*:53–59, 1978.
5. Parker, W.: Modern approaches to dizziness and vertigo. Drug Ther., 53–64, August 1980.

CHAPTER 13

MANAGEMENT OF POSTMENOPAUSAL WOMEN

Morris Notelovitz and Marsha Ware

Menopause refers to the cessation of menstruation secondary to aging of the ovary and is often the first sign that a woman is undergoing the transition from the reproductive to the nonreproductive stage of life. However, the menopause is just one facet of the larger climacteric, which encompasses endocrine, somatic, and psychologic changes and usually precedes the more obvious and dramatic event of menopause by several years. The distinction between the menopause and the climacteric is important, because changes related to failing ovarian hormone production can occur in women who are still menstruating.

The age at which menopause is reached and the manner in which it occurs are variable. In Western societies it usually occurs at about 50 years of age. Menopause before age 40 is said to be "premature" and occurs in about 8 per cent of women.[1] In most women ovulation and menstruation occur sporadically throughout the climacteric; menopause is defined following a one year period of amenorrhea. Constituting a special class of menopausal women are those who have undergone bilateral oophorectomies prior to the onset of natural menopause. Surgical menopause clinically resembles natural menopause but occurs in a much reduced time frame and mandates long term estrogen replacement therapy.

The transition from fertile to nonfertile status is a physiologic process not to be considered a medical condition requiring treatment. For most women this transition is smooth and uncomplicated, the cessation of menstruation being the only dramatic "symptom." For a significant minority of women, estrogen deprivation can produce debilitating symptoms, which interfere with daily living. For these women estrogen replacement therapy is indicated to alleviate symptoms and improve the quality of life.

In the past a myriad of symptoms have been incorrectly attributed to the menopause, resulting in the indiscriminate use of exogenous estrogens. With the inherent risks of administering any pharmacologic preparation and the evidence linking estrogens with endometrial cancer, careful selection of patients for estrogen replacement therapy is crucial. In addition to considering all contraindications, one must be certain that the symptoms are indeed estrogen related and not due to aging or an undiagnosed disease.

As with any decision concerning drug therapy, the relative benefits and risks of estrogen replacement therapy must be weighed individually for each patient. This evaluation must include considerations of the often clinically silent metabolic effects of estrogen lack, which can be manifested many years after the menopause, threatening the health of the aging woman. For example, osteoporosis has been linked to estrogen lack and is often preventable with long term estrogen replacement therapy if commenced within three years after the menopause.[2,3] The question in regard to estrogen replacement therapy and atherosclerosis is not as clear; estrogens appear to restore the increased ratio of high to low density lipoproteins found in premenopausal women. This lipid profile is thought to confer some protection against atherosclerosis.[4]

ENDOCRINOLOGY OF THE CLIMACTERIC

Each stage of a woman's reproductive life is maintained by an intricate relationship between ovarian and hypothalamic-pituitary factors. Aging of the ovary, diminished follicular activity, and reduced steroidogenesis affect this relationship, resulting in the altered endocrine profile and loss of reproductive capability of the menopausal woman. Physiologic aging of the hypothalamic-pituitary unit may also contribute to the changes.

The most striking endocrine change of the climacteric is the reduction in ovarian estrogen production to about 20 per cent of premenopausal values. This change results in a dramatic rise in the levels of the gonadotropins, follicle stimulating hormone and luteinizing hormone. The reason for this is twofold. With increasing age and decreasing ovulation, the ovary becomes less responsive to the stimulatory actions of follicle stimulating hormone and luteinizing hormone, and their production is accelerated in an attempt to compensate for the diminished response. In addition, both hormones are regulated by a negative feedback mechanism in which estrogen inhibits their production. During the climacteric when estrogen levels decline, this inhibition does not occur, and high follicle stimulating hormone and luteinizing hormone levels, characteristic of the postmenopausal endocrine profile, result.

These high gonadotropin levels are suppressed after administration of exogenous estrogens. A role for follicle stimulating hormone and luteinizing hormone and their hypothalamic releasing factors in the manifestation of climacteric symptoms (particularly hot flashes) has been suggested.[5] Suppression of gonadotropin production may be one mechanism by which estrogens exert their therapeutic effects.

The postmenopausal ovary is commonly misconceived as being an inert organ. Although follicular activity after age 50 is rare, the stroma of the ovary continues production of androstenedione, testosterone, and, to a small extent, estrogen. Androstenedione is peripherally converted to estrogen in skin and fat and is the primary source of postmenopausal estrogen. Loss of the ovarian source of estradiol results in a shift from estradiol to estrone (the product of androstenedione conversion) as the predominant estrogen. Not only are postmenopausal estrogen levels greatly diminished, but estrone has less biologic potency than the premenopausal estrogen, estradiol.

When choosing the type, dose, and duration of estrogen replacement therapy, the existing endocrine status and the effects of estrogen on that status must be considered. This is particularly true of prolactin and progesterone levels, both of which decline in the menopause. Prolactin continues its life-long pattern of paralleling estrogen by declining in direct proportion to estrogen in the climacteric. High prolactin levels are associated with an increased risk of breast cancer; for this reason serum prolactin levels should probably be assayed before initiating long term estrogen therapy.[6]

Progesterone levels decline as well during and after the menopause. Because unopposed estrogen activity can lead to overstimulation of the endometrium with resulting hyperplasia or cancer, the cyclic use of progestogens in women with intact uteri is strongly recommended when estrogen therapy is indicated.

CLIMACTERIC RELATED CHANGES: DIAGNOSIS AND TREATMENT

Manifestations of the endocrine events of the climacteric vary considerably among women. Not all women experience a symptomatic menopause: only 25 to 30 per cent seek medical attention for their complaints. One reason for this variation may be that comparable variation in the degree of peripheral conversion of androstenedione to estrogen exists, resulting in varying levels of endogenous estrogens.

Changes in Estrogen Target Tissues

Vulva

Many of the changes in genital tissue result from diminishing estrogen mediated maintenance of epidermal integrity. Perineal skin is particularly active in estrogen uptake and metabolism and with decreasing estrogen, begins to atrophy, losing its normal lubrication and elasticity.[7] Pathologic atrophy can lead to shrinkage and contracture of the introitus, resulting in dyspareunia—one of the most distressful symptoms for some postmenopausal women. Vulval dystrophies (kraurosis vulvae, leukoplakia, and lichen sclerosus) and pruritus vulvae are more common than in the premenopause, but a causal link with estrogen lack has not been established. Treatment requires identification of the etiologic factors and specific therapy. This can be achieved only by biopsy of suspicious areas.

In practical terms, only two types of lesions are found, each of which requires specific treatment. The histologic picture may be one of atrophy; these patients are best treated with testosterone proprionate in a petroleum base. Hyperplastic vulval dystrophies respond best to a topically applied mixture of a corticosteroid and an antipruritic drug; an excellent combination is cream containing seven parts of betamethasone valerate and three parts of crotamiton (Eurax).[8] Such creams should be applied twice a day, if necessary, with an occlusive dressing. Hyperplastic lesions usually respond within two to three weeks, after which time treatment should be stopped. Unfortunately atrophic dystrophies have a much greater tendency to relapse, and treatment must be continued for months to years. Broad spectrum antibiotics should be used for local secondary infections and the patient counseled as to the chronicity of various vulval dystrophies.

Because of a small but direct association between vulval dystrophies and squamous carcinoma, all vulval lesions should be regarded with suspicion, and adequate biopsy performed and a firm histologic diagnosis obtained.[9]

Vagina

Postmenopausal changes in the vagina are exceptionally responsive to estrogen therapy—a reflection of their direct relationship to estrogen lack. Decreased elasticity and increased submucosal connective tissue result in the gradual shortening and narrowing of the vagina with loss of its usual rugosity. The thinning vaginal epithelium is susceptible to ulceration and infection and may bleed easily to the touch. The presence of parabasal cells shed from the deeper epithelial layers indicates an atrophic epithelium and can be used as a guide to diagnosis and treatment.

Vaginitis is more common in the postmenopause period and may result from alterations of vaginal acidity and bacterial profile. However, the possibility that pathogens are responsible for vaginitis in premenopausal women should not be ruled out. Vaginitis associated with an overgrowth of several bacterial species (characterized by a thin gray discharge) or not attributable to known pathogens should be treated with antibacterial creams or estrogens (local or systemic administration). By improving the texture of vaginal tissue and enhancing lubrication, estrogen therapy alleviates associated dyspareunia and in most instances is the preferred approach.

An active sexual life is an important but infrequently noted determinant of vaginal pliability, as abstinence is often associated with progressive vaginal shrinkage. If sexual activity is resumed after lengthy abstinence, graduated vaginal dilators may be necessary and, when indicated, should be prescribed along with an estrogen cream.

Cervix

Postmenopausal changes in the cervix occur relatively later in the climacteric and for the most part are asymptomatic. As the uterus and cervix undergo atrophy, the portio vaginalis of the cervix no longer projects into the vagina and the external os becomes flush with the vaginal wall. Colposcopic examination reveals withdrawal of the squamocolumnar junction zone into the cervical canal. The covering squamous epithelium becomes thin and is easily traumatized. Speculum examination may cause slight bleeding, which must be distinguished from pathologic hemorrhage. Endocervical polyps (usually benign) are often found.

Although the average age at which cervical carcinoma in situ occurs is 38 years, the highest incidence of the invasive stage of cervical cancer is in the 45 and older age group. The need for careful cervical examination and regular Papanicolaou smears is obvious. Colposcopic assessment of atypical cytologic findings may be hampered by migration of the metaplastic area into the cervical canal and the frequently associated cervical stenosis. If visualization is limited, cervical curettage and diagnostic cone biopsy may be required.

Uterus

The early climacteric is most often characterized by irregular bleeding, making diagnosis of abnormal bleeding difficult. However, each patient must be thoroughly investigated because of the increased incidence of premalignant and malignant neoplasia during this time. In the absence of organic lesions, the usual cause of abnormal bleeding is unopposed estrogen activity (endogenous or exogenous) with incomplete shedding. This can lead to endometrial hyperplasia and possibly adenocarcinoma. Since progestogens can reverse most endometrial hyperplasia to normal, cyclic usage of these drugs is advocated. With time, as endogenous estrogen production declines, withdrawal bleeding no longer occurs. A postmenopausal uterus should not bleed; the clinician should beware of one that does.

Ovaries

Ovarian function begins to slowly decline early in life (about age 25) and in the climacteric is characterized by reduced steroidogenesis and follicular activity. This is followed by thinning of the cortex and a relative increase in the thickness of the medulla. Pregnancy after age 50 is rare, but ovulation can occur sporadically up to and occasionally beyond the menopause, ovulatory cycles occurring even after a period of amenorrhea. For this reason women are well advised to continue contraceptive practices for one year after the last menstrual period.

Orally administered combination contraceptives are not recommended, because their use in women over 40 is associated with increased cardiovascular complications. This may not be true for the newer generation of low dose orally administered estrogen-progestogen contraceptives. Recent data have demonstrated a dramatic fall in venous thrombosis related mortality associated with their usage.[10] Selective use of orally administered contraceptives containing 35 μg. of ethinyl estradiol and 0.35 to 0.4 mg. of norethindrone, for example, may be justified in certain instances. Oral doses of progestogens (norgestrel or norethindrone) and intrauterine contraceptive devices are effective but are often associated with irregular bleeding, which must frequently be investigated to exclude neoplasia. Barrier contraception (diaphragms, condoms, jellies, or foams) is free from this disadvantage, but patient acceptability may be low and decreased vaginal elasticity with time may make insertion of a diaphragm difficult and uncomfortable.

The progesterone intrauterine contraceptive device may be of some value. Its contraceptive action is apparently localized to the endometrium, since little progesterone derived from the device can be detected systemically. Apart from its contraceptive action, it may also protect the endometrium from the stimulatory effect of estrogen given for climacteric symptoms.

Urinary Tract

The epithelium of the urinary tract also responds to the hormonal changes of the climacteric, which is not surprising given its common embryologic origin with genital tissue. The distal urethra becomes rigid and inelastic, with a thin and easily traumatized or inflamed epithelium. These changes can interfere with bladder function by producing a distal obstruction to urethral outflow, leading to increased residual urine. The urethritis and inadequate flow rate and pattern (eddying instead of a spiral flow) allow ascent of organisms from the introitus, resulting in local urethral discomfort and secondary cystitis. Both are manifested as the urethral syndrome.

Urinary and vaginal smears can be compared for the assessment of abacterial cystitis (urethral syndrome) and identification of estrogen related symptoms. Comparison may also be useful as a guide to effective estrogen replacement therapy. Nocturnal frequency, dysuria, and incontinence are other common complaints in the postmenopause. Many times these symptoms are not related to estrogen lack, and only careful objective evaluation clearly defines the causes. Estrogen therapy should be used exclusively for estrogen related symptoms, chiefly those of abacterial urethritis. Estrogens also can be used as a supplement to the antibiotic treatment of recurrent cystitis and stress urinary incontinence, provided estrogen lack is a contributing factor.

Breasts

In most postmenopausal women the breasts involute, although in some instances they may actually hypertrophy. Deprived of the cyclic stimulation of estrogen and progesterone, the alveoli (progesterone dependent) begin to disappear and the mammary ducts (estrogen dependent) decrease in number. The epithelium of the secretory compartment atrophies, and connective tissue obliterates the lumina of the ducts. Regression occurs in most women in whom fibrocystic changes have occurred. Breast atrophy is never an indication for estrogen replacement therapy.

Although the cause of breast cancer is probably multifactorial, there is much circumstantial evidence to support a role of sex steroids in the pathogenesis or progress of breast cancer. For example, removal of the ovaries before age 35 results in a 70 per cent reduction in the incidence of breast cancer.[11] The administration of estrogen to postmenopausal women may increase or decrease the rate of growth of a cancer, depending upon the presence or absence of estrogen receptors. At this time a causal relationship between estrogens and breast cancer in healthy women has not been established.

One problem associated with estrogen therapy is that an increase in breast size and tissue turgor may preclude palpation of a suspicious nodule. Reduction of the estrogen dose or the addition of a small dose of testosterone—5 mg. of methyltestosterone twice daily for one week—will alleviate much of the accompanying mastalgia and ensure a more accurate examination.

Changes in Sexuality

Menopause signals the cessation of menstruation and the loss of reproductive capability of the female but by no means marks the end of an active sexual life. Indeed Masters and Johnson report that the aging female is capable of full sexual performance and pleasure, provided she is regularly exposed to effective stimulation.[12] Continuation of sexual activity throughout the climacteric may delay and even prevent some atrophic vaginal changes and associated discomfort.

Many women report menopausal changes in the libido, but it is important to realize that the menopause or aging per se is not the cause. Assessment of the sexuality of menopausal women in terms of frequency of coitus or orgasm risks overlooking important factors such as increasing age or the nonavailability of sexual partners, the presence or absence of dyspareunia, and the host of psychosocial variables influencing both pre- and postmenopausal sexuality.

Even in the absence of dyspareunia, atrophic changes in vaginal tissues often bring a reduction in the amount and speed with which lubrication is produced during sexual stimulation. For the sexually active menopausal woman, estrogen therapy can bring relief from vaginal soreness and dryness and can indirectly benefit by alleviating distressing hot flashes and by its well recognized mental tonic effect.

Increasing menopausal libido may be due to several factors. The lifting of "at home" restraints, such as busy households and workloads, and an increase in leisure time may have positive effects on sexuality. The effects of testosterone on sexual interest and function are well documented, and a role for testosterone in libido elevation has been suggested by several investigators. Elevated androgen-estrogen ratios in postmenopausal women suggest, on a strictly biologic basis, that menopausal libido would increase. However, the aforementioned variables appear to play more important roles in determining the sexual interests of menopausal women. Nonetheless subcutaneous pellet implants containing 100 mg. of testosterone and 50 mg. of estradiol have been suggested for treating psychosexual dysfunction during the climacteric.[13] As with other endocrine manipulations, these patients must be carefully followed by regular clinical examination and, if possible, biannual plasma testosterone assays.

The elderly female patient should be watched carefully for symptoms or signs of virilization secondary to androgen therapy, such as hoarseness or deepening of the voice and hirsutism. Hypercalcemia is more likely to occur in immobilized patients and in patients with breast cancer. Finally, prolonged androgen therapy may result in sodium and fluid retention, which may produce significant complications in the elderly patient with compromised cardiac reserve or renal disease.

Changes in Psyche

Depression, anxiety, irritability, and insomnia are common complaints and major sources of distress for many menopausal women. Attributing a psychosomatic origin to these complaints, as is often done, ignores the potent effects of hormones on emotional states and prevents many women from obtaining much needed relief. Whether these symptoms are indeed manifestations of climacteric changes or simply exacerbations of existing problems is still widely contested, but recent studies indicate a relationship between estrogen levels, depression, and insomnia. Evidence of such a relationship for other psychogenic complaints is not as strong.

The relationship between estrogen, depression, and insomnia appears to be mediated by changes in free tryptophan levels in the blood.[14] Menopausal women complaining of insomnia or depression have lower tryptophan levels than matched controls, and treatment with estrogen brings relief of symptoms with a concomitant rise in the blood tryptophan level. As a precursor to the neurotransmitter serotonin and as the rate determining factor in serotonin synthesis, tryptophan is not unexpectedly involved with depression and insomnia. Low serotonin levels are classically associated with depression, and high serotonin levels lead to somnolence. Estrogen is believed to increase free tryptophan levels by dissociating the binding of tryptophan with albumin, thereby increasing the amount of free tryptophan available for serotonin synthesis.

The treatment of psychogenic complaints during the menopause requires a careful evaluation of etiologic factors. A premenopausal history of depression or insomnia suggests that the complaints are not related to climacteric changes and therefore contraindicates estrogen replacement therapy. However, if the onset of symptoms coincides with the menopause, and underlying central nervous system disorders are excluded, treatment with estrogens may be appropriate.

Vasomotor Symptoms

Hot flashes, night sweats, and palpitations are the most common menopausal symptoms and the reasons many women seek medical attention. Recent investigations of the pathogenesis of hot flashes have revealed a close synchrony with luteinizing hormone secretion, implicating the hypothalamic-pituitary unit in the appearance of these symptoms.[5] Luteinizing hormone levels per se are not the determining factor, for hot flashes occur in hypophysectomized women.[15] Mechanisms governing luteinizing hormone releasing factors of the hypothalamus appear to be the key, and the close proximity of luteinizing hormone releasing factor neurons to the thermoregulatory centers of the hypothalamus make this hypothesis even more attractive. Functional changes in these neurons as a result of estrogen depletion after long term exposure have been suggested as the neuroanatomic substrate of vasomotor symptoms, making hot flashes a type of "withdrawal" symptom of estrogen lack.

The capacity of adrenergic alpha-blocking drugs (e.g., clonidine) to inhibit hot flashes further supports this idea, since catecholamines are closely associated with thermoregulation.[16] Naloxone, a potent opiate receptor antagonist, is also effective in preventing hot flashes.[17] The mechanism of action is not clear, but further investigations promise exciting insights into both the pharmacology of climacteric symptoms and the role of endogenous opiates in female endocrinology.

Estrogen therapy is still the most effective and most widely used treatment for vasomotor symptoms and offers an advantage over the previously mentioned experimental treatments in that it relieves other climacteric symptoms as well. More recently progestogens have also been found to be effective in alleviating hot flashes. Medroxyprogesterone acetate (Provera), titrated in dosages up to 30 to 50 mg. per day, significantly reduces the number of hot flashes, as do three-monthly intramuscular injections of Depo-Provera, 150 mg.[18] Although estrogen replacement therapy is probably the treatment of choice, progestogens can be used to advantage in women in whom there are absolute contraindications to the use of estrogen.

THE SYMPTOMATIC MENOPAUSE: WHEN TO TREAT

When deciding whether estrogen replacement therapy is indicated for a particular patient, the physician first must identify a valid indication for estrogen therapy and then make a risk-benefit assessment based on the severity of the symptoms, the health of the patient, and any contraindications to estrogen therapy.

In order to determine the clinical significance of reported symptoms, the patient should be asked to subjectively rate each estrogen related symptom on a four point "climacteric well-being" scale on the basis of severity and the need for treatment.[19] Letters of the alphabet can be used, "A" representing no symptoms, "B" representing mild symptoms that the patient can tolerate without treatment, "C" representing moderate symptoms for which treatment is requested but not essential, and "D" representing severe symptoms for which treatment is essential. For purposes of management and classification, the symptom complex with the most severe grade is used as the primary indication for treatment.

Having identified a valid indication, the physician must make an objective assessment of menopausal health on the basis of a thorough history and examination. Contraindications to estrogen replacement therapy can be identified by taking an appropriate history. Relative contraindications include existing hypertension, diabetes (overt, latent, or family history), liver disease, gallbladder disease, epilepsy, migraine, gross obesity, asymptomatic fibroids, previous endometrial hyperplasia (no atypia or cancer), cystic breast disease, a history of a single episode of phlebitis-thrombophlebitis, and a history of heavy smoking. Absolute contraindications include recent myocardial infarction, venous thrombosis-embolism, stroke, known or suspected estrogen sensitive cancer (e.g., breast or endometrial), pancreatitis or cholelithiasis associated with previous estrogen treatment, and undiagnosed abnormal genital bleeding.

A full physical examination—including a Papanicolaou smear, endometrial biopsy, and breast and pelvic examination—enables one to determine whether the patient is in good health and free from the stigmata of recent or chronic disease. Regardless of whether aspiration or curettage is used to obtain endometrial tissue, the endocervical canal should first be curetted, followed by circumferential sampling of endometrial cavity tissue from the fundus to the lower segment. Instillation of 5.0 ml. of 4 per cent lidocaine adds considerable comfort to the procedure.[20]

One of four grades of menopausal health is assigned on the basis of the history and examinations: "1" to individuals with normal results in all examinations and no associated disease; "2" to those in good health, with a negative Papanicolaou smear and endometrial biopsy findings but with some abnormal correctable feature (e.g., atrophic vaginitis, urethral syndrome, or moderate obesity); "3" to individuals with previous endometrial hyperplasia without atypia or any other chronic relative contraindication; and "4" to those with endometrial atypia or cancer or any other absolute contraindication.

A guide to the need for and suitability of estrogen replacement therapy is obtained by combining the patient's subjective assessment (A to D) with the objective results of the medical examination (1 to 4), thus providing a therapeutic index. For example, 1-B would represent a healthy patient with mild menopausal symptoms who would probably respond to explanation, psychologic support, and other nondrug measures. Individual assessment and judgment are required for grade 3 patients since they have some relative contraindication to estrogen replacement therapy. Thorough discussion with the patient regarding the benefits and risks of therapy, the type, dose, and duration of estrogen to be used, and the reliability and cooperation required by the patient to reduce certain risk factors (such as smoking) will determine whether estrogen replacement therapy should be prescribed. Estrogen replacement therapy is never prescribed for grade 4 patients, since in these cases there is some absolute contraindication to the use of estrogen. The suggested approach to estrogen replacement therapy for climacteric symptoms is summarized in Table 13–1.

ESTROGEN THERAPY: A CLINICAL GUIDE

Once the need for estrogen replacement has been defined in a particular patient, the questions of how much estrogen should be given, how estrogens are to be administered, how long therapy should be continued, the

TABLE 13–1. Menopausal Therapeutic Index

Menopausal Well-being (Patient Self-rating)	Menopausal Health (History and Examination)	Estrogen Replacement Therapy
A	1–4	None
B	1–4	None
C	1 and 2	Treat
	3	Individual assessment
	4	None
D	1 and 2	Treat
	3	Individual assessment
	4	None

A = no symptoms.
B = mild symptoms; can manage without treatment.
C = moderate symptoms; treatment requested but not essential.
D = severe symptoms; treatment essential.
1 = good health; no contraindications.
2 = good health, with some nonlife threatening features (e.g., atrophic vaginitis); no contraindications.
3 = endometrial hyperplasia without atypia or any other relative contraindication.
4 = endometrial atypia or cancer or any other absolute contraindication.

risks of estrogen therapy, and whether they should be used in women over 60 are addressed.

The Estrogen Dosage

The lowest effective dosage of estrogen should be given; this varies with the indication (Table 13–2). If the therapeutic objective is to alleviate hot flashes, the dosage would be titrated to the level at which maximal relief is achieved with minimal side effects. With atrophic vaginitis, suitable markers are the disappearance of symptoms and the absence of parabasal cells from the vaginal smear. Determination of plasma estrogen levels is advocated, for this allows for a more objective assessment of the amount actually absorbed. Plasma estrone and estradiol values of 60 to 80 pg. per ml. should be aimed for.[21] Persistence of symptoms in the presence of high plasma estrogen values indicates either excessive binding with globulin (thereby inactivating the estrogen) or that the symptom is not estrogen related.

Overdosage of estrogen is signaled by engorged and tender breasts, excessive weight gain, leukorrhea, and abnormal uterine bleeding. Dosage reduction is the primary approach after endometrial abnormalities have been excluded. Additional relief of symptoms may be achieved with judicious use of diuretics, the addition of a progestogen for the last 10 days of the treatment cycle, or both. Less obvious signs of overdosage or hyper-responsiveness to

TABLE 13–2. Estrogen Therapy—A Pharmacologic Guide

Condition	Type	Route	Estrogen Dose	Duration	Progestogen
Vasomotor and psychogenic symptoms	Natural				
	Estrone sulfate (Premarin, Ogen)	Oral	0.3–0.625 gm. daily	6–18 months	4 day cycles* of Provera, 5 mg., or Norlutate 2.5–5 mg.
	Estradiol (Estrace)	Oral	1–2 mg. daily	6–18 months	4 day cycles* of Provera, 5 mg., or Norlutate, 2.5–5 mg.
	Nonsteroidal Ethinyl estradiol	Oral	0.01–0.02 mg. daily	6–18 months	4 day cycles* of Provera, 5 mg., or Norlutate, 2.5–5 mg.
Atrophic vaginitis and urethral syndrome	Natural				
	Estrone sulfate (Premarin, Ogen)	Vaginal	1 gm. at bedtime	1 week	Nil
			1 gm. biweekly or	2–3 months	
		Oral	0.3–0.625 mg. daily	2–3 months	Nil
	Estradiol (Estrace)	Oral	1–2 mg. daily	2–3 months	Nil
	Nonsteroidal Ethinyl estradiol	Oral	0.01–0.02 mg. daily or	2–3 months	Nil
	Dienestrol cream	Vaginal	1 applicator at bedtime	1 week	
			1 applicator biweekly or	2–3 months	
	Diethylstilbestrol	Vaginal	0.1 mg. daily	1 week	Nil
		Suppository	0.1 mg. alternate days	2–3 months	

*Only required with intact uterus. Taken last 4 days of 21 day estrogen cycle.

estrogen therapy may include asymptomatic blood pressure elevation and alterations of coagulation and lipid and carbohydrate profiles.

As a clinical guide, 1.25 mg. of conjugated estrogen (Premarin) is biologically equivalent to 2 mg. of micronized estradiol (Estrace) or 0.01 mg. of ethinyl estradiol. In the absence of biologic monitoring, 0.3 to 0.625 mg. of Premarin per day or its equivalent is recommended, the dosage being titrated according to the patient's response.

The Route of Administration

Orally administered preparations of estrogen are preferred, because they allow for easy adjustment of dosage and easy withdrawal, if required. The usual practice is to administer the estrogen in three-week cycles, allowing the target organs (breasts and endometrium) a week of rest. Many patients complain of an increase in vasomotor symptoms during this break, and an alternative approach is to prescribe estrogen on a Monday through Friday basis (never on weekends). This is of particular value in the woman who has undergone a hysterectomy. For the woman with an intact uterus, a progestational drug should routinely be incorporated during the two weeks of estrogen therapy. Suitable preparations are 5 mg. of norethindrone, 10 mg. medroxyprogesterone (Provera), or 0.5 mg. of ethynodiol diacetate daily. In the perimenopausal period this regimen results in endometrial shedding, and the patient must be willing to accept menstruation as part of the treatment.

The traditional approach to treatment of atrophic vaginitis is the topical application of estrogen creams. It is now known that plasma levels of estrogen rise rapidly after application of the cream and may reach levels far in excess of those normally seen in reproductive women.[22] Serum hormone levels usually return to baseline values in 48 to 72 hours.[23] Commercially available creams or suppositories contain either natural or synthetic estrogens; the lowest effective dosage of these preparations has not been established. On the basis of plasma levels achieved with oral doses of estrogen, it would be more appropriate to use, for example, 1 gm. of conjugated estrogen cream (0.625 mg. of estrogens) or its equivalent, rather than the 2 to 4 gm. per day currently recommended. Once nightly applications for one week should restore the epithelial integrity without excessively raising serum estrogen levels. Thereafter, twice weekly applications should keep the vagina healthy. The physician should demonstrate the correct use of the applicator when estrogen cream therapy is to be started.

The Duration of Therapy

The duration of therapy varies with the indication. Vasomotor or psychogenic symptoms usually require treatment for six months to one year, after which time the patient should be gradually weaned from therapy. Intermittent treatment of one to three months' duration may be required to deal with recurrent episodes of urogenital symptoms. Long term therapy—measured in years—is required if excessive bone loss is to be prevented in osteoporosis prone individuals. A complete physical examination should be performed annually.

The Risks of Therapy

Endometrial cancer, hypertension, gallbladder disease, thromboembolism, decreased glucose tolerance, and hepatic adenoma are potential risks of estrogen therapy. There is no satisfactory evidence that estrogens given to postmenopausal women increase the risk of cancer of the breast, although recent animal data suggest this possibility. With proper screening to exclude patients at high risk and with careful follow-up of all patients given estrogen replacement therapy, the risk of these complications can be greatly reduced. With regard to endometrial cancer, the risk is related less to plasma levels of estrogen than to the duration of exposure and the presence or absence of progestogens. The cyclic use of progestogens with estrogen therapy promotes endometrial shedding, thereby reducing the risk of hyperstimulation of endometrial tissue.[24] Table 13–3 indicates the adverse effects most commonly associated with estrogen therapy.

Apparently normal women may respond in an idiosyncratic fashion to standard dosages of estrogen. It is recommended that patients be seen three and nine months after the start of therapy and at annual intervals thereafter. Care should be taken to perform a full clinical examination, including a thorough pelvic and

TABLE 13–3. Selected Adverse Effects Associated with Estrogen Therapy

Target Tissue	Adverse Effects
Genitourinary system	Vaginal candidiasis, change in cervical eversion and degree of cervical secretion, cystitis-like syndrome
Breast	Tenderness, enlargement, secretion
Gastrointestinal	Nausea, vomiting, abdominal cramps, bloating, cholestatic jaundice, gall bladder disease, hepatic adenoma
Skin	Chloasma or melasma, erythema multiforme, erythema nodosum, hemorrhagic eruption, loss of scalp hair
Eyes	Steepening of corneal curvature, intolerance to contact lenses
Endocrine	Decreased glucose tolerance
Central nervous system	Headache, migraine, dizziness, mental depression, chorea
Miscellaneous	Fluid retention, body weight fluctuations (increase or decrease), reduced carbohydrate tolerance, edema, change in libido, endometrial cancer, thromboembolism, hypertension

breast examination. Fasting plasma glucose, cholesterol, triglyceride, and high density lipoprotein levels should be measured. Papanicolaou smears and endometrial biopsy should be repeated annually. Episodes of intermenstrual or abnormal bleeding should be investigated by dilatation and curettage.

Use in Elderly Women

Estrogen lack is associated with relatively few symptoms that necessitate long term replacement therapy. By age 60 most women have adapted to the vasomotor and psychogenic symptoms, and in patients being treated for these symptoms therapy should be tapered off after 12 to 18 months. The dosage should be reduced over a period of a few months. Except in the case of potential and established bone loss, estrogens should be necessary only for limited periods when one is dealing with target tissue-related disorders (e.g., atrophic vaginitis and the urethral syndrome). Repeated short term (two to three month) courses may be required.

Patients aged 60 or more who have been taking long term estrogen replacement therapy compose a separate category of elderly women whose needs and suitability for such therapy must be reviewed and evaluated. Although estrogen replacement therapy has been shown to prevent development of osteoporosis, the usefulness of estrogens in treating established osteoporotic disease has not been clearly defined and is an issue the physician may have to confront in a previously untreated 60 year old woman. Progestogens should be added to the regime in any patient given long term estrogen replacement therapy. Although endometrial shedding is less likely in this population, the possibility of its occurrence must be carefully explained to the patient before starting treatment. Addition of progestogens is necessary only in women with an intact uterus and is not required for short term therapy.

An additional consideration in either continuing or instituting estrogen therapy in elderly women is the increased incidence of contraindications in this population. Certain physical changes are associated with aging, e.g., a gradual increase in blood pressure, diminution of glucose tolerance, and an increase in blood coagulation factors. The dividing line between "normal" and "pathologic" change is often ill defined, and this distinction becomes particularly significant when the potential risk of estrogen replacement therapy in these disorders is considered. These conditions are more prevalent in the elderly and may pose a real threat to their well-being. The physician must ensure that the benefits of estrogen replacement therapy outweigh the potential risks.

OSTEOPOROSIS, ATHEROSCLEROSIS, AND THE MENOPAUSE

The physician must be aware of the potential harmful effects of osteoporosis and atherosclerosis. Both conditions are asymptomatic early in their course. To a certain extent both can be prevented or ameliorated by early diagnosis and suitable therapeutic intervention.

Osteoporosis

Osteoporosis afflicts 25 per cent of "natural menopausal" women and 40 to 50 per cent of "surgical menopausal" women not receiving estrogen replacement therapy. Long term estrogen replacement therapy, commenced within three years of the menopause (and immediately after surgical menopause) and before osteoporosis has developed, retards bone resorption greatly and prevents subsequent liability to pathologic fractures. The problem lies in identifying the women predisposed to the disorder, for at present there is no definitive test to identify the early stages of osteoporosis. For the present, the identification of osteoporosis is largely an exercise in exclusion, for the etiology and predisposing factors have not been clearly defined.

Osteoporosis must be distinguished from osteopenia, the asymptomatic physiologic bone loss occurring with age. Osteoporosis is a pathologic exaggeration of osteopenia, which in its early stages is asymptomatic but if left untreated progresses to a stage characterized by pain, deformity, and fracture. An association between the estrogen status and the rate of bone resorption and formation has long been recognized. However, estrogens are one of many factors affecting bone mass; osteoporosis also is a multifactorial disease. Study of osteoporotic bone has provided little insight into the pathogenesis other than an observed increase in bone resorption with normal or slightly decreased bone formation. In view of the foregoing, postmenopausal osteoporosis may be related to an interplay of the following factors:

Alterations of Calcium Homeostasis

Parathyroid hormone is instrumental in maintaining appropriate blood levels of ionized calcium. Secreted in response to decreasing blood calcium, it acts on the kidney to increase calcium reabsorption. In cases of calcium dietary deficiency or inadequate absorption from the gut, parathyroid hormone continues to exert its effects in maintaining proper calcium levels at the expense of skeletal calcium (90 per cent of the body total) by increasing bone resorption. In addition, parathyroid hormone stimulates conversion of vitamin D to its active form, calcitriol—one of the most potent human steroid hormones. Calcitriol acts on the gut to increase calcium absorption and together with parathyroid hormone induces mobilization of bone calcium. Calcitonin, a "calcium sparing" hormone produced by the thyroid, antagonizes various functions of parathyroid hormone and inhibits production of calcitriol. Its major effect is inhibition of bone resorption.

Several studies show that osteoporotic patients consume less calcium than matched control subjects. Further, calcium absorption declines with age, starting at age 55 to 60 in women. Lactose intolerance is also more prevalent in the elderly population, leading to reduced intake of dairy products—the principal dietary source of calcium. When the foregoing is coupled with the fact that the absorptive mechanism becomes less sensitive to vitamin D with aging and that older individuals are usually less frequently exposed to sunlight, it would seem logical that calcium and vitamin D supplements should effectively prevent and be effective in the treatment of osteoporosis. However, studies indicate that such supplements are not a "cure" for bone loss but rather an important adjunct to treatment.[25]

Considerations of dietary phosphorus are also important, for a phosphorus-calcium ratio greater than unity results in bone loss. The average ratio in the American diet is 1.5 : 2.0, largely because of the high phosphorus-calcium ratio of red meat containing diets. The high sulfur content of meat also affects the body's acid-base balance, inducing acidosis and subsequent urinary excretion of calcium. It is well established that bone is mobilized in many types of acidosis and that chronic alkali ingestion increases bone formation.

Hormonal Status

Evidence of the importance of estrogen in osteoporosis is strong. Young oophorectomized women lose bone rapidly: a woman in whom ovarian function is lost at age 35, by age 45 has as little bone as a woman at age 60 who underwent natural menopause 10 years earlier. By contrast, in women who are still menstruating in their fifties the normal premenopausal bone mass is maintained.

It has been proposed that low estrogen levels sensitize the skeleton to the resorbing action of parathyroid hormone, thereby increasing calcium levels, which in turn results in a slight fall in parathyroid hormone production.[26] Consequently the kidney and gut are less effective in calcium conservation, leading to skeletal resorption, hypercalcemia, and calcium malabsorption. Clinically this hypothesis has been supported by the finding that osteoporotic women have low to normal levels of parathyroid hormone levels, low calcitriol levels, and fasting hypercalcemia.

However, lack of estrogen alone cannot

explain why only 25 per cent of postmenopausal women develop osteoporosis and why blood estrogen levels do not differentiate normal from osteoporotic-prone populations. Part of the explanation may be in differences in the degree of androstenedione conversion to estrogen. Obesity and increasing age are known stimulants of this process. Thus, obese women rarely develop osteoporosis, and the rate of bone loss in women decreases significantly after age 65. In a recent study plasma androstenedione levels were significantly lower in postmenopausal osteoporotic women than in equally matched control subjects.[27] This suggests that plasma androstenedione may be useful in a screening profile of asymptomatic osteoporosis and emphasizes the need to preserve postmenopausal ovarian function, for a significant amount of the androstenedione produced at this time comes from the ovary.

It should be remembered that postmenopausal ovarian atrophy (or oophorectomy) involves the loss of progesterone as well as estrogen. Progesterone has been shown to prevent bone loss by increasing bone formation, rather than decreasing resorption.[28] The mechanism of this action is unknown.

Physical Activity

Immobilization is associated with a significant alteration of bone mineral homeostasis and loss of structural integrity. Exercise has a conserving effect on the bone mineral content and matrix, with denser, stronger, and usually thicker bones the result. However, there is still a need to define the type, degree, and duration of exercise that will maintain or increase bone mass.

Personal Habits

Heavy smokers, on the average, reach menopause earlier than matched controls. This has been related to a greater incidence of cardiovascular disease and an increase in bone loss. It is not clear whether there is a direct causality between smoking and increased bone loss or whether the latter is mediated via an earlier menopause and longer exposure to estrogen deficiency. Until the exact nature of the relationship is defined, it can be concluded that heavy smoking enhances the rate of bone loss in postmenopausal women.

Excessive alcohol intake is associated with low calcium levels and increased liability to osteoporosis. As with smoking, excessive alcohol intake has an additive effect, rather than an initiating role, in an individual predisposed to osteoporosis.

Race

Certain ethnic or racial groups are more susceptible to osteoporosis (women and descendents from the British Isles, northern Europe, Scandinavia, China, and Japan) than others (blacks and, to a lesser degree, whites from southern and central Europe). Postmenopausal osteoporosis is uncommon in black women, and osteoporosis almost never develops in black men. The reason for this "ethnic" immunity is not entirely clear, but differences in muscle and bone mass and hormone milieu between black and white women may account in part for the difference.

Diagnosis

Detection of osteoporosis is difficult given the asymptomatic nature of the disease in its early stages. However, there are certain clinical and biochemical indicators that can be used in a screening profile.

Certain generalizations can preselect women who are more likely to develop osteoporosis. Thus a frail, inactive, white woman of Scandinavian origin is more likely to develop osteoporosis than an obese, physically active black woman. Bilaterally oophorectomized women are at similar risk, especially if the procedure was performed premenopausally. A history of long term corticosteroid, antiepileptic, or anticoagulation (heparin) therapy is of significance, as is alcohol abuse and smoking. Medical and surgical histories may reveal information leading one to suspect and look for osteoporosis. Finally, a thorough dietary history should be taken to determine the daily intake of calcium, the relative ratio of phosphorus-rich and acidic foods, and exposure to both dietary and environmental sources of vitamin D.

Loss of height is probably the most important early physical sign of pathologic bone loss in the vertebral column. Arm span measurements serve as an excellent estimation of height at bone maturity and can be used to measure the degree of vertebral bone loss. The normal decrease in height in women is estimated to be ± 1.5 cm. per decade. The presence of "thin" skin may also be indicative of early osteoporosis: "thin" skin is often associated with "thin" bones. The skin in some osteoporotic women appears to be transparent, indicating collagen breakdown paralleling similar changes in osteoporotic bone.

Symptomatic osteoporosis is invariably caused by collapse of one or more vertebral bodies and presents as nonradiating back pain, localized to the weight bearing vertebrae below T7. The pain can be exacerbated by direct pressure and is not associated with generalized bone pain.

Photon absorptiometry of the distal end and midshaft of the radius is possibly the most cost-effective means of screening for bone loss. However, the cost of the instrument prohibits its routine use in other than specially equipped centers. An alternative is metacarpal radiogrammetry. Radiologic measurement of the metacarpals is of value in quantitating bone loss at a given time or longitudinally. Because of the architecture of the bone, this method reflects cortical bone loss as measured by changes in cortical width (the difference between total metacarpal width and medullary width). The normal decrease in cortical width is about 0.05 mm. per year. The midpoint of the second metacarpal (some workers include the third and fourth metacarpals as well) is usually used because of its low morphologic variability. Precision calipers are used to measure the total and medullary widths, from which cortical thickness and area can be derived. The nondominant hand should be used.

Once an osteopenic state has been determined, a battery of plasma and urine tests should be performed to determine whether the bone loss is "idiopathic" or secondary to an established metabolic or malignant process. Postmenopausal osteoporosis is characterized by a normal or slightly elevated plasma calcium level and a normal alkaline phosphatase level. The urinary hydroxyproline-creatinine and calcium-creatinine ratios are also normal or slightly elevated. With this confirmatory biochemical profile and documentation of decreased bone mineral content or density, one can safely treat the patient for postmenopausal osteoporosis.[79] Measurement of androstenedione levels may also be helpful, as indicated previously. When the screening profile suggests secondary disease, additional tests should be ordered to define the etiologic factor. These patients are best treated by specialists in bone metabolism and disease.

Because of the potentially high cost of osteoporosis in terms of morbidity and sometimes mortality, it is strongly suggested that this screening profile be incorporated into every postmenopausal (natural or surgical) woman's annual examination. The most crucial time is within the first three years after the menopause.

Treatment

Significant bone loss can be prevented or bone mass re-established if therapy is commenced within three years after the menopause. Once an exaggerated rate of bone loss is established, specific measures can be used to slow the rate. All postmenopausal women, however, benefit from the recommendations regarding diet, smoking, drug intake, physical activity, and exposure to sunlight.

Diet. The recommended daily allowance of calcium is now estimated to be 1400 mg. rather than the previous 800 mg. All patients with established disease should receive calcium supplements, especially if they are receiving treatment that inhibits bone resorption (e.g., estrogens). Os-Cal tablets (two to four per day) can be used to supplement both calcium and vitamin D; each tablet contains 250 mg. of calcium and 125 units of vitamin D.

If calcium loss continues despite oral supplementation, a failure of absorptive mechanisms can be assumed, and measures should be instituted to reduce the intake of foodstuffs known to interfere with the process (e.g., phosphorus rich meats, high fiber vegetables, vegetables high in oxalates, and the outer husks of cereal). Absorption can also be enhanced with vitamin D supplements or estrogens.

The recommended daily allowance of vitamin D is 400 units. In the absence of osteomalacia, a maximum of 1000 units of vitamin D should be added to the diet in osteoporosis prone women, especially those who are not exposed to sunlight. Depending upon the amount of Os-Cal taken for calcium supplementation, the balance of the vitamin D requirement can be supplied with multivitamin tablets, each of which contains upwards of 400 units. In addition, the acidity of the diet should be considered and the intake of soft drinks and red meats reduced.

Physical Activity. Regular exercise helps postpone or slow osteoporotic bone loss. Although maximal benefit is achieved by weight bearing pressure on the bones, most forms of exercise are beneficial. Some patients with long established or severe osteoporosis may actually be harmed, however, if too strenuous an exercise program is instituted. The objective must be to reduce rather than increase the compressive forces on the spine. Further, the exercise chosen should match the physical fitness and interests of the individual.

Back braces are useful in the early stages of vertebral collapse, for they provide support and enable the patient to walk. However, in the long term, braces may actually worsen osteoporosis by reducing the weight bearing stimulus on the spine. Some recommend a girdle as an acceptable substitute.

Estrogen Therapy. The dosages and types of estrogens that have been effectively used in the prophylaxis and treatment of osteoporosis are summarized in Table 13–4. Excessive estrogen should be avoided, since there is little evidence that increasing the dosage increases the osteogenic action; however, there is abundant proof that side effects, such as endometrial hyperplasia, will be increased.

The goal of estrogen replacement therapy for osteoporosis should be to suppress bone loss until advent of the adrenopause (approximately age 65), at which time the rate of bone loss decreases because of the diminished activity of osteolytic adrenal steroids. At this point adequate bone mass should be achieved and the osteopenia of old age should not (it is hoped) progress to senile osteoporosis. Annual monitoring of bone loss should be maintained and estrogen replacement therapy reinstituted if the rate of bone loss exceeds the norm for that age group.

One concern in regard to long term estrogen replacement therapy is that diminished bone resorption will be followed by decreased bone formation, since new bone formation is dependent upon bone resorption. Therefore, all women given estrogen replacement therapy for osteoporosis should receive supplemental calcium to guard against a possible negative calcium balance.

As experience with estrogen is gained and its mechanisms of action defined, it is likely that lower dosages and combinations of different estrogens will be found that decrease side effects, enhance the calcium retentive capacity, and reduce the bone formation inhibition that presently complicates this form of treatment.

Progestogens. Whether a combination of estrogen and progesterone will provide the "ideal" situation of concurrent slowing down of bone resorption and acceleration of new bone formation remains to be seen. Long term use of progestogens would overcome the problem of estrogen induced endometrial hyperplasia. Unfortunately prolonged use of progestogens may decrease the formation of high density lipoprotein (thought to be protective to vascular intima) and, in theory, may enhance the development of atherosclerosis.[30]

Judging from the experience and relative safety of contraceptive progestogens, it is suggested that patients in whom there are con-

TABLE 13–4. Estrogen Therapy for the Prevention and Treatment of Postmenopausal Osteoporosis

Condition	Type	Route	Estrogen Dosage	Duration	Progestogen
Osteoporosis prophylaxis	Estrone sulfate (Premarin, Ogen)	Oral	0.3–0.625 mg.*†	±10 years	4 day cycles of Provera, 5 mg.,‡ or Norlutate, 2.5–5 mg.
	Estradiol (Estrace)	Oral	1–2 mg.*†	±10 years	4 day cycles of Provera, 5 mg.,‡ or Norlutate, 2.5–5 mg.
	Ethinyl estradiol	Oral	0.02 mg.*†	±10 years	4 day cycles of Provera, 5 mg.,‡ or Norlutate, 2.5–5 mg.
Established disease	Estrone sulfate (Premarin, Ogen)	Oral	1.25 mg.*†	±10 years	4 day cycles of Provera, 5 mg.,‡ or Norlutate, 2.5–5 mg.
	Ethinyl estradiol	Oral	0.05 mg.*†	±10 years	4 day cycles of Provera, 5 mg.,‡ or Norlutate, 2.5–5 mg.

*Uterus intact: 21 days per month.
†Hysterectomy: daily, Monday–Friday, or daily continuously.
‡Required only with intact uterus. Taken last 4 days of 21 day estrogen cycle.

traindications to estrogen therapy and who require adjunctive hormonal therapy be treated with 125 to 150 mg. of Depo-Provera intramuscularly every three months. The usual pretherapy diagnostic work-up is required, and these patients must be followed-up every three to six months for evaluations of blood pressure and lipid profile. Two orally administered forms of progestogen have been evaluated to date—Lynestrenol, 5 mg. daily, given continuously, and medroxyprogesterone acetate, 10 mg. in one week cycles each month. No adverse side effects were reported, and both appeared to be effective in maintaining bone density.

Calcitonin. Calcitonin has been shown to inhibit bone resorption in early administration, but its potential long term usefulness is limited by the fact that bone formation diminishes with time and may lead to a negative bone balance.[31] As yet, its use has not been associated with a decrease in the incidence of fractures. The recommended dosage is 50 to 100 MRS units daily, or three times per week, and it must be given subcutaneously. Calcitonin does not seem to offer any real advantage other than its availability as a safe alternative for women in whom estrogens or other hormones are contraindicated.

Treatment of Advanced Disease

Unfortunately there is no truly effective treatment for advanced osteoporosis other than prevention of further bone loss by nutritional adjustments, graduated exercise, and estrogen therapy. Definitive orthopedic management of long bone fractures is self-evident. Stabilization of the vertebral column is more problematic, because a balance must be struck between the need for immobilization and the risk of accelerating bone loss.

The only definitive therapy that has been reported is the use of larger dosages of estrogen. In a prospective study of women with advanced osteoporosis, 1.25 mg. of conjugated estrogens per day was found to reduce the incidence of fractures to three per 1000 women-years, whereas a daily dosage of 0.625 mg. reduced the incidence to 25 per 1000 women-years.[32] The following dosages of estrogen have been suggested as effective "anti-fracture" measures: 1.25 mg. of conjugated estrogen (Premarin); 50 μg. of ethinyl estradiol, and 1 mg. of diethylstilbestrol. In addition, adequate calcium and vitamin D supplements should be prescribed.

Low doses of parathyroid hormone offer an exciting new possibility in the treatment of established osteoporosis. Researchers, realizing that new bone formation has to be activated by bone resorption, have used small quantities of parathyroid hormone in an attempt to stimulate new bone formation and thereby increase bone density in women with osteoporosis. It is hoped that this hormone may prove useful for the treatment of the "crush fracture syndrome." Together with estrogens, calcitonin, or some other drug that increases overall bone formation, parathyroid hormone therapy could herald an exciting and positive future for the treatment of overt osteoporosis.[33]

Atherosclerosis

The lower incidence of atherosclerosis and associated vascular diseases in premenopausal women than in men of the same age has led to the theory that endogenous estrogens impart some protective effect in the pathogenesis of these disorders. This theory is supported by the increased incidence of atherosclerosis in cases of premature or early surgical menopause. Estrogen replacement therapy in these women is associated with decreased morbidity and mortality from atheroma or related diseases.

Whether estrogen replacement therapy in postmenopausal women will restore the protection against atherosclerosis is unclear. Serum cholesterol and triglyceride levels increase after the menopause, suggesting a decrease in the ratio of high density to low density lipoproteins (because high density lipoprotein levels are inversely related to triglyceride levels).[34,35] An increased high density/low density lipoprotein ratio, as found in premenopausal women, is associated with a reduced risk of atherosclerosis; conversely a decreased ratio is associated with increased risk.[36] Estrogen mediated maintenance of the premenopausal lipid profile may be responsible for the lower incidence of atherosclerosis in women under 50. Estrogen replacement therapy in postmenopausal women, by restoring the increased high density/low density lipoprotein ratio, may in theory reduce the risk of atherosclerosis in this population.

Since atherosclerosis is a multifactorial disease, it would be simplistic to suggest that this disease could be prevented or induced by the use or misuse of estrogens. Important factors such as smoking, stress, and the potential role of estrogen induced hypertension and increased coagulability need to be considered. In addition, the beneficial effects of diet and exercise cannot be overemphasized. However, the effect of estrogens on the lipid component of atherogenic disease is also important and is best summarized by this excerpt from a leading article:

> ... the net effect of estrogens in coronary atherosclerosis might be largely determined by the pre-existing state of the vessels and, therefore, by the age of the subject. Increased endogenous estrogen production from an early age, as in normal females, might protect against the development of the disease, whereas increased production or exogenous administration much later in life might predispose to thrombosis over existing complicated lesions.[37]

In this context, the need to preserve endogenous ovarian steroidogenesis by limiting the practice of premenopausal oophorectomy cannot be overemphasized. The protective effect of estrogen replacement therapy still must be proved, although there is evidence to support the use of estrogen replacement therapy in agonadol females and in women who are subject to an early menopause. The optimal dosage of estrogen has not been evaluated for this indication. Until this has been clearly defined, daily treatment with 0.625 mg. of conjugated estrogen or its equivalent is recommended. The usefulness of estrogen replacement therapy in older postmenopausal women is more controversial and is difficult to assess because the risk-benefit of this treatment depends on the presence of pre-existing atherogenic disease and other at-risk factors.

There is a close corrollary between estrogen replacement therapy and coronary heart disease and between estrogen replacement therapy and osteoporosis. In the latter, estrogen is effective in preventing osteoporosis but not in treating the condition once it has developed. The same might be true for estrogens and coronary heart disease.

CONCLUSIONS

As the median age of the American population continues to rise, more women are entering the over-50 age group. With a life expectancy of 28 years beyond the menopause, these women expect and deserve safe and efficacious treatment of menopausal problems to ensure the quality of their later years. Although estrogen therapy will probably continue to be the mainstay of menopause management, new therapeutic modalities developed from investigations of neuroendocrine correlates and steroid analogues may provide these women with effective alternatives to estrogen in the future.

Until the long term safety and efficacy of these experimental treatments are demonstrated, clinicians should concentrate on using estrogens to the safest maximal benefit. Before prescribing estrogens, the physician must distinguish symptoms of aging from those of estrogen lack. The latter respond to estrogen therapy, whereas the former do not and in some cases may serve as contraindications to estrogen replacement therapy. Proper screening of patients at risk and careful periodic evaluations of patients receiving estrogens will minimize the chance of estrogen related complications. For patients with intact uteri who are given estrogen replacement therapy, the cyclic addition of progestogens will reduce the associated risk of endometrial cancer.

REFERENCES

1. Keetel, W.C., and Bradburg, J.T.: Premature ovarian failure, permanent and temporary. Am. J. Obstet. Gynecol., 9:83–96, 1964.
2. Nordin, B.E.C., Horsman, A., Marshall, D.H., Hanes, F., and Jakeman W.: The treatment of postmenopausal osteoporosis. In Barzel, U.S., (Editor): Osteoporosis II. New York, Grune & Stratton, Inc., 1979, pp. 183–203.
3. Lindsay, R., et al.: Long-term prevention of postmenopausal osteoporosis by oestrogen. Evidence for an increased bone mass after delayed onset of oestrogen therapy. Lancet, 1:1038–1041, 1976.
4. Editorial. HDL and CHD. Lancet, 2:131, 1976.
5. Casper, R.F., Yen, S.S., and Wilkes, M.M.: Menopausal flushes: a neuroendocrine link with pulsatile luteinizing hormone secretion. Science, 205:823–825, 1979.
6. Furth, J.: The role of prolactin in mammary carcinogenesis. In Pasteel, J.L., and Robyn, C. (Editors): Human Prolactin. New York, American Elsevier Publishing Company, 1973, pp. 223–248.
7. Stumpf, W.E., Sar, M., and Joshi, S.G.: Estrogen target cells in the skin. Experientia, 30:196–198, 1974.
8. Friedrich, E.G.: Vulvar Disease, Philadelphia, W.B. Saunders Company, 1976, p. 55.
9. Jeffcoate, T.N.A.: Principles of Gynecology. London, Butterworth & Company (Publishers) Ltd., 1975, p. 329.
10. Stolley, P.D., et al.: Thrombosis with low-estrogen oral contraceptives. Am. J. Epidemiol., 102:197–208, 1975.

11. MacMahon, B., Cole, P., and Brown, J.: Etiology of human breast cancer: a review. J. Natl. Cancer Inst., 50:21–42, 1973.
12. Masters, V.H., and Johnson, V.E.: Human Sexual Response. Boston, Little, Brown and Company, 1966.
13. Greenblatt, R.B., and Suran, R.R.: Indications for hormonal pellets in the therapy of endocrine and gynecologic disorders. Am. J. Obstet. Gynecol., 57:294–301, 1949.
14. Aylward, M.: Estrogen, plasma tryptophan levels in perimenopausal patients. In Campbell, S. (Editor): The Management of the Menopause and Postmenopausal Years. Baltimore, University Park Press, 1976, pp. 135–147.
15. Mulley, G., Mitchell, J.R.H., and Tattersall, R.B.: Hot flushes after hypophysectomy. Br. Med. J., 2:1062, 1977.
16. Clayden, J.R., Bell, J.W., and Pollard, P.: Menopausal flushing: double-blind trial of a non-hormonal medication. Br. Med. J., 1:409–412, 1974.
17. Lightman, S.L., and Jacobs, H.S.: Naloxone: nonsteroidal treatment for postmenopausal flushing? Lancet, 2:1071, 1979 (letter).
18. Morrison, J.C., et al.: The use of medroxyprogesterone acetate for relief of climacteric symptoms. Am. J. Obstet. Gynecol. 138:99–105, 1980.
19. Notelovitz, M.: Menopause—when to treat. Hosp. Med. 16:9–21, 1980.
20. Hofmeister, F.J.: The pros and cons of estrogen therapy. Ob/Gyn Digest, 21:37–42, 1979.
21. Lauritzen, C.H.: Estrogen deficiency syndrome and management of the patient. In van Keep, P.A., Greenblatt, R.B., and Alveaux-Fernet, M. (Editors): Consensus on Menopause Research. Lancaster, MTP Press, 1976, pp. 37–43.
22. Martin, P.L., Yen, S.S.C., Burnier, A.M., and Hermann, H.: Systemic absorption and sustained effects of vaginal estrogen creams. J.A.M.A., 242:2700, 1979.
23. Katz, M., and Roux, J.P.: Oestrogen cream for the older vagina. South Afr. Med. J., 55:236, 1979 (letter).
24. Campbell, R.C.: The role of hormones in endometrial cancer. South. Med. J., 10:80–1286, 1978.
25. Thomson, D.L., and Frame, B.: Involutional osteopenia: current concepts. Ann. Intern. Med., 85:789–803, 1976.
26. Heaney, R.P.: A unified concept of osteoporosis. Am. J. Med., 39:877–880, 1965 (editorial).
27. Crilly, R., Cawood, M., Marshall, D.H., and Nordin, B.E.C.: Hormonal status in normal, osteoporotic and corticosteroid-treated postmenopausal women. J. Roy. Soc. Med., 71:733–736, 1978.
28. Lindsay, R., Hart, D.M., Purdie, D., Ferguson, M.M., Clark, A.S., and Kraszewski, A.: Comparative effects of oestrogen and a progestogen on bone loss in postmenopausal women. Clin. Sci. Mol. Med., 54:193–195, 1978.
29. Nordin, B.E.C., Horsman, A., and Aaron J.: Diagnostic procedures. In Nordin, B.E.C. (Editor): Calcium, Phosphate and Magnesium Metabolism. New York, Churchill Livingstone, 1976, pp. 469–524.
30. Bradley, D., Wingerd, J., Petitti, D., Krauss, R., and Ramcharan, S.: Serum high-density-lipoprotein cholesterol in women using oral contraceptives, estrogens and progestins. N. Engl. J. Med., 299:17, 1978.
31. Wallace, S.: Management of osteoporosis. Hosp. Pract., 13:91–98, 1978.
32. Gordan, G.S., Picchi, J., and Roof, B.S.: Antifracture efficacy of long-term estrogens for osteoporosis. Trans. Assoc. Am. Physicians, 6:326–332, 1973.
33. Reeve, J., et al.: Anabolic effect of parathyroid hormone fragment on trabelcular bone in involutional osteoporosis: a multi-centre trial. Br. Med. J., 2:1340–1344, 1980.
34. Shibata, H., Marsuzaki, T., and Hatano, S.: Relationship of relevant factors of atherosclerosis to menopause in Japanese women. Am. J. Epidemiol., 109:420–424, 1979.
35. Hulley, S.B., Cohen, R., and Widdowson, G.: Plasma high-density lipoprotein cholesterol level. Influence of risk factor intervention. J.A.M.A., 238:2269–2271, 1977.
36. Gordon, T., et al.: High-density lipoprotein as a protective factor against coronary heart disease. The Framington Study. Am. J. Med., 62:707–714, 1977.
37. Editorial. Oestrogens and atheroma. Lancet, 2:508–509, 1978.

… CHAPTER 14

PAIN MANAGEMENT
Allan A. Maltbie

Pain is perhaps the most dreaded of all human experiences, and indeed the common experience of those who suffer. This is particularly true for the aging population as a simple function of their increased incidence of chronic illnesses. Pain stands pre-eminent among all sensory experiences by which man judges the existence of disease within himself.[1] Since there are few illnesses of man that are not in some way and at some time experienced painfully, pain presents a major diagnostic tool for the physician. Therefore, a careful description of pain, its mode of onset, duration, location, quality, time of occurrence, and provoking and relieving factors are all diagnostically significant.

Acute pain is typically experienced during an active illness or injury, and disappears as the individual recovers from his primary condition. In its acute form, pain serves the individual by providing a warning signal or alert to the presence of something wrong.[2-4] The presence of acute pain in one individual has enormous impact on others.[5] In the face of acute pain, friends and family invariably suffer along with the patient. The apparent severity of pain is equated with the seriousness of the illness. Pain itself is perceived as a threat to life. Death, should it occur, would be somehow better if painless.

Protracted or chronic pain presents a situation that is quite different from acute pain.[2-4] The perception of pain no longer serves as a warning function, but rather has become a burden for the individual involved and represents something to live with. No longer does the patient's suffering evoke the same response from others, since now it is protracted and not perceived as a threat to life. When the source of chronic pain is physically apparent, concern and empathy by others may continue once all efforts to relieve or salve the suffering have failed, but such concern may be characterized by guilt ridden attentiveness and periodic angry outbursts between the patient with chronic pain and his family. Friends may eventually avoid the patient and in time fade from the picture altogether. Often the medical management of the patient with chronic pain follows a gradual escalation of progressively more potent analgesics, sedatives, and tranquilizers. If the patient's pain persists, various surgical procedures may be attempted. If surgery fails to relieve pain, as it often does, it serves only to further escalate the frustration and disillusionment shared by physician, patient, and family alike.

Pain is not a diagnosis, but a symptom that requires diagnostic explanation. Many patients with chronic pain have no obvious lesion to explain the pain, or, perhaps more commonly, the severity of their suffering is not explainable by the detectable disease. Such a patient may be accused of laziness or malingering, may be dismissed from employment as being unproductive, and may be declared ineligible for disability benefits, since there is no readily apparent medical justification. Patients with "functional" pain or a considerable "functional overlay" are often found in the geriatric population and present very special therapeutic problems for the physician.

It is essential for the physician to formulate a clear differential diagnosis in an effort to specifically characterize the pain complaints of the elderly patient. When pain is acute, little other consideration exists beyond the accurate diagnosis and treatment of the primary condition generating the pain. Additionally, the physician attempts to render the patient as comfortable as possible while the primary disorder is effectively diagnosed and treated. For patients with chronic pain, the situation becomes more complex, since in this situation, cure of the primary disorder is no longer a likelihood, and efforts toward palliative long term management become the primary medical focus.

PSYCHOLOGIC ASPECTS OF PAIN

Since there is no effective way to directly measure the afferent stimulus of pain, the physician must always rely upon a subjective complaint. Inherent in that subjective complaint is the affective elaboration by the patient of the perceived pain. Freud defined pain as an affective response to an actual loss or injury.[6] He noted in chronic pain the presence of an emotional investment or preoccupation with the pain, which in some patients may be so all-consuming that it can drain the individual of the capacity to function. He equated the process of mourning, in which there is an actual loss, with pain, in which there is an actual injury. In both situations the individual is forced to adapt to a new situation. With the loss of a loved one, the loss is clearly irreversible and requires an active adaptational grieving process or a pathologic, and relatively apparent, denial of reality. Unfortunately for the patient with chronic pain, it is often easier to deny the reality of chronicity and persistently search for the total or complete cure. Although this is an effective defensive posture in the face of acute pain when recovery is expectable, with chronic disorders lasting many years, such persistent expectation of cure serves only to maintain a denial of the reality of a chronic disorder and retards active adaptational efforts toward living with the pain.

Sternbach presents the concept of stimulus, perception, and response in his definition of pain, which he sees as an abstraction that incorporates the following three components: a harmful stimulus that signals current or impending tissue damage, a personal, private sensation of hurt, and a pattern of responses that operates to protect the organism from harm.[4] Kapp notes that pain as an experience involves a fusion of mind and body, serving normally as a signal of danger to body tissue.[7] He adds that the experience requires consciousness, attention, and self-concern, noting the common observation of distractability when the individual is subjected to other intense stimulation. For example, athletes in the course of intense competition or soldiers in battle may exhibit no evidence of pain despite serious injury. Conversely, the experience of pain may become nagging and persistent, impairing the individual's ability to work, think, or sleep, to the point that it may destroy his will to live, at times resulting in suicidal preoccupation.

According to Rangell, the ability to tolerate and utilize small amounts of pain as warning signals, taking the appropriate measures to avoid pain, and reacting appropriately in kind and degree to pain that is unavoidable, are the normal responses of persons to pain.[8] In considering deviation from the normal, he observed that there are individuals who seek or produce pain rather than avoid it. This group comprises those with psychogenic pain problems in which unconscious motivations may involve the seeking of pain for itself. An example is masochism, in which there is a neurotic component to the experience, or in which the pain satisfies a feeling of guilt and a need for punishment. An individual may also seek and suffer pain to enjoy an associated gratification, such as increased affection or attention from others, financial reward resulting from disability status, or elevation in self-esteem accomplished by excusing one's shortcomings as being the result of the painful disorder.

Rangell observed that a patient's pain adaptation is a function of his previous historical development as reflected by his personality structure.[8] Pain or illness may precipitate a neurotic reaction or become incorporated as a symptom in a pre-existing neurotic or psychotic process. Some individuals may use the symptom of chronic pain to maintain a psychologic equilibrium. For these individuals, relinquishing the pain symptom would pose a potential threat.

Patients with chronic pain, for example, may develop a psychotic reaction or attempt suicide after a successful pain relieving procedure, or at times simply in response to an impending threat of relief.[9]

In his classic article on psychogenic pain, Engle identified six characteristics tending to make a patient more vulnerable to protracted pain.[10] These characteristics include the following: prominence of guilt and the use of pain to expiate guilt; a history of harsh and punitive childhood experiences in which pain was regularly inflicted for discipline; a chronic inability to directly express anger, in which instead anger is turned on the self; a long history of suffering and defeat with an apparent inability to tolerate success; strong conflicts over sexual impulses, which in combination with aggressive and guilt feelings are symbolically expressed as pain; and pain that serves to reflect the loss or potential loss of another person. In a later article, Engle addressed the issue of pain occurring with inadequate grief or mourning.[11] Cavenar and associates likewise reported cases in which pain was the presenting complaint of unresolved grief reactions, sometimes occurring many years after the loss, on the occasion of a specific anniversary.[12] Pain complaints in these patients include headache, back pain, chest pain, and abdominal pain, all occurring at the anniversary of a significant loss.

It is not uncommon to find an elderly patient with chronic pain (with or without an organic component) in whom the experience of pain is fused with the affects associated with multiple losses, including the loss of friends, loved ones, health, and status. The elderly patient can more readily focus on the physical symptoms than on the distressing feelings of loss. In this way a fabric of physical sensation of pain becomes integrally woven into issues of mourning and loss.

A MULTILEVEL APPROACH TO THE DIAGNOSIS AND TREATMENT OF CHRONIC PAIN

In a previous publication the author suggested a multilevel approach as being helpful, both diagnostically and therapeutically, in managing chronic pain.[13] First to be considered is a physical reality of the noxious stimulus generating pain in the individual. This, of course, is the traditional medical evaluation focusing on accurate diagnosis and proper treatment of the physical disorder generating the afferent painful stimulus.

The second level to be considered diagnostically is the patient's affective cognitive reaction to the chronically persistent and painful stimulus. Often a cycle of affective escalation may be noted in which the patient becomes preoccupied with pain, incorporating memories of painful experiences and responses and anxiously anticipating additional pain. In time this affective reaction can become all-consuming and interfere with the patient's capacity to function. Consequently the physician must carefully consider the presence of secondary affective reactions with either persistent symptoms of anxiety or vegetative symptoms of depression. In the elderly a pseudodementia may be the presenting symptom complex of an affective disorder precipitated by the struggle with chronic pain. Recognition of the secondary affective reaction to pain and the proper therapeutic management of these reactions can greatly enhance the overall treatment of such patients. For example, the judicious administration of tricyclic antidepressants, as discussed later in this chapter, may greatly relieve this affective component.

The third level of consideration is the coping reaction utilized by the patient in the struggle to adapt to chronic pain. Although for acute pain the appropriate psychologic defense is one of action to avoid or eliminate pain, when pain is chronic, a persistent struggle for relief in lieu of "coping" would itself suggest disease. In such an instance the patient's refusal to accept the reality of chronicity and its required life adjustments is a maladaptation. Thus the persistent searching for nothing but absolute cure prevents effective adaptation to a chronic disorder. Additionally, chronic pain may result in the emergence of more infantile and more dependent modes of behavior in the elderly patient.

With protracted pain over an extended interval (many years), some form of fixed adaptation would be expected, regardless of whether the individual continues to seek pain relief and whether an afferent source of the pain stimulus can be located. The individual would also be expected to have psychologically incorporated and handled the pain defensively. The best measurement of the success of the patient's psychologic defenses is not through the patient's direct expression of the experience of pain; rather it is reflected by the patient's real life adaptation to his medical condition. Consequently an evaluation in terms of maintenance of self-esteem, degree of independent function, and effectiveness of interpersonal relationships provides a good indication of pain adaptation. The working quality of family and sexual relationships and the ability to sleep all reflect the patient's success in adaptation. When the patient with chronic pain is working up to his physical and intellectual capability, actively involved with friends and family, and eating and sleeping consistently despite the presence of chronic pain, a satisfactory adaptation has indeed been accomplished.

When adaptation to chronic pain is not satisfactory, abnormal patterns and responses become ingrained and feed on longstanding maladaptive personality traits. Once ingrained, a maladaptive response to chronic pain can be changed only when the individual specifically seeks and desires such change and participates actively in a behavioral or psychotherapeutic regimen designed to assist in adaptational change. Various modalities have been developed for such patients and may involve inpatient or outpatient techniques. Individual psychotherapy, group psychotherapy, family approaches, and behavioral approaches may all be useful or effective for the elderly patient with chronic pain who desires to learn more effective ways of living with the pain.

For many patients with chronic pain the regular visit to the family physician can be most helpful. The simple act of expressing to an empathetic physician the frustrations associated with a persistent chronic physical disorder and the physical losses accompanying the aging process can have substantial meaning to the elderly patient. For many such patients the office visit itself may have far more utility than any efforts to adjust, change, or enlarge upon analgesic programs. Paying attention to the patient's sources of psychologic support and self-esteem may be quite helpful in overall management. Work, family, social, recreational, and religious activities have long aided the patient in defining himself, and the physician is wise to continually monitor the patient's activities in these spheres and encourage as much involvement as the patient is able to accomplish. Clearly the more involved the patient is in these established interests, the less involved he will be in matters of illness and pain.

PHARMACOLOGIC CONSIDERATIONS IN THE MANAGEMENT OF CHRONIC PAIN IN THE ELDERLY

A common and thorny management problem for the physician is that presented by the elderly patient with intractable cancer pain. The reader is referred elsewhere in this text for detailed management considerations regarding arthritic, rheumatic, neurologic, cardiovascular, orthopedic, genitourinary, gastrointestinal, and other specific painful disorders affecting the elderly.

For the patient suffering cancer pain, a thorough medical evaluation will be necessary to define whether the pain management program should also include surgical, chemotherapeutic, radiotherapeutic, or anesthesiologic procedures. In addition, despite the presence of diagnosed cancer, psychologic assessment is essential. All the considerations mentioned previously in this chapter must be taken into consideration for the patient suffering cancer pain. Furthermore, the patient's reaction to the knowledge of the terminal illness should be closely scrutinized, as this reaction will be an integral part of his adaptational struggle with the pain syndrome generated by the malignant disease.

Analgesic Drugs

Narcotics

A significant development in neurochemistry occurred in 1973 with the localization and demonstration of narcotic receptors. Since that time we have learned much about the properties of these receptors, their distribution throughout the body, and their specific interaction with agonists and antagonists. Of equal note was the discovery of endogenous substances, the endorphins and enkephalins, which possess morphine-like qualities and bind with the opiate receptor. With such developments, the search for the long sought after nonaddictive narcotic has been accelerated.

For the management of pain in the cancer patient, the mainstay continues to be the narcotic analgesics.[14,15] These drugs are structurally and pharmacologically related, sharing similar qualitative effects, yet with widely differing potencies and durations of action (Tables 14–1, 14–2). Although narcotics vary widely in potency, by adjusting the dosage,

TABLE 14-1. Narcotic Agonist Analgesics

Generic Name	Trade Name	Dose (Subcutaneous)*	Dose (Oral)*	Duration (Hours)	Distinguishing Features
Morphine	—	10	60	4–5	Wide range or oral absorption
Hydromorphone	Dilaudid	1.5	7.5	4–5	
Hydrocodone	Dicodid	—	15	4–6	
Codeine	—	120	200	4–6	Idiosyncratic dissociative reaction
Oxymorphone	Numorphan	1	6	4–6	
Oxycodone	(in Percodan and Tylox)	15	30	4–5	
Levorphanol	Levodromoran	2	4	4–5	
Methadone	Dolophine	10	20	4–5	Longer analgesic action due to cumulative effects
Meperidine	Demerol	75	300	2–4	Little constipation or biliary spasm
Alphaprodine	Nisentyl	45	—	1–2	

*Dose in milligrams producing same analgesic effect as morphine, 10 mg. subcutaneously.

equianalgesic results are obtainable. Thus, they are equal in efficacy, and by increasing the dose of a less potent narcotic, the physician can obtain the same analgesic effect produced by a more potent narcotic. Also of note, different types of pain are relieved by different dosages of narcotics—dull, continuous pain being much more readily managed than colicky pain. Moreover narcotics do not block the perception of pain, but rather alter the affective interpretation of the pain sensation in such a way that the individual is aware of pain, but its quality is far less distressing. Narcotics differ widely in their oral/parenteral potency ratio (Tables 14–1, 14–2). In this regard, morphine is inferior to other drugs.

Besides potency variations, which can be corrected by dosage adjustment, the greatest difference among the narcotics is in duration of action, which ranges from as little as two hours with meperidine (Demerol) to as much as 12 hours with methadone. By increasing the duration of narcotic action by using methadone, a longer pain-free interval results, allowing enhanced freedom of daily activities and uninterrupted sleep for those responding effectively to this drug. Patients with such a regimen may also have a greater feeling of control over their pain and illness, since they require less frequent doses of medication.

Belleville et al. in a report in 1971 noted that for patients over 60 years of age, as compared with the younger adult population, there seemed to be both a decrease in the sensitivity to pain and an increase in analgesic response to narcotic drugs.[16] This observation is consistent with the general observation of Bender regarding an increasing sensitivity to drug effect in older age groups.[17] Thus, although each patient must be clinically treated to maximize the analgesic response, the elderly patient is likely to require a somewhat smaller

TABLE 14-2. Narcotic Agonist-Antagonist Analgesics*

Generic Name	Trade Name	Dose (Subcutaneous)†	Dose (Oral)†	Duration (Hours)	Distinguishing Features
Butorphanol	Stadol	2–3	—	3–4	Narcotic antagonist activity 30x pentazocine and 1/40 naloxone
Nalbuphine	Nubain	10	—	3–6	Narcotic antagonist activity 10x pentazocine
Pentazocine	Talwin	30–60	150–180	2–3	Weak narcotic antagonist

*The narcotic agonist-antagonist analgesics are potent analgesic drugs with lower abuse potential than pure narcotic agonists. Because of their narcotic antagonist activity, these drugs may precipitate withdrawal symptoms in patients with narcotic dependency (addiction).
†Dose in milligrams producing same analgesic effect as morphine, 10 mg. subcutaneously.

dosage than the same patient would have required for an equianalgesic effect during his younger adult years.

Belleville et al. in the same article considered a possible explanation of the increased effectiveness of narcotic drugs in the older population. They questioned whether the observed differences represented a shift in the body's absorption, distribution, metabolism, and elimination of the drug with age, which might result in a net increase of available active drug at the same dosage. To test this hypothesis, the same population of patients was examined in reference to analgesic side effects. They considered that if the increased analgesic responses were due solely to altered absorption or distribution, an increased incidence of side effects should also be observed, corresponding to the net gain in drug effect. They found no such increased incidence. For example, when they evaluated the degree of sedation, they found that despite increased analgesic effect at the same dosage in the 60-plus age group versus the younger adult age group, the degree of sedation remained constant throughout. Thus, it would appear from this finding that although the elderly patient may expect an enhanced analgesic response to narcotic drugs, there is no readily apparent additional liability of side effects beyond those experienced by the population at large, all other things being equal (e.g., cardiovascular status, renal status, hepatic status, gastrointestinal status, genitourinary status).

The treatment of chronic pain in a rational and therapeutically appropriate manner is very desirable in the cancer patient because pain is often the most feared manifestation of the disease. Chronic pain is characterized by a pain-anxiety-pain continuum rather than the typical mild-moderate-severe description of acute pain for which there are definite beginnings and ends. Lack of knowledge about narcotic analgesics on the part of health professionals and the attitudes and social conditioning of the patient may interfere with rational treatment of chronic pain. The following section enumerates 10 principles of the management of chronic pain that, if recognized and applied, can contribute substantially to improved therapeutic outcomes in pain management.

Ten Principles in the Management of Chronic Pain

1. The patient is the best judge of his pain. This is the most important concept and has to be accepted by all involved health professionals, patients, and families if proper management of chronic pain is to be achieved. Pain is what, and occurs when, the experiencing person says.

2. Placebos have no place in the treatment of chronic pain. If we are convinced that the patient is in fact the best judge of the pain, it is obvious that there is no need for placebos in treating that pain. Using placebos reveals more about our own attitudes than about the patient's comfort.

3. All narcotic analgesics are equivalent if equivalent dosages are given. Several sources of drug information contain charts of the relative potencies of narcotic analgesics. Given in appropriate dosages, drugs given either orally or by injection can relieve chronic pain effectively.

4. All narcotic analgesics have similar side effects. Few patients with chronic pain exhibit evidence of the usual side effects of narcotic analgesics, including respiratory depression or gastrointestinal and dermatologic side effects.

5. Around the clock dosing is preferred over as-needed dosing. If chronic pain is thought of as a continuum, several problems exist when an analgesic is given on demand rather than on a regular schedule. It is discouraging to the patient when relief is not available until the pain recurs. Patients are often hesitant to ask for pain relief for a variety of reasons, including fear that complaining about pain is a sign of a weak or bothersome patient. Nurses may encourage patients to wait until the pain becomes unbearable before giving a dose of a strong analgesic because they fear drug dependence.

6. When changing from one narcotic analgesic to another, one should keep the old drug available on an as-needed basis for a short while. It is very comforting for the patient to keep the old analgesic available on a whenever-necessary basis when a different drug is used on an around the clock schedule. Often within one to two days the call for the old drug ends, and the patient has adequate control of pain.

7. Analgesic drugs should not be switched without an adequate trial. To treat chronic pain appropriately, it is necessary to have a treatment plan and follow it. Indiscriminate switching of drugs will only result in a diminution of trust on the part of the patient and the family, since none of the drugs is given adequate time to produce relief. When drugs must

be switched, an equivalent dosing chart should be used.

8. One should think of analgesic orders in terms of daily equivalent dosages. It would be useful for all health professionals dealing with chronic pain management to think of the equivalent daily dosage of analgesic given to a patient.

9. The dosage and frequency of administration of narcotic analgesics generally should not be changed at the same time. A small change in the dosage and frequency of administration can result in a substantial reduction in the daily dosage of pain medication. For example, changing the administration of hydromorphone from 4 mg. every three hours to 2 mg. every four hours results in a large reduction in the daily dosage.

10. Oral dosage forms are preferred over injectable drugs. Since the object is to treat chronic pain properly, it is hoped that many patients will then be able to return home. An oral regimen will facilitate this.

Side Effects. Perhaps the most worrisome and most significant side effect resulting from narcotic administration is respiratory depression.[14] This is produced by decreases in the sensitivity of brain stem respiratory centers to increasing levels of carbon dioxide. Additionally the brain stem centers responsible for respiratory rhythmicity are depressed. As a result of these influences, with overdosage one finds a slow periodic irregular respiratory pattern often characterized by a decrease in tidal volume, retention of carbon dioxide, and even coma. With the increased carbon dioxide retention, the respiratory drive becomes oxygen dependent. In such a situation the paradoxical phenomenon of the administration of oxygen resulting in apnea can occur. When excessive oxygen is administered in the absence of respiratory assistance, the oxygen dependent respiratory centers become saturated, with a resultant cessation in respiration. A constant feature of the narcotics, respiratory depression, may be expected at equianalgesic doses for all these drugs. Although respiratory depression is a constant concern, the careful use of narcotics within appropriate dosage ranges should result in the relief of pain without a significant threat to respiratory function.

Other central nervous system side effects may occur with the narcotics. The seizure threshold may be lowered, especially in patients with a history of a seizure disorder. Sedation and alterations in mood have been reported. Euphoria may occur with all these drugs and is generally equal in degree at equianalgesic dosages. More worrisome are the dysphorias, which range from vague apprehensions to fulminant deliria. These are most common with codeine and pentazocine hydrochloride (Talwin).[18] When dysphorias occur, they are best treated by changing to a different narcotic drug. Other central nervous system side effects include dizziness, miosis, mental clouding, lack of coordination, transient hallucinations, and confusion.

Gastrointestinal side effects occur frequently with the narcotics. Nausea and vomiting may occur and are produced by the drug stimulation effect on the chemoreceptor trigger zone of the medulla. This can be effectively managed by prochlorperazine (Compazine), trimethobenzamide hydrochloride (Tigan), or thiethylperazine maleate (Torecan).

An almost constant side effect seen with narcotics is constipation secondary to decreased intestinal peristalsis and increased intestinal tone. Owing to the frequency of occurrence of constipation in the older patient receiving narcotic drugs, a preventative approach is recommended. The active well hydrated patient is less likely to have problems with constipation. For this reason exercise programs and minimal daily fluid requirements should be provided for these patients. The use of various stool softeners and intestinal stimulants is also recommended. Such drugs as dioctyl sodium sulfosuccinate (Colace), 100 mg. two to three times a day, combined with an irritant laxative (senna, cascara, phenolphthalein, danthron) at bedtime is one useful remedy. Narcotic drugs also increase pressure in the biliary tract. Such an increase in pressure may result in symptoms ranging from epigastric distress to typical biliary colic.

Since narcotic drugs have the effect of increasing smooth muscle tone, genitourinary symptoms may occasionally result. Bladder spasm may occur, as may urinary retention, as a result of the increase in urinary sphincter tone. Should such symptoms occur, a reduction in dosage or a change to a different narcotic drug generally relieves this complication.

Adverse cardiovascular effects are most common after the intravenous administration of narcotics. Such effects include flushing of the face, tachycardia, bradycardia, palpitation, faintness, hypotension, and syncope. Allergic manifestations occur rarely and may be systemic or local. Miscellaneous adverse effects include diaphoresis, pain at the injection site, and laryngospasm.

Precautions and Warnings. Numerous

precautions and warnings are associated with narcotic use. Patients who receive narcotics for medical reasons seldom develop physical dependency or a compulsion to abuse narcotics. The narcotics are addictive, however, with repeated administration and should be administered with caution. Narcotics should be used with caution in patients with head injuries, a brain tumor, or other intracranial lesions because the drugs may elevate cerebrospinal fluid pressure or obscure the assessment of neurologic deficit induced by the intracranial lesion. Since the narcotics may decrease respiratory drive, they should be administered with extreme caution in patients with asthma, chronic obstructive pulmonary disease, or previously existing respiratory depression. In individuals with compromised capacity to maintain the blood pressure, narcotic administration may lead to episodes of orthostatic hypotension, which can lead to dizziness, disorientation, and subsequent falls and fractures. These drugs suppress the cough reflex and may retard expectoration in patients who require elimination of tracheobronchial debris. The narcotics should be used with caution in patients with atrial flutter and other supraventricular tachycardias because they may produce a vagolytic action. In patients with renal or hepatic dysfunction the narcotics may exhibit a prolonged duration of action.

Drug Interactions. Narcotics should be used with caution and in reduced dosages in patients concurrently receiving other narcotic analgesics, general anesthetics, antihistamines, phenothiazines, alcohol, barbiturates, antianxiety drugs, nonbarbiturate sedative-hypnotics, tricyclic antidepressants, and other central nervous system depressants. Respiratory depression, hypotension, profound sedation, or coma may result. The narcotics, particularly meperidine, have precipitated severe reactions in patients receiving monoamine oxidase inhibitors. This interaction is of significance in cancer patients, for the antineoplastic drug procarbazine inhibits monoamine oxidase. The concurrent administration of rifampin or phenytoin (Dilantin) has been shown to decrease the serum concentration of methadone to the point of inducing withdrawal symptoms. The concurrent administration of narcotics with furosemide (Lasix) or ethacrynic acid (Edecrin) may produce or aggravate orthostatic hypotension. Morphine has been shown to increase the activity of coumarin anticoagulants (e.g., Coumadin).

Tolerance and Physical Dependence. Development of a physiologic tolerance to narcotic drugs is a well established phenomenon. In patients being treated by a stabilized analgesic narcotic regimen, the sudden cessation of the narcotic medication would precipitate the onset of a classic narcotic withdrawal syndrome. This should be guarded against by insuring that the patient does not run out of medications abruptly. Although these drugs have potential for misuse and abuse, this is seldom of significant concern in the elderly population, particularly in patients being treated for cancer pain. When a history of drug abuse exists, or the physician is concerned about the possibility of abuse in a particular patient, the problem is best managed by limiting the total amount of narcotic available. This is accomplished through more frequent prescribing of smaller quantities per prescription and by involving another family member or an additional responsible party to assist in a dispensing plan. In this way drug consumption is closely monitored and the distribution of the medication is controlled.

Perhaps more serious in the management of the elderly patient with cancer is the situation in which the physician withholds effective narcotic analgesia for fear of addicting the patient.[19] Although a few patients misuse or abuse narcotics, most follow their doctor's recommendations. Perhaps more important, many patients are reluctant to take even small amounts of narcotics for fear of addiction, and in fact need encouragement from their physician to agree to an analgesic regimen that will provide relief.

A frequent concern of physicians contemplating the extended treatment of chronic cancer pain is the progressive escalation of the narcotic dosage such that by the time the illness has progressed to a point at which pain would be expectedly most severe, narcotic tolerance levels are so high that the analgesic effectiveness of the drug is severely limited. Although this can occur, the opposite situation also has been observed, in which a steady or even decreasing analgesic requirement is maintained over many months.[20]

When it is necessary to change from one narcotic drug to another in a dependent person, the physician should remember the relative potencies and durations of action of the drugs involved, such that equianalgesic dosages are administered with appropriate regularity. The physician should also be aware that the abrupt transition from a traditional narcotic regimen to an analgesic regimen of pentazocine (Talwin), butorphanol (Stadol), or nalbuphine (Nubain) could result in precipitation of acute narcotic withdrawal as a result of the narcotic antagonist activity of these drugs (Table 14–2). The physician is advised to be familiar with the details on the package insert of the synthetic narcotic analgesic drugs in regard to their antagonistic effects.

Management of Acute Narcotic Overdosage. Serious overdosage is characterized by respiratory depression, somnolence progressing to stupor or coma, maximally constricted pupils, muscle flaccidity, cold clammy skin, and possibly bradycardia and hypotension. If not effectively treated, such symptoms could progress to circulatory collapse, cardiac arrest, and death.

Primary attention should be given to the re-establishment of adequate respiratory exchange through provision of a patent airway and institution of assisted or controlled ventilation. The narcotic antagonists are specific antidotes, and naloxone (Narcan), a drug devoid of agonist action, is the antagonist of choice. Naloxone should be administered, preferably by the intravenous route, simultaneously with efforts at respiratory resuscitation. The usual initial adult dose of naloxone is 0.4 mg. intravenously. If the desired degree of respiratory improvement is not obtained immediately, the intravenous dose should be repeated at two to three minute intervals. Failure to obtain improvement after two or three doses suggests that the condition may be due to a disease process or a non-narcotic drug. If the patient responds to naloxone, repeated doses may be necessary because the duration of action of the narcotic may exceed that of naloxone. Oxygen, the intravenous administration of fluids, vasopressors, and other supportive measures should be employed as indicated. If the overdose was ingested by the oral route, the stomach should be evacuated by emesis or lavage if treatment can be instituted within two hours following ingestion. The patient should be observed for a rise in temperature or pulmonary complications that may signal an infection and the need for antibiotic therapy.

Management of the Acute Abstinence (Withdrawal) Syndrome. Acute withdrawal symptoms from narcotics include yawning, excessive perspiration, lacrimation, rhinorrhea, sneezing, involuntary motor movements, restlessness, irritability, tremor, gooseflesh, chills and fever, dilated pupils, tachycardia, body aches, nausea, vomiting, diarrhea, and abdominal cramps. The severity of the withdrawal syndrome is related to the degree of dependence, the abruptness of withdrawal, and the drug used.

The treatment of the withdrawal syndrome is primarily supportive and symptomatic. Treatment includes the maintenance of proper fluid and electrolyte balance and the administration of a tranquilizer to suppress anxiety.

Other Centrally Acting Analgesics

Special mention is in order in regard to propoxyphene (Darvon) and methotrimeprazine (Levoprome), for they are in a unique pharmacologic class. They are not pure narcotic agonists or narcotic agonist-antagonists and do not act peripherally and therefore are distinct from the salicylates and other nonsteroidal anti-inflammatory drugs. Propoxyphene is chemically related to the narcotics but not comparable with the narcotics in terms of analgesic potency or abuse potential. Methotrimeprazine is a phenothiazine derivative.

Propoxyphene is 1/50 to 1/25 as potent as morphine and approximately 2/3 as potent as codeine in analgesic effect. Administered alone in usual analgesic doses (32 to 65 mg. of the hydrochloride and 50 to 100 mg. of the napsylate salt), propoxyphene is no more effective and possibly less effective than 30 to 60 mg. of codeine sulfate or 650 mg. of aspirin or acetaminophen. Despite its mild analgesic properties, however, many patients have responded well to this drug, and it may be beneficial for selected cancer patients.

There is no conclusive evidence that combining propoxyphene with other analgesics will potentiate the analgesic response. When taken in higher than recommended dosages over long periods of time, propoxyphene may produce drug dependence. Its potential for producing drug dependency appears to be somewhat less than that of codeine. Adverse effects are similar to those induced by narcotics, but the margin of safety between therapeutic dose and toxic dose is greater with propoxyphene.

Methotrimeprazine (Levoprome), a phenothiazine derivative and potent central nervous system depressant, produces suppression of sensory impulses, reduction of motor activity, sedation, and tranquilization. The drug has a tendency to produce amnesia; possesses antihistaminic, anticholinergic and antiadrenergic effects, may induce orthostatic hypotension, must be injected intramuscularly, and generally produces excessive sedation. In view of the incidence and severity of adverse effects, the fact that many elderly patients demonstrate hypersensitivity to phenothiazines, and the intramuscular injection requirement, this drug is a poor choice for use in the elderly, even though it produces analgesic effects comparable with those of morphine and meperidine, with little potential for depressing respiration or inducing physical dependency at the usual dosages.

Non-narcotic Analgesics

The antipyretic anti-inflammatory analgesic drugs, including aspirin, indomethacin, ibuprofen, and related substances, are considered elsewhere in this text, but deserve special mention in reference to the treatment of cancer pain. In a double blind crossover trial that included aspirin, propoxyphene hydrochloride, and placebo, Moertel and associates demonstrated that aspirin was the most effective of these drugs in relieving cancer pain.[22] They demonstrated that two aspirin tablets were as effective as the standard dose of codeine in relieving moderate cancer pain. Brodie demonstrated the usefulness of indomethacin in the treatment of cancer pain.[23]

These drugs have several advantages over narcotics for the management of cancer pain when they are effective. Aspirin, for instance, is inexpensive and readily available without a prescription. All these drugs are nonaddictive, are not euphoragenic, and do not have the property of depressing respiration. They also, in some circumstances, may provide an additive analgesic effect in combination with narcotic drugs.

Psychoactive Drugs

In recent years the application of psychoactive drugs in the adjunctive treatment of the pain of cancer has begun to be discussed in the clinical literature. In 1967 Dalessio noted that the tricyclic antidepressants might be effective in the treatment of severe pain syndromes.[23] In 1972, Merskey and Hessler reported a clinical trial including 30 patients with chronic pain in whom a combination of phenothiazines, tricyclic antidepressants, and antihistamines resulted in "moderately good" relief of pain, and added that the best results seemed to occur in the patients taking phenothiazines.[24] Taub and Collins reported that 34 of 39 patients with denervation dysesthesia were improved by a combination of fluphenazine (Prolixin) and amitriptyline (Elavil).[25] Unfortunately most clinical reports to date regarding the application of psychoactive drugs in the treatment of various pain syndromes have not been controlled studies.

Antipsychotic Drugs. Antipsychotic drugs or neuroleptics of the phenothiazine group have long been known to potentiate the effects of narcotics and alcohol. This particular synergistic effect has been utilized clinically, as, for example, when promethazine (Phenergan) is used to potentiate the effect of meperidine (Demerol). Ban observed the same potentiating effect for haloperidol as an intensifier of anesthetic, narcotic, and alcohol actions.[26] The present author has further elaborated this action in the clinical application of haloperidol as an adjunctive treatment of cancer pain.[27]

Antipsychotic drugs have properties that may make them useful in the management of cancer pain. Although larger dosages tend to produce sedation, the judicious use of smaller dosages may be helpful in calming an agitated patient. Additionally many of these drugs have an antiemetic effect, useful because cancer patients often suffer from nausea or vomiting.

The use of antipsychotic drugs in combination with narcotics for analgesia is common but until recently has been infrequently reported. Kocher reviewed several studies reporting the effects of neuroleptic drugs in the management of chronic pain of various origins.[28] Maltbie et al. reported the analgesic properties of haloperidol, with particular emphasis on its usefulness in the treatment of cancer pain.[29,30] The administration of haloperidol seemed either to eliminate the need for narcotic analgesics or more commonly resulted in a significant reduction in the narcotic dosage in patients with cancer pain. The apparent explanation for the analgesic properties of haloperidol include its isomeric similarity to meperidine and its established and demonstrated affinity for the opiate receptor.[27,31] Dosages ranging from 2 to 15 mg given in a single nightly dose should be sufficient for the elderly patient. This bedtime regimen tends to enhance sleep, maximize nocturnal analgesia, and minimize extrapyramidal complications. Patients may be somewhat sedated at these dosages but are easily arousable, and often their analgesic requirements can be reduced dramatically. The resultant reduced narcotic dosage diminishes the risk of constipation, addiction, respiratory depression, and other side effects.

Extrapyramidal complications occur frequently with haloperidol use and are best prevented in the elderly cancer patient rather than treated. Trihexyphenidyl hydrochloride (Artane), 2 mg. two to three times a day, or a comparable dosage of another anticholinergic antiparkinsonian drug is recommended. Once the pain regimen has been stabilized, antiparkinsonian drugs should be discontinued or made available to the patient on a whenever-necessary basis for extrapyramidal complications. This precaution should minimize the likelihood of tardive dyskinesia.

Other antipsychotic drugs may be equally as effective as haloperidol. Chlorpromazine (Thorazine), thioridazine (Mellaril), and fluphenazine (Prolixin) all have been reported to be effective in this regard. The physician is advised to utilize a regimen with these drugs similar to that with haloperidol, utilizing small to moderate dosage ranges in a single nightly dose. Chlorpromazine and thioridazine, having anticholinergic properties of their own, should not require prophylactic antiparkinsonian management. These drugs are more sedative than other antipsychotic drugs and may better enhance the sleep of the patient with chronic cancer pain who has insomnia.

Tricyclic Antidepressants. The second major class of psychoactive drugs that have shown considerable promise in the treatment of pain are the tricyclic antidepressants. Gingras compared imipramine to a placebo in a crossover study involving a population of arthritic patients who were being treated by antiinflammatory drugs.[32] Imipramine was demonstrated to be superior to placebo in regard to the degree of relief of pain, grip strength, joint stiffness, and patient preference. Tricyclics in combination with antipsychotic drugs have been shown by multiple observers to be efficacious in the treatment of pain of cancer, as well as other chronically painful conditions.[23-25, 28]

The analgesic effect of the tricyclic antidepressants is most likely a function of a combination of factors, including a possible direct analgesic effect of the drug, its capacity to potentiate other analgesics, and the antidepressant effect itself, which would expectedly lessen the severity of the perceived pain. The recommended dosages of the tricyclic antidepressants would be comparable with those suggested elsewhere in this text for an antidepressant effect in an elderly patient. The specific choice of a tricyclic drug likewise would be determined on grounds as detailed in Chapter 3.

Although most published data to date have dealt with imipramine, amytriptyline, or doxepin, no evidence has supported one tricyclic antidepressant over another as being more efficacious in the treatment of pain. As with therapeutic intervention with depression, a reasonable trial of tricyclic antidepressants for analgesic effects would be a minimum of three weeks, although an analgesic response often may be apparent during the initial week of treatment.

Antianxiety Drugs. As a general rule, the antianxiety drugs, primarily the benzodiazepine subclass of medications, have been of little or no use in the treatment of chronic cancer pain. The exceptional patient who presents with a marked anxiety component to the pain symptomatology might expectedly respond to benzodiazepine adjunctive care.

Patients who are sleep deprived as a result of chronic cancer pain merit an increase in analgesic dosage. In patients with sleep disturbance despite adequate analgesia, the addition of a sedative-hypnotic such as flurazepam hydrochloride (Dalmane) or chloral hydrate would be of use. Because the sedative-hypnotics synergize the opiate induced respiratory depression, these medications must be used cautiously together. As an adjunct in sleep disturbances, sedative-hypnotics should be used for only brief intervals, since tolerance develops. Impaired sleep may reflect a symptomatic depression, which, if present, is far more responsive to the nightly administration of a tricyclic antidepressant in therapeutic dosages.

Use of the Brompton Mixture

An oral narcotic mixture initially utilized by the British was made popular through the work of Saunders and Twycross at St. Christopher's Hospice.[20] The standard Brompton mixture contains a variable amount of morphine sulfate, ranging from as little as 2.5 mg. to as much as 100 mg., mixed with 10 mg. of cocaine, 2.5 ml. of ethyl alcohol (98 per cent), 5 ml. of flavoring syrup, and a variable amount of chloroform water—a total of 20 ml. per dose.[33] Some centers are abandoning inclusion of the cocaine component, as well as the alcohol in the mixture, with no change in the efficacy of the analgesic effect. Most cancer patients respond to a morphine dosage ranging from 5 to 20 mg. per dose of the mixture. Elderly patients often respond to somewhat smaller dosages and in fact may respond to as little as 2.5 mg. per dose. It should be noted that the Brompton mixture is usually given with a phenothiazine. The phenothiazine is given for both the antiemetic effect as well as the potentiation of the narcotic analgesic effect.[33] Prochlorperazine (Compazine), 5 mg., or chlorpromazine (Thorazine), 10 to 25 mg., is usually utilized for this purpose. It is recommended that the mixture be given every four hours around the clock in 20 ml. doses on a fixed rather than a whenever-necessary basis. By sequentially increasing the narcotic dosage level per dose, a pain-free state generally can be achieved. Mount recommends that only one variable in the mixture be adjusted at a time, so that either the morphine dose can be adjusted singly or the dose of phenothiazine can be adjusted singly.[33] He further recommends a dosage adjustment at intervals ranging from 48 to 72 hours. With the initial application of narcotic therapy, sedation may be expected and generally disappears within the first two to three days.

GENERAL PRINCIPLES OF CANCER PAIN MANAGEMENT

For most patients experiencing cancer pain the use of analgesics given on a regular basis, generally every four hours, has been demonstrated to be far more effective than whenever-necessary administration. The regular fixed interval protocol eliminates the struggle between the patient and the nurse or family member administering the drug and also eliminates any potential guilt about taking the medication. It also eliminates the anticipatory anxiety of expected pain.

The choice of analgesic drugs should reflect the severity of the pain complaint. For mild to moderate pain, an initial trial with aspirin or acetaminophen on a three to four hour basis is recommended. If this regimen fails to control the pain symptoms, aspirin or acetaminophen can be combined with codeine. For some patients who cannot tolerate codeine, a combination of aspirin or acetaminophen with oxycodone (Percodan or Tylox) might be tried. When sleep disturbances are considerable and depressive elements are apparent, the tricyclic antidepressants merit a trial. They should be administered in a single nightly dose. For more severe pain, hydromorphone (Dilaudid) or the Brompton mixture might be considered. When the duration of analgesic response is inadequate and pain breakthrough is occurring between doses of a drug, methadone might be substituted because of its long biologic half-life. The addition of haloperidol or other antipsychotic drugs might be useful in lengthening the duration of the dose response. It is recommended that oral medication be utilized whenever possible to avoid the many complications of intramuscular or subcutaneous administration. The elderly patient with chronic cancer pain requires an individualized treatment plan, taking into account the patient's particular circumstances. With care, most patients with cancer pain can be kept essentially pain free and maintained in a relatively comfortable and alert state throughout the terminal phase of their illness.

REFERENCES

1. Adams, R.D., and Resnick, W.H.: Cardinal manifestations of disease. In Harrison, T.R., et al. (Editors): Principles of Internal Medicine. Ed. 5. New York, McGraw-Hill Book Company, 1966, pp. 10–17.
2. Bonica, J.J.: Introduction to symposium on pain. Arch. Surg., 112:749, 1977.
3. Bonica, J.J.: Neurophysiologic and pathologic aspects of acute and chronic pain. Arch. Surg., 112:750–761, 1977.
4. Sternbach, R.H.: Pain: A Psychophysiological Analysis. New York, Academic Press, Inc., 1968.
5. Wilson, W.P., and Nashold, B.S., Jr.: Pain and emotion. Postgrad. Med., 46:183–187, 1970.
6. Freud, S.: Inhibitions, symptoms, and anxiety. In Starchy, J. (Translator): Complete Psychological Works of Sigmund Freud. London, Hogarth Press, 1955, Vol. 20, pp. 169–172.
7. Kapp, F.T.: Psychogenic pain. In Freedman, A.M., Kaplan, H.I., and Sadock, B.J. (Editors): Comprehensive Textbook of Psychiatry. II. Baltimore, The Williams & Wilkins Company, 1975, pp. 1704–1708.
8. Rangell, L.: Psychiatric aspects of pain. Psychosom. Med., 15:22–37, 1953.
9. Delaney, J.F.: Atypical facial pain as a defense against psychosis. Am. J. Psychiatry, 133:1151–1154, 1976.
10. Engle, G.L.: Psychogenic pain and the pain prone patient. Am. J. Med., 26:899–918, 1959.
11. Engle, G.L.: The death of a twin: mourning and anniversary reactions. Int. J. Psychoanal., 56:24–40, 1975.
12. Cavenar, J.O., Jr., Nash, J.L., and Maltbie, A.A.: Anniversary reactions presenting as physical complaints. Dis. Nerv. Syst., 39:369–372, 1978.
13. Maltbie, A.A., Cavenar, J.O., Jr., Hammett, E.B., and Sullivan, J.L.: A diagnostic approach to pain. Psychosomatics, 19:359–366, 1978.

14. Jaffe, J., Martin, W.: Narcotic analgesics and antagonists. *In* Goodman, L.S., and Gilman, A. (Editors): The Pharmacological Basis of Therapeutics. Ed. 5. New York, Macmillan Publishing Co., Inc., 1975, pp. 245-283.
15. Shimm, D.S., Logue, G.L., Maltbie, A.A., and Dugan, S.: Medical management of chronic cancer pain. J.A.M.A., *241*:2408-2412, 1979.
16. Belleville, J., Forrest, W., Miller, E., and Brown, B.: Influence of age on pain relief from analgesics. J.A.M.A., *217*:1835-1841, 1971.
17. Bender, A.: Pharmacologic aspects of aging: a survey of the effect of increasing age on drug activity in adults. J. Am. Geriatr. Soc., *12*:114-134, 1964.
18. Paddock, R., Beer, E., Belleville, J., Ciliberti, B., Forrest, W., and Miller, E.: Analgesic and side effects of pentazocine and morphine in a large population of postoperative patients. Clin. Pharmacol. Ther., *10*:355-365, 1969.
19. Marks, R.M., and Sachar, E.J.: Undertreatment of medical inpatients with narcotic analgesics. Ann. Intern. Med., *78*:173-181, 1973.
20. Twycross, R.G., and Wald, S.J.: Long-term use of diamorphine in advanced cancer. *In* Bonica, J.J., and Albe-Fessard, D. (Editors): Advances in Pain Research and Therapy. New York, Raven Press, 1976, Vol. 1, pp. 653-661.
21. Moertel, C.G., Ahmann, D.L., Taylor, W.F., and Schwartau, N.: A comparative evaluation of marketed analgesic drugs. N. Engl. J. Med., *286*:813-815, 1972.
22. Brodie, G.N.: Indomethacin and bone pain. Lancet, *2*:1160, 1974 (letter).
23. Dalessio, D.J.: Chronic pain syndromes and disordered cortical inhibition: effects of tricyclic compounds. Dis. Nerv. Syst., *28*:325, 1967.
24. Merskey, H., and Hessler, R.A.: The treatment of chronic pain with psychotropic drugs. Postgrad. Med. J., *48*:594, 1972.
25. Taub, R.A., and Collins, W.F., Jr.: Observations on the treatment of denervation dysesthesia with psychotropic drugs: postherpetic neuralgia, anesthesia dolorosa, peripheral neuropathy, Adv. Neurol., *4*:309, 1974.
26. Ban, T.A.: Psychopharmacology. Baltimore, The Williams & Wilkins Company, 1969, p. 248.
27. Maltbie, A.A., Cavenar, J.O., Jr., Sullivan, J.L., Hammett, E.B., and Zung, W.W.K.: Analgesia and haloperidol: a hypothesis. J. Clin. Psychol., *40*:323-326, 1979.
28. Kocher, R.: The use of psychotropic drugs in treatment of chronic severe pains. Eur. Neurol., *14*:458-464, 1976.
29. Maltbie, A., and Cavenar, J.: Haloperidol and analgesia. Milit. Med., *142*:946-948, 1977.
30. Cavenar, J., and Maltbie, A.: Another indication for haloperidol. Psychosomatics, *17*:128-130, 1976.
31. Creese, I., Feinberg, A.P., and Synder, S.H.: Butyrophenone influences on the opiate receptor. Eur. J. Pharmacol., *36*:231, 1976.
32. Gingras, M.: A clinical trial of Tofranil in rheumatic pain in general practice. J. Int. Med. Res., *4* (Suppl. 2):41-49, 1976.
33. Mount, B., Ajimian, I., and Scott, J.: Use of the Brompton mixture in treating the chronic pain of malignant disease. Can. Med. Assoc. J., *115*:122-124, 1976.

CHAPTER 15

OPHTHALMIC DISORDERS

Frank J. Weinstock

By virtue of their frequency and serious consequences, diseases of the eye assume a major significance in the elderly. The aging eye, especially sensitive to topically administered medication, is vulnerable to local insult from ocular drugs; likewise the systemic actions of topically administered medications can compromise the elderly patient. Furthermore, the diverse composition of the eye with its specialized vascular, epithelial, collagenous, neural, and pigmentary tissues mandates a careful understanding of drug therapy. In this chapter a consideration of general concepts of treatment of eye disease is followed by an overview of ocular medications; some practical suggestions for their use in aging patients are given. A discussion of specific disease entities concludes the chapter.

GENERAL CONCEPTS OF OCULAR TREATMENT IN THE ELDERLY

With changes in body weight, absorption rate, excretion rate, and metabolic activity in the elderly, the topical or systemic use of medication that might be well tolerated by a younger individual can seriously compromise the health of an older patient. For example, an elderly individual in a borderline nutritional state, with the addition of drugs with an osmotic action or carbonic anhydrase inhibitors for antiglaucoma therapy, might progress to a state of electrolyte imbalance and dehydration, which could result in great morbidity and even mortality. With the rapid absorption of medications through the aging conjunctiva, merely one drop of a potent medication may have a marked systemic effect. Because of the variation in dosage forms, the clinician must carefully prescribe the topically applied preparation with the least potential systemic side effects. For example, in the elderly patient there is a vast difference in the effect of one drop of 4 per cent pilocarpine (which contains approximately 2 mg. of pilocarpine per drop) and one drop of 10 per cent phenylephrine (which contains approximately 5 mg. of phenylephrine per drop).

Whatever preparation is used, the admonition, "One drop is safer than two," bodes well for the elderly. Instructing the elderly patient to occlude the punctum by pressing the inner aspect of the lower lid with a finger for several minutes can markedly reduce the amount of systemic dissemination of an eyedrop, further enhancing the safe topical use of medication.

Because of the need for exact control of concentration and delivery vehicles, generic topically applied medications are usually not recommended in the elderly. Studies of generic drugs containing 2 per cent pilocarpine have shown wide ranges of concentration variations. Likewise a patient may be unable to tolerate a drop from a generic manufacturer but might be able to successfully use a brand name medication owing to the choice of preservative or other formulation component of the preparation. Generic prescribing of ophthalmic preparations in the elderly rarely provides any significant cost saving and may complicate management of the ophthalmic disorder.

Because of the marked variation in "generic equivalents," brand name medications are preferred. Obtaining a price list of frequently used brand name medications from local pharmacies and ordering the least expensive medication that is effective can help contain cost. Although at times less expensive per bottle, generic drugs often cost the patient more eventually, because irritating medications may require more physician visits, longer use of medications, and change to a more effective medication.

Because an informed patient is a better patient, actions as well as undesirable side effects should be discussed with elderly patients. For example, an awareness by the patient that miotic drops for the treatment of glaucoma may cause headache and blurred or dim vision, or that acetazolamide for glaucoma may cause paresthesias, anorexia, and depression, will alert the patient to call the ophthalmologist if these symptoms occur, thus avoiding the possibility of involving another physician who might not understand the circumstances.

An additional concern in the geriatric population is the confusion of eye medications with other medications. For example, acetazolamide (Diamox) and acetohexamide (Dymelor) tablets resemble each other in name and appearance. Substances such as the newer superstrength glues are available in small containers similar to those containing contact lens solution. Poor vision or decreased alertness may result in use of the wrong product in the eye.

The patient should be instructed to tell his personal physician or emergency room physician of any eye medications being used if other conditions arise that require medical evaluation. For example, a physician's unawareness that a patient is using atropine drops might lead to an extensive neurologic work-up because of a dilated pupil. Likewise, a lack of awareness that a patient undergoing general anesthesia has been using anticholinesterase (e.g., phospholene iodide) eyedrops may lead to prolonged apnea and death if succinylcholine is used during anesthesia. Unfortunately patients often fail to mention eyedrops that they are using unless specifically asked by the physician. Occasionally the patient may mention the use of eyedrops but be unable to remember the name of the medication. In this case the physician can ask about the color of the eye container top.

Green top bottles contain miotic drops, which constrict the pupil and are usually used in the treatment of glaucoma; red top bottles are cycloplegics, which relax the muscles of accommodation (focusing) and dilate the pupil.

HAZARDS OF TOPICAL ADMINISTRATION

The administration of ophthalmic drops may cause reactions that mimic other illnesses, causing potential diagnostic problems for the physician. Ophthalmic medications may be administered by drop or ointment or by placement of an ocular insert, injected beneath the conjunctiva or Tenon's capsule, injected through the skin behind the eye (retrobulbar), or injected directly into the anterior chamber or vitreous cavity of the eye. Whatever the route, anxiety on the part of the patient over the administration of the medication may lead to unrelated syncope requiring appropriate care and differentiation from a toxic reaction. Likewise eyedrops may cause local irritation or allergy, which may be confused with infection; stopping the medication usually clears up both the eye disorder and the diagnostic dilemma. Another frequent diagnostic problem concerns the patient who uses over-the-counter eyedrops to treat a scratched or self-abraded cornea. Many of these preparations contain 0.125 per cent phenylephrine, which may dilate the pupil. Without a careful history, the physician might pursue a heroic and expensive diagnostic work-up to seek the cause of dilation of the pupil.

The topical use of drugs in the eye can produce serious illness. Ten per cent phenylephrine eyedrops used to dilate the pupil for an adequate fundus examination have been implicated as a possible cause of myocardial infarction, pulmonary edema, and death in a number of instances. Of 33 cases of adverse effects possibly related to 10 per cent phenylephrine ophthalmic drops reported to the National Registry of Drug-Induced Ocular Side Effects, there were 15 myocardial infarctions (10 of which were terminal), two cases requiring cardiopulmonary resuscitation, and a number of cases of elevated blood pressure. Thus, to decrease the possibility of serious adverse reactions, 2.5 per cent phenylephrine is preferred over 10 per cent phenylephrine. Additionally, punctal occlusion after instillation may decrease systemic absorption.

All dilating drugs, in the susceptible individual, may precipitate angle closure glaucoma. The history is usually of little value since the patient who states that he has glaucoma usually has some type of chronic open angle glaucoma in which dilation rarely causes harm. The patient who is susceptible to angle closure glaucoma rarely knows of this predisposition until the glaucoma is precipitated. Angle closure glaucoma precipitated by dilating drugs may require laser iridotomy or surgical iridectomy for correction.

Four patients have developed aplastic anemia after prolonged topical use of chloramphenicol. The ophthalmic dosage form remains an excellent medication for short term use in many clinical situations, however.

With the increasing use of intraocular implants after cataract surgery, pupil dilation in certain patients can lead to dislocation of the implant, damage to the cornea, and loss of vision. Therefore, prior to dilating the eyes of any patient, a history of cataract extraction and use of an intraocular implant should be sought as well as questioning to determine previous adverse reactions to eyedrops or past symptoms of angle closure glaucoma (rainbow colored halos, eye pain, red eye, blurred vision, and dilated pupil).

AN OVERVIEW OF OCULAR MEDICATIONS

Topically Applied Anesthetics

Topically applied anesthetics should be used only to allow an examination of a painful eye or to anesthetize a normal eye for tonometry. Since prolonged use of these drugs can cause permanent corneal damage and blindness, they should not be prescribed for use outside the physician's office or hospital. If the eye pain is sufficiently severe, other medications, including systemically administered analgesics, are more appropriate.

Dilating and Cycloplegic Drugs

For routine use in dilating the pupil, 2.5 per cent phenylephrine, which does not severely affect accommodation or blur near vision, is the medication of choice. Cycloplegic drugs (e.g., tropicamide, atropine, cyclopentolate, homatropine, scopolamine, and hydroxyamphetamine), because they blur near vision by interfering with accommodation, are inferior products for routine pupil dilation.

In addition to the dilating effect for eye examination, the ophthalmologist uses dilating and cycloplegic drugs after some intraocular operations and for the treatment of iritis and anterior uveitis. The duration of pupillary dilation following the use of drops varies from two to 14 days with atropine, scopolamine, and homatropine to several hours with phenylephrine, tropicamide, and cyclopentolate.

Administration of these cycloplegic drugs should be discontinued when possible prior to the use of anesthetics that sensitize the myocardium to sympathomimetic drugs (e.g., halothane, cyclopropane). These drugs should be used with caution in patients with hypertension, diabetes, hyperthyroidism, heart disease, or longstanding bronchial asthma. Because of the strong action of these drugs on the dilator musculature, the elderly are prone to develop transient pigmentary floaters, which may mimic anterior uveitis. The pressor response from these sympathomimetic drugs may be markedly exaggerated in patients who are receiving or have received monoamine oxidase inhibitors, tricyclic antidepressants, propranolol, reserpine, guanethidine, methyldopa, and anticholinergic drugs. Careful supervision and adjustment of dosages may be required.

Fluorescein

Fluorescein is used topically to reveal corneal abrasions or ulcers. It is rare for problems to occur with the commonly used fluorescein impregnated paper strips. Since fluorescein drops easily become contaminated with pathogenic Pseudomonas species, they have no place in modern medical practice.

Fluorescein is used intravenously by the ophthalmologist to evaluate the vascular system of the eye. Often carried out as an office procedure, this special examination is usually well tolerated, although reactions ranging from slight nausea and headache to syncope, bronchospasm, pulmonary edema, hypotension, anaphylaxis, cardiac arrest, and death have been reported.

Antibiotics

A culture and sensitivity determination is rarely performed before choosing an antibiotic for topical use. In empirical use, the topically applied antibiotics of choice are 0.5

per cent chloramphenicol or 10 per cent sulfacetamide, one drop in the affected eye every one or two hours while awake for two days and then one drop four times a day. To prevent recurrence of the infection, the antibiotic should be used for three to four days after the infection has cleared. Although some physicians prescribe drops for daytime use and ointments at bedtime, ointments are rarely necessary.

In conditions that fail to respond rather quickly to the topical use of antibiotics, a culture and sensitivity determination should be done and appropriate systemically administered antibiotics used. For cellulitis and other serious ocular and periocular infections, medications should be given intramuscularly or intravenously in the appropriate high dosages for the suspected or proven organism.

Antiviral Drugs

Idoxuridine, vidarabine, and trifluridine are the principal antiviral ophthalmic drugs and are clinically effective against herpes simplex virus, types 1 and 2. The exact mechanism by which these drugs exert their antiviral action is not known, but they appear to block reproduction of the herpes simplex virus by interfering with DNA synthesis.

Adverse effects associated with the use of these ophthalmic drugs include mild local irritation, pruritus, inflammation, edema, photophobia, lacrimation, and superficial punctate keratopathy. Corticosteroids may accelerate the spread of a viral infection and are usually contraindicated in the treatment of herpes simplex keratitis.

A response is usually seen in seven or eight days. Re-epithelialization requires several additional days, however. After re-epithelialization has occurred, treatment should be continued for an additional seven days at a reduced dosage to minimize recurrence.

The usual dosage of the 0.1 per cent idoxuridine ophthalmic solution is one drop in each infected eye every hour during the day and every two hours at night until improvement evidenced by loss of staining with fluorescein occurs. The dosage then may be reduced to one drop every two hours during the day and every four hours at night. Reduced dosing should occur for seven days after healing appears to be complete. The 0.5 per cent ophthalmic ointment should be administered five times daily approximately four hours apart, with the last dose at bedtime.

A ½ inch aliquot of 3.0 per cent vidarabine ointment is placed into the lower conjunctival sac five times daily at three hour intervals. If there is no sign of improvement after seven days and complete re-epithelialization has not occurred after 21 days, other forms of therapy should be considered.

The 1.0 per cent trifluridine solution should be instilled onto the cornea of the affected eye as a one drop dose every two hours while awake—a maximal daily dosage of nine drops—until the ulcer has completely re-epithelialized. The dosage following complete re-epithelialization should be reduced to one drop every four hours while awake, a minimum of five doses per day for an additional seven days.

Topically Applied Steroids

Topical steroid therapy is used for the treatment of acute ocular inflammation of the cornea, sclera, conjunctiva, and anterior uveal tract. Unfortunately these drugs are overprescribed for nonspecific irritation or prescribed without proper monitoring. Cataracts and an open angle type of glaucoma may be produced by the topical use of steroids, and thus patients taking such medication require periodic intraocular measurements and funduscopic evaluation.

Topically applied ophthalmic steroids are contraindicated in fungal diseases of ocular structures, herpes simplex keratitis, vaccinia, varicella, and most other viral diseases of the cornea and conjunctiva. Prolonged use is generally inappropriate and may result in glaucoma, damage to the optic nerve, defects in visual acuity and fields of vision, and posterior subcapsular cataract formation and may contribute to secondary ocular infections.

Other Medications Used Systemically

Several other medications that are given systemically can cause ocular toxicity. Phenothiazines may aggravate glaucoma secondary to their anticholinergic properties and produce photophobia, blurred vision, myosis, mydriasis, and ptosis. Prolonged phenothiazine therapy may result in pigment deposition in the lens and cornea, star shaped lenticular opacities, epithelial keratopathies, and pigmentary retinopathy. Pigmentary retinopathy is associated with diminished visual acuity, brownish coloring of vision, and impairment of night vision. Phenothiazines should be discontinued, if at all possible, if retinal changes develop.

The antitubercular drugs, isoniazid and ethambutol, may produce decreases in visual acuity, apparently as a result of optic neuritis and seemingly related to the dosage and duration of treatment. Change in color perception is an early sign of toxicity. Patients should be encouraged to report such an event to their physician, for ocular toxicity is generally reversible if the drug is discontinued promptly.

The antimalarial drugs, quinacrine, chloroquine, and hydroxychloroquine, may produce visual disturbances such as blurred vision and difficulty in focusing that are reversible upon discontinuation of therapy. More severe ocular toxicity is associated with long term therapy and is manifested as retinal changes (e.g., narrowing of the arterioles, macular lesions, pallor of the optic disc, optic atrophy, and patchy pigmentation). Retinal changes may be irreversible. When prolonged therapy with antimalarial drugs is contemplated, baseline and periodic ophthalmologic examinations should be performed.

Diuretics, especially chlorthalidone, the sulfonamides, and tetracycline have been implicated as being capable of causing severe but transient myopia. Optic atrophy has been associated with the use of iodochlorhydroxyquin.

SPECIFIC DISEASE ENTITIES AND THEIR TREATMENT

Blepharitis

Inflammation of the lids may be due to irritation, allergy, or infection. Irritation and allergy may result from medication (local or systemic), foods, chemicals, plants, or bacterial toxins. Infection may be bacterial, viral, or fungal. The insulting agent causes localized inflammation, which may be associated with a varying amount of edema.

Redness and itching of the lids signal allergy or irritation. Bacterial infection is marked by a purulent discharge with varying degrees of edema of the lids. A unilateral rash is characteristic of herpes zoster.

If allergy or irritation is suspected, the offending agent must first be eliminated. If symptoms are significant, the systemic administration of an antihistamine may be used three to four times a day. Rarely a topically applied steroid cream may be massaged into the lids three to four times a day. The systemic administration of steroids would be indicated rarely.

Infectious blepharitis is most commonly due to *Staphylococcus aureus* and is treated topically with 15 per cent sulfacetamide drops, or 0.5 per cent chloramphenicol, one drop every two hours for two days and then one drop four times a day, the excess being massaged over the lid margins. In addition, lid cleansing with plain warm water is carried out when discharge accumulates on the lids. Warm compresses using a hot water bottle over a clean moist washcloth are often effective. Chronic blepharitis often develops an allergic component requiring the topical use of steroids.

If the infection fails to respond to empirical treatment, it is wise to discontinue all medications for one to three days followed by cultures and scrapings to search for a specific agent. On rare occasions appropriate antibiotics may be used systemically three to four times per day, using the most specific drug for the suspected organism.

Viral conditions, except for herpes simplex (discussed on page 442), are treated symptomatically. Antibiotic drops (0.5 per cent chloramphenicol or 10 per cent sulfacetamide) are often used four times a day to prevent secondary bacterial infection.

Edema of the Lids

Edema of the lids, whether due to irritation, allergy, or infection, is marked by edematous transudates collecting in the loose lid tissues, causing significant swelling. Lid swelling, without redness or pain, occurs more frequently with allergies than with infection. Noninfectious edema is treated by the systemic administration of antihistamines three to four times a day. Only rarely is the systemic use of steroids necessary in treatment. Infectious conditions are treated in the same way as for blepharitis.

Lid Cellulitis

The entire spectrum of infectious agents may be encountered in lid cellulitis. Sinus infections must always be considered as the probable source of lid cellulitis. The infectious agent causes a significant cellular reaction with a combination of edema and a purulent exudate in the lids, which may extend to adjacent structures. Clinical manifestations include lid swelling with redness and warmth and induration of the lids associated with fever and systemic lassitude. The local infection may progress to involve the cavernous sinus with paralysis of the extraocular muscles, causing diplopia and possibly loss of vision.

Minor degrees of lid cellulitis may respond to warm compresses. Greater involvement requires careful evaluation including x-ray examination, computed tomographic scanning, the use of ultrasound, and blood cultures. Depending on the gravity of the situation, the oral, intramuscular, or intravenous use of antibiotics is indicated to treat the infection. If cultures indicate a specific agent or sensitivity, the appropriate antibiotic should be selected.

Chalazion

The chalazion probably results from a staphylococcal infection of the meibomian glands. Inflammation of the meibomian glands progresses from an acute to a chronic process of lipogranuloma formation. At the outset there is a diffuse tender inflammation of the palpebral conjunctiva forming a pealike swelling, which becomes visible on the skin surface of the lid. A chalazion has no significant effect on vision.

Continual warm compresses are probably the most effective therapy. In the early stages the topical use of antibiotics such as chloramphenicol may help. If the chalazion persists for three to four weeks and is unsightly, surgical excision via the conjunctival approach may be carried out.

Herpes Zoster

The herpes zoster virus typically infects the gasserian ganglion or the ophthalmic division of the fifth cranial nerve. The virus may directly invade the neural tissue to interfere with the function of the involved nerves and the structures in the distribution of the nerve. In addition to the characteristic rash, which does not cross the midline, keratitis, conjunctivitis, blepharitis, pupillary dilation, and oculomotor paralysis may occur.

The topical application of 0.5 per cent chloramphenicol or 10 per cent sodium sulfacetamide drops is used empirically four times a day. With the skin involvement secondary infection may complicate the situation, requiring the systemic use of antibiotics. The systemic use of steroids in severe cases is controversial, but they seem to help alleviate the symptoms. Prednisone, 10 to 15 mg. orally four times daily, can be used for two days then the dosage can be tapered gradually. Antibiotics may be used systemically on the basis of the theory that the patient's resistance is low and that the skin is infected. Postherpetic neuralgia defies treatment.

Uveitis secondary to herpes zoster infection is marked by significant pain and photophobia. One per cent atropine or 5 per cent homatropine drops are used four times daily to relieve some of the discomfort. Prednisolone or dexamethasone drops may be used every two hours while awake for two days and then administration can be decreased to four times a day until there is clearing. The antiviral drugs fail to help in herpes zoster but may be required if superinfection with herpes simplex occurs.

Conjunctivitis

Conjunctivitis is a nonspecific term referring to inflammation of the conjunctiva. Although conjunctivitis may be associated with viral, bacterial, or fungal infections, it may also be secondary to trauma, corneal disease, a foreign body, surgery, intraocular disease, systemic disease, or local or systemic allergy. Practically speaking, conjunctivitis should be differentiated from acute glaucoma, uveitis, and keratitis, since it is only secondarily involved in those conditions.

Bacterial Conjunctivitis

Although *Staphylococcus aureus* and *Diplococcus pneumoniae* are the most common causes of bacterial conjunctivitis, any bacterium may be responsible. The responsible bacterium incites an acute inflammatory response with the production of a mucopurulent exudate. The mild to marked injection of the conjunctiva is usually more pronounced in the fornix and on the palpebral conjunctiva, the area near the limbus being less involved. The mucopurulent discharge causing sticking of the lids may cause slight blurring of vision if it gets on the cornea; there is relatively little photophobia. Progression to corneal and intraocular involvement may rarely lead to loss of vision.

The topical administration of antibiotics is used empirically. If no improvement occurs, another antibiotic may be tried. If the condition persists, the antibiotic should be discontinued for several days and cultures and sensitivity studies should be done. Occasionally chronic conjunctivitis may require the addition of an antibiotic given orally to bring the infection under control.

Allergic Conjunctivitis

Almost any allergen may involve the conjunctiva. The allergen induces a vasomotor response, which causes hyperemia and edema of the conjunctiva. Conjunctival injection is present, with tearing and mild irritation but there is no photophobia or visual disturbance. Occasionally the conjunctiva may be extremely edematous to the point of appearing like a sac of clear fluid protruding between the lids.

Usually allergic conjunctivitis is self-limited, with no treatment necessary. Cool compresses provide symptomatic relief. Topically applied steroids have a marked beneficial effect and are used in the weakest strength possible and discontinued when improvement occurs. Because of their potential side effects, steroids should not be prescribed routinely. If there are associated systemic allergic signs and symptoms, the oral administration of antihistamines or steroids may be required in rare cases.

Viral Conjunctivitis

Most viral organisms may cause viral conjunctivitis. The virus attacks the conjunctival epithelium directly or via hematogenous spread, causing a local follicular reaction, which may spread to deeper layers or to other parts of the eye. If the infection is localized to the conjunctiva, there is bulbar injection, which is more marked in the fornix, with a nonpurulent discharge. There may be follicular hypertrophy. With corneal or more extensive involvement there may be severe photophobia and blurring of vision.

Except for herpes simplex and trachoma, there is no specific therapy for viral conjunctivitis. Cool compresses and bland drops may provide some relief. Topically applied steroids constitute a dual edged sword, which may be employed cautiously by the ophthalmologist. Meticulous hygiene is necessary to avoid transmission of viral conjunctivitis. Handwashing by the physician and patient is essential to assist in avoiding transmission of this contagious condition.

Subconjunctival Hemorrhage

Trauma, systemic hypertension, blood dyscrasias, coughing, or sneezing may cause subconjunctival hemorrhages, but usually no inciting cause is found. A fragile conjunctival vessel typically ruptures, causing hemorrhage beneath the surface, producing an asymptomatic, bright red, sharply demarcated area on the external surface of the eye.

There is no treatment for subconjunctival hemorrhage, which spontaneously resorbs in 10 to 14 days. With recurrent hemorrhages, an underlying systemic cause should be sought.

Keratitis

Inflammatory disease of the cornea is caused by the same bacterial and viral organisms that produce conjunctivitis. Trauma, tumors, and cerebrovascular accidents may precipitate exposure keratitis. A break in the corneal epithelium incites an inflammatory response in the normally clear cornea, enabling edema and vascularization to take place. Microorganisms may enter the damaged epithelium and spread their ravages throughout the cornea.

Keratitis is accompanied by significant pain, photophobia, and decreased vision. The epithelial defect is seen as a bright green area when fluorescein dye is placed on the eye with a moistened fluorescein impregnated paper strip and viewed with a blue light. Often the defect can be seen only under the high magnification of the ophthalmologist's biomicroscope (slit lamp).

Bacterial Keratitis

A broad spectrum of bacteria may be implicated in bacterial keratitis. In addition to pain, photophobia, and decreased vision, a marginal corneal ulcer or inferior punctate corneal staining may be visible. The presence of a hypopyon (pus in the anterior chamber) is an extremely grave sign.

Cultures and sensitivity studies should be

done to permit usage of the most appropriate antibiotic. Since bacterial keratitis is often due to Staphylococcus, intensive topical therapy should be quickly instituted with chloramphenicol or gentamicin drops every one to two hours while the patient is awake, for one to two days and then four times a day. In the patient with a hypopyon, the ophthalmologist may institute the intravenous, subconjunctival, or intracameral administration of antibiotics.

Herpes Simplex (Dendritic) Keratitis

The herpes simplex virus is the responsible organism in herpes simplex keratitis. Invasion of the corneal epithelium occurs externally from contact or with viral organisms present in the conjunctiva or lacrimal gland. Epithelial vesicles may progress to ulcers with significant epithelial and stromal scarring. The chracteristic dendritic pattern is evident with fluorescein staining. Later the lesion progresses to a geographic ulcer with corneal scarring, thus placing herpes simplex keratitis in the forefront as a condition requiring corneal transplants. Descementocele formation and corneal perforation may occur, especially if steroids have been used topically at the wrong time. In about 20 per cent of the cases there is a recurrence of the lesion, which may become chronic.

Ophthalmologists are fortunate to have antiviral drugs that are quite effective against herpes simplex. These drugs apparently interfere with viral DNA synthesis, thereby preventing virus replication. Several topically useful medications are available. Those include idoxuridine, vidarabine (Ara-A), and trifluridine. Some ophthalmologists prefer to debride the epithelial lesion with a moist cotton applicator prior to instituting medication. Dosage guidelines are presented in the previous section entitled "An Overview of Ocular Medications—Antiviral Drugs." Concurrent use of chloramphenicol or sodium sulfacetamide drops four times a day is a common practice. Despite therapy, there is a 20 per cent incidence of recurrence.

Fungal Keratitis

Fungi infections of the cornea may occur following trauma, via contaminated solutions such as those used in the care of contact lenses or as a complication of extended steroid treatment. The fungus and its toxins induce a severely destructive inflammatory reaction of the cornea and the conjunctiva. A fluffy white lesion on the cornea, associated with marked conjunctival hyperemia, may persist. There may be a significant reduction in vision with marked pain.

Topically applied amphotericin B drops (1.5 to 5 mg. per ml.), Nystatin drops (5000–10,000 units per ml.), natamycin suspension (5 per cent), or gentamicin drops may be used intensively as one drop every hour until improvement occurs, after which the frequency of administration is decreased gradually. If progression occurs, a thin conjunctival flap may be pulled over the cornea surgically. If no positive response to one of the foregoing drugs is seen within seven to 10 days after therapy was initiated, the fungus is not likely to be susceptible and a new regimen should be initiated.

Exposure Keratitis

Inability to close the eye secondary to a stroke, Bell's palsy, or trauma leaves the eye constantly exposed. Desiccation and opacification of the cornea with secondary infection occur with exposure. The cornea becomes hazy with corresponding conjunctival hyperemia without a significant amount of associated pain.

Efforts to lubricate the cornea and to keep it moist should be carried out. Artificial tears and ointments may be used hourly if necessary. The use of hydroxypropyl methylcellulose drops (made for gonioscopic eye examinations) every two to four hours has eliminated protective lid closure. Drops are preferable to ointments, especially in patients who have sustained a stroke, since these enable periodic ophthalmoscopic examinations to be carried out. In some patients the cornea may be kept lubricated and moist by taping the lids closed.

Neuroparalytic or Neurotrophic Keratitis

Interference with trigeminal nerve function by trauma or following neurosurgical intervention involving the fifth cranial nerve (especially operations on the gasserian ganglion for tic douloureux) may lead to neurotrophic keratitis. Anesthesia of the cornea leads to drying and ulceration of the cornea in an unknown manner. The corneal anesthesia leaves the patient unaware of foreign bodies or trauma and prevents the normal protective lid closure. A moderate amount of conjunctival hyperemia is associated with a central corneal ulceration. There may be a marked visual loss, especially if corneal perforation occurs. Drug management is the same as for exposure keratitis.

Recurrent Erosion

A minor corneal abrasion, especially following a fingernail scratch, may be complicated by a recurrent corneal breakdown. For poorly understood reasons, the corneal epithelium regenerates but fails to adhere strongly to the underlying Bowman membrane, making possible periodic recurrence of corneal erosion. Classically, upon awakening in the morning, days to years following the original abrasion, the patient experiences a pulling or sticking sensation followed by tearing, photophobia, and a varying amount of pain. With proper magnification the abnormal epithelium usually may be demonstrated by fluorescent staining.

Treatment requires debriding of the loose epithelium with a moist applicator, patching the eye overnight, and then applying bacitracin eye ointment to the eye in the morning and at night for four to six weeks. This procedure may have to be repeated several times and is usually very painful, requiring the systemic administration of analgesics for 24 hours. Occasionally a bandage soft contact lens is necessary to allow proper corneal regeneration to take place.

Trachoma

The trachoma virus, which is spread by poor hygienic conditions, is the leading cause of blindness in the world. The trachoma virus invades the cells of the conjunctiva, cornea, and lids, causing the devastating inflammatory response.

Conjunctivitis is followed by corneal vascularization, leading to scarring and scar retracture. This involves the conjunctiva, cornea, and lids and leads to blindness by opacification and possible perforation of the cornea.

Proper hygiene and cleanliness must be instituted, with avoidance of use of another person's towels, washcloths, or cosmetics. Tetracycline or sulfonamide ointment applied topically to the eyes three times a day for six weeks should cure the patient. Occasionally systemic administration of tetracycline or sulfonamides, four times a day for six weeks, may be required.

Epidemic Keratoconjunctivitis

Epidemic keratoconjunctivitis is caused by type 8 adenovirus. This is a highly virulent adenovirus, which directly affects the cornea and conjunctiva. It is spread primarily from person to person by the hands and instruments of medical personnel to the eyes. Marked persistent conjunctivitis, which may be complicated by corneal involvement (keratitis), is associated with pain and photophobia, which may last for many weeks. Corneal scarring may lead to a significant reduction in vision.

Meticulous cleanliness is essential to avoid spreading this highly contagious disease. There is no specific treatment for this self-limited condition. Most ophthalmologists prescribe an antibiotic drop, such as 10 per cent sulfacetamide or 0.5 per cent chloramphenicol, one drop four times a day. With significant pain, 5 per cent homatropine or 1 per cent atropine drops, by their cycloplegic action, give some relief when administered as one drop three to four times a day. Topically applied steroids such as fluoromethalone, hydrocortisone, prednisolone, or dexamethasone also give some relief when used as one drop four times a day with careful slit lamp and pressure examinations to avoid harmful side effects.

Keratoconjunctivitis Sicca (Sjögren's Syndrome)

As part of a generalized connective tissue disorder, which may involve lymphocytic and plasma cell infiltration of the lacrimal glands, keratoconjunctivitis sicca (Sjögren's syndrome) is marked by a reduction in tear production and an alteration in the composition of the tears. The clinical manifestations of the complete syndrome consist of decreased tear production, dryness of the mouth, and arthritis. In the most severe form, vision is impaired.

Treatment is empirical. Bland nonprescription artificial tear substitutes used every two to four hours provide relief in most cases.

Although most drops contain varying concentrations of methylcellulose, there are a multitude of substances that may be used as drops. Patients may respond to one artificial tear substitute but not to others. Slow, continuous release lubricants such as Lacrisert may also be utilized. Often 2.5 per cent hydroxpropyl methylcellulose (Goniosol) is effective when all other drops have failed to provide relief.

Retinal Artery Occlusion

Emboli or thrombi from the carotid system or cardiac valves may occlude the retinal artery or one of its branches. The occluding material interrupts the retinal artery circulation, resulting in edema and swelling of the inner retinal layers. There is a sudden painless loss of vision and a dilated fixed pupil.

Transient loss of vision in one eye (amaurosis fugax or transient ischemic attacks) may occur as a symptom of carotid artery occlusive disease. On funduscopic examination the retinal arteries are found to be thin, with segmentation of the blood column. The macula appears as a cherry red spot. Plaque may be seen in the arterial tree.

Initially intermittent digital massage of the eye for five to 10 second periods should be caried out in an attempt to move the embolus to a smaller, more peripheral arteriole. Inhalation of 5 per cent carbon dioxide for five to 10 minute periods may induce some dilation of the arterioles. Acetazolamide, 500 mg. given orally, may lower the intraocular pressure to decrease resistance to arterial blood flow. Other methods that may be used by the ophthalmologist are a retrobulbar lidocaine block or paracentesis of the anterior chamber. The use of anticoagulants is recommended by some clinicians (see Chapter 10).

Senile Macular Degeneration

Senile macular degeneration probably results from a decrease in the vascular supply to the macula from the lamina choriocapillaris. The etiology of senile macular degeneration is unknown in most cases, although it may occur secondary to trauma or inflammatory disease. Alterations of the retinal pigment epithelium and Bruch's membrane occur with dissemination of pigment in the macular area, resulting in the formation of drusen and atrophy of the cone cells.

Clinically senile macular degeneration is marked by loss of the foveal light reflex. Macular pigmentation, often associated with a flat serous retinal detachment, causes a variable loss of vision. Macular hemorrhage may be present in some cases. Because the peripheral retina remains intact, complete blindness does not occur.

Although vasodilators, vitamins, and many other medications have been used, there is no definitive treatment for senile macular degeneration. Laser photocoagulation is an effective treatment in some cases.

Uveitis

The vascular uveal tract serves to absorb shock and is involved in many inflammatory conditions. The most common conditions causing uveitis are histoplasmosis, toxoplasmosis, and sarcoidosis. In addition, uveitis may follow ophthalmic surgical procedures, ocular trauma, bacterial infections, traumatic keratitis, herpes simplex keratitis, and herpes zoster infection.

Uveitis results when a relatively direct irritation of the uveal tract or an indirect insult secondary to an immunologic reaction sets up an inflammatory process, with breakdown of the blood-aqueous barrier. Inflammatory exudative cells and fibrin enter the anterior chamber and cause clogging of the trabecular meshwork. This inflammatory exudative process in turn can produce cataract and posterior opacification of the vitreous with scarring, macular edema, and inflammatory changes of the posterior pole of the eye. Posterior synechiae can result from adherence of the iris on the lens. Occasionally glaucoma can be produced by uveitis.

Anterior uveitis is associated with circumcorneal injection, photophobia, decreased vision, miosis, and marked pain. Fine nongranulomatous cells (plasma cells and lymphocytes) or thick granulomatous clumps of cells (macrophages and pigment) are visible on biomicroscopy. These cells may collect on the corneal endothelium as keratic precipitates.

Posterior uveitis produces a painless blurring of vision. Cells can be seen in the vitreous, inflammation may be seen in the retina or in the area of the pars plana, and macular edema may be present.

Prior to instituting therapy, a general medical examination should be performed and a chest film obtained to help rule out toxoplasmosis, histoplasmosis, sarcoidosis, rheumatoid problems, sinusitis, and dental disease. In most cases of anterior uveitis, no etiologic agent can be found and empirical treatment is necessary. Cycloplegia reduces pain by relieving ciliary spasm. Pupillary dilation can be obtained with 1 per cent atropine or 2 or 5 per cent homatropine eyedrops used two to four times a day; 10 per cent Neo-Synephrine eyedrops four times a day produce movement of the iris and additional dilation. Steroids can be applied topically every one to two hours for one to two days and then four times a day until resolution of uveitis in order to reduce inflammation. If the topical application of steroids is ineffective, their systemic administration may be required.

Systemic steroids are necessary in cases of posterior uveitis that impairs vision. The usual dosage of steroids for posterior uveitis is 15 mg. of prednisone four times daily. This dosage can be tapered gradually after the acute condition clears. Chronic posterior uveitis may require the prolonged systemic use of steroids. In these cases alternate day dosage of prednisone should be used.

Angle Closure Glaucoma

Angle closure glaucoma results from forward displacement of the iris against the cornea and obstruction of flow of aqueous humor into the chamber angle and the spaces of Fontana. In patients in whom the distance between the posterior surface of the cornea and the anterior surface of the iris is slight, the entrance to the chamber angle is narrow and more susceptible to closure than in the normal individual. In these patients sudden dilation of the pupil, swelling of the iris from inflammation, or swelling of the lens may produce a sudden and complete obstruction to outflow of the aqueous humor. A family history of angle closure glaucoma alerts the physician to the possibility of this process.

Acute attacks of angle closure glaucoma produce blurred vision, rainbow colored halos, headaches or eye pain, redness of the eye, and a semidilated fixed pupil. On examination, the intraocular pressure is found to be elevated (often over 70 mm. Hg) and the eye is red, with corneal edema. Direct observation of the angle closure is seen with gonioscopy. Intermittent angle closure attacks that resolve spontaneously without treatment may be misdiagnosed as sinus attacks, neuroses, or migraine headaches.

Angle closure glaucoma is treated by lowering the intraocular pressure medically, followed by curative laser iridotomy or surgical iridectomy. Miotics, carbonic anhydrase inhibitors, and systemically administered hyperosmotic drugs are used in the medical treatment of glaucoma.

During acute attacks of angle closure glaucoma, 4 per cent pilocarpine drops should be used every 10 to 15 minutes for four to six doses.

If there are no medical contraindications, rapid lowering of the intraocular pressure may be obtained by the use of the osmotic drug, 50 per cent glycerin. Glycerin is given orally in a dosage of 1.0 to 1.5 gm. per kg. of body weight in a mixture with equal parts of iced lemon juice. Occasionally, the hyperosmotic drug mannitol, given as an intravenous infusion in a dose of 6 to 8 ml. per kg. of body weight of a 20 per cent solution over a 20 to 30 minute period, may be necessary to lower the intraocular pressure. These methods cause great stress on the biologic system and should be used with caution in the elderly.

Additional lowering of intraocular pressure may be obtained by the use of the carbonic anhydrase inhibiting drug, acetazolamide. An initial dose of 250 to 500 mg. of acetazolamide given either orally or intravenously may be followed by the administration of 125 to 250 mg. of Diamox orally every six hours. As the acute attack becomes controlled, medical therapy is reduced but maintained at a level that controls the intraocular pressure and permits congestion to subside. Following medical control, laser iridotomy or surgical iridectomy should be performed on the involved eye, often followed by laser iridotomy or iridectomy on the other eye, since similar acute attacks are likely to occur in the uninvolved eye if surgery is not performed.

Chronic Simple Open Angle Glaucoma

A multifactorial genetic trait makes blood relatives of patients with glaucoma more susceptible to the development of chronic simple open angle glaucoma. Aqueous humor is produced in the ciliary body and flows from the posterior chamber around the pupil and out through the canal of Schlemm into the drainage system. In the trabecular meshwork there is a poorly understood block to the outflow of the aqueous humor. With continued production of aqueous humor the intraocular pressure increases and causes damage to the optic nerve with a resulting decrease in the visual field and late loss of central, macular vision.

The term chronic simple open angle glaucoma is used when optic nerve damage and visual field loss result from elevated intraocular pressure in an eye with an open angle (as determined by gonioscopy) and no etiology is found. Symptoms are usually absent until optic nerve damage and resulting visual field loss occur, thereby making the early diagnosis of this preventable condition essential. In a patient with an elevated intraocular pressure but normal optic nerve and visual field, it is impossible to predict whether the condition will progess to optic nerve damage. Patients with elevated intraocular pressure, therefore, require careful periodic observation to determine whether it is necessary to institute therapy. Because only 5 to 10 per cent of the patients with ocular hypertension (intraocular pressure greater than 21 mm. Hg) develop open angle glaucoma, most patients with ocular hypertension should be observed without therapy to avoid therapeutic complications.

Chronic simple open angle glaucoma develops gradually. The eye usually appears perfectly normal externally. The pupil may be slightly dilated and reacts sluggishly to light. After the disease has progressed, ophthalmoscopic examination reveals glaucomatous cupping of the disc and atrophy of the optic nerve.

The goal of treatment for simple open angle glaucoma is to preserve visual function and prevent visual damage in the safest way possible. Often a trial of therapy is carried out. This technique consists of treating one eye to determine the effectiveness of the medication, using the untreated eye as a control.

Whatever treatment is used, the goal of therapy should be to use the lowest concentration of medication that will produce the lowest incidence of side effects in order to reduce the intraocular pressure enough to preserve visual function. The medications available for the treatment of open angle glaucoma, each with specific actions, indications, and side effects, include parasympathomimetic (cholinergic) drops (pilocarpine, carbachol, and cholinesterase inhibitors), sympathetic (adrenergic) drops (epinephrine) and adrenergic blocking drugs (timolol), and carbonic anhydrase inhibitors.

Parasympathomimetic Drugs. The parasympathomimetic drugs improve the aqueous outflow from the eye in a very effective manner. Except for the long acting cholinesterase inhibitors (echothiophate iodide, demecarium bromide, and isoflurophate), these drops have an action that lasts for about six hours. In sustained release form, pilocarpine (Ocusert) is delivered via contact lens type of membrane placed on the conjunctiva and replaced each week. The major complaints of patients given miotic drops are blurring due to accommodative spasm and decreased vision due to miosis, especially in patients with cataracts. When such medication is used in more frequent doses or in susceptible individuals, adverse parasympathetic effects may include diarrhea, muscle cramps, nausea, vomiting, perspiration, abdominal cramps, headache, bradycardia, and respiratory distress. The anticholinesterase drops, in addition to the foregoing effects, may be responsible for the development of cataracts, conjunctivitis, blurred vision, and retinal detachment as well as a decrease in the blood cell cholinesterase level, which makes the patient susceptible to prolonged apnea when succinylcholine is used during general anesthesia.

The frequency of instillation of drops and the concentration of the drug are determined by the severity of the glaucoma and the patient's response. The usual concentrations of pilocarpine employed are between 0.5 and 4.0 per cent in a dosage of one drop four to five times daily. Other parasympathetic drugs are considered second line drugs and may be employed if pilocarpine fails.

Epinephrine. The sympathetic drug, epinephrine, stimulates both alpha and beta adrenergic receptors, producing both a decrease in aqueous humor production and an increase in outflow. Epinephrine is of primary value as an adjunct to parasympathomimetic therapy, but may be used alone in the elderly patient with lens opacities. The usual dose is one to two drops of a 0.1 per cent solution with frequency individualized to patient response.

Epinephrine has several adverse local and systemic effects. Adverse local effects include blepharitis, conjunctivitis, and tearing. Adverse systemic effects that are possible with the topical use of drops include headache, tachycardia, palpitations, extrasystoles, and arrhythmias.

The new prodrug, dipivefrin, may be used as the initial therapy of open angle glaucoma. The drug appears to have fewer adverse effects than epinephrine.

Timolol. The adrenergic blocking drug, timolol, as a 0.25 or 0.5 per cent solution, decreases aqueous production and may increase outflow by an as yet unknown mechanism. It is extremely effective in many individuals singly or in combination with miotics or epinephrine drops. The adverse effects associated with timolol therapy are more frequent and more severe than those associated with pilocarpine and epinephrine. Mild ocular irritation is occasionally reported. A slight reduction in the resting heart rate has been observed. It has been implicated as a causative agent in pulmonary edema, exacerbation of asthma, and death. It is contraindicated in patients with asthma and serious pulmonary disorders.

The usual starting dosage is one drop of a 0.25 per cent solution twice daily. If an adequate response is not obtained, the concentration of the solution is increased to 0.5 per cent and administered twice daily. A maintenance dose of one drop once daily may be adequate. The long action and infrequent local hypersensitivity reactions foster good compliance in the elderly patient.

Carbonic Anhydrase Inhibitors. Carbonic anhydrase inhibitors (acetazolamide, methazolamide, ethoxzolamide, and dichlorphenamide), given in pill form two to four times a day, lower aqueous production. Most patients respond to doses of 250 mg. given every six hours. Side effects range from transient myopia to confusion, depression, paresthesias, loss of appetite, impotence, and severe electrolyte and acid-base disturbances. Other adverse effects include nausea, confusion, weight loss, rash, tinnitus, renal calculi, and bone marrow depression.

When, despite maximally tolerated medical therapy, the intraocular pressure cannot be lowered sufficiently to prevent optic nerve damage and progressive visual field loss, pressure lowering filtration surgical procedures such as trabeculectomy, trabeculotomy, and sclerotomy may be necessary. Prior laser trabeculoplasty may eliminate the need for surgical treatment. These procedures create an additional aqueous outflow drainage path to help preserve vision.

In a patient with systemic hypertension, the optic nerve is adapted to a particular level of blood pressure. If the blood pressure is lowered too rapidly in a patient with ocular hypertension or glaucoma, the vascular supply of the optic nerve may suddenly be decompensated, causing a rapid loss of vision. This phenomenon may also occur with severe hemorrhage or shock.

Cataracts

A cataract is an opacification on the crystalline lens of the eye. Most cataracts are idiopathic. They diminish vision by altering the refractive power of the lens and causing a decrease in the transparency of the lens. A small number of patients develop cataracts following trauma. The most common cause of human cataract formation is aging. The most common pharmacologic cause of cataracts, steroid usage, can occur with systemic or, less commonly, topical usage. The steroid cataract is usually of the posterior subcapsular type, is most likely in patients taking steroids at dosages of 15 mg. of prednisone per day for one year or more, and responds well to surgical treatment. The topical application of anticholinesterase drops and the systemic use of MER 29 have been implicated in the etiology of cataracts.

Although cataracts are most prevalent in the geriatric population, they can occur any time in life. Cataracts may be unilateral or bilateral and progress at uniform or sporadic rates. Ninety per cent of the patients do not require surgery when the diagnosis is made.

The first clinical manifestation of a cataract consists of a dimming of vision; bright lights or dimly lit situations may intensify the symptom. Cataracts are not associated with headaches or pain. The reduction in vision increases with the progress of the cataract until finally only light is perceived. Occasionally there is annoying diplopia or polyopia due to irregular refraction of the lens. There are no medications that have any direct beneficial effect upon cataract formation or progression. With certain central cataracts, dilation of the pupil with mydriatic or cycloplegic drops may enlarge the pupil sufficiently to improve vision by allowing light to enter the eye around the cataract. These drops may improve vision sufficiently to enable patients to function for years without surgery.

When vision is decreased to the point of interfering with the individual's ability to function, or if the cataract becomes hypermature to the point of causing glaucoma, surgical intervention becomes necessary. Surgical intervention, with a 90 to 95 per cent success rate, is the only definitive treatment for cataracts. Removal of the cataractous lens requires postoperative correction of vision with glasses, contact lenses, or more commonly an intraocular lens implant. Cataract surgery in the elderly, however, is not without hazard. Even with the reduced amount of preoperative medication, the delicate balance in a geriatric patient can be upset by surgery causing major vascular, cardiac, and other systemic complications. Preoperative sedation and hyperosmotic drugs can cause electrolyte imbalance, respiratory changes, and alterations in the cardiac rate and rhythm. For these reasons preoperative medications should be kept to a minimum. Because cardiac problems can occur at any time, electrocardiographic monitoring should be used in all cases and the blood pressure and pulse frequently monitored.

With the use of local anesthesia, minimal preoperative medication, and ambulatory surgery, morbidity is decreased to a minimum.

The postoperative administration of analgesics can cause respiratory depression. A major cause of disorientation and electrolyte imbalance is dehydration. The most frequent problems after discharge from cataract surgery are allergy and irritation due to eyedrops. The most serious complication of cataract surgery is postoperative infection (endophthalmitis)—an emergency situation that requires intensive antibiotic treatment, often combined with vitrectomy.

SUGGESTED READINGS

1. Bergaust, B., and Westby, R.K.: Zoster ophthalmicus; local treatment with cortisone. Acta Ophthalmol., 45:787, 1967.
2. Blaricom, L.S., and Hurrax, G.: Chronic postherpetic neuralgia. J.A.M.A., 161:511, 1956.
3. Boyd, B.: Ocular infection. Mini-highlights of ophthalmology. Monthly Letter, 7:4, 5, 6, 1979.
4. Diabetic Retinopathy Study Group: Four risk factors for severe visual loss in diabetic retinopathy. 3rd report from the Diabetic Retinopathy Study. Arch. Ophthalmol., 97:654–655, 1979.
5. Duane, T.: Clinical Ophthalmology. Hagerstown, Harper & Row, 1976.
6. Eaglstein, W.H., Katz, R., and Brown, J.A.: The effects of early corticosteroid therapy on the skin eruption and pain of herpes zoster. J.A.M.A., 211:1681, 1970.
7. Ellis, P.P.: Ocular Therapeutics and Pharmacology. St. Louis, The C.V. Mosby Company, 1977.
8. Ernest, J.T.: Pathogenesis of glaucomatous optic nerve disease. Trans. Am. Ophthalmol. Soc., 73:366–388, 1975.
9. Frank, R.N.: Treating diabetic retinopathy. Surg. Rounds, 33–39, April 1980.
10. National Institutes of Health: New standards for classification and diagnosis of diabetes. J.A.M.A., 243:2296–2297, 1980.
11. Grayston, J.T., Wang, S.P., Woolridge, R.L., Yang, Y.F., and Johnson, P.B.: Trachoma—studies of etiology, laboratory diagnosis and prevention. J.A.M.A., 172:1577, 1960.
12. Havener, W.H.: Ocular Pharmacology. St. Louis, The C.V. Mosby Company, 1978.
13. Kaufman, H.E.: Herpetic keratitis. Invest. Ophthalmol. Vis. Sci., 17:941–957, 1978.
14. Kohn, A.N., Moss, A.P., Hargett, N.A., Ritch, R., Smith, H., Jr., and Podos, S.M.: Clinical comparison of dipivalyl epinephrine and epinephrine in treatment of glaucoma. Am. J. Ophthalmol., 87:196–201, 1979.
15. Laibson, P.R., and Dupre-Strachan, S.: Community and hospital outbreak of epidemic keratoconjunctivitis. Arch. Ophthalmol., 80:467, 1968.
16. Leopold, I., and Mosier, M.: Diabetes and the eye. Geriatrics, 35:67–73, 1980.
17. Macular Photocoagulation Study (MPS), National Eye Institute.
18. Maichuk, Y.F.: Some aspects of rational trachoma therapy. Am. J. Ophthalmol., 74:694, 1972.
19. McMahon, C.D., Shaffer, R.N., Hoskins, D.H., Jr., and Hetherington, J., Jr.: Adverse effects experienced by patients taking timolol. Am. J. Ophthalmol., 88:736–738, 1979.
20. Newell, F.W., and Ernest, J.: Ophthalmology—Principles and Concepts. Ed. 3. St. Louis, The C.V. Mosby Company, 1974.
21. O'Malley, B.C.: Recent advances in managing the complications of diabetes. Geriatrics, 51–55, June 1980. vol. 35.
22. Pavan-Langston, D.: Acrylic antimetabolite therapy of experimental herpes simplex keratitis. Am. J. Ophthalmol., 86:618–623, 1978.
23. Physicians' Desk Reference for Ophthalmology (PDR). Oradell, Medical Economics Company, 1979/1980.
24. Podolsky, S., and L'Esperance, F.: Diabetic retinopathy: update on therapeutic advances. Geriatrics, 35:67–73, 1980.
25. Reddy, V.: Dynamics of transport systems in the eye. Invest. Ophthalmol. Vis. Sci., 18:1000–1018, 1979.
26. Waring, G.: Viewpoints—initial therapy of suspected marginal corneal ulcers. Surv. Ophthalmol., 24:97–116, 1979.
27. Weinstock, F.J.: Simple treatment of neurotrophic keratitis. Am. J. Ophthalmol., 67:150–151, 1969.
28. Weinstock, F.J.: Glaucoma: how to treat and when to refer. Geriatrics, 33:31–38, 1978.
29. Weinstock, F.J.: What your aging patient may want to know about cataracts. Geriatrics, 33:57–64, 1978.
30. Weinstock, F.J.: Management of ocular hypertension. Glaucoma, 2:465–467, 1980.
31. Wilson, F.: Adverse external ocular effects of topical ophthalmic medications. Surv. Ophthalmol., 24:97–116, 1979.
32. Yates, D.: Syncope and visual hallucinations, apparently from timolol (letters to the editor). J.A.M.A., 244:768–769, 1980.
33. Zimmerman, T.J., and Kaufman, H.E.: Timolol: dose response and duration of action. Arch. Ophthalmol., 95:605–607, 1977.
34. Van Buskirk, E.M.: Side effects from glaucoma therapy. Ann. Ophthalmol., 12:964–965, 1980.
35. Adverse systemic effects from ophthalmic drugs. Med. Letter 24:53–54, 1982.

36. Wilson, R.P., Spaeth, G.L., and Poryzees, E.: The place of timolol in the practice of ophthalmology. Ophthalmology, *87:*451–454, 1980.
37. Van Buskirk, E.M.: Hazards of medical glaucoma therapy in the cataract patient. Ophthalmology, *89:*238–241, 1982.
38. LeBlanc, R.P., and Krip, G.: Timolol: Canadian multicenter study. Ophthalmology, *88:*244–248, 1981.
39. Lockey, S.D.: Bronchospasm precipitated by ophthalmic instillations of timolol. Ann. Allergy, *46:*267, 1981.
40. Vonwil, A., et al.: Bronchoconstrictive side effects of timolol eye drops in patients with obstructive lung diseases. Schweiz. Med. Wochenschr., *111:*665–669, 1981.

INDEX

Page numbers in *italics* refer to illustrations; page numbers followed by "t" refer to tables.

Absorption, of drugs, 19, 20, 30, 31t. See also *Pharmacokinetics.*
  variations with age, 42–46, *43,* 44t, 46t
of food, inhibition of, obesity and, 362
Acetohexamide (Dymelor), 18t, 343, 343t
Acidosis, metabolic, chronic renal failure and, 378
Adrenergic inhibiting drugs, 143–147, 144t, 148, 149
Advertising, and drug use, 7
Affective disorders. See *Psychiatric disorders, affective; Depression.*
Aging, and antiarrhythmic therapy, 163
  and creatinine clearance, 158, *159,* 159t
  and estrogen therapy, 414
  and hypertension, 140
  and psychotropic drugs, 75
  and sleep, 100
Agitation, 79
Akathisia, 79
Albumin, plasma, drugs binding to, 47–49, 48t
Albuterol, 114t, 115
Alcohol, drug interactions and, 93t, 242t
  hepatotoxicity of, 18t, 93t
Alcoholism, 15, 97
Allergy, and eye disease, 439, 441
  to drugs, 17
Alzheimer's disease, 397, 398
Amantadine, 395
Amebiasis, 210
Aminoglycoside(s), adverse effects of, 18t, 22t, 242t, 250
  doses for, 241t, 244t, 249, 250, 250t, *251*
  pharmacokinetics of, 241t
Amphotericin B, 18t, 241t, 242t, 244t, 258
Amyl nitrite, 150, 151t
Analgesics. See also *Pain, chronic.*
  and hemolysis, 17t
  narcotic. See *Narcotics.*
  non-narcotic, 431
  toxic effects of, 18t, 132t, 133t
Androgens, 333
Anemia(s), 307–327, 307t, *308,* 309t, 315t, *317,* 321t
  aplastic, 307t, 324–326
  blood loss, 307t, 308–315, *308,* 309t
    due to acute hemorrhage, 307t, 308, *308*

Anemia(s) (*Continued*)
  due to hemolysis, 307t, 309–315, 309t
    acquired, 309t, 311–315
    autoimmune, 309t, 311–313
    chemical factors and, 309t, 314
    diagnosis of, 309, 310
    drug-induced, 17, 17t, 309t, 313
    glucose-6-phosphate deficiency and, 17, 17t
    hereditary, 309t, 310, 311
    infection and, 309t, 314
    mechanical factors and, 309t, 314
    paroxysmal nocturnal hemoglobinuria and, 309t, 315
    physical factors and, 309t, 314
    splenomegaly and, 309t, 315
  definition of, 307
  etiologic classification of, 307, 307t
  folate deficiency and, 307t, 319, 323
  hypoplastic, 307t, 324–326
  iron deficiency, 307t, 315–318, 315t, *317*
  megaloblastic, 307t, 319–324, 321t
    causes of, 321, 321t
    diagnosis of, 321, 321t
    pathophysiology of, 320
    treatment of, 322
    vitamin B_{12} deficiency and, 319, 322
  pernicious, and depression, 86, 86t
  renal failure and, 379
  secondary to chronic disease, 327
  vitamin B_{12} deficiency and, 307t, 319, 323
Anesthetics, drug interaction with, 93t
  ophthalmic, topical, 437
  pulmonary toxicity and, 132t
Aneurysms, cerebral hemorrhage and, 390
Angina, Prinzmetal's, 150, 154
Angina pectoris, 149–156
  prevention of, 150
  treatment of, 150–156
    beta blockers for, 153
    calcium channel blockers for, 154–156, 154t
    nitrates for, 150–153, 151t, 152t, 153t
Ankylosing spondylitis, antimalarial drugs for, 288t, 294
  corticosteroids for, 288t, 295
  cytotoxic drugs for, 288t, 295
  indenes for, 287t, 290
  indole for, 287t, 290

451

Ankylosing spondylitis (*Continued*)
   oxicams for, 287t, 292
   penicillamine for, 287t, 294
   phenylanthranilic acids for, 287t, 292
   phenylpropionic acids for, 287t, 290
   pyrazolones for, 287t, 291
   salicylates for, 287t, 288–290
   pathophysiology of, 278t, 280
   treatment of, guidelines for, 298
     principles for, 283–286, 284t
Antacids, and drug absorption, 193, 194t
   drug interactions and, 242t
   for peptic ulcer disease, 187–193, 189t, 190t, 191t, 194t
   neutralizing capacity of, 188–191, 189t, 190t
   neutralizing ingredients in, 189t, 190t, 191–193
   saccharin content of, 191, 191t
   sodium content of, 189t, 190, 190t, 193
   sugar content of, 191, 191t
Antiadrenergic drugs, 143–149, 144t. See also *Hypertension*.
Antianxiety drugs, 432
Antiarrhythmic therapy, effects of aging on, 163. See also *Cardiac arrhythmia(s)*.
Antiarthritic drugs. See specific arthritides.
   and depression, 86, 86t
Antibiotics. See *Antimicrobial drugs* and specific infections.
Anticholinergic drugs, 80
   drug interactions with, 22t, 87t, 90t, 93t, 394
   for gastric ulcer disease, 194
   for nausea, 215–217, 216t
   for obstructive airway diseases, 106, 117
   for Parkinson's disease, 394
   for peptic ulcer disease, 194
   for ulcerative colitis, 231
   for vomiting, 215–217, 216t
Anticoagulants, drug interactions with, 22t, 90t, 388, 389
   for cerebral thrombosis, 386, 387, 387t
   for dementia, 96
   for pulmonary embolism, 127–132, 129t. See also *Embolism, pulmonary*.
   for transient ischemic attacks, 387
   pulmonary toxicity and, 132t, 133t
Anticonvulsants, and depression, 86, 86t
   for epilepsy, 399–402
   pulmonary toxicity and, 132, 132t, 133t
Antidepressant(s), tetracyclic, 90
   tricyclic, 87–90, 87t, 88t, 89t, 90t
     dosage for, 88, 88t
     drug interactions with, 24t, 89, 90t, 93t
     for anxiety, 99
     for chronic pain, 432
     plasma levels of, 88, 89t
     side effects of, 87t, 88
     toxicity of, 87, 89, 132t
Antidiabetics, 22t, 242t, 342–344, 343t
Antidiarrheal drugs, 179, 211, 212t, 231
Antidopaminergic drugs, 216t, 217–220
Antiemetic drugs. See *Nausea; Vomiting*.
Antifungal drugs, 241t, 258–260
   pulmonary toxicity and, 132t, 133t
Antigout drugs, 288t, 296–298
Antihistamines, drug interactions with, 90t
   for nausea and vomiting, 216t, 217
Antihypertensive drugs, 142–149, 142t, 144t. See *Hypertension, diuretic therapy for*.

Antihypertensive drugs (*Continued*)
   and depression, 86, 86t
   and pulmonary toxicity, 132t
   drug interactions with, 89, 90t
Anti-infectives, 17t, 20t, 86, 86t, 132t. See also *Antimicrobial drugs; Infection(s);* and specific drugs and organs.
Anti-inflammatory drugs. See specific disease processes and drugs.
Antimalarial drugs, for arthritides, 288t, 294
   hemolysis and, 17, 17t
Antimicrobial drugs, 242–260
   aminoglycosides, adverse effects of, 18t, 22t, 242t, 250
     doses for, 241t, 244t, 249, 250, 250t, *251*
     pharmacokinetics of, 241t
   cephalosporins, 241t, 242t, 244t, 247–249
   chloramphenicol, 17t, 18t, 241t, 242t, 244t, 253
   clindamycin, 18t, 241t, 242t, 244t, 252
   creatinine clearance and, 239, 240, *240*, 240t
   doses for, 241t
     programmed, 64
     renal failure and, 244, 244t
   drug interactions with, 242t
   elimination of, 63, 63t
   erythromycin, 18t, 241t, 250–252
   for fungi, 241t, 258–260
   for tuberculosis, 241t, 256–258
   for urinary tract infections, 254, 255
   lincomycin, 241t, 242t, 252
   penicillins, 243–249. See *Penicillin(s)*.
   pharmacokinetics of, 239–242, *240*, 240t, 241t
   pulmonary toxicity and, 132t, 133t
   sulfonamides, 17t, 18t, 20t, 242t, 244t, 254
   tetracyclines, 242t, 252
   trimethoprim, 254
   vancomycin, 241t, 256
Antiparkinson drugs, 392–396
   and depression, 86, 86t
   drug interactions with, 90t, 93t
Antiplatelet drugs, 389
Antipsychotic drugs, 76–82, 77t, 78t
   and enzyme activity, 20t, 76
   anticholinergic effect of, 78t, 81
   chlorpromazine (Thorazine), 18t, 39t, 75, 77t, 78, 78t, 82
   chronic pain and, 431
   classes of, 76, 77t, 78, 79
   dopamine blockage by, 76, 79
   dosages of, 77t, 78, 79
   electrocardiographic changes and, 78t, 81
   extrapyramidal disorders and, 78t, 79
   for dementia, 97
   for depression, 94
   half-life of, 77
   initiation of, 76
   orthostatic hypotension and, 78t, 81
   sedation by, 78t, 81
   side effects of, 77, 78, 78t, 79–82
   tardive dyskinesia and, 78t, 80
   thioridazine (Mellaril), 18t, 75, 77t, 78, 78t
   trifluoperazine (Stelazine), 75, 78t, 79
   withdrawal of, 77
Antirheumatic drugs, 18t, 286–298, 287. See specific arthritides and drugs.
Antithyroid drugs, 90t, 350–352
Anxiety, 98–100, 98t. See also *Psychiatric disorders*.
Aplastic anemia, 307t, 324–326

Appetite, drugs for suppression of, 360, 361
Arrhythmias, cardiac, 162–176. See also *Cardiac arrhythmias.*
Arthritides, 277–299. See also *Ankylosing spondylitis; Arthritis; Gouty arthritis; Osteoarthritis; Rheumatoid arthritis.*
  antimalarial drugs for, 288t, 294
  corticosteroids for, 288t, 295
  cytotoxic drugs for, 288t, 295
  nondrug therapy for, 286
  oxicams for, 287t, 292
  pathophysiology of, 277–283, 278t
  penicillamine for, 287t, 294
  phenylanthranilic acids for, 287t, 292
  phenylpropionic acids for, 287t, 290
  principles of treatment for, 283–286, 284t
  pyrazolones for, 287t, 291
Arthritis. See also *Ankylosing spondylitis; Gouty arthritis; Osteoarthritis; Rheumatoid arthritis.*
  infectious, 268
  quack cures for, 8
Aspiration, pulmonary, 133
Aspirin, 17t, 18t. See also *Salicylates.*
Asthma, 104, 105, 122–125, *123*. See also *Lung(s), obstructive airway diseases of.*
Atherosclerosis, 419
  diabetes mellitus and, 334, 340
  postmenopausal, 419
Atrial fibrillation, 164, 166t
Atrial flutter, 164, 166t
Atrial premature beats, 164, 166t
Atrioventricular block, 165
Atrophy, of disuse, prescribing and, 35
Azathioprine, 230

Bacitracin, 18t, 231
Bacteremia, 271
Bacteria, associated with systemic diseases, 274t. See also entries for organs and systems.
Barbiturates, drug interactions with, 22t, 93t, 242t
  for epilepsy, 400
Beclomethasone dipropionate, 120, 124
Behavior modification, 359
Benzodiazepine(s), drug interactions with, 22t
  for anxiety, 98, 98t
  for depression, 94
  pharmacokinetics of, 98, 98t
Benzquinamide, 216t, 220
Beta blockers, 153
Beta$_2$ receptor-selective drugs, 113–117, 113t, 114t, 115t, 123, 124
Bile duct stones, 208
Biliary tract disease, 205–208
Bioavailability, of drugs, 57, *57*
Bioequivalence, of drugs, 57, *57*
Bleeding, increased tendency to, drug interactions and, 22t
Blepharitis, 439
Blood flow, mesenteric, effects on drug absorption of, 45, 46t
Blood loss anemia(s). See *Anemia(s), blood loss.*
Blood serum laboratory values, drug interactions and, 26–28t
Blood transfusion, for hemolytic anemia, 309t, 313

Blood vessels, infections of, 271
Body, composition of, changes with age, 46, 46t
Bone, disorders of, 277–299. See also *Ankylosing spondylitis; Arthritis; Gouty arthritis; Osteoarthritis; Rheumatoid arthritis.*
  infection of, 268–270
Brain. See also *Cerebrovascular disease.*
  abscess of, 265
  edema of, 386, 390, 391
  embolism in, 389
  hemorrhage in, 390
  neoplasms of, 392
  thrombosis of, 385–389, 387t
  trauma to, 391
Bran, for constipation, 179, 180
  for diverticular disease, 203
Breasts, reduced estrogen and, 408
Bretylium, 166t, 168t, 174
Bromocriptine, 395
Brompton mixture, 432. See also *Narcotics; Pain, chronic.*
Bronchitis, 104, 105, 125, 261. See also *Lung, obstructive airway diseases of.*
Bronchodilators, 106
Bronchospasm, 132, 133t. See also *Asthma.*
Bulk-forming laxatives, 179, 182t, 183t
Butyrophenone(s), for nausea and vomiting, 216t, 218
  for psychoses, 77t, 78t, 79

Calcitonin, 333, 419
Calcium, and osteoporosis, 328, 330, 331, 332, 415
  concentration of, chronic renal failure and, 378
  effect of drugs on, 26t
Calcium channel blockers, 154–156, 154t
Calculi, renal, 370–373
Cancer, and depression, 86, 86t
  management of pain in. See *Pain, chronic.*
  quackery and, 8
Captopril, 149
Carbamazepine (Tegretol), 391, 401
Carbidopa, 393
Carbonic anhydrase inhibitors, 18t, 447
Cardiac. See also *Heart.*
Cardiac arrhythmia(s), 162–176
  antiarrhythmic drugs for, 166–176, 166t–169t
    dosages for, 167t–169t
    efficacy of, 166, 166t
    pharmacokinetics of, 167, 167t
  bretylium for, 166t, 168t, 174
  digitalis glycosides for, 166t, 167t, 169, 169t
  digoxin for, 166t, 167t, 169, 169t. See also *Digoxin.*
  disopyramide for, 166t, 167t, 169t, 172
  lidocaine for, 166t, 168t, 172
  phenytoin for, 166t, 173
  procainamide for, 166t, 167t, 169t, 171
  propranolol (Inderal) for, 166t, 168t, 173
  quinidine for, 166t, 167t, 170
  types of, 163–166, 166t
  verapamil (Calan, Isoptin) for, 168t, 175
Cardiac output, drug activity and, 75
Cardiovascular disorders. See specific diseases such as *Angina pectoris; Cardiac arrhythmia(s); Congestive heart failure;* and *Hypertension.*

Carotid endarterectomy, 387
Cataracts, 437, 447
Causalgia, 404
Cellulitis, 270, 274t, 439
Central anticholinergic syndrome, antipsychotic drugs and, 78t, 81
Cephalosporins, 241t, 242t, 244t, 247–249
Cephalothin (Keflin), hemolysis and, 314
Cerebral embolism, 389
Cerebral thrombosis, 385–389, 387t
Cerebrovascular disease, 385–391, 387t
 and dementia, 398t
 cerebral edema, 386, 390, 391
 cerebral embolism, 389
 cerebral thrombosis, 385–389, 387t
 hypertensive intracerebral hemorrhage, 390
 infectious complications of, 274t
 stroke, 386, 387t
 transient ischemic attacks, 387–389
Cervix, estrogen and, 407
Chalazion, 440
Chenodeoxycholic acid (cheno), 206
Chinese herbal remedies, 9
Chloramphenicol, 17t, 18t, 241t, 242t, 244t, 253
Chlorpromazine (Thorazine), 18t, 39t, 75, 77t, 78, 78t, 82
Chlorpropamide (Diabinese), 17t, 18t, 343, 343t
Cholangitis, 207
Cholecystitis, 205–208
Cholelithiasis, 205–208
Cholinergic drugs, 132t
Chorea, senile, 396
Cimetidine, 188, 194t, 195–199, 196t, 198t
Climacteric, endocrinology of, 406
 estrogen target-tissue changes during, 406–409
 treatment of, 410, 411
  estrogen therapy for, 411–414, 412t, 414t
 vasomotor symptoms during, 410
Clindamycin, 18t, 241t, 242t, 244t, 252
Clonidine, 144t, 145
Clotrimazole, 259
Codeine, 14
Coffee enema, 9
Colitis, drug-induced, 225, 225t
 ulcerative, 224–232, 225, 225t
  anticholinergic drugs for, 231
  antidiarrheal drugs for, 231
  azathioprine for, 230
  bacitracin for, 231
  causes of, 225, 225t
  corticosteroids for, 226
  cromolyn sodium (Intal) for, 230
  nutritional supplements for, 231
  pathophysiology of, 224–226, 225
  sulfasalazine for, 227–230
  vancomycin for, 231
Colon, changes in, drug absorption and, 45, 46t
 physiology of, 179
Colonic diverticular disease, 200–205, 201, 203t, 204. See Diverticular disease.
Coma, diabetes mellitus type II and, 341, 345
 myxedema, hypothyroidism and, 348, 349
Congestive heart failure, 156–162
 and chronic obstructive pulmonary disease, 126
 digitalis glycosides for, 157–161, 159, 159t
 digoxin for, 157–161, 159, 159t
 diuretics for, 161
 infectious complications of, 274t
 inotropic drugs for, 162

Congestive heart failure (Continued)
 nondrug treatment of, 157
 pathophysiology of, 156, 156
 treatment of, 157–162
 vasodilators for, 162
Conjunctivitis, 440
Constipation, 178–182, 182t, 183t
Cor pulmonale, 126
Cornea, 441–443
Corticosteroids, adverse effects of, 18t, 20t, 121, 121t
 and depression, 86, 86t
 clinical characteristics of, 119, 119t
 drug interactions with, 23t
 for arthritides, 288t, 295
 for cerebral edema, 386, 390, 391
 for chronic renal failure, 377
 for eye infections, 438
 for idiopathic autoimmune hemolytic anemias, 309t, 311
 for obstructive airway diseases, 119–122, 119t, 121t, 124
 for ulcerative colitis, 226
 gastrointestinal system and, 121t, 122
Coumadin (warfarin sodium), 388
Coumarin, 128–130, 129t
Craniocerebral trauma, 391, 398t
Creatinine clearance, aging and, 158, 159, 159t
 antimicrobial drugs and, 239, 240, 240, 240t
 kidney function and, 239, 240, 240, 240t, 367
Cromolyn sodium (Intal), for obstructive airway diseases, 118, 123
 for ulcerative colitis, 230
Cushing's disease, and depression, 86, 86t
Cycloplegic drugs, 436, 437
Cytotoxic drugs, for arthritides, 288t, 295

Decubitus ulcers, 270, 274t
Degenerative diseases, and dementia, 398
 of joints. See Osteoarthritis.
Dehydration, 47
 hyponatremia and, 366, 368
Dementia, 86, 95–97, 397–399, 398t
Depression, 85–95, 86t. See also Antidepressants; Psychiatric disorders.
 and drug absorption, 43, 44
 diagnosis of, 86
 drug-precipitated, 86, 86t
 estrogen level and, 409
 incidence of, 85
 manifestations of, 86
 physical illnesses and, 86, 86t, 398
 treatment of, antipsychotic drugs for, 94. See also Antipsychotic drugs.
  benzodiazepines for, 94
  electroconvulsive therapy for, 94
  monoamine oxidase inhibitors for, 92, 93t
  stimulants for, 94
  trazodone hydrochloride (Desyrel) for, 91
  tetracyclic antidepressants for, 90
  tricyclic antidepressants for, 87–90, 87t, 88t, 89t, 90t
Dexamethasone, 119, 119t
Diabetes insipidus-like syndrome, lithium use and, 85
Diabetes mellitus, 333–345, 338t, 343t
 antacid use and, 191, 191t
 constipation and, 180

Diabetes mellitus (*Continued*)
  depression and, 86, 86t
  diagnosis of, 333
  infections associated with, 274t
  insulin-dependent. See *type I.*
    laxative use and, 180
  noninsulin-dependent. See *type II.*
  obesity and, 340, 342, 357
  type I, 333–339, 338t
    complications of, 334–336
    diet for, 336
    etiology of, 334
    therapy for, 335–339, 338t
  type II, 339–345, 343t
    coma and, 341, 345
    complications of, 340
    diet for, 342
    etiology of, 340
    therapy for, 342–345, 343t
Diagnosis, problems in, drug therapy and, 3, 5, 37, 37t
Dialysis, 379–382
Diarrhea, 208–213, 212t
  diagnosis of, 209
  drug-induced, 210
  micro-organisms and, 209, 210
  pathophysiology of, 208
  treatment of, 179, 211, 212t
Diet, and osteoporosis, 328, 330, 417
  for diabetes mellitus, 336, 342
    laxative use and, 180
  for obesity, 359
  for quack cures, 8
  high-fiber, for diverticular disease, 203, 203t
  sodium-restricted, antacid use and, 189t, 190, 190t, 193
  laxative use and, 180
Digitalis glycosides. See also *Digoxin.*
  drug interactions with, 23t, 242t
  for cardiac arrhythmias, 166t, 167t, 169, 169t
  for congestive heart failure, 157–161, *159,* 159t
Digoxin, absorption of, effect of antacids on, 194t
  dosage of, 64, 64t, 65–67, 66t, 67t
  drug interactions with, 23t, 242t
  for cardiac arrhythmias, 166t, 167t, 169, 169t
  for congestive heart failure, 157–161, *159,* 159t
  therapeutic plasma range of, 39t
Dilator(s), for pupil, 436, 437
Diltiazem (Cardizem), 154, 154t, 155
Dimethylsulfoxide (DMSO), 9
Diphenidol, 216t, 220
Diphtheria immunization, 260
Disability, incidence of, age and, 36, *36*
Disease, chronic, incidence of, with age, 36, *36*
Disopyramide, 166t, 167t, 169t, 172
Diuretics, drug interactions with, 84, 84t, 93t
  for congestive heart failure, 161
  for hypertension, 142–149, 142t, 144t. See also *Hypertension, diuretic therapy for.*
  ototoxicity and, 18t
Diverticular disease, 200–205, *201,* 203t, *204*
  complications of, 204, *204*
  diagnosis of, 201, *201,* 202
  pathophysiology of, 201
  treatment of, 202–205, 203t
Diverticulitis, 201, 204, 205. See also *Diverticular disease.*

Diverticulosis, 201, *201.* See also *Diverticular disease.*
Domperidone, 216t, 220
Dopamine, blockage of, by antipsychotic drugs, 76, 79
  replacement of, 392–394
Duodenal ulcer, 185–187. See *Peptic ulcer disease.*
Duodenum, changes in, drug absorption and, 44, 46t
Dyskinesia, tardive, 80, 396
Dystonia, 79
Drug(s). See also specific conditions, preparations, and types.
  absorption of, 19, 20, 30, 31t, 42–46, *43,* 44t, 46t
  abuse of, 14
    food and, 30, 31t
  administration of, improper, 10t, 11
  adverse reactions to, 15–19, 17t–19t
    classification of, 16
    Food and Drug Administration program for, 16
    incidence of, 16
    mechanisms of, 17
  advertising and, 6
  and acute intermittent porphyria, 17, 17t
  and hemolysis, 17, 17t, 314
  atrophy of disuse and, 35
  bioavailability of, 57, *57*
  bioequivalence of, 57, *57*
  chronic use of, 36
  diagnosis and, 3, 37, 37t
  disposition of, effect of age on, 58t
  distribution of, 20, 46–49, 46t. See also *Pharmacokinetics.*
  dosage modification of, 58–65, 58t, *60,* 244, 244t
    computer programs for, 64, 64t
    kidney function and, 60, 61t
    methods for, 62
    regimens for, 61
    precautions in, 63, 63t
  elimination of, 49–57, *50,* 51t, 52t, 54t, 56t, 58, 58t. See also *Pharmacokinetics.*
  excretion of, 20
  generic vs. brand name, 435, 436
  hepatotoxic, 18, 18t
  ideal, characteristics of, 67t
  idiosyncratic reactions to, 17, 17t
  illicit, 14
  inappropriate, reasons for, 10t, 11
  interactions of, 19–33, 19t, 20t, 22t–24t, 26t–30t, 31t
    drug-drug, 19–21, 19t, 20t, 22t–24t
      management of, 21
      mechanisms of, 19–21, 20t
      with antimicrobials, 242t
      with lithium, 84, 84t
    drug-food, 25, 30–32, 31t
    drug-laboratory test, 21, 24, 25t, 26t–30t
      hematology values, 28t
      serum values, 26–29t
      urine values, 29t
  malnutrition and, 36
  metabolism of, 20, 20t
  microsomal enzyme activity and, 20, 20t
  monitoring of, 33
  multimorbidity and, 36, *36*

INDEX/**455**

Drug(s) (*Continued*)
  multiple use of, 3, 4–6, 5t
  nephrotoxic, 18, 18t
  ototoxic, 18, 18t
  overprescribing of, 5
  over-the-counter, 7
  paradox of use of, 4
  patient expectations and, 6
  patterns of consumption of, 4–15
    compliance aids for, 13
    drug-dependence, 14
    noncompliance, 9–14, 10t, 11t, 13t
      clinical consequences of, 11
      correlates of, 11, 11t
      education materials for, 13, 13t
      intelligent, 13
      medication errors in, 10, 10t
      premature discontinuation and, 10t, 11
      treatment of, 12
    polypharmacotherapy, 4–6, 5t
    self-medication, 6–9
  pharmacokinetics of. See *Pharmacokinetics.*
  pharmacologic reactions to, 17
  placebo, 5
  plasma protein binding of, 47–49, 48t
  prescribing difficulties with, 35–37, *36,* 37t
  quackery and, 7–9
  sex differences and, 35
  side effects of, 17
  therapeutic goal and, 38, *39,* 39t
  therapeutic plasma concentration ranges of, 38, 39t
  timing of, 10, 10t
  toxic effects of, 17, 17t, 18, 18t

Ear(s), drugs potentially toxic to, 18, 18t
Edema, effect of, on furosemide, 56, 56t
  of brain, 386, 390, 391
  of eyelids, 439
  of lung, drug-induced, 133t
Electrocardiographic changes, antipsychotic drugs and, 78t, 81
Electroconvulsive therapy, 94
Electromagnetic devices, for quack cures, 8
Electronic devices, for quack cures, 8
Elimination, of drugs, variations with age, 49–57, *50,* 51t, 52t, 54t, 56t
Embolism, cerebral, 389
  pulmonary, 126–132
    anticoagulants for, 127–132, 129t
      coumarin derivatives, 128–130, 129t
      heparin, 127
      indanedione derivatives, 128–130, 129t
      oral, 128–130, 129t
      thrombolytic enzymes, 130–132
    supportive management of, 127
Emollient laxatives, 181, 182t, 183t
Emphysema, 105, 125. See also *Lung(s), obstructive airway diseases of.*
Endocarditis, 272–274
Endocrine disorders, 328–362. See also entries for specific disorders.
  diabetes mellitus, 333–345, 338t, 343t
  obesity, 352–362
  osteoporosis, 328–333
  of thyroid, 345–352
Endocrine system, effects of corticosteroids on, 121t, 122

Endocrine system (*Continued*)
  obesity and, 358
Endocrinology, climacteric and, 405
Enema, coffee, 9
  for quack cancer cures, 8
Enzymes, for pulmonary embolism, 130–132
  for quack cancer cures, 8
  microsomal, drug inhibition of, 20, 20t
Epilepsy, 399–402
Epinephrine, for, 446
Erysipelas, 270
Erythromycin, 18t, 241t, 244t, 250–252
Esophagus, changes in, and drug absorption, 43, 46t
Estrogen, reduction of, changes in target tissues and, 406–409
  effects of, 406–410
  therapy with, 411–414, 411t, 412t, 414t
    atherosclerosis treatment and, 419
    osteoporosis and, 331, 415, 418, 418t
Ethambutol, 241t, 244, 257
Ethosuximide (Zarontin), for epilepsy, 402
  therapeutic plasma range of, 39t
Euhydration, hyponatremia and, 368
Exercise, diabetes mellitus type I and, 337
  obesity and, 361
  osteoporosis and, 332, 416, 417
Eye(s), 439–448
  bacterial infection of, 439, 440, 441, 444
  blepharitis of, 439
  cataracts of, 437, 447
  cellulitis of lids of, 439
  chalazion of, 440
  conjunctivitis of, 440
  corneal erosion of, recurrent, 443
  diabetes mellitus and, 334, 335, 336, 337
  dilation of, 436, 437
  drugs for, diseases associated with use of, 435, 436
    generic vs. brand name, 435, 436
    hazards in administration of, 436
    interactions with, 436
    systemic effects of, 435
    types of, 436, 437–439
  edema of lids of, 439
  effects of systemic medications on, 82, 121t, 438
  fungal infection of, 442
  glaucoma of, 82, 437, 445–447
  herpes zoster of, 440
  keratitis of, 441–443
  keratoconjunctivitis of, 443
  occlusion of retinal artery of, 444
  senile macular degneration of, 444
  subconjunctival hemorrhage of, 441
  trachoma of, 443
  treatment of, general concepts, 435. See also specific conditions.
  uveitis of, 444
  viral diseases of, 438, 439, 440, 441, 442, 443
Eyelids, diseases of, 439

Fenoterol, 114, 114t, 115
Fever, of undetermined origin, 276
Fibrillation, 164, 165, 166t
Flucytosine, 241t, 244t, 259
Fluorescein, 437
Fluoride, 332
Folates, deficiency, anemia and, 307t, 319, 323

Food, and interactions with drugs, 25, 30–32, 31t, 93t
Food and Drug Administration (FDA), adverse drug reaction program of, 16
Fractures, osteoporosis and, 328, 329
Fungus, 241t, 258–260, 442
Furosemide, drug interactions and, 23t
  effect of edema on, 56, 56t
  toxic effects of, 18t
Furunculosis, 270

Gallstones, 205–208
Gastric ulcer, 184–187. See *Peptic ulcer disease.*
Gastrointestinal disorders, 178–234. See also entries for *Colitis, ulcerative; Diverticular disease; Diarrhea; Nausea; Peptic ulcer disease; Vomiting.*
  cholecystitis, 205–208
  cholelithiasis, 205–208
  colitis, ulcerative, 224–232, *225,* 225t
  colonic diverticular disease, 200–205, *201,* 203t, *204*
  constipation, 178–182, 182t, 183t
  diarrhea, 179, 208–213, 212t
  drug-induced hepatitis, 232–234
  nausea, 213–224, 213t, 216t
  peptic ulcer disease, 182–200, 189t, 191t, 194t, 196t, 198t
  vomiting, 213–224, *213,* 213t, *215,* 216t
Gastrointestinal system, corticosteroids and, 121t, 122
Guanethidine, 148
Gerovital H3, 9, 96
Giardiasis, 210
Glaucoma, 82, 437, 445–447
Glomerulonephritis, acute renal failure and, 375
Glucose-6-phosphate dehydrogenase deficiency, hemolytic anemia and, 309t, 311
  precipitation of, 17, 17t
Glucose tolerance test, diabetes mellitus and, 333
Glycolysis, interference in, hemolytic anemia and, 309t, 311
Goiter, hyperthyroidism and, 349
Gold salts, for arthritides, 287t, 293
  toxic effects of, 18t
Gouty arthritis, antigout drugs for, 288t, 296–298
  antimalarial drugs for, 288t, 294
  corticosteroids for, 288t, 295
  cytotoxic drugs for, 288t, 295
  indenes for, 287t, 290
  indole for, 287t, 290
  oxicams for, 287t, 292
  pathophysiology of, 278t, 281
  penicillamine for, 287t, 294
  phenylanthranilic acids for, 287t, 292
  phenylpropionic acids for, 287t, 290
  pyrazolones for, 287t, 291
  salicylates for, 287t, 288–290
  treatment of, guidelines for, 298, 299
    principles for, 283–286, 284t
  uricosuric drugs for, 288t, 296
Grafts, vascular, infection of, 276
Graves' disease, 349
Griseofulvin, 17t, 242t, 260
Guanabenz, 144t, 146
Guanethidine, 23t, 148

Half-life, 40, 40t
Haloperidol (Haldol), 77t, 78t, 79
Heart. See also *Cardiac arrhythmia(s); Congestive heart failure.*
  disease of, hypothyroidism and, 347, 348
    infectious complications of, 274t
  palpitations of, menopause and, 410
  premature beats of, 164, 165, 166t
Hemiballismus, 397
Hemodialysis, 379–382
Hemoglobinopathies, hereditary, hemolytic anemia and, 309t, 311
Hemoglobinuria, nocturnal, paroxysmal, hemolytic anemia and, 309t, 315
Hemolysis, drug-induced, in patients with glucose-6-phosphate deficiency, 17, 17t
  mechanisms of, 314
Hemolytic anemias. See *Anemia(s), blood loss, due to hemolysis.*
Hemorrhage, acute, anemia and, 307t, 308, *308*
  drug interactions and, 22t
  intracerebral, hypertensive, 390
  parenchymal, drug-induced, 133t
  subarachnoid, 390
  subconjunctival, 441
Heparin, for cerebral thrombosis, 386, 387, 387t
  for pulmonary embolism, 127
  for stroke, 387, 387t
Hepatic. See *Liver.*
Hepatitis, and depression, 86, 86t
  drug-induced, 232–234
Hepatotoxins, 18t, 82, 232–234
Herbs, Chinese, 9
Hereditary glycolytic enzyme deficiencies, hemolytic anemia and, 309t, 311
Hereditary hemoglobinopathies, hemolytic anemia and, 309t, 311
Hereditary spherocytosis, hemolytic anemia and, 309t, 310
Herpes simplex virus, of eye, 442
Herpes zoster virus, of eye, 440
  of skin, 271
  shingles and, 404
High-fiber diet, for diverticular disease, 203, 203t
Hip, fracture of, 329. See also *Osteoporosis.*
Hormone(s). See also *Endocrine disorders; Estrogen.*
  and depression, 86, 86t
  obesity and, 358
  osteoporosis and, 333, 415, 418, 418t
  quack arthritis cures and, 8
Hot flashes, menopause and, 410
Huntington's disease, 396
Hydralazine, 18t, 147
Hydrocortisone, 119, 119t
Hyperbaric oxygen, 95
Hyperglycemia, 336–339, 338t
Hyperkalemia, 378
Hyperosmolar hyperglycemic nonketotic coma, 341, 345
Hyperosmotic laxatives, 181, 182t, 183t
Hyperparathyroidism, 86, 86t
Hypersensitivity, to drugs, 17
Hypertension, aging and, 140
  cerebrovascular disease and, 385, 386
  diagnosis of, 141
  diuretic therapy for, 142–149, 142t, 144t
    pharmacokinetics and, 142

INDEX/457

Hypertension (*Continued*)
  diuretic therapy for, precautions in, 143
    with adrenergic inhibiting drugs, 143-147, 144t
      and captopril, 149
      and guanethidine, 148
      and hydralazine, 147
      and minoxidil, 148
    with thiazides, 142, 142t, 143
  drug-induced, 133t
  life style changes and, 141
  obesity and, 357
  treatment objectives in, 141
  vasodilators for, 147
Hyperthyroidism, 86t, 349-352
Hyperuricemia, pathophysiology of, 282
  treatment guidelines for, 299
  uricosuric drugs for, 288t, 296
Hypokalemia, 27t, 143, 378
Hyponatremia, 161, 366, 367-370
Hypoplastic anemia, 307t, 324-326
Hypotension, drug-induced, 78t, 81
Hypothyroidism, 86, 86t, 346-349
Hypovolemia, 161

Idiopathic autoimmune hemolytic anemias, 309t, 311-313
Idiosyncratic reactions, 17, 17t
Imidazole drugs, 259
Immunization, 260
Immunohemolytic anemias, drug-induced, 309t, 313
Immunosuppressive drugs, 309t, 312
Impetigo, 270
Indanedione derivatives, 128-130, 129t
Indenes, 287t, 290
Indole, 77t, 78t, 287t, 290
Infections, 239-276. See also *Antimicrobial drug(s); Penicillin(s);* and affected organs.
  and dementia, 398t
  and fever of undetermined origin, 275
  and hemolytic anemia, 309t, 314
  chronic diseases and, 274, 274t
  in compromised host, 274, 274t
  intravascular, 271
  of bone, 268-270
  of brain, 265
  of endocardium, 272-274, 274t
  of eyes, 439, 440, 441, 444
    medications for, 437, 438, 439, 440. See also *Eye(s).*
  of joint, 268-270
  of leptomeninges, 264
  of prostate, 267
  of respiratory tract, 261-263, 274t
  of skin, 270, 274t
  of urinary tract, 245t, 254, 255, 265-267, 274t
  of vagina, 267
  pacemaker and, 276
  resistance to, 274, 274t
  tubercular, 263, 274t
  vascular grafts and, 275
Influenza, 260, 261
Inotropic drugs, 162
Insomnia, 100
Insulin, 337-339, 338t, 344
Insulin-dependent diabetes. See *Diabetes mellitus, type I.*

Intravascular infections, 271
Iodine, 350-352
Iron deficiency anemia, 307t, 315-318, 315t, *317*
Isoniazid, 241t, 256, 257
  drug interactions with, 242t
  hepatotoxicity of, 18t
  kidney failure and, 244t
Isoetharine, 114t, 115
Isosorbide dinitrate, 150, 151t

Jaundice, 18t, 82, 232-234
Joint(s), disorders of, 277-299. See also *Ankylosing spondylitis; Arthritides; Gouty arthritis; Osteoarthritis; Rheumatoid arthritis.*
  infection of, 268-270

Keratitis, 441-443
Keratoconjunctivitis, 443
Keratoconjunctivitis sicca (Sjögren's syndrome), 443
Ketoconazole, 260
Kidney(s), aging and, 366
  calculi of, 370-373
  creatinine clearance and, 239, 240, *240*, 240t, 367
  diabetes mellitus and, 334, 335
  drugs toxic to, 18, 18t
  elimination of drugs and, 53-57, 54t, 56t
    rates of, 58, 58t
  failure of, acute, 373-375, 374t
    chronic, 376-379
      corticosteroids for, 377
    cimetidine use during, 196, 196t
    drug doses and, 244, 244t
    evaluation of, 367
    glomerulonephritis-induced, 375
    iatrogenic, 375
    incidence of, 366
  function of, dose adjustment based on, 60, 61t
  glomerular filtration rate, effect of changes in, 55, 56t
  hyponatremia and, 366, 367-370
  hemodialysis and, 379-382
  home dialysis for, 381
  impairment of, classification of, 240, 240t
  lithiasis of, 370-373
  peritoneal dialysis and, 379, 382
  psychotropic medication and, 75, 83, 85
  stones of, 370-373

Laboratory tests, hematologic, drug interactions and, 28t
  serum, drug interactions and, 21, 25, 26t-28t
  urine, drug interactions and, 28t
Laetrile, 8
Laxatives, 179-181, 182t, 183t
Leptomeninges, 264
Levodopa (Larodopa), drug interactions with, 23t, 393
  for Parkinson's disease, 392-394
Lidocaine, 166t, 168t, 172
  therapeutic plasma range of, 39t
Lincomycin, 241t, 242t, 252
Lithiasis, renal, 370-373
Lithium, drug interactions with, 84, 84t
  for bipolar disorders, 83-85, 84t, 85t
  for mania, 83-85, 84t, 85t

Lithium (*Continued*)
   kidney function and, 83, 85
   side effects of, 85
   therapeutic plasma range of, 39t
   toxicity of, 83, 84, 85t
Liver, drug elimination by, 50–53, *50,* 51t, 52t
   rates of, 58, 58t
   inflammation of, 86, 86t, 232–234
   toxic effects and, 18t, 232–234
Lung(s), disorders of, susceptibility to, 104, 274t, 357
   drug-induced disease of, 132, 132t, 133t
   embolism of, 126–132. See *Embolism, pulmonary.*
   infection of, 261–263
   heart failure and, 126
   nonpharmacologic treatment of, 104
   obstructive airway diseases of, 104–126
     asthma, 104, 105
     bronchitis, 104, 105, 261
     emphysema, 105
   pharmacologic treatment of, 106–122
     anticholinergic drugs for, 106, 117
     corticosteroids for, 119–122, 119t, 121t, 124
     cromolyn sodium (Intal) for, 118, 123
     dexamethasone for, 119, 119t
     mechanism of action of bronchodilators in, 106
     sympathomimetic drugs for, 106, 113–117, 113t, 114t, 115t, 123, 124
     theophylline for, 107–113, 108t, 109t, 110, 110t, 112t. See also *Theophylline.*
   treatment of, special considerations in, 122–126, *123*
   toxicity and, 132, 132t, 133t
Lupus-like syndrome, 132, 133t

Macula, senile degeneration of, 444
Malnutrition, prescribing drugs and, 36
Mania, 82, 83t
   lithium for, 83–85, 84t, 85t
Maprotiline (Ludiomil), 39t, 90
Marie-Strumpell disease. See *Ankylosing spondylitis.*
Marijuana, 216t, 221–224
Megaloblastic anemia, 307, 319–324, 321t. See also *Anemia(s), megaloblastic.*
Meningitis, 264
Menopause, management of women after, 405–421. See also *Atherosclerosis; Climacteric; Estrogen; Osteoporosis.*
Metabolic acidosis, chronic renal failure and, 378
Metabolism, of drugs, 20, 20t. See also *Pharmacokinetics.*
Metaproterenol, 114t, 115
Methotrimeprazine (Levoprome), 430
Methyldopa, 144t, 145
   and hemolysis, 314
   drug interactions and, 23t, 93t
   hepatotoxicity of, 18t
Methylprednisolone, 119, 119t
Metoclopramide, 216t, 218–220
Metoprolol, 144t, 146
Miconazole, 241t, 244t, 260
Microsomal enzymes, hepatic, and drug activity, 20, 20t
Mineral oil, 181, 182t, 183t

Minoxidil, 148
Monoamine oxidase (MAO) inhibitors, and microsomal enzyme activity, 20t
   characteristics of, 93t
   drug interactions with, 22t, 23t, 90t, 93t
   food containing tyramine and, 31, 31t
   for depression, 92, 93t
Morphine, 14. See also *Narcotics.*
Movement disorders, 392–397
   drug-induced, 396
   hemiballismus, 397
   Huntington's disease, 396
   Parkinson's disease, 392–397. See also *Parkinson's disease.*
   senile tremor, 397
Multi-infarct dementia, 386, 398t
Myxedema coma, hypothyroidism and, 348, 349

Nadolol, 153, 154
Nalidixic acid, 17t, 242t, 244t, 255
Narcotics, 23t, 425–430, 426t, 432
   Brompton mixture, 432
   dose of, 425, 426t
   drug interactions with, 23t, 429
   effectiveness of, 426, 427
   overdosage of, 430
   physical dependence on, 429
   precautions in use of, 428
   principles of use of, 427
   side effects of, 428
   tolerance of, 429
   types of, 426, 426t
   warnings in use of, 428
   withdrawal from, 430
Nausea, 213–224, 213t, 216t
   anticholinergic drugs for, 215–217, 216t
   antidopaminergic drugs for, 216t, 217–220
   antihistamines for, 216t, 217
   benzquinamide for, 216t, 220
   causes of, 213, 213t
   diphenidol for, 216t, 220
   marijuana for, 216t, 221–224
   treatment of, 214–224, 216t. See specific drugs.
   trimethobenzamide for, 216t, 221
Neoplasms, and dementia, 398t
   of brain, 392
Nephropathy, diabetes mellitus and, 334, 335
Nephrotoxicity, drugs associated with, 18, 18t, 242t
Nervous system, central, disorders of. See *Cerebrovascular disorders; Movement disorders; Neurologic disorders; Parkinson's disease.*
   changes in, psychotropic drugs and, 76
   diabetes mellitus and, 334, 335, 336
   peripheral, disorders of, 403
Neuralgia, 271, 404
Neurologic disorders, 385–404
   affecting movement, 392–397. See also *Movement disorders; Parkinson's disease.*
   cerebrovascular disease, 385–391. See also *Cerebrovascular disease.*
   craniocerebral trauma, 391
   dementia, 86, 95–97, 397–399, 398t
   epilepsy, 399–402
   neoplasms, 392
   neuralgia, 271, 404
   neuropathy, 334, 335, 336, 403

Neurologic disorders (*Continued*)
  status epilepticus, 402
  vertigo, 403
Neuropathy, 334, 335, 336, 403
Neuropeptides, 97
Neurotransmitters, 97
Nifedipine (Procardia), 154, 154t, 155
Night sweats, menopause and, 410
Nitrates, for angina pectoris, 150–153, 151t, 152t, 153t
Nitroglycerin, 150–153, 151t, 152t, 153t
Noncompliance, 9–14, 10t, 11t, 13t. See also *Drug(s), pattern of consumption of.*
Nootropics, 96
Nurse, responsibilities of, in drug therapy, 3
Nutritional supplements, for ulcerative colitis, 231

Obesity, 352–362
  and arthritis, 358
  and diabetes mellitus, 340, 342, 357
  and osteoporosis, 358
  complications of, 356–358
  definition of, 352
  etiology of, 353–356
  therapy for, 358–362
Obstructive airway disease. See *Lung(s), obstructive airway diseases of.*
Occlusive disease. See *Cerebrovascular disease.*
Ophthalmic disorders, 435–449. See *Eye(s).*
Oral cavity, changes in, and drug absorption, 42, 46t
Osteoarthritis, antimalarial drugs for, 288t, 294
  corticosteroids for, 288t, 295
  cytotoxic drugs for, 288t, 295
  indenes for, 287t, 290
  indole for, 287t, 290
  obesity and, 358
  oxicams for, 287t, 292
  pathophysiology of, 277–279, 278t
  penicillamine for, 287t, 294
  phenylanthranilic acids for, 287t, 292
  phenylpropionic acids for, 287t, 290
  pyrazolones for, 287t, 291
  salicylates for, 287t, 288–290
  treatment of, drug therapy for, 286–298, 287–288t
    guidelines for, 298
    principles of, 283–286, 284t
Osteomyelitis, 269, 274t
Osteoporosis, 328–333, 414–419, 418t
  advanced, 419
  alcohol intake and, 416
  calcium and, 328, 330, 331, 332, 415
  clinical presentation of, 328
  diagnosis of, 329, 416
  etiology of, 330
  hormonal status and, 415
  obesity and, 358
  physical activity and, 416
  prevention of, 415, 418, 418t
  race and, 416
  smoking and, 416
  therapy for, 331–333, 405, 417–419, 418t
Ototoxicity, drugs involved in, 18, 18t, 242t
Ovaries, reduced estrogen and, 408
Overhydration, hyponatremia and, 366, 369
Oxicams, 287t, 292

Oxycodone (Percodan), abuse of, 14. See also *Narcotics.*
Oxygen, hyperbaric, for dementia, 95

Pacemakers, infection around, 276
Pain, 422–433
  acute, 422
  chronic, 424–433
    antianxiety drugs for, 433
    Brompton mixture for, 432
    diagnosis of, 423, 424
    methotrimeprazine (Levoprome) for, 430
    narcotics for, 425–430, 426t, 432. See also *Narcotics.*
    non-narcotic drugs for, 431
    principles of management in, 433
    propoxyphene (Darvon) for, 430
    psychoactive drugs for, 431
    treatment of, approach to, 424
  functional, 423
  herpes zoster and, 271
  peripheral neuropathy and, 404
  psychological aspects of, 423
  types of, 422, 423, 424
Paralysis agitans. See *Parkinson's disease.*
Paranoid disorders, functional, treatment of, 76–82, 77t. See also *Antipsychotic drugs; Psychiatric disorders.*
Parkinsonism, 392, 396
Parkinson-like syndrome, 79
Parkinson's disease, 392–396
  and depression, 86, 86t
  drugs for, interaction of, 90t, 93t
Penicillamine, for arthritides, 287t, 294
  nephrotoxicity and, 18t
Penicillin(s), 243–249, 243t, 244t, 245t, 246t
  action of, 243, 244, 244t
  adverse effects of, 18t, 242t, 314
  characteristics of, 243, 243t
  cost of, 246, 246t
  doses of, 241t, 244, 244t, 245t
  pharmacokinetics of, 241t
Peptic ulcer disease, 182–200, 189t, 191t, 194t, 196t, 198t
  antacids for, 187–193, 189t, 190t, 191t, 194t. See also *Antacids.*
  anticholinergic drugs for, 194
  cimetidine for, 195–199, 196t, 198t
  duodenal ulcer, 185–187
  gastric ulcer, 184–187
  pathophysiology of, 183–187
  ranitidine for, 199
  sucralfate (Carafate) for, 193
  treatment of, 187–200. See also names of specific drugs.
Peritoneal dialysis, 379, 382
pH, urinary, effect of food on, 31, 31t
Pharmacist, responsibilities of, in drug therapy, 3
Pharmacokinetics, absorption, 19, 20, 30, 31t, 42–46, *43*, 44t, 46t
  clinical, 39–42, *40*, 40t, 41t
  distribution, 20, 46–49, 46t
  elimination, 49–57, 51t, 52t, 54t, 56t
    one-compartment calculations and, 63, 63t
    hepatic metabolism and, 50–53, *50*, 51t, 52t
    kidney and, 53–57, 54t, 56t
  elimination constant, 41
  half-life, 40, 40t

Pharmacokinetics (*Continued*)
  of aminoglycosides, 241t
  of antiarrhythmics, 167, 167t
  of antimicrobial drugs, 239-242, 240, 240t, 241t, 247-249
  of benzodiazepines, 98, 98t
  of calcium channel blockers, 154, 154t
  of diuretics, 142
  of theophylline, 107-109, 108t
  programmed dosing regimens and, 64, 64t
  variations in, with age, kidney and, 53-57, 54t, 56t
    liver and, 50-53, 50, 51t, 52t
Phenobarbital, for epilepsy, 400
  hepatotoxicity of, 18t
  therapeutic plasma range of, 39t
Phenothiazines, drug interactions of, 90t, 93t
  for nausea and vomiting, 216t, 217
  for psychoses, 77t, 78, 78t, 79
  side effects of, 78t, 81
Phenylanthranilic acids, 287t, 292
Phenylpropionic acids, 287t, 290
Phenytoin (Dilantin), drug interactions and, 24t, 242t, 400
  for cardiac arrhythmias, 166t, 173
  for epilepsy, 399
  toxic effects of, 17t, 18t
Physicians, responsibilities of, in drug therapy, 3, 5, 5t
Placebo, 5
Plasma, drugs in, optimal concentration range of, 38, 39t
  tricyclic antidepressant levels in, 88, 89t
Plasma albumin, drugs binding to, 47-49, 48t
Plasma glucose level, in diagnosis of diabetes mellitus, 333
  monitoring of, 339
Plasma protein, drugs binding to, 47-49, 48t
Pneumonia, 261, 262
Polypharmacotherapy, 3, 4-6, 5t
Polyvalent pneumococcal polysaccharide vaccine, 261
Porphyria, acute, intermittent, drugs precipitating, 17, 17t
Potassium, concentration of, chronic renal failure and, 162, 378
  diuretics and, 143
  effect of drugs on, 27t
Prazosin, 144t, 145
Prednisone. See also *Corticosteroid(s)*.
  for idiopathic autoimmune hemolytic anemias, 309t, 311
  for obstructive airway diseases, 119t, 120
Priacetam, 96
Primidone (Mysoline), for epilepsy, 401
  therapeutic plasma range of, 39t
Prinzmetal's angina, 150, 154
Procainamide, adverse effects of, 17t, 18t
  for cardiac arrhythmias, 166t, 167t, 169t, 171
  therapeutic plasma range of, 39t
Procaine, 96
Progestogens, 418, 418t
Propoxyphene (Darvon), for chronic pain, 430
  hepatotoxicity of, 18t
Propranolol (Inderal), for angina pectoris, 153, 154
  for anxiety, 99
  for cardiac arrhythmias, 166t, 168t, 173
  ototoxicity and, 18, 18t

Propranolol (*Continued*)
  therapeutic plasma range of, 39t
"PROven," 9
Prostatitis, 267
Prosthesis, valvular, hemolysis and, 314
Psyche, estrogen level and, 409
Psychiatric disorders, 75-100
  affective, 82-95
    bipolar, 82, 83t
    depression, 85-95. See also *Depression*.
    lithium treatment for, 83-85, 84t, 85t
    mania, 82, 83t
    types of, 82, 83t
  alcohol withdrawal, 97
  anxiety, 98-100, 98t
  dementia, 86, 95-97, 397-399, 398t
  paranoid, functional, 76-82, 77t. See also *Antipsychotic drugs*.
  schizophrenia, 76-82, 77t, 78t. See also *Antipsychotic drugs*.
  sleep disturbances, 100
Psychotropic drugs, 5, 75. See also *Antidepressants; Antipsychotic drugs*.
Pulmonary. See *Lung(s)*.
Pulmonary aspiration, 133
Pulmonary disease, drug-induced, 132, 132t, 133
Pulmonary embolism, 126-132. See also *Embolism, pulmonary*.
Pyrazolones, for 287t, 291

Quackery, 7-9
Quinidine, drug interactions with, 24t
  for cardiac arrhythmias, 166t, 167t, 170
  therapeutic plasma range of, 39t
  toxic effects of, 18t

Race, and osteoporosis, 416
Radius, fracture of, 328, 329
Ranitidine, 199
Renal disease, 366-383. See also *Kidney(s)*.
Reserpine, 144t, 145
Respiration, disorders of. See also *Lung(s)*.
  drug-induced, 132, 132t, 133t
Respiratory disease, susceptibility to, 104, 274t, 357
Retina, occlusion of artery to, 444
Retinopathy, diabetes mellitus and, 334, 335, 336, 337
Rheumatoid arthritis, antimalarial drugs for, 288t, 294
  corticosteroids for, 288t, 295
  cytotoxic drugs for, 288t, 295
  gold salts for, 287t, 293
  indenes for, 287t, 290
  indole for, 287t, 290
  oxicams for, 287t, 292
  pathophysiology of, 278t, 279
  penicillamine for, 287t, 294
  phenylanthranilic acids for, 287t, 292
  phenylpropionic acids for, 287t, 290
  pyrazolones for, 287t, 291
  salicylates for, 287t, 288-290
  treatment of, guidelines for, 298
  principles of, 283-286, 284t
Rheumatologic diseases. See *Arthritides; Ankylosing spondylitis; Gouty arthritis; Osteoarthritis; Rheumatoid arthritis*.
Rifampin, 18t, 241t, 242t, 244t, 257

Salicylates, adverse effects of, 17t, 18t
  for arthritides, 287t, 288–290
  therapeutic plasma range of, 39t
Saline laxatives, 180, 182t, 183t
Salmonellosis, 210
Schizophrenia, 76–82, 77t, 78t. See also *Antipsychotic drugs; Psychiatric disorders.*
Scopolamine, 215–217, 216t
Sedation, anticholinergic drugs and, 78t, 81
  antidepressants and, 87, 87t
Seizures, antipsychotic drugs and, 82
Self-medication, 6–9
Senile macular degeneration, 444
Senile tremor, 397
Septicemia, 271
Serum laboratory values, drug interactions with, 26t–28t
Sex differences, prescribing and, 35
Sexuality, estrogen level and, 409
Shigellosis, 210
Shingles, 404
Sinus bradycardia, 163, 166t
Sinus tachycardia, 164, 166t
Sinusitis, 261
Sjögren's syndrome (keratoconjunctivitis sicca), 443
Skin, effects of antipsychotic drugs on, 82
  effects of corticosteroids on, 121t
  infection of, 270
    diseases associated with, 274t
    treatment for, 241t, 258–260
Sleep, 100. See also *Psychiatric disorders.*
Smoking, osteoporosis and, 416
Sodium, concentration of, chronic renal failure and, 378
  decreased, 161, 366, 367–370
  effect of drugs of, 27t, 161
  restriction of, antacid use and, 189t, 190, 190t, 193
    laxative use and, 180
Spine, compression fracture of, 328, 329. See also *Osteoporosis.*
Splenectomy, for hereditary spherocytosis, 309t, 310
  for idiopathic autoimmune hemolytic anemia, 309t, 312
Splenomegaly, hemolytic anemia and, 309t, 315
Spherocytosis, hereditary, hemolytic anemia and, 309t, 310
Spondyloarthritis. See *Ankylosing spondylitis.*
Status epilepticus, 402
Steroids. See *Corticosteroids.*
Stibophen (Fuadin), 314
Stimulant(s), for depression, 94
  for dementia, 96
Stimulant laxatives, 180, 182t, 183t
Stomach, changes in, drug absorption and, 43, 44, 46t
  emptying of, delay in, 44, 44t, 45
Stroke, 386, 387t. See also *Cerebrovascular disease.*
Sty, 440
Sucralfate (Carafate), 193
Sulfasalazine, 227–230
Sulfonamides, 17t, 18t, 20t, 242t, 244t, 254
Sulfonylurea, 342–344, 343t
Supraventricular arrhythmias, 164, 165, 166t. See also *Cardiac arrhythmia(s).*
Surfactant laxatives, 181, 182t, 183t

Surgery, for anemias, 309t, 310, 312
  for hyperthyroidism, 350–352
  for obesity, 361
  for transient ischemic attacks, 387
  for ulcerative colitis, 231
Sympathomimetic drugs, drug interactions with, 90t, 93t
  for obstructive airway diseases, 106, 113–117, 113t, 114t, 115t, 123, 124
  pulmonary toxicity and, 132t
Systemic lupus erythematosus, and depression, 86, 86t

Tachyarrhythmias, 164, 166t. See also *Cardiac arrhythmia(s).*
Tachycardia, 164, 165, 166t
Tardive dyskinesia, 80, 396
Terbutaline, 114, 114t, 115, 115t
Tetanus immunization, 260
Tetracyclines, 242t, 252
Tetrahydrocannabinol (THC), 216t, 221–224
Theophylline, for obstructive airway diseases, 106, 107–113, 108t, 109t, *110*, 110t, 112t. See also *Lung(s).*
  administration of, 110–112, 110t, 112t
  interaction potential of, 109
  mechanism of action of, 106
  pharmacokinetics of, 107–109, 108t
  therapeutic level of, 39t, 109, 109t, *110*, 122, 123, *123*
  toxicity of, 109, 109t, *110*
Therapy, drug. See *Drug(s)* and specific conditions and drugs.
  goals of, 38, *39*, 39t
Thiazides, 18t, 24t, 93t, 142, 142t, 143
Thioridazine (Mellaril), 18t, 75, 77t, 78, 78t
Thioxanthines, 77, 77t, 78, 78t
Thrombolytic enzymes, 130–132
Thrombosis, cerebral, 385–389, 387t
Thyroid disorders, 345–352
  drugs for, 90t, 350–352
  hyperthyroidism, 349–352
  hypothyroidism, 346–349
  lithium and, 85
Thyroxine, 348, 349
Timolol, 447
Tolazamide (Tolinase), 343, 343t
Tolbutamide (Orinase), 17t, 18t, 20t, 343, 343t
Trachoma virus, 443
Transfusion, blood, 309t, 313
Transient ischemic attacks, 387–389. See also *Cerebrovascular disease.*
Trazodone hydrochloride (Desyrel), 91
Tremor, 397. See also *Parkinson's disease.*
Tricyclic antidepressants. See *Antidepressant(s), tricyclic.*
Trifluoperazine (Stelazine), 75, 78t, 79
Trigeminal nerve, interference of, and keratitis, 442
Triiodothyronine, 28t, 348, 349
Trimethobenzamide, 216t, 221
Trimethoprim, 254
Tuberculosis, 241t, 256–258, 263, 274t
Tyramine, monoamine oxidase (MAO) inhibitors and, 31, 31t, 93t

Ulcer(s), decubitis, 270, 274t
  duodenal, 185–187

Ulcer(s) (*Continued*)
  gastric, 184–187
  peptic, 182–200. See also *Peptic ulcer disease.*
Ulcerative colitis, 224–232, *225,* 225t. See also *Colitis, ulcerative.*
Uremic syndrome, 379
Uric acid, 28t, 29t, 282
Uricosuric drugs, 288t, 296
Urinary tract, infection of, 245t, 254, 255, 265–267, 274t
  reduced estrogen and, 408
Urine, effect of drugs on laboratory values of, 29t
  pH of, effect of food on, 31, 31t
Uterus, reduced estrogen and, 407
Uveitis, 444

Vagina, reduced estrogen and, 407
Vaginitis, 267, 274t
Valproic acid (Depakene), for epilepsy, 402
  therapeutic plasma range of, 39t
Valvular prosthesis, hemolysis and, 314
Vancomycin, for infection, 241t, 256
  for ulcerative colitis, 231
  kidney failure and, 244t
  toxicity of, 18t
Vasodilator(s), for congestive heart failure, 162
  for dementia, 95
  for hypertension, 147
Ventricular fibrillation, 165, 166t
Ventricular premature beats, 165, 166t

Ventricular tachycardia, 165, 166t. See also *Cardiac arrhythmia(s).*
Verapamil (Calan, Isoptin), for angina, 154, 154t, 155
  for cardiac arrhythmias, 168t, 175
Vertigo, 403
Viral diseases, herpetic, 271, 404, 440, 442
  ocular, 439, 440, 441, 442, 443
Vitamin(s), 8, 17t, 18t
Vitamin B_{12}, deficiency of, anemia and, 307t, 319, 322
Vomiting, 213–224, *213,* 213t, *215,* 216t
  anticholinergic drugs for, 215–217, 216t
  antidopaminergic drugs for, 216t, 217–220
  antihistaminic drugs for, 216t, 217
  benzquinamide for, 216t, 220
  causes of, 213, 213t
  marijuana for, 216t, 221–224
  metabolic consequences of, 213, 213t, 214
  treatment of, 214–224, 216t
  trimethobenzamide for, 216t, 221
Vomiting center, 214, *215*
Vulva, reduced estrogen and, 406

Warfarin sodium (Coumadin), drug interactions with, 242t
  for transient ischemic attacks, 388
Weight, aging and, effects on drug distribution, 46, 46t
Women, postmenopausal. See *Atherosclerosis; Climacteric; Estrogen; Osteoporosis.*